Gastrointestinal Diseases: A Multidisciplinary Approach

Editorial Advisor

JOEL J. HEIDELBAUGH

ELSEVIER

1600 John F. Kennedy Boulevard • Suite 1800 • Philadelphia, Pennsylvania, 19103-2899

http://www.theclinics.com

CLINICS COLLECTIONS
ISSN 2352-7986, ISBN-13: 978-0-323-42826-2

Editor: John Vassallo (j.vassallo@elsevier.com)
Developmental Editor: Patrick Manley (p.manley@elsevier.com)

Clinics Collections (ISSN 2352-7986) is published by Elsevier Inc., 360 Park Avenue South, New York, NY 10010-1710. Business and editorial offices: 1600 John F. Kennedy Boulevard, Suite 1800, Philadelphia, PA 19103-2899. **POSTMASTER:** Send address changes to *Clinics Collections*, Elsevier Health Sciences Division, Subscription Customer Service, 3251 Riverport Lane, Maryland Heights, MO 63043. **Customer Service: Telephone: 1-800-654-2452** (U.S. and Canada); **1-314-447-8871** (outside U.S. and Canada). **Fax: 314-447-8029. E-mail: journalscustomerserviceusa@elsevier.com** (for print support); **journalsonlinesupport-usa@ elsevier.com** (for online support).

Reprints. For copies of 100 or more of articles in this publication, please contact the Commercial Reprints Department, Elsevier Inc., 360 Park Avenue South, New York, NY 10010-1710. Tel.: 212-633-3874; Fax: 212-633-3820; E-mail: reprints@elsevier.com.

Contributors

EDITORIAL ADVISOR

JOEL J. HEIDELBAUGH, MD, FAAFP, FACG
Clinical Associate Professor, Departments of Family Medicine and Urology; Clerkship
Director, University of Michigan Medical School, Ann Arbor; Ypsilanti Health Center,
Ypsilanti, Michigan

AUTHORS

JULIAN A. ABRAMS, MD, MS
Assistant Professor of Medicine and Epidemiology, Division of Digestive and Liver
Diseases, Columbia University Medical Center, New York, New York

ANDRES ACOSTA, MD, PhD
Clinical Enteric Neuroscience Translational and Epidemiological Research (C.E.N.T.E.R.);
Fellow, Division of Gastroenterology and Hepatology, Mayo Clinic, Rochester, Minnesota

AMAN ALI, MD
Assistant Professor of Gastroenterology, Southern Illinois University School of Medicine,
Springfield, Illinois

RICHARD W. ARNOLD, MD, FACP
Clinical Professor of Medicine, Department of Medicine, University of Washington, Seattle,
Washington

PREET BAGI, MD
Division of Gastroenterology, University of California, San Diego, La Jolla, California

MARK E. BAKER, MD, FARS, FSCBT/MR
Professor of Radiology, Cleveland Clinic Lerner College of Medicine, Case Western
Reserve University; Staff Radiologist, Abdominal Imaging, Imaging Institute; Digestive
Disease Institute and Cancer Institute, Cleveland Clinic, Cleveland, Ohio

MARC BARDOU, MD, PhD
Gastroenterology Department & Centre d'Investigations Clinique, France

ALAN N. BARKUN, MD, MSc
Divisions of Gastroenterology and Clinical Epidemiology, McGill University Health Center,
McGill University, Montré al, Canada

MAYAN BOMSZTYK, MD
Acting Instructor, Department of Medicine, University of Washington, Seattle, Washington

MICHAEL CAMILLERI, MD
Clinical Enteric Neuroscience Translational and Epidemiological Research (C.E.N.T.E.R.);
Professor of Medicine, Pharmacology and Physiology, Mayo Clinic, Rochester, Minnesota

RICHARD CARMONA, BA
New York University School of Medicine, New York, New York

IBRAHIM BULENT CETINDAG, MD
Assistant Professor of Surgery, Southern Illinois University School of Medicine, Springfield, Illinois

YEN-I CHEN, MD
Division of Gastroenterology, McGill University Health Center, McGill University, Montréal, Canada

VANESSA C. COSTILLA, MD
Resident, Department of Internal Medicine, Mayo Clinic in Arizona, Scottsdale, Arizona

GEERT R. D'HAENS, MD, PhD
Robarts Clinical Trials Inc., London, Ontario, Canada; Department of Gastroenterology, Academic Medical Centre, Amsterdam, The Netherlands

VENKATA S.P.B. DURVASULA, MD, FRCS ENT
Clinical Fellow, Departments of Pediatric Otolaryngology and Head and Neck Surgery, Arkansas Children's Hospital, Little Rock, Arkansas

DAVID M. EINSTEIN, MD, FARS
Clinical Professor of Radiology, Cleveland Clinic Lerner College of Medicine, Case Western Reserve University; Vice-Chairman, Education, and Staff Radiologist, Abdominal Imaging, Imaging Institute, Cleveland Clinic, Cleveland, Ohio

STEVE EUBANKS, MD
Director of Academic Surgery; Medical Director of the Institute for Surgical Advancement, Center for Interventional Endoscopy, Florida Hospital Institute for Minimally Invasive Therapy; Professor of Surgery, University of Central Florida, Orlando, Florida

GARY W. FALK, MD, MS
Professor of Medicine, Division of Gastroenterology, University of Pennsylvania Perelman School of Medicine, Philadelphia, Pennsylvania

MARCIE FEINMAN, MD
Assistant in Surgery, Division of Acute Care Surgery, Department of Surgery, Anesthesiology/Critical Care Medicine (ACCM), Emergency Medicine, The Johns Hopkins University School of Medicine, Baltimore, Maryland

KYLE J. FORTINSKY, MD
Department of Medicine, Toronto General Hospital, University of Toronto, Canada

AMY E. FOXX-ORENSTEIN, DO, FACG, FACP
Associate Professor of Medicine, Division of Gastroenterology, Mayo Clinic in Arizona, Scottsdale, Arizona

LAURA M. GOBER, MD
Division of Allergy, Immunology, and Infectious Diseases; Attending Physician, Center for Pediatric Eosinophilic Disorders, The Children's Hospital of Philadelphia, Philadelphia, Pennsylvania

NANCY S. GRAVES, MD
Assistant Professor, Department of Family and Community Medicine, Milton S. Hershey Medical Center, Penn State Hershey, Hershey, Pennsylvania

CINDY HA, MD
Resident in General Surgery, Southern Illinois University School of Medicine, Springfield, Illinois

JASON F. HALL, MD, MPH, FACS
Senior Surgeon, Department of Colon and Rectal Surgery, Lahey Clinic, Burlington; Assistant Professor, Department of Surgery, Tufts University School of Medicine, Boston, Massachusetts

MICHELLE S. HAN, MD
Research Fellow, Department of Surgery, University of Rochester Medical Center, University of Rochester, Rochester, New York

WILLIAM L. HASLER, MD
Professor, Division of Gastroenterology, University of Michigan Health System, Ann Arbor, Michigan

CESARE HASSAN, MD
Digestive Endoscopy Unit, IRCCS Istituto Clinico Humanitas, Rozzano, Milan, Italy

ELLIOTT R. HAUT, MD, FACS
Associate Professor of Surgery, Division of Acute Care Surgery, Department of Surgery, Anesthesiology/Critical Care Medicine (ACCM), Emergency Medicine, The Johns Hopkins University School of Medicine, Baltimore, Maryland

IKUO HIRANO, MD
Director, Esophageal Center; Professor of Medicine, Division of Gastroenterology, Northwestern University Feinberg School of Medicine, Chicago, Illinois

I. LISANNE HOLSTER, MD, PhD
Department of Gastroenterology and Hepatology, Erasmus MC University Medical Centre, Rotterdam, The Netherlands

HU JIANZHONG, PhD
Assistant Professor, Department of Genetics and Genomic Sciences, Icahn School of Medicine at Mount Sinai, New York, New York

MATTHEW F. KALADY, MD
Digestive Disease Institute, Cleveland Clinic Foundation, Cleveland, Ohio

VIJAY KANAKADANDI, MD
Division of Gastroenterology and Hepatology, Veterans Affairs Medical Center, University of Kansas School of Medicine, Kansas City, Kansas

DAVID A. KATZKA, MD
Professor of Medicine, Division of Gastroenterology and Hepatology, Mayo Clinic, Rochester, Minnesota

ABRAHAM KHAN, MD
Clinical Instructor of Medicine, Division of Gastroenterology, Department of Medicine, Center for Esophageal Disease, New York University School of Medicine, New York, New York

ALOK A. KHORANA, MD
Taussig Cancer Institute, Cleveland Clinic Foundation, Cleveland, Ohio

CHRISTOPHER L. KNIGHT, MD
Associate Professor of Medicine, Division of General Internal Medicine, Department of Medicine, University of Washington School of Medicine, Seattle, Washington

ERNST J. KUIPERS, MD, PhD
Department of Gastroenterology and Hepatology, Erasmus MC University Medical Centre, Rotterdam, The Netherlands

BARRETT G. LEVESQUE, MS, MD
Robarts Clinical Trials Inc., London, Ontario, Canada; Division of Gastroenterology, University of California, San Diego, La Jolla, California

CHRIS A. LIACOURAS, MD
Co-Director of the Center for Pediatric Eosinophilic Disorders; Division of Gastroenterology, Hepatology and Nutrition, The Children's Hospital of Philadelphia; Professor of Pediatrics, Perelman School of Medicine, University of Pennsylvania, Philadelphia, Pennsylvania

YIDAN LU, MD
Division of Gastroenterology, McGill University Health Center, McGill University, Montréal, Canada

JOHN D. MELLINGER, MD, FACS
Professor of Surgery, J. Roland Folse Endowed Chair in Surgery, Chair of General Surgery, Residency Program Director, Southern Illinois University School of Medicine, Springfield, Illinois

KAIHONG MI, MD, PhD
Taussig Cancer Institute, Cleveland Clinic Foundation, Cleveland, Ohio

UDAYAKUMAR NAVANEETHAN, MD
Assistant Professor of Internal Medicine, University of Central Florida; Center for Interventional Endoscopy, Florida Hospital Institute for Minimally Invasive Therapy, Orlando, Florida

LINDA ANH NGUYEN, MD
Division of Gastroenterology, Department of Medicine, Stanford University, Palo Alto, California

RAMINDER NIRULA, MD, MPH
Associate Professor, Department of Surgery, University of Utah, Salt Lake City, Utah

ASHLEY C. O'NEILL, MS
Speech-Language Pathologist, Departments of Audiology and Speech Pathology, Arkansas Children's Hospital, Little Rock, Arkansas

MARYANN KATHERINE OVERLAND, MD
Acting Instructor, Division of General Internal Medicine, Primary Care Clinic, VA Puget Sound Health Care System, University of Washington, Seattle, Washington

DARRELL S. PARDI, MD, MS
Professor of Medicine, Vice Chair, Division of Gastroenterology and Hepatology, Inflammatory Bowel Disease Clinic, Mayo Clinic College of Medicine, Rochester, Minnesota

CAROL REES PARRISH, MS, RD
Nutrition Support Specialist, Digestive Health Center, University of Virginia Health System, Charlottesville, Virginia

JEFFREY H. PETERS, MD, FACS
Chief Operating Officer, Department of Surgery, University Hospitals, Cleveland, Ohio

EAMONN M.M. QUIGLEY, MD, FRCP, FACP, FACG, FRCPI
David M Underwood Chair of Medicine in Digestive Disorders; Professor of Medicine, Weill Cornell Medical College; Chief, Division of Gastroenterology and Hepatology, Houston Methodist Hospital, Weill Cornell Medical College, Houston, Texas

CRISTIANO QUINTINI, MD
Digestive Disease Institute, Cleveland Clinic Foundation, Cleveland, Ohio

JAMES REGAN, MD
Resident in General Surgery, Southern Illinois University School of Medicine, Springfield, Illinois

ALESSANDRO REPICI, MD
Digestive Endoscopy Unit, IRCCS Istituto Clinico Humanitas, Rozzano, Milan, Italy

GRESHAM T. RICHTER, MD
Associate Professor, Department of Pediatric Otolaryngology and Head and Neck Surgery, Arkansas Children's Hospital, Little Rock, Arkansas

GIANLUCA ROTONDANO, MD, FASGE, FACG
Division of Gastroenterology and Digestive Endoscopy, Hospital Maresca, Azienda Sanitaria Locale Napoli 3 Sud, Torre del Greco, Italy

JOEL H. RUBENSTEIN, MD, MSc
Veterans Affairs Center for Clinical Management Research; Barrett's Esophagus Program, Division of Gastroenterology, University of Michigan Medical School, Ann Arbor, Michigan

THOMAS M. RUNGE, MD, MPH
Gastroenterology Research Fellow, Division of Gastroenterology and Hepatology, Center for Esophageal Diseases and Swallowing, University of North Carolina School of Medicine, University of North Carolina at Chapel Hill, Chapel Hill, North Carolina

MARK A. SAMAAN, MBBS
Robarts Clinical Trials Inc., London, Ontario, Canada; Department of Gastroenterology, Academic Medical Centre, Amsterdam, The Netherlands

ALAIN M. SCHOEPFER, MD
Division of Gastroenterology and Hepatology, Centre Hospitalier Universitaire Vaudois/
CHUV, Lausanne, Switzerland

NICHOLAS J. SHAHEEN, MD, MPH
Professor of Medicine and Epidemiology; Chief, Division of Gastroenterology and
Hepatology, Center for Esophageal Diseases and Swallowing, University of North
Carolina School of Medicine, University of North Carolina at Chapel Hill, Chapel Hill,
North Carolina

VIRENDER K. SHARMA, MD, FACG, AGAF, FASGE
Director, Arizona Digestive Health, Gilbert, Arizona

PRATEEK SHARMA, MD
Division of Gastroenterology and Hepatology, Veterans Affairs Medical Center,
University of Kansas School of Medicine, Kansas City, Kansas

DANIEL SIFRIM, MD, PhD
Centre for Digestive Diseases, Barts and the London School of Medicine and Dentistry,
Queen Mary University of London; Gastrointestinal Physiology Unit, Barts Health NHS
Trust, Royal London Hospital, London, United Kingdom

SIDDHARTH SINGH, MD
Fellow, Inflammatory Bowel Disease Clinic, Division of Gastroenterology and Hepatology,
Department of Internal Medicine, Mayo Clinic, Rochester, Minnesota

C. DANIEL SMITH, MD
Professor of Surgery, Mayo Clinic, Atlanta, Georgia

WILLIAM J. SNAPE Jr, MD
Division of Gastroenterology, Department of Medicine, California Pacific Medical
Center, San Francisco, California

JONATHAN SPERGEL, MD
Co-Director of the Center for Pediatric Eosinophilic Disorders; Division of Allergy,
Immunology, and Infectious Diseases, The Children's Hospital of Philadelphia;
Professor of Pediatrics, Perelman School of Medicine, University of Pennsylvania,
Philadelphia, Pennsylvania

THEODORE STEINER, MD
Associate Professor, Infectious Diseases, University of British Columbia, Vancouver,
British Columbia, Canada

CHRISTINA M. SURAWICZ, MD
Professor of Medicine, Division of Gastroenterology, Department of Medicine,
University of Washington School of Medicine, Seattle, Washington

ERIC T.T.L. TJWA, MD, PhD
Department of Gastroenterology and Hepatology, Erasmus MC University Medical
Centre, Rotterdam, The Netherlands

MORRIS TRAUBE, MD, JD
Professor of Medicine, Division of Gastroenterology, Department of Medicine;
Director, Center for Esophageal Disease, New York University School of Medicine,
New York, New York

NIELS VANDE CASTEELE, PharmD, PhD
Robarts Clinical Trials Inc., London, Ontario, Canada; Division of Gastroenterology, University of California, San Diego, La Jolla, California; Department of Pharmaceutical and Pharmacological Sciences, KU Leuven, Leuven, Belgium

MARCELO F. VELA, MD, MSCR
Associate Professor of Medicine, Division of Gastroenterology, Mayo Clinic Arizona, Scottsdale, Arizona

MATTHEW J. WHITSON, MD
Fellow, Division of Gastroenterology, Hospital of the University of Pennsylvania, University of Pennsylvania Perelman School of Medicine, Philadelphia, Pennsylvania

PHILIP WOODLAND, MBBS, PhD
Centre for Digestive Diseases, Barts and the London School of Medicine and Dentistry, Queen Mary University of London; Gastrointestinal Physiology Unit, Barts Health NHS Trust, Royal London Hospital, London, United Kingdom

ETSURO YAZAKI, PhD, MAGIP
Centre for Digestive Diseases, Barts and the London School of Medicine and Dentistry, Queen Mary University of London; Gastrointestinal Physiology Unit, Barts Health NHS Trust, Royal London Hospital, London, United Kingdom

ANGELO ZULLO, MD
Digestive Endoscopy Unit, IRCCS Istituto Clinico Humanitas, Rozzano, Milan, Italy

Contents

Upper Gastrointestinal Diseases

Gastroesophageal Reflux Disease

Gastroesophageal reflux disease (GERD) is frequently diagnosed by symptoms and good response to acid suppression with proton pump inhibitors. Further work up is required when the diagnosis of GERD is uncertain, for alarm symptoms, PPI-refractoriness, and often for extraesophageal presentations. Useful tools include endoscopy for mucosal assessment and reflux monitoring (pH or impedance-pH) to quantify reflux burden. Objective documentation of pathological reflux is mandatory prior to anti-reflux surgery. In some patients, symptoms that can be attributed to GERD may have other causes; in these patients, testing that excludes GERD helps direct the diagnostic and treatment efforts to other causes.

The barium esophagram is an integral part of the assessment and management of patients with gastroesophageal reflux disease (GERD) before, and especially after, antireflux procedures. While many of the findings on the examination can be identified with endosocopy, a gastric emptying study and an esophageal motility examination, the barium esophagram is better at demonstrating the anatomic findings after antireflux surgery, especially in symptomatic patients. These complementary examinations, when taken as a whole, fully evaluate a patient with suspected GERD as well as symptomatic patients after antireflux procedures.

The development and advancement of ambulatory esophageal pH monitoring has provided a key tool with which pathologic esophageal acid exposure can be objectively measured; although not perfect, it provides the clinician with arguably the most important piece of information in the diagnosis and management of patients with gastroesophageal reflux disease. It is also important to emphasize that, although esophageal pH monitoring can reliably measure esophageal acid exposure, assessing the relationship of abnormal findings and the patients' symptoms is a much more complex matter and, of course, the key to successful treatment outcomes.

Barrett's Esophagus

development of esophageal adenocarcinoma. There are multiple clinical, endoscopic, and pathologic factors that increase the risk of neoplastic progression to high-grade dysplasia or esophageal adenocarcinoma in Barrett's esophagus. This article reviews both risk and protective factors for neoplastic progression in patients with Barrett's esophagus.

Joel H. Rubenstein

Surveillance of Barrett's esophagus for preventing death from esophageal adenocarcinoma is attractive and widely practiced. However, empirical evidence supporting its effectiveness is weak. Longer intervals between surveillance examinations are being recommended, supported by computer simulation analyses. If surveillance is performed, an adequate number of biopsies should be performed or the effect of surveillance would be squandered.

Upper Gastrointestinal Bleeding

Gianluca Rotondano

Acute upper gastrointestinal bleeding (UGIB) is a common gastroenterological emergency. A vast majority of these bleeds have nonvariceal causes, in particular gastroduodenal peptic ulcers. Nonsteroidal antiinflammatory drugs, low-dose aspirin use, and Helicobacter pylori infection are the main risk factors for UGIB. Current epidemiologic data suggest that patients most affected are older with medical comorbidit. Widespread use of potentially gastroerosive medications underscores the importance of adopting gastroprotective pharamacologic strategies. Endoscopy is the mainstay for diagnosis and treatment of acute UGIB. It should be performed within 24 hours of presentation by skilled operators in adequately equipped settings, using a multidisciplinary team approach.

Raminder Nirula

The cause and management of gastroduodenal perforation have changed as a result of increasing use of nonsteroidal antiinflammatories and improved pharmacologic treatment of acid hypersecretion as well as the recognition and treatment of Helicobacter pylori. As a result of the reduction in ulcer recurrence with medical therapy, the surgical approach to patients with gastroduodenal perforation has also changed over the last 3 decades, with ulcer-reducing surgery being performed infrequently.

Eric T.T.L. Tjwa, I. Lisanne Holster and Ernst J. Kuipers

Upper gastrointestinal bleeding (UGIB) is the most common emergency condition in gastroenterology. Although peptic ulcer and esophagogastric varices are the predominant causes, other conditions account for up to 50% of UGIBs. These conditions, among others, include angiodysplasia,

Dieulafoy and Mallory-Weiss lesions, gastric antral vascular ectasia, and Cameron lesions. Upper GI cancer as well as lesions of the biliary tract and pancreas may also result in severe UGIB. This article provides an overview of the endoscopic management of these lesions, including the role of novel therapeutic modalities such as hemostatic powder and over-the-scope-clips.

This review discusses the indications, technical aspects, and comparative effectiveness of the endoscopic treatment of upper gastrointestinal bleeding caused by peptic ulcer. Pre-endoscopic considerations, such as the use of prokinetics and timing of endoscopy, are reviewed. In addition, this article examines aspects of postendoscopic care such as the effectiveness, dosing, and duration of postendoscopic proton-pump inhibitors, Helicobacter pylori testing, and benefits of treatment in terms of preventing rebleeding; and the use of nonsteroidal anti-inflammatory drugs, antiplatelet agents, and oral anticoagulants, including direct thrombin and Xa inhibitors, following acute peptic ulcer bleeding.

Nonvariceal upper gastrointestinal bleeding (UGIB) is a major cause of morbidity and mortality worldwide. Mortality from UGIB has remained 5-10% over the past decade. This article presents current evidence-based recommendations for the medical management of UGIB. Pre-endoscopic management includes initial resuscitation, risk stratification, appropriate use of blood products, and consideration of nasogastric tube insertion, erythromycin, and proton pump inhibitor therapy. The use of post-endoscopic intravenous proton pump inhibitors is strongly recommended for certain patient populations. Post-endoscopic management also includes the diagnosis and treatment of Helicobacter pylori, appropriate use of proton pump inhibitors and iron replacement therapy.

Dyspepsia

Dyspepsia is a common and complex condition consisting of chronic upper gastrointestinal symptoms. A rational approach to diagnosis and treatment of dyspepsia includes identifying those patients with alarm symptoms and referring them for prompt endoscopy. Those without alarm symptoms can be differentiated into patients who do and do not have symptoms consistent with gastroesophageal reflux disease. In the absence of predominant heartburn and regurgitation, patients should be tested and treated for Helicobacter pylori. Functional (nonulcer) dyspepsia is a multifactorial disorder with several possible pathophysiologic mechanisms, but no clear guidelines for therapy. There is some evidence of efficacy of proton pump inhibitors, antisecretory agents, antidepressants, and psychotherapy for functional dyspepsia.

Eosinophilic Esophagitis

A validated disease-specific symptom-assessment tool for eosinophilic esophagitis (EoE) has yet to be approved by regulatory authorities for use in clinical trials. Relevant end points for daily practice include EoE-related symptoms and esophageal eosinophilic inflammation. Endoscopic features should also be taken into account when establishing a therapy plan. A reasonable clinical goal is to achieve a reduction in EoE-related symptoms and esophageal eosinophilic inflammation. Evidence is increasing to support an anti-inflammatory maintenance therapy, as this can reduce esophageal remodeling. In EoE patients in clinical remission, annual disease monitoring with symptom, endoscopic, and histologic assessments of sustained treatment response is recommended.

Eosinophilic esophagitis (EoE) is increasing in western nations. Symptoms in infants and young children include feeding difficulties, failure to thrive, and gastroesophageal reflux. School-aged children may present with vomiting, abdominal pain, and regurgitation; adolescents and adults with dysphagia and food impaction. Delayed diagnosis increases risk of stricture formation. Children with untreated EoE have tissue changes resembling airway remodeling. Endoscopy does not always correlate. Management centers on food elimination. Approaches include skin prick and patch testing, removal of foods, or an amino acid formula diet. Long-term elimination diets can produce nutritional deficiencies and have poor adherence.

Gastroparesis

Gastroparesis is a heterogeneous disorder defined by delay in gastric emptying. Symptoms of gastroparesis are nonspecific, including nausea, vomiting, early satiety, bloating, and/or abdominal pain. Normal gastric motor function and sensory function depend on a complex coordination between the enteric and central nervous system. This article discusses the pathophysiology of delayed gastric emptying and the symptoms of gastroparesis, including antropyloroduodenal dysmotility, impaired gastric accommodation, visceral hypersensitivity, and autonomic dysfunction. The underlying pathophysiology of gastroparesis is complex and multifactorial. The article discusses how a combination of these factors leads to symptoms of gastroparesis.

Although many surgical procedures originally associated with gastroparesis are less commonly performed nowadays, several more recently developed upper abdominal procedures may be complicated by the development of gastroparesis. Gastroparesis has been described in association with neurologic disorders ranging from Parkinson disease to muscular dystrophy, and its presence may have important implications for patient management and prognosis. Although scleroderma is most frequently linked with gastrointestinal motility disorder, gastroparesis has been linked to several other connective tissue disorders. The management of these patients presents several challenges, and is best conducted in the context of a dedicated and skilled multidisciplinary team.

Although prokinetic agents typically are used for gastroparesis, antiemetic, analgesic, and neuromodulatory medications may help manage nausea, vomiting, pain, or discomfort. Antiemetic benefits are supported by few case reports. An open series reported symptom reductions with transdermal granisetron in gastroparesis. Opiates are not advocated in gastroparesis because they worsen nausea and delay emptying. Neuromodulators have theoretical utility, but the tricyclic agent nortriptyline showed no benefits over placebo in an idiopathic gastroparesis study raising doubts about this strategy. Neurologic and cardiac toxicities of these medications are recognized. Additional controlled study is warranted to define antiemetic, analgesic, and neuromodulator usefulness in gastroparesis.

Prokinetic agents are medications that enhance coordinated gastrointestinal motility and transit of content in the gastrointestinal tract, mainly by amplifying and coordinating the gastrointestinal muscular contractions. In addition to dietary therapy, prokinetic therapy should be considered as a means to improve gastric emptying and symptoms of gastroparesis, balancing benefits and risks of treatment. In the United States, metoclopramide remains the first-line prokinetic therapy, because it is the only approved medication for gastroparesis. Newer agents are being developed for the management of gastroparesis. This article provides detailed information about prokinetic agents for the treatment of gastroparesis.

Gastroparesis, or delayed gastric emptying, has many origins and can wax and wane depending on the underlying cause. Not only do the symptoms significantly alter quality of life, but the clinical consequences can also be life threatening. Once a patient develops protracted nausea and vomiting, providing adequate nutrition, hydration, and access to therapeutics such as prokinetics and antiemetics can present an exceptional challenge to clinicians. This article reviews the limited evidence available for oral nutrition, as well as enteral and parenteral nutritional support therapies. Practical strategies are provided to improve the nutritional depletion that often accompanies this debilitating condition.

Dysphagia

Patients frequently present to a physician with complaints of difficulty swallowing. The approach to systematically evaluating these problems can be challenging for those who do not manage this type of patient regularly. The potential for life threatening malignancies is present and makes this evaluation a priority. Numerous excellent tools are available to aid with the determination of the cause of dysphagia and assist with the formulation of a logical treatment algorithm.

Oropharyngeal dysphagia (OPD) is a challenging and relatively common condition in children. Both developmentally normal and delayed children may be affected. The etiology of OPD is frequently multifactorial with neurologic, inflammatory, and anatomic conditions contributing to discoordination of the pharyngeal phase of swallowing. Depending on the severity and source, OPD may persist for several years with significant burden to a patient's health and family. This article details current understanding of the mechanism and potential sources of OPD in children while providing an algorithm for managing it in the acute and chronic setting.

Dysphagia, or difficulty swallowing, is a common problem in the elderly. Based on the initial clinical history and physical examination, the dysphagia is assessed as either primarily oropharyngeal or esophageal in origin. Most oropharyngeal dysphagia are of neurologic origin, and management is coordinated with a clinical swallow specialist in conjunction with an ear, nose, and throat (ENT) physician if warning signs imply malignancy. Several structural and functional esophageal disorders can cause dysphagia. If a patient has likely esophageal dysphagia, a video barium esophagram is a good initial test, and referral to a gastroenterologist is generally warranted leading to appropriate treatment.

Esophageal function testing should be used for differential diagnosis of dysphagia. Dysphagia can be the consequence of hypermotility or hypomotility of the muscles of the esophagus. Decreased esophageal or esophagogastric junction distensibility can provoke dysphagia. The most well established esophageal dysmotility is achalasia. Other motility disorders can also cause dysphagia. High-resolution manometry (HRM) is the gold standard investigation for esophageal motility disorders. Simultaneous measurement of HRM and intraluminal impedance can be useful to assess motility and bolus transit. Impedance planimetry measures distensibility of the esophageal body and gastroesophageal junction in patients with achalasia and eosinophilic esophagitis.

Esophageal Tumor

Benign esophageal and paraesophageal masses and cysts are a rare but important group of pathologies. Although often asymptomatic, these lesions can cause a variety of symptoms and, in some cases, demonstrate variable biological behavior. Contemporary categorization relies heavily on endoscopic ultrasound and other imaging modalities and immunohistochemical analysis when appropriate. Minimally invasive options including endoscopic, laparoscopic, and thoracoscopic methods are increasingly used for symptomatic or indeterminate lesions.

Lower Gastrointestinal Diseases

Colon Polyps/Cancer

Colorectal cancer represents a major cause of mortality in Western countries, and population-based colonoscopy screening is supported by official guidelines. A significant determinant of the cost of colonoscopy screening/surveillance is driven by polypectomy of diminutive ($\leq$5 mm) lesions. When considering the low prevalence of advanced neoplasia within diminutive polyps, the additional cost of pathologic examination is mainly justified by the need to differentiate between precancerous adenomatous versus hyperplastic polyps. The aim of this review is to summarize the data supporting the clinical application of a resect and discard strategy, also addressing the potential pitfalls associated with this approach.

Multiple new treatment options for metastatic colorectal cancer have been developed over the past 2 decades, including conventional chemotherapy and agents directed against vascular endothelial growth factor and epidermal growth factor receptor. Combination regimens, integrated with surgical approaches, have led to an increase in median survival, and a minority of patients with resectable disease can survive for years. Clinical decision-making therefore requires a strategic, biomarker-based multidisciplinary approach to maximize life expectancy and quality of life. This review describes systemic approaches to the treatment of patients with metastatic colorectal cancer, including integration with liver resection, other liver-directed therapies, and primary resection.

Constipation

Constipation is a frequently diagnosed gastrointestinal disorder. Symptoms of constipation are common, with the greatest prevalence in the elderly. Evaluation of constipation begins with a detailed medical history and a focused anorectal examination. Diagnostic testing for constipation is not routinely recommended in the initial evaluation in the absence of alarm signs. Key self-management strategies include increased exercise, a high-fiber diet, and toilet training. High-fiber diets can worsen symptoms in some patients who have chronic constipation. Biofeedback is an effective treatment option for patients who have constipation caused by outlet obstruction defecation. A variety of medications are available to remedy constipation.

Inflammatory Bowel Disease

Extensive genetic studies have identified more than 140 loci predisposing to Crohn disease (CD). Several major CD susceptibility genes have been shown to impair biological function with regard to immune response to recognizing and clearance of bacterial infection. Recent human microbiome studies suggest that the gut microbiome composition is differentiated in carriers of many risk variants of major CD susceptibility genes. This interplay between host genetics and its associated gut microbiome may play an essential role in the pathogenesis of CD. The ongoing microbiome research is aimed to investigate the detailed host genetics-microbiome interacting mechanism.

Microscopic colitis is a frequent cause of chronic watery diarrhea, especially in older persons. Common associated symptoms include abdominal pain, arthralgias, and weight loss. The incidence of microscopic colitis had been increasing, although more recent studies have shown a stabilization of incidence rates. The diagnosis is based on characteristic histologic findings in a patient with diarrhea. Microscopic colitis can occur at any age, including in children, but it is primarily seen in the elderly. Several treatment options exist to treat the symptoms of microscopic colitis, although only budesonide has been well studied in randomized clinical trials.

Anti-tumor necrosis factor-α (TNF) agents, including infliximab, adalimumab, and certolizumab pegol, are effective medications for the

Gastroenteritis

Travel medicine continues to grow as international tourism and patient medical complexity increases. This article reflects the state of the current field, but new recommendations on immunizations, resistance patterns, and treatment modalities constantly change. The US Centers for Disease Control and the World Health Organization maintain helpful Web sites for both patient and physician. With thoughtful preparation and prevention, risks can be minimized and travel can continue as safely as possible.

Clostridium difficile is emerging as a common cause of infectious diarrhea. Incidence has increased dramatically since 2000, associated with a new strain that features both increased toxin production and increased resistance to antibiotics. For patients with mild to moderate disease, oral metronidazole is usually the first choice of treatment, and those with severe disease should be treated with vancomycin, with additional intravenous metronidazole in some cases. Fecal microbiota transplantation is a potentially promising therapy for patients with multiple recurrences of *C difficile* infection. Prevention of nosocomial transmission is crucial to reducing disease outbreaks in health care settings.

Lower Gastrointestinal Bleeding

This article examines causes of occult, moderate and severe lower gastrointestinal (GI) bleeding. The difference in the workup of stable vs unstable patients is stressed. Treatment options ranging from minimally invasive techniques to open surgery are explored.

Hemorrhoids

Complaints secondary to hemorrhoidal disease have been treated by health care providers for centuries. Most symptoms referable to hemorrhoidal disease can be managed nonoperatively. When symptoms do not respond to medical therapy, procedural intervention is recommended. Surgical hemorrhoidectomy is usually reserved for patients who are refractory to or unable to tolerate office procedures. This article reviews the pathophysiology of hemorrhoidal disease and the most commonly used techniques for the nonoperative and operative palliation of hemorrhoidal complaints.

Preface

Each year, Elsevier's prestigious *Clinics Review Articles* series publishes more than 250 issues (3000 plus articles) encompassing over 50 medical and surgical disciplines. This curated collection of articles, devoted to gastrointestinal diseases, draws from the robust *Clinics'* database to provide multidisciplinary teams with practical clinical advice on comorbidities and complications of these highly prevalent diseases.

Featured articles from the *Gastroenterology Clinics of North America, Gastrointestinal Endoscopy Clinics of North America, Medical Clinics of North America, Clinics in Geriatric Medicine, Surgical Oncology Clinics of North America*, and *Surgical Clinics of North America* reflect the wide range of clinicians who manage the GI patient. This multidisciplinary perspective is essential to successful team-based management.

I hope you share this volume with your colleagues and that it spurs more collaboration, deeper understanding, and safer, more effective care for your patients.

Joel J. Heidelbaugh, MD, FAAFP, FACG
Ypsilanti, MI
July 2015

http://dx.doi.org/10.1016/j.ccol.2015.06.001
2352-7986/15/$ – see front matter © 2015 Published by Elsevier Inc.

Diagnostic Work-Up of GERD

Marcelo F. Vela, MD, MSCR

KEYWORDS

- Gastroesophageal reflux disease (GERD) • Heartburn • Proton pump inhibitor test
- Endoscopy • pH monitoring • Impedance-pH monitoring

KEY POINTS

- Gastroesophageal reflux disease (GERD) may be diagnosed by symptoms and a positive PPI test in some settings; however, it is important to be aware of the limited sensitivity and specificity of this approach as a diagnostic intervention.
- The finding of erosive esophagitis on endoscopy provides robust evidence of GERD but endoscopy is normal in most patients with GERD.
- Ambulatory reflux monitoring is the gold standard for diagnosing GERD.
- In some patients without good response to PPI, the reported symptoms are due to non-GERD causes; a negative work up can exclude GERD and help direct the diagnostic and treatment efforts toward other causes.
- Work up of patients with PPI-refractory symptoms should proceed in this order: optimization of PPI therapy; investigation for non-GERD causes by endoscopy for typical symptoms as well as ears-nose-throat, allergy, and pulmonary evaluation for atypical presentations; and, finally, reflux monitoring if the reason for refractoriness remains unclear.

INTRODUCTION

Gastroesophageal reflux disease (GERD) is a very common clinical problem. Heartburn or acid regurgitation is experienced on a weekly basis by nearly 20% of the US population, with an annual prevalence of up to 59%.[1] GERD may be diagnosed by symptom assessment through patient history or GERD questionnaires, response to a trial of proton pump inhibitors (PPIs), findings of reflux-related esophageal mucosal damage by endoscopy, or by establishing the presence of pathologic reflux on prolonged ambulatory monitoring with pH or impedance-pH. In routine clinical practice, GERD is frequently diagnosed by symptom presentation along with a good response to a PPI trial. Although this constitutes a simple and reasonable approach in the appropriate setting (eg, primary care of uncomplicated patients), it is important to bear in mind its limitations.

This article originally appeared in Gastrointestinal Endoscopy Clinics, Volume 24, Issue 4, October 2014.

Division of Gastroenterology, Mayo Clinic Arizona, 13400 East Shea Boulevard, Scottsdale, AZ 85259, USA

E-mail address: Vela.Marcelo@mayo.edu

In addition to careful history-taking for typical symptoms of GERD, validated questionnaires are available to measure specific symptoms and GERD-related quality of life scales. These instruments can be helpful but they generally have similar specificity and sensitivity compared with clinical examination by a gastroenterologist. Therefore, they are most commonly used in clinical trials.

Upper endoscopy is indicated for patients with alarm features such as dysphagia, bleeding, or weight loss, and in patients with typical symptoms that do not respond appropriately to PPI therapy. The finding of erosive esophagitis on endoscopy provides robust evidence of GERD, but this lesion is present in only one-third of untreated patients[2] and it is uncommon in those that are in treatment with a PPI. Random biopsies to document GERD in patients with normal endoscopy are not advised because of the limited diagnostic capabilities of conventional histology for this purpose.

When endoscopy is negative in patients with an uncertain diagnosis of GERD or a suboptimal response to PPI, further work up involves objective quantification of gastroesophageal reflux. This can be accomplished through pH monitoring (catheter-based or wireless), which can establish whether a pathologic amount of acid reflux is present and may provide insight regarding the association between reflux episodes and reported symptoms. Impedance-pH monitoring enables measurement of not only acid, but also nonacid (with a pH >4) reflux episodes. Nonacid reflux may be important in patients with PPI-refractory symptoms. Objective documentation of GERD by endoscopy or reflux monitoring is mandatory before antireflux surgery. Of note, barium esophagram and esophageal manometry cannot establish whether GERD is present and are not useful to diagnose it. However, these tests, especially manometry, may enable a diagnosis of non-GERD causes of esophageal symptoms in PPI-refractory patients (ie, achalasia or rumination). It is important to keep in mind the possibility of non-GERD causes (eg, achalasia, eosinophilic esophagitis [EoE], or a functional disorder) in PPI-refractory patients. In this context, endoscopy and reflux monitoring can be valuable tools to exclude GERD. The pros and cons of diagnostic modalities for GERD are summarized in **Table 1**. This article focuses primarily on patients with typical symptoms (heartburn or regurgitation) and discusses different modalities for the work up of GERD. A section summarizing the diagnostic approach for PPI-refractory symptoms, a common clinical problem, is also included.

DIAGNOSING GERD BY SYMPTOMS AND RESPONSE TO ACID SUPPRESSION

Heartburn and regurgitation are considered the most reliable symptoms for making a history-based diagnosis of GERD but are far from perfect in this respect.[3] In fact, these symptoms actually have variable sensitivity and specificity for diagnosing GERD.[4] Although heartburn is the most typical symptom of GERD, patients with heartburn represent a heterogeneous group; even if many or most of them have GERD, others may experience heartburn as a result of other esophageal disorders such as EoE or achalasia. Furthermore, some patients may have no organic cause for this symptom and are thus diagnosed with functional heartburn, one of the recognized functional gastrointestinal disorders.[5] GERD patients may also present with dysphagia, one of the alarm symptoms that warrants endoscopic evaluation to exclude a complication including malignancy. However, other potential causes for dysphagia must not be ignored. Chest pain may also be reported by GERD patients but this symptom requires thorough evaluation for cardiac disease before GERD is considered.

Recently, the spectrum of clinical presentations attributed to GERD has expanded beyond the typical esophageal symptoms of heartburn and regurgitation and now

Table 1
Pros and cons of diagnostic modalities for gastroesophageal reflux disease

Diagnostic Modality	Pros	Cons
PPI test	• Widely available • Simple • Noninvasive • Inexpensive	• Administration of test not standardized (PPI dose and duration vary) • Definition of response (partial vs complete) not standardized • Limited sensitivity and specificity
Endoscopy	• GERD can be diagnosed confidently when erosive esophagitis is present • Can diagnose non-GERD disorders such as EoE	• Invasive, often requiring sedation • A normal endoscopy (found in 2/3 of GERD patients) does not rule out GERD • Esophageal biopsies obtained during endoscopy are not useful to diagnose GERD
Reflux monitoring		
Catheter-based pH	• The gold standard for GERD diagnosis by assessing esophageal acid exposure • Positive test predicts response to therapy	• Catheter discomfort may limit diet and activities • Study restricted to 24 h • Unable to detect nonacid reflux (with pH>4)
Wireless pH	• Like catheter-pH, measures esophageal acid exposure • Better tolerability • Prolonged monitoring (up to 96 h)	• More costly than catheter-based techniques • Requires endoscopy for placement • Unable to detect nonacid reflux (with pH>4)
Impedance-pH	• Measures esophageal acid exposure • Can detect nonacid reflux	• Catheter discomfort may limit activities • Study restricted to 24 h • Analysis of tracings more laborious than pH alone

includes various extraesophageal manifestations, including asthma, chronic cough, and laryngitis.[6,7] However, a causal relationship between reflux and these extraesophageal presentations has been difficult to prove and these atypical symptoms frequently have multifactorial causes in which gastroesophageal reflux may be a cofactor instead of a cause. Extraesophageal syndromes rarely occur in isolation without concomitant typical symptoms of GERD.[8]

A variety of validated questionnaires have been developed for GERD, including specific symptom scales, quality of life scales, and those which combine the two. A comprehensive discussion of these instruments is outside the scope of this article. Although these instruments may be helpful, they have similar specificity and sensitivity to a clinical examination by a gastroenterologist and are usually reserved for screening large numbers of patients by personnel who are not specialists or as part of clinical trials.[9]

Although the limitations of heartburn and regurgitation for making a diagnosis of GERD should be recognized, it is not necessary to conduct a diagnostic evaluation in all patients with typical symptoms and no alarm features. For these patients, a short trial of acid suppression with a PPI represents a noninvasive, simple, and reasonable option for supporting a diagnosis of GERD. If the patient has a clear response to therapy, it can be assumed that GERD is present. That is not to say that the PPI test is without shortcomings. The manner in which this test is administered is not standard-ized, with differing PPI doses (once vs twice daily), variable duration of treatment (from 1 to 4 weeks), and different definitions of a positive response to PPI (either partial or complete). Moreover, a meta-analysis of several studies that evaluated the diagnostic capability of a short course of PPI compared with other diagnostic interventions, found a sensitivity of 78% and specificity of 54% for the PPI test.[10]

ESOPHAGRAM AND ESOPHAGEAL MANOMETRY

A diagnosis of GERD cannot be made based on the results of an esophagram or esoph-ageal manometry. However, it is important to briefly discuss these tests because they are often used in the work-up of patients with symptoms suggestive of GERD.

The presence of erosive esophagitis may be documented through a high-quality barium esophagram but the overall sensitivity of this test for esophagitis is low.[11] The finding of reflux of barium from stomach to esophagus is frequently included in esophagram reports, with or without provocative maneuvers. However, this finding may be absent in GERD patients and it can be elicited with provocative maneuvers in some healthy patients.[12,13] An esophagram can be helpful when a patient has dysphagia because it may reveal a structural abnormality such as a stricture or ring; however, endoscopy has a higher yield for this purpose. In summary, a diagnosis of GERD cannot be made through esophagram.

GERD patients may show evidence of impaired peristalsis or a hypotensive lower esophageal sphincter during esophageal manometry[14] but these findings are not spe-cific and may be found in the absence of GERD. In patients with esophageal symp-toms (heartburn, regurgitation, chest pain, and dysphagia) attributed to GERD who do not respond to PPI therapy, manometry should be performed to rule out achalasia or other motor disorders.[3] Before antireflux surgery, esophageal manometry is mandatory to rule out achalasia or scleroderma-like esophagus because these condi-tions represent contraindications to fundoplication. The presence of decreased peri-stalsis before surgery is less important because this has not been found to reliably predict dysphagia following fundoplication.[15]

ENDOSCOPIC EVALUATION AND ROLE OF ESOPHAGEAL BIOPSIES

Upper endoscopy enables direct visualization of the esophageal mucosa and may reveal erosive esophagitis as well as stricture and Barrett esophagus. The most widely used system for grading the severity of esophagitis is the Los Angeles classification, which has been well validated in terms of interobserver variability.[16] GERD can be diagnosed with confidence when erosive esophagitis is found; however, endoscopy is normal in approximately two-thirds of patients with heartburn and regurgitation, and the absence of esophagitis does not rule out GERD.[17] Obtaining random esoph-ageal biopsies as a means of diagnosing GERD in patients with normal endoscopy is not recommended because the so-called classic histologic findings of GERD (basal cell hyperplasia, papillary elongation, and infiltration with neutrophils or eosinophils) have poor diagnostic performance characteristics. These findings may be absent in disease, and present in non-GERD controls.[18,19] In the current era of increasing prev-alence of EoE, random distal and proximal esophageal biopsies may be useful in pa-tients without a clear diagnosis because EoE patients may present with symptoms that are similar to those experienced by GERD patients (heartburn, dysphagia, and chest pain). Importantly, endoscopy may appear normal (without the typical rings or linear furrows) in up to 10% of EoE patients.[20]

REFLUX MONITORING

Direct quantification of reflux is only possible by ambulatory, prolonged (at least 24 hours) reflux monitoring techniques, which represent the gold standard in the diagnosis of GERD. The main goal of a reflux monitoring test is to establish whether an abnormal, pathologic amount of reflux is present by measuring esophageal acid exposure or the number or reflux episodes. In addition, reflux monitoring offers an opportunity to assess the temporal relationship between reflux episodes and reported symptoms. Traditionally, reflux monitoring was performed through catheter-based pH measurements. Recent advances include the development of a wireless pH capsule that allows catheter-free monitoring and impedance-pH measurement, a catheter-based technique that enables detection of acid, as well as nonacid reflux (ie, with pH >4). Esophageal bilirubin monitoring has been used but is not routinely used in clinical practice and not widely available.[21] There are several catheters that incorporate pH monitoring at the level of the pharynx. However, pharyngeal pH monitoring has important shortcomings and it generally does not predict response to treatment.[22] A new transnasal pharyngeal catheter that is capable of detecting acid in liquid or aerosolized form has been developed[23] but data supporting its use are limited.

Catheter-Based and Wireless pH Monitoring

For many years the standard approach to ambulatory pH monitoring was to use a transnasal catheter to measure esophageal pH in the distal esophagus for 24 hours with a pH electrode positioned 5 cm above the proximal border of the lower esophageal sphincter. A reflux episode is defined by a drop in pH to below 4.0. A study of this nature enables several measurements, including the percentage of time during which esophageal pH is below 4 (acid exposure time), the number of reflux episodes, number of reflux episodes longer than 5 minutes, and longest reflux episode.[24] Of these, esophageal acid exposure is thought to be the most useful indicator of pathologic acid reflux.[25] A positive pH test can establish a diagnosis of GERD in a patient with normal endoscopy; it may also help to confirm or exclude GERD in patients who do not respond to PPI therapy. Although the sensitivity and specificity of this test are above 90% in some studies,[26,27] other data point to lower sensitivity.[28]

The presence of a transnasal catheter may result in changes in patient behavior such as altered eating habits and decreased activity.[29] To circumvent this issue and to allow for longer monitoring periods, a wireless pH monitoring capsule was developed. This capsule, which is attached to the distal esophagus during endoscopy, transmits pH data via radiofrequency signals to an external recording device worn on the patient's belt. Wireless pH monitoring has similar and possibly improved accuracy compared with catheter-based pH monitoring.[30] Not surprisingly, it is better tolerated than a transnasal catheter and results in less interference with diet and acitivity.[31,32] Furthermore, with the wireless pH capsule the standard is to perform monitoring for 48 hours and the test can be extended to up to 96 hours.[33] This prolonged monitoring period has been shown to improve sensitivity for distinguishing controls from subjects with GERD.[34]

Impedance-pH Monitoring

Both catheter-based and wireless capsule pH monitoring are focused on measuring acid reflux (ie, drops in pH to <4.0). However, these techniques do not allow assessment of nonacid reflux (ie, with pH >4), which may occur when the gastric contents are buffered (during pharmacologic acid suppression or in the postprandial period).

Impedance-pH monitoring is the only available test that can measure acid as well as nonacid reflux. By measuring intraesophageal impedance in a series of conducting electrodes placed in a catheter that spans the length of the esophagus it is possible to detect movement of intraesophageal material in either antegrade or retrograde direction.[35] When coupled with a pH electrode (thus the term impedance-pH), these catheters enable very detailed characterization of gastroesophageal reflux episodes, including acidity (acid, nonacid), composition (air, liquid, or mixed), proximal extent (height), velocity, and clearance time. Impedance-pH is currently the most accurate and detailed method to measure gastroesophageal reflux.[36] During combined impedance and pH monitoring, impedance is used to detect retrograde bolus movement (ie, reflux), whereas pH measurement establishes the acidity of the reflux episode (acid if pH <4.0, nonacid otherwise). Nonacid reflux may be further classified as either weakly acidic (pH $\geq$4 but <7) or weakly alkaline (pH $\geq$7). During impedance-pH monitoring, reflux burden can be ascertained by measuring distal esophageal acid exposure or by the number of reflux episodes. Symptom association studies are performed by assessing the relationship between symptoms and all forms of reflux (acid and nonacid).

The main advantage of impedance-pH monitoring is the ability to detect nonacid reflux because acid reflux can be reliably measured by catheter-based or wireless pH monitoring. Therefore, the usefulness of impedance-pH monitoring is directly linked to the clinical relevance of nonacid reflux. It has been shown that nonacid reflux can cause symptoms that are indistinguishable from those caused by acid reflux.[37] As noted previously, nonacid reflux occurs only when the gastric contents are buffered, which is seen in the postprandial period or in patients who are receiving acid-suppressing medication. A recent systematic review found that in subjects on PPI therapy, most reflux episodes have a pH above 4. Furthermore, nonacid reflux is responsible for most reflux-related symptoms in subjects on PPI treatment.[38] Nonacid reflux can be treated by pharmacologic inhibition of transient lower esophageal sphincter relaxations[39] or through fundoplication.[40] However, there is a paucity of controlled studies examining the benefit of treating nonacid reflux. Therefore, although impedance-pH is considered the most accurate method for reflux detection, the clinical indications for its use and its role in managing GERD patients are still evolving while the merits of finding and treating nonacid reflux await confirmation by high-quality trials. Finally, even with available software, interpretation of impedance-pH tracings is usually more time consuming compared with pH monitoring tracings.

Beyond Reflux Burden: Symptom Association Studies During Reflux Monitoring

The main goal of reflux monitoring is to establish whether an abnormal amount of reflux is present. An additional goal may be to determine whether the patient's symptoms are indeed being caused by reflux episodes. The two most common methods to evaluate the temporal association between reflux episodes and symptoms are the symptom index (SI)[41] and the symptom association probability (SAP).[42] The SI is defined as the percentage of symptom events that are temporally related to a reflux episode (number of reflux-related symptom events/total number of symptom events $\times$ 100%). An SI of 50% is considered positive, meaning that the symptom is related to reflux. Although this value was derived from receiver operating characteristic (ROC) curves that found this threshold to be sensitive and specific for heartburn,[43] the SI is used to analyze any symptom that may be attributed to GERD. The SAP is calculated by dividing the pH or impedance-pH tracing in 2-minute segments and determining whether a reflux episode and/or a symptom occurred in each 2-minute segment. A 2 $\times$ 2 contingency table with the number of segments with and without symptoms and with and without reflux is built; the probability that a positive association between reflux and symptoms occurred by more than chance is evaluated through a modified chi-square test, with an SAP greater than 95% considered positive.

An in-depth discussion of the advantages and disadvantages of the SI and the SAP is beyond the scope of this article; however, it is important for clinicians to know that both have methodological shortcomings[44] and that symptom association studies are the least robust measure obtained during reflux monitoring. Regardless of whether SI or SAP is used, precise and timely symptom recording by the patient is needed along with accurate reflux detection by the testing device. Furthermore, prospective data to validate the ability of these symptom association measures to predict response to treatment are scarce. Nevertheless, during patient management, a strongly positive SI or SAP may suggest the need for a therapeutic intervention and a negative result supports the notion that the patient's symptoms are unlikely to be due to reflux. However, given the limitations of these measures, recent guidelines recommend that the SI and SAP should not be used in isolation and other reflux monitoring parameters, as well as the patient's overall presentation, should be taken into account.[3]

WORK UP OF PATIENTS WITH PPI-REFRACTORY SYMPTOMS

A frequent reason for consultation to gastroenterology is failure to achieve satisfactory symptom improvement after treatment with PPI. PPI-refractory patients are heterogeneous but may fall into one of four general categories: (1) true PPI failure with ongoing symptoms due to persistent reflux of acidic gastric material (acid reflux), (2) adequate acid gastric suppression by the PPI but frequent reflux of nonacidic material as the cause of the symptoms, (3) symptoms due to other disorders (eg, EoE or achalasia), (4) no organic cause for the symptoms (ie, a functional gastrointestinal disorder such as functional heartburn). Because, clearly, not all patients who fail to respond to PPIs have GERD, a very important goal of the diagnostic evaluation in these patients is to differentiate those with persistent reflux as the cause of the ongoing symptoms from those with non-GERD etiologies.

The first step in the management of PPI-refractory patients is to confirm compliance and ensure that dosing and timing of medication are adequate. Once compliance and appropriate dosing are ensured, a single trial of a different PPI can be considered. A randomized controlled trial in subjects with persistent GERD symptoms despite a single daily dose of PPI, showed that increasing PPI to twice daily or switching to another PPI resulted in symptomatic improvement in roughly 20% of subjects, without a clear advantage for either strategy.[45]

Patients with persistent symptoms despite optimization of PPI therapy require further work-up. Endoscopy is recommended for typical esophageal symptoms to look for erosive esophagitis (rare in acid-suppressed patients) and exclude nonreflux esophageal disorders such as EoE. If endoscopy is negative, as is frequently the case, reflux monitoring is indicated. Reflux monitoring should also be considered in patients with extraesophageal symptoms that persist despite PPI optimization and in whom non-GERD causes have been ruled out through pulmonary, ears-nose-throat, and allergy evaluation.

Two important issues to weigh when preparing to perform reflux monitoring are whether the test should be done while on PPI therapy or after cessation of this medication, and what tool to use (catheter-based pH, wireless pH, or impedance-pH). Reflux monitoring off PPI (7 days after stopping therapy) can be performed with any of the available techniques (catheter, wireless pH, or impedance-pH) because the main goal is to measure acid reflux. Reflux monitoring on PPI should be performed with impedance-pH monitoring to enable measurement of nonacid reflux. The yield of pH monitoring without impedance in a patient taking a PPI is very low because in acid-suppressed patients reflux becomes predominantly nonacid.[37]

Studies comparing the yield of off-therapy with on-therapy reflux monitoring in refractory GERD patients are limited and inconclusive. For instance, Hemmink and colleagues[46] concluded that testing should be performed off PPI; in contrast, Pritchett and colleagues[47] found that reflux monitoring on PPI may be the preferred strategy. Not surprisingly, there is no clear consensus regarding the optimal testing approach for patients with PPI-refractory symptoms. One option is to stop medication in all such patients so that GERD can be either confirmed or ruled out. Patients without GERD can go on to testing and treatment of other causes, including functional disorders, whereas those with confirmed GERD can undergo escalation of therapy and further diagnostic interventions, possibly including reflux monitoring while on PPI to assess for ongoing acid or nonacid reflux. A second option, suggested in recent guidelines,[3,25] is to base the approach to testing on the patient's clinical presentation and pretest likelihood of GERD (**Fig. 1**). Patients with low likelihood of GERD (eg, complete absence of response to PPI, extraesophageal presentations without concomitant typical symptoms) may be tested off therapy. If the test is negative, GERD is excluded and other causes are pursued. Patients with high likelihood of GERD (eg, at least partial response to PPI, typical symptoms, other features to suggest GERD such as large hiatus hernia) may be tested while on therapy in search of reflux (acid or nonacid) that persists despite acid suppression. In the latter patients, off-PPI reflux monitoring has reasonable likelihood to be positive but this finding will not provide information regarding the reason for the ongoing symptoms. In some patients, testing both off as well as on therapy is necessary to clarify the reason for PPI-refractoriness.

Finally, it is important to stress the importance of stopping PPI therapy in patients with refractory symptoms in whom all testing is negative. In a recent study, after a

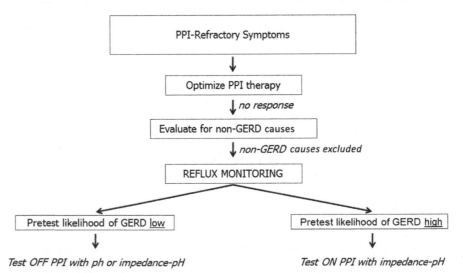

Fig. 1. Suggested work up for patients with PPI-refractory symptoms. (*Adapted from* Katz PO, Gerson L, Vela MF. Guidelines for the diagnosis and management of gastroesophageal reflux disease. Am J Gastroenterol 2013;108:322; with permission.)

negative evaluation for refractory GERD that included normal endoscopy and impedance-pH monitoring, 42% of 90 subjects reported continued use of PPI despite negative results.[48] This study highlights the importance of educating the patient about the need to stop PPIs after the work-up is negative for GERD.

SUMMARY

GERD may be diagnosed based on symptoms and a positive response to acid suppression (the PPI test) in patients with typical presentations and no alarm features. However, it is important to be aware of the limited sensitivity and specificity of this approach as a diagnostic intervention. Patients with alarm features such as dysphagia or weight loss and those with typical symptoms and incomplete response to PPI, should undergo endoscopy. When endoscopy reveals erosive esophagitis, GERD can be diagnosed confidently; however, most patients have normal endoscopic evaluation. Esophageal biopsies to diagnose GERD based on histologic findings are not recommended because of the poor diagnostic capability of these findings. Reflux monitoring can document the presence of pathologic reflux and may shed light on the relationship between reflux episodes and reported symptoms. Monitoring by pH relies on detecting acid reflux, either by catheter technique or with a wireless capsule. Impedance-pH monitoring is required when there is a need to measure nonacid reflux (ie, with a pH >4), which may be clinically important in patients who do not improve with PPI therapy. Patients with persistent symptoms despite PPI are a heterogeneous group. These patients may have ongoing reflux (acid or nonacid) as the cause of their symptoms, they may have non-GERD disorders such as EoE or achalasia, or they may have a functional gastrointestinal disorder. There is no consensus regarding whether testing of refractory patients should be performed on versus off therapy. One option is to use the pretest likelihood of GERD to guide testing: those with low likelihood of GERD should be tested off therapy, whereas those with high likelihood of GERD should be tested on PPI. For PPI-refractory patients in whom GERD is ruled out, PPI should be discontinued and other causes need to be investigated.

REFERENCES

1. Locke GR III, Talley NJ, Fett SL, et al. Prevalence and clinical spectrum of gastro-esophageal reflux: a population-based study in Olmsted County, Minnesota. Gastroenterology 1997;112:1448–56.
2. Lind T, Havelund T, Carlsson R, et al. Heartburn without esophagitis: efficacy of omeprazole therapy and features determining therapeutic response. Scand J Gastroenterol 1997;32:974–9.
3. Katz PO, Gerson L, Vela MF. Guidelines for the diagnosis and management of gastroesophageal reflux disease. Am J Gastroenterol 2013;108:308–28.
4. Klauser AG, Shcindelbeck NE, Muller-Lissner SA. Symptoms in gastro-oesophageal reflux disease. Lancet 1990;335:205.
5. Zerbib F, Bruley de Varannes S, Simon M, et al. Functional heartburn: definition and management strategies. Curr Gastroenterol Rep 2012;14:181–8.
6. Irwin RS, Curley FJ, French CL. Chronic cough. The spectrum and frequency of causes, key components of the diagnostic evaluation, and outcome of specific therapy. Am Rev Respir Dis 1990;141:640–7.
7. El-Serag HB, Sonnenberg A. Comorbid occurrence of laryngeal or pulmonary disease with esophagitis in United States military veterans. Gastroenterology 1997;113:755–60.

8. Vakil N, van Zanten SV, Kahrilas P, et al. The Montreal definition and classification of gastroesophageal reflux disease: a global evidence-based consensus. Am J Gastroenterol 2006;101:1900.
9. Stanghellini V, Arsmtrong D, Monnikes H, et al. Systematic review; do we need a new gastroesophageal diseases questionnaire. Digestion 2007;75(suppl 1): 3–16.
10. Numans ME, Lau J, de Wit NK, et al. Short-term treatment with proton-pump inhibitors as a test for gastroesophageal reflux disease. Ann Intern Med 2004;140: 518–52.
11. Johnston BT, Troshinsky MB, Castell JA, et al. Comparison of barium radiology with esophageal pH monitoring in the diagnosis of gastroesophageal reflux disease. Am J Gastroenterol 1996;91:1181–5.
12. Thompson JK, Koehler RE, Richter JE. Detection of gastroesophageal reflux: value of barium studies compared with 24-hr pH monitoring. Am J Roentgenol 1994;162:621–6.
13. Richter JE, Castell DO. Gastroesophageal reflux. Pathogenesis, diagnosis, and therapy. Ann Intern Med 1982;97:93–103.
14. Savarino E, Gemignani L, Pohl D, et al. Oesophageal motility and bolus transit abnormalities increase in parallel with the severity of gastro-oesophageal reflux disease. Aliment Pharmacol Ther 2011;34:476–86.
15. Shaw JM, Bornman PC, Callanan MD, et al. Long-term outcome of laparoscopic Nissen and laparoscopic Toupet fundoplication for gastroesophageal reflux disease: a prospective, randomized trial. Surg Endosc 2010;24:924–32.
16. Lundell LR, Dent J, Bennett JR, et al. Endoscopic assessment of oesophagitis: clinical and functional correlates and further validation of the Los Angeles classification. Gut 1999;45:172–80.
17. Johnsson F, Joelsson B, Gudmundsson K, et al. Symptoms and endoscopic findings in the diagnosis of gastroesophageal reflux disease. Scand J Gastroenterol 1987;22:714–8.
18. Nandurkar S, Talley NJ, Martin CJ, et al. Esophageal histology does not provide additional useful information over clinical assessment in identifying reflux patients presenting for esophagogastroduodenoscopy. Dig Dis Sci 2000;2000(45): 217–24.
19. Tytgat G. The value of esophageal histology in the diagnosis of gastroesophageal reflux disease in patients with heartburn and normal endoscopy. Curr Gastroenterol Rep 2008;10:231–4.
20. Prasad GA, Talley NJ, Romero Y, et al. Prevalence and predictive factors of eosinophilic esophagitis in patients presenting with dysphagia: a prospective study. Am J Gastroenterol 2007;102:2627.
21. Vaezi MF, Richter JE. Role of acid and duodenogastroesophageal reflux in gastroesophageal reflux disease. Gastroenterology 1996;111:1192–9.
22. Vaezi MF, Hicks DM, Abelson TI, et al. Laryngeal signs and symptoms of gastroesophageal reflux disease (GERD): a critical assessment of cause and effect association. Clin Gastroenterol Hepatol 2003;1:333–44.
23. Sun G, Muddana S, Slaughter JC, et al. A new pH catheter for laryngopharyngeal reflux: Normal values. Laryngoscope 2009;119:1639–43.
24. Johnson LF, Demeester TR. Twenty-four-hour pH monitoring of the distal esophagus. A quantitative measure of gastroesophageal reflux. Am J Gastroenterol 1974;62:325–32.
25. Pandolfino JE, Vela MF. Esophageal reflux monitoring. Gastrointest Endosc 2009; 69:917–30.

26. Jamieson JR, Stein HJ, DeMeester TR, et al. Ambulatory 24-h esophageal pH monitoring: normal values, optimal thresholds, specificity, sensitivity, and reproducibility. Am J Gastroenterol 1992;87:1102–11.

27. Richter JE, Bradley LA, DeMeester TR, et al. Normal 24-hr ambulatory esophageal pH values. Influence of study center, pH electrode, age, and gender. Dig Dis Soi 1992;37:849–56.

28. Schlesinger PK, Donahue PE, Schmid B, et al. Limitations of 24-hour intraesophageal pH monitoring in the hospital setting. Gastroenterology 1985;894:797–804.

29. Fass R, Hell R, Sampliner RE, et al. Effect of ambulatory 24-h esophageal pH monitoring on reflux-provoking activities. Dig Dis Sci 1999;44:2263–9.

30. Pandolfino J, Zhang Q, Schreiner M, et al. Acid reflux event detection using the Bravo™ wireless vs the Slimline™ catheter pH systems: why are the numbers so different? Gut 2005;54:1687–92.

31. Wenner J, Jonsson F, Johansson J, et al. Wireless esophageal pH monitoring is better tolerated than the catheter-based technique: results from a randomized cross-over trial. Am J Gastroenterol 2007;102:239–45.

32. Ward EM, Devault KR, Bouras EP, et al. Successful oesophageal pH monitoring with a catheter-free system. Aliment Pharmacol Ther 2004;19:449–54.

33. Hirano I, Zhang Q, Pandolfino JE, et al. Four-day Bravo pH capsule monitoring with and without proton pump inhibitor therapy. Clin Gastroenterol Hepatol 2005;3:1083–8.

34. Pandolfino JE, Richter JE, Ours T, et al. Ambulatory esophageal pH monitoring using a wireless system. Am J Gastroenterol 2003;984:740–9.

35. Vela MF. Non-acid reflux: detection by multichannel intraluminal impedance and pH, clinical significance and management. Am J Gastroenterol 2009;104:277–80.

36. Sifrim D, Castell D, Dent J, et al. Gastro-oesophageal reflux monitoring: reflux and consensus report on detection and definitions of acid, non-acid, and gas reflux. Gut 2004;53:1024–31.

37. Vela MF, Camacho-Lobato L, Srinivasan R, et al. Intraesophageal impedance and pH measurement of acid and non-acid reflux: effect of omeprazole. Gastroenterology 2001;96:647–55.

38. Boeckxstaens GE, Smout A. Systematic review: role of acid, weakly acidic and weakly alkaline reflux in gastro-oesophageal reflux disease. Aliment Pharmacol ther 2010;32:334–43.

39. Vela MF, Tutuian R, Katz PO, et al. Baclofen decreases acid and non-acid postprandial gastro-oesophageal reflux measured by combined multichannel intraluminal impedance and pH. Aliment Pharmacol Ther 2003;17:243–51.

40. Frazzoni M, Conigliaro R, Melotti G. Reflux parameters as modified by laparoscopic fundoplication in 40 patients with heartburn/regurgitation persisting despite PPI therapy: a study using impedance-pH monitoring. Dig Dis Sci 2011;56:1099–106.

41. Wiener GJ, Richter JE, Copper JB, et al. The symptom index: a clinically important parameter of ambulatory 24-hour esophageal pH monitoring. Am J Gastroenterol 1988;83:358–61.

42. Weusten BL, Roelofs JM, Akkermans LM, et al. The symptom-association probability: an improved method for symptom analysis of 24-hour esophageal pH data. Gastroenterology 1994;107:1741–5.

43. Singh S, Richter JE, Bradley LA, et al. The symptom index. Differential usefulness in suspected acid-related complaints of heartburn and chest pain. Dig Dis Sci 1993;34:309–16.

44. Connor J, Richter J. Increasing yield also increases false positives and best serves to exclude GERD. Am J Gastroenterol 2006;101:460–3.
45. Fass R, Murthy U, Hayden CW, et al. Omeprazole 40 mg once a day is equally effective as lansoprazole 30 mg twice a day in symptom control of patients with gastro-oesophageal reflux disease (GERD) who are resistant to conventional-dose lansoprazole therapy-a prospective, randomized, multi-centre study. Aliment Pharmacol Ther 2000;14:1595–603.
46. Hemmink GJ, Bredenoord AJ, Weusten BL, et al. Esophageal pH-impedance monitoring in patients with therapy-resistant reflux symptoms: 'on' or 'off' proton pump inhibitor? Am J Gastroenterol 2008;103:2446–53.
47. Pritchett JM, Aslam M, Slaughter JC, et al. Efficacy of esophageal impedance/pH monitoring in patients with refractory gastroesophageal reflux disease, on and off therapy. Clin Gastroenterol Hepatol 2009;7:743–8.
48. Gawron AJ, Rothe J, Fought AJ, et al. Many patients continue using proton pump inhibitors after negative results from tests for reflux disease. Clin Gastroenterol Hepatol 2012;10:620–5.

Barium Esophagram

Does It Have a Role in Gastroesophageal Reflux Disease?

Mark E. Baker, MD, FARS, FSCBT/MR[a,b,c,d,*],
David M. Einstein, MD, FARS[a,b]

KEYWORDS

- Barium esophagogram • Gastroesophageal reflux disease
- Post-fundoplication barium appearance

KEY POINTS

- The barium esophagram is an integral part of the assessment and management of patients with gastroesophageal reflux disease (GERD) before, and especially after, antireflux procedures.
- While many of the findings on the examination can be identified with endoscooopy, a gastric emptying study and an esophageal motility examination, the barium esophagram is better at demonstrating the anatomic findings after antireflux surgery, especially in symptomatic patients.
- These complementary examinations, when taken as a whole, fully evaluate a patient with suspected GERD as well as symptomatic patients after antireflux procedures.

In the age of endoscopy, pH studies, and high-resolution manometry and impedance, the barium esophagram has been deemphasized in the diagnosis and management of patients with suspected gastroesophageal reflux disease (GERD). Unfortunately, as a result, as in most luminal gastrointestinal radiology, training for this important examination has suffered, resulting in the inability of recently trained radiologists to perform an adequate examination. Nevertheless, this examination is a vital part of a patient's workup when GERD is suspected.[1–4] This examination helps define both the morphology and function of the esophagus, identifying important findings relevant to treatment as well as suggesting diagnoses other than GERD. The authors believe

This article originally appeared in Gastroenterology Clinics, Volume 43, Issue 1, March 2014.
[a] Cleveland Clinic Lerner College of Medicine, Case Western Reserve University, 9500 Euclid Avenue, Cleveland, OH 44195, USA; [b] Abdominal Imaging, Imaging Institute, Cleveland Clinic, 9500 Euclid Avenue, Cleveland, OH 44195, USA; [c] Digestive Disease Institute, Cleveland Clinic, 9500 Euclid Avenue, Cleveland, OH 44195, USA; [d] Cancer Institute, Cleveland Clinic, 9500 Euclid Avenue, Cleveland, OH 44195, USA
* Corresponding author. Abdominal Imaging, Imaging Institute, Cleveland Clinic, 9500 Euclid Avenue, Cleveland, OH 44195.
E-mail address: bakerm@ccf.org

that the examination is essential in defining the anatomic causes of symptoms after antireflux surgery. At the Cleveland Clinic many, if not most patients with suspected GERD are evaluated with a barium esophagram, especially if antireflux surgery is contemplated. Furthermore, all symptomatic patients after antireflux procedures are also evaluated with a barium esophagram.

ESOPHAGRAM: IMPORTANT GENERAL ELEMENTS OF THE EXAMINATION

Several factors are important to the success of a well-performed barium esophagram. First, the complete examination should be recorded in some fashion. A DVD recorder directly set up to the fluoroscopy unit will burn a DVD of the examination. With modern PACS (picture archiving and communication system), it is now possible to capture the fluoroscopic examination directly in DICOM (digital imaging and communications in medicine) format, and save the study without the hard-copy problems of a disk. Second, to reduce radiation exposure a pulsed-fluoroscopy unit is best, generally at 15 pulses per second, to reduce frame flickering. Third, if the patient has a specific complaint, such as dysphagia, before the start of the examination, the radiologist should encourage the patient to voice these symptoms when they occur during the examination.

Just before the examination, a brief history should be elicited from the patient including the presence of dysphagia, regurgitation, chest pain, and heartburn, as well as duration of symptoms and significant weight loss. Symptoms of GERD are often similar to those of a severe dysmotility disorder, most commonly achalasia and less commonly diffuse esophageal spasm. Therefore, when a patient complains of dysphagia, the examiner must know whether it is to solids alone or to both solids and liquids. When liquid dysphagia is a significant part of the history, the patient starts in the upright position, swallowing a small amount of low-density barium. If there is any delay in emptying, or findings suggesting achalasia, such as a dilated esophagus or a bird-beak appearance of the distal esophagus, the patient proceeds to a timed barium swallow.[5] If the examiner starts the study of a patient with unsuspected achalasia with the routine, air-contrast examination, using gas-producing crystals and high-density barium, the subsequent study is largely ruined.

There are multiple phases of a barium esophagram, not all of which need be performed (**Box 1**). It is important to tailor the examination to the patient based on

---

Box 1
Phases of a barium esophagram

- Timed barium swallow (assesses esophageal emptying with the patient in the upright position)
- Upright phase (most often performed using air-contrast techniques)
- Motility phase performed primarily in the right anterior oblique position (performed in the semiprone position)
- Distended or full-column phase performed primarily in the right anterior oblique position (performed in the semiprone position with the patient rapidly drinking)
- Mucosal relief phase (observed at the end of the distended or full-column phase of the examination)
- Reflux assessment (after esophagus has emptied, with the patient in the supine or left posterior oblique position)
- "Solid" food assessment (13 mm barium tablet, marshmallow, or offending food)
- Gastric findings, including emptying (observing the gastric motility fluoroscopically)

condition, signs and symptoms, and ability to ingest various densities of barium, a barium tablet, or various foodstuffs.

THE PREOPERATIVE BARIUM ESOPHAGRAM
Initial Upright Phase

If there is liquid dysphagia, an initial timed barium swallow is performed (**Fig. 1**).[5] With the patient in the upright position, the patient is asked to ingest up to 250 mL of

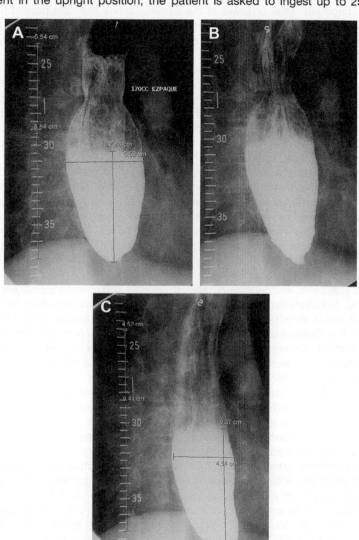

Fig. 1. Timed barium swallow in a patient with type I achalasia. (*A*) One-minute, upright film, with measurements after the patient ingested 170 mL of low-density barium. (*B*) Two-minute, upright film, without measurements. (*C*) Five-minute, upright film, with measurements. There is very little emptying between the 1- and 5 minute films. Unless there has been complete emptying at 2 minutes, the height and width of the barium column is reported at 1 and 5 minutes.

low-density barium. The patient is told that the volume is entirely self-regulated and based on his or her tolerance level. The patient is allowed to ingest the barium over 45 seconds after which an upright spot film is taken, attempting to include the entire barium column on this film. If the column is too high, 2 spot films are take, 1 lower and 1 upper. If barium does not empty, the authors then take 2- and 5-minute films. Unless the barium has emptied in the interval, the 1- and 5-minute films are compared, measuring the height and width of the barium column on both. It is important to keep the image intensifier or tower at the same distance from the patient for all the spot films, so as not to alter the level of magnification. The amount of barium ingested is also recorded. A normal esophagus should empty 250 mL of low-density barium within seconds.

If there is no significant liquid dysphagia, the examination should start with the patient in the upright position, preferably using an air-contrast technique.[2,4] In the authors' practice, the upright position helps in identifying a foreshortened or short esophagus (also known as a fixed, hiatal hernia) (**Fig. 2**).[6–8] Many surgeons, especially thoracic surgeons, consider it important to preoperatively identify a foreshortened esophagus, as this often leads to the addition of a Collis gastroplasty or lengthening procedure, rather than a Nissen fundoplication alone. Their belief is that with a short esophagus the hernia often cannot be completely mobilized and reduced below the diaphragm, especially using abdominal, laparoscopic techniques. If the esophagus is not adequately mobilized and the hernia reduced, the hernia repair is under tension, given the propensity of the foreshortened esophagus to pull back into the mediastinum; this often leads not only to disruption of the hiatus repair and a recurrence of the hernia, but also to a disruption of the fundoplication.[9] It should be noted that not all surgeons believe in the concept of a short esophagus.

In most practices, endoscopy is used to identify reflux esophagitis and Barrett esophagus. Nonetheless, the air-contrast portion of the examination can identify findings of reflux esophagitis and Barrett esophagus, although with much lower sensitivity. The findings of mild reflux esophagitis include a fine nodular or granular mucosal pattern. Changes of moderate to severe reflux esophagitis vary from shallow ulcers and erosions to longitudinal fold thickening and submucosal ridging. Peptic stricture formation is the most significant finding of severe esophagitis.[10] A high esophageal stricture or ulcer and a reticular pattern are strongly associated with Barrett esophagus (**Fig. 3**). Using meticulous technique, the air-contrast portion of the examination can identify patients at low, moderate, or high risk for Barrett esophagitis. In a blinded retrospective study of 200 patients with severe reflux symptoms examined with double-contrast esophagrams and endoscopy, moderate risk was considered present when there was a distal stricture or esophagitis, and high risk if there was a high stricture or ulcer or a reticular pattern.[11] The sensitivity of the esophagram for moderate or severe esophagitis was 71% and for severe esophagitis 85%, with endoscopy detecting only 20 of 46 (43%) of radiographically diagnosed strictures, and with endoscopy failing to identify any stricture not identified on esophagography. Using the esophagram as a method of selecting patients based on moderate or high risk for Barrett esophagus, the overall radiologic sensitivity was 95% (21 of 22) but the specificity was only 65% (116 of 178). The positive predictive value was only 25% (21 of 83) but the negative predictive value was 99% (116 of 117).

If the air-contrast phase cannot be performed, it is still essential to attempt to examine the patient in the upright position with low-density barium to identify a fixed hiatal hernia (ie, foreshortened esophagus).

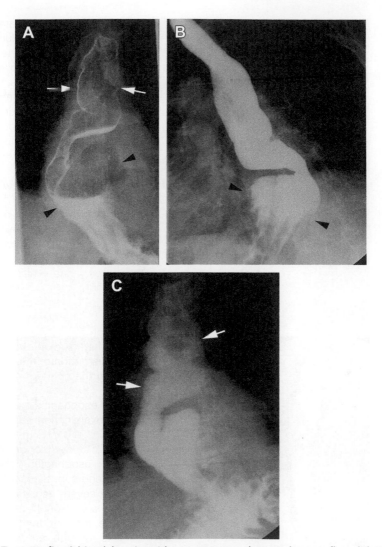

Fig. 2. Type III, fixed hiatal hernia with spontaneous, large-volume reflux. (*A*) Upright, air-contrast spot film showing a large, fixed (nonreducible) hiatal hernia (*black arrowheads*) and a tortuous, patulous esophagus (*white arrows*). (*B*) The large hiatal hernia filled with barium on the full column, semiprone view (*arrowheads*). (*C*) Spontaneous, continuous reflux in the supine position (*white arrows*).

Semiprone or Right Anterior Oblique Phase

The motility portion of the examination is important because it demonstrates the presence and state of peristalsis and bolus transfer, something that only impedance can show.[12] Seminal work by Ott and Richter showed that if 4 of 5 single swallows on a barium esophagram were normal, showing normal bolus transfer in an aboral fashion, then the manometry was normal as well.[13,14] The examiner must focus attention on the inverted V of the tail end of the barium column to properly assess the motility (this corresponds to the upstroke of the pressure wave identified on manometry) (**Fig. 4**). In

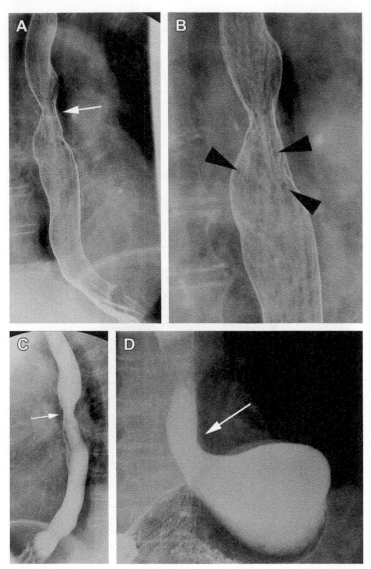

Fig. 3. Barrett stricture in a patient with long-standing GERD and solid-food dysphagia. (*A*) Smooth, tapered narrowing (*white arrow*) at the level of the left pulmonary artery (mid esophagus) on the air-contrast portion of the examination. (*B*) A smaller field-of-view spot film of the air-contrast portion showing nodular folds (*black arrowheads*). (*C*) Persistent, smooth narrowing (*white arrow*) on the semiprone, full-column portion of the examination. (*D*) Spontaneous and continuous reflux (*white arrow*) in the supine portion of the examination. This continuous reflux was present to the level of the cervical esophagus and never cleared.

one retrospective series of 151 patients, the frequency of dysmotility (defined by intermittent weakened or absent peristalsis without or with multiple transient indentations on the barium column as the peristaltic wave traversed the esophagus) was much higher in patients with GERD than in those without.[15]

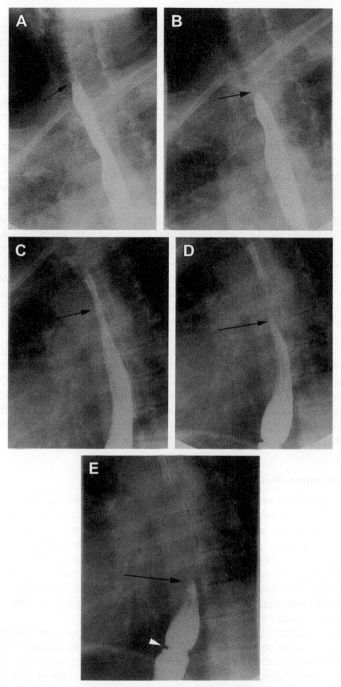

Fig. 4. Esophageal motility. (*A–E*) Freeze frames from a video esophagram demonstrating aboral transmission of the pressure wave distally from the cervical esophagus to the epiphrenic ampulla. The inverted V (*black arrow*) corresponds to the upstroke of the pressure wave. There is some retrograde escape of barium above the inverted V at the juncture of the proximal and middle third of the esophagus (at the juncture of the skeletal and smooth muscle) (*C, D*). This finding is generally not clinically significant unless a large amount escapes above the pressure wave. There is also a distal mucosal ring (*white arrowhead in E*).

With the full implementation of high-resolution manometry and the concurrent use of high-resolution impedance with high-resolution manometry, the impact of the barium assessment of motility has been reduced.[16] The combination of these 2 techniques will show whether low-amplitude peristalsis will have any effect on bolus transit. Regardless, unsuspected and severe motility disorders can be identified during the esophagram, leading to a more detailed analysis with these new techniques. Conversely, if 4 of 5 separate swallows are normal, it is very unlikely that a motility disorder exists.

The full-column, distended, or rapid-drinking phase of the examination identifies overall esophageal distensibility, extrinsic compression or narrowing, strictures, and distal mucosal rings. It may be difficult for patients with long-standing, significant dysphagia to rapidly drink, as they have mentally accommodated over time to not do so. It is important for the examiner to encourage the patient to drink as rapidly as tolerable. During this phase, the authors often slowly pan down the entire course of the esophagus during fluoroscopy, not taking spot films, to identify contour abnormalities and assess the distensibility of the lumen. Special attention should be focused on the distal esophagus, in the region of the epiphrenic ampulla and gastroesophageal junction, a common site of disease. Diffuse, subtle narrowing of the esophagus can result from GERD, but other causes must be considered, especially eosinophilic esophagitis (EOE). EOE is increasingly recognized as a common cause of dysphagia, but unfortunately many of the patients have been misdiagnosed with GERD, as EOE and GERD symptoms overlap.

Directly after the cessation of the rapid drinking is the start of the mucosal relief portion of the examination. This underutilized part of the evaluation is important in several respects. First, the ringed esophagus sometimes present in EOE is often only identified during this phase.[17] Second, thickened esophageal folds from esophagitis are best identified during this phase. If one is unable to adequately coat the esophagus with high-density barium, the only other way to diagnose mild to moderate esophagitis is by identifying fold thickening.

Reflux Identification Phase

The next phase of the examination is to identify gastroesophageal reflux. While the patient remains in the semiprone position, after the mucosal relief stage the esophagus is fluoroscopically assessed for retained barium. If present, the table is raised to the semierect position and the patient is given some water to clear the esophagus of barium. Then, after resuming the horizontal position, the patient is turned to the supine position and the esophagus is examined fluoroscopically. If barium is present in the esophagus, it must have refluxed with motion. If barium is not present the authors proceed with a series of maneuvers starting with a cough or Valsalva maneuver, and then to a water siphon test.

This graded approach in a well-performed investigation increased the sensitivity of identifying reflux when compared with 24-hour pH monitoring studies.[18] When reflux occurs the authors record the cause, if not spontaneous, the height of the reflux (distal, mid, and proximal thoracic and cervical) as well as the length of time the barium remains in the esophagus (<30 or >30 seconds).

This phase of the examination is less important vis-à-vis continuous pH monitoring using a catheter or capsule. However, it is important when there is repeated, continuous, and spontaneous reflux to the cervical esophagus. Trace, intermittent, or low-volume reflux identified on barium studies has little to no clinical significance.

Solid Food Ingestion Phase

The next part of the examination is to assess for the passage of solid food. The authors generally use a 13-mm barium tablet and have the patient ingest the tablet with water. If tablet passage is impaired, the patient ingests low-density barium to identify the precise site and cause, and whether symptoms were elicited (again, before the examination, the patient should be encouraged to voice symptoms if such symptoms occur during the examination). It is common for the tablet to transiently hang up at the level of the transverse aorta and at the level of the gastroesophageal junction. Some institutions administer a standard 30 × 30-mm or a smaller 13 × 12-mm marshmallow (sometimes used in hot chocolate) rather than a 13-mm barium tablet in patients with a distal mucosal ring.[19]

If the patient has consistent dysphagia with a particular food, it is best for the referring physician to have the patient bring that food to the fluoroscopy suite. Ingesting the food, combined with barium paste, can be instructive in 2 ways. First it can show the site and cause of obstruction. More often in the authors' experience, it shows that there is no obstruction. When patients view the examination and sees that there is nothing causing obstruction their anxiety is often relieved, and their often chronic symptoms may resolve.

Feline Esophagus

The feline esophagus is a transient finding on barium esophagrams, most often fleetingly seen during the air-contrast portion of the examination when the esophagus is collapsing. The finding is that of narrowly spaced, transverse folds, giving a crenulated or accordion appearance, a finding caused by contraction of the longitudinal muscles in the esophagus. The cat esophagus has a similar appearance, hence the naming of this finding.

There is controversy as to whether this finding is caused by GERD or is merely associated with GERD. In a recent investigation from the University of Pennsylvania, during a 2-year period 20 of 224 patients examined with a barium esophagram had a feline esophagus,[20] which was detected during barium reflux in 17 of these 20 patients. Gastroesophageal reflux (GER) of barium was present in all 20 patients, of whom 10 had marked GER and 7 moderate GER (marked GER as defined by reflux of barium to or above the thoracic inlet; moderate GER as defined by reflux of barium to the level of the midthoracic esophagus or aortic arch). From this and other investigations, it seems prudent to investigate patients with this finding for the presence of GERD.

Distal Mucosal Ring (Schatzki Ring)

A distal mucosal ring is an idiopathic ridge of tissue composed of mucosa and submucosa located at the gastroesophageal junction (**Fig. 5**). It is often only identified during the semiprone distended phase of the examination,[21] and by definition is associated with a small, often sliding type I hiatal hernia. It was first described by Templeton in 1944, and later reported by Schatzki and Gary and Ingelfinger and Kramer in 1953.[22] Later reports just identify the ring as the Schatzki ring. Because multiple investigators have described the ring, the authors prefer to use the term distal mucosal ring. There is controversy as to the etiology of this redundant tissue, but the finding, like the feline esophagus, is strongly correlated with GERD. Some gastroenterologists recommend that patients with this finding be evaluated for GERD with pH monitoring.[22]

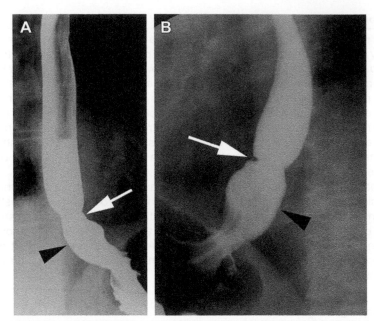

Fig. 5. Small, fixed hiatal hernia with distal mucosal ring in a patient with intermittent solid-food dysphagia. (*A*) Persistent hernia (*black arrowhead*) and narrowing caused at the gastroesophageal junction (*white arrow*) on the upright, air-contrast portion of the examination. (*B*) The same hernia (*black arrowhead*) with the narrowing caused by a mucosal ring (*white arrow*) on the semiprone, full-column portion of the examination.

OUTCOME OF THE PREOPERATIVE EXAMINATION

At the end of the examination, gastroenterologists and esophageal surgeons expect that the radiologist has assessed the level of esophageal emptying in patients with liquid dysphagia (**Box 2**).[3] The presence and type of hiatal hernia should be identified.[23] Type I hernias are sliding-type, small hernias present only in the semiprone position. There is a large degree of subjectivity in the criteria defining a sliding-type or type I hernia using radiography. The radiographic definition is more than a 2 cm separation between the B ring and the diaphragmatic hiatus.[24] Separation less than

---

Box 2
What the gastroenterologist and esophageal surgeon want to know from the preoperative examination

- Assessment of esophageal emptying
- Presence and type of hiatal hernia
- Foreshortening of the esophagus (ie, a hiatal hernia that does not reduce in the upright position)
- Motility: ineffective or absent pump
- Stricture or distal mucosal ring
- Presence, cause, height, and persistence of reflux
- Does the patient have an alternative diagnosis to GERD?

2 cm has been attributed to physiologic herniation. Unfortunately, the B ring is not visible in many patients. In addition, the esophageal gastric junction moves during deglutition because of longitudinal muscle contraction. As a result, the esophagus can shorten approximately 2 cm. Thus, the radiographic identification of a type I hernia is considered unreliable, as is endoscopic identification. Clinically this is not as important as recognizing a fixed hernia.

Type II hernias are rare and are true paraesophageal hernias, with the gastroesophageal junction below the diaphragm and a portion of the fundus herniated through a rent in the diaphragm separate from the hiatus. Type III hernias are the most common paraesophageal hernia and are complex, often large, and associated with a foreshortened esophagus, when a large portion of the fundus is present in the posterior, inferior mediastinum. The herniated stomach may rotate along the vertical (mesoaxial) or horizontal (organoaxial) planes. Type IV hernias are large, complex paraesophageal hernias, which contain not only the stomach but also other organs such as the transverse colon, small bowel, and pancreas. There is a strong association between the size of the hiatal hernia and the presence of reflux.[25]

The presence of a foreshortened esophagus (most often with a fixed or nonreducible hiatal hernia) should be noted. Findings that suggest a short esophagus include a large hernia (>5 cm), a fixed or nonreducible hernia in the upright position, the presence of an esophageal stricture, and nondistensibility of the distal esophagus/epiphrenic ampulla.

A qualitative assessment of the motility should be stated. The most important findings are an ineffective or absent peristalsis. Ineffective motility is suggested by the presence of a primary peristaltic wave but with significant retrograde escape. Retrograde escape is relatively common, and occurs at the juncture of the proximal and middle third of the esophagus, at the level of the transverse aorta. Anatomically this is at the juncture of the skeletal and smooth muscle. Significant retrograde escape is a qualitative judgment, but generally is present when more than half of the barium bolus is not transferred and escapes proximally past this site. When there is no propagation of the primary wave, there is aperistalsis.

The presence and significance of a distal mucosal ring or stricture should also be noted, as well as whether an ingested barium tablet or food has caused obstruction at the level of the narrowing and whether the obstructed tablet or food has caused symptoms. There is a strong relationship between the degree of narrowing of a distal mucosal ring and the presence of symptoms.[19] As the luminal diameter decreases from 20 mm to 9 mm, the likelihood of symptoms from an ingested marshmallow increases. In general, distal mucosal rings larger than 20 mm rarely, if ever, cause symptoms. Rings 13 to 20 mm in diameter variably cause symptoms, with symptoms increasing based on the increasing size of the food bolus. Rings less than 13 mm in diameter invariably cause symptoms regardless of the size of the food bolus.

The presence, cause, height, and persistence (<30 or >30 seconds) of reflux should be noted. Lastly, alternative diagnoses other than GERD should be raised. Two important categories are a severe dysmotility disorder and EOE.

ALTERNATIVE DIAGNOSES TO GERD

The most common severe dysmotility disorders are achalasia and diffuse esophageal spasm. It may be difficult to distinguish the two, but generally achalasia is more easily identified. The barium findings of achalasia include a dilated, aperistaltic esophagus containing foam/saliva, food, and fluid.[26,27] The region of the lower esophageal sphincter can have a bird-beak appearance. Thus, the 2 basic findings of achalasia can be identified: aperistalsis and abnormal relaxation of the lower esophageal sphincter. These findings are typical of the newly classified type I or classic achalasia (based on high-resolution manometry) (impaired relaxation with esophageal dilation and negligible esophageal pressurization).[28] Other findings include vigorous esophageal contractions along with aperistalsis, generally in a normal-caliber esophagus (often type II [panesophageal pressurization] or type III [spastic, contractions of the distal esophageal segment] achalasia). It is often impossible to distinguish achalasia from diffuse esophageal spasm in a patient with these radiographic findings. Furthermore, a normal esophagram may not identify any abnormalities in patients with early achalasia. It is interesting that in a relatively recent investigation from the University of Pennsylvania, 7 of 21 patients with radiographic findings of achalasia on barium esophagrams had complete relaxation of the lower esophageal sphincter (manometry performed was not high-resolution manometry).[27]

EOE is increasingly identified as a common cause of dysphagia, and is more common in men and Caucasian patients. In the authors' experience many patients with EOE have been misidentified as having GERD or a psychogenic cause of their symptoms. Unless the findings on the barium esophagram are identified and confirmed by endoscopy and biopsy, the patients continue to suffer. The findings of EOE on the barium esophagram include: focal esophageal strictures (either single or multiple and relatively equally present in the proximal, mid, and distal esophagus); a ringed esophagus (**Fig. 6**), most commonly identified on collapsed or partially collapsed esophagus; and a small-caliber or diffusely narrowed esophagus.[17,29–32] Any of these findings, especially in the absence of a hiatal hernia, changes of reflux esophagitis, and/or absence of identifiable reflux on the barium examination, should prompt the examiner to consider EOE as the cause.

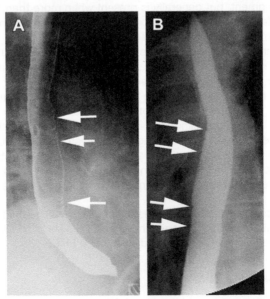

Fig. 6. Ringed esophagus in a young man with solid-food dysphagia. (*A*) Subtle rings (*white arrows*) in the upright, air-contrast portion of the examination. (*B*) These rings (*white arrows*) persist during the semiprone, full-column portion of the examination. Biopsies confirm the presence of eosinophilic esophagitis.

DIAGNOSIS OF ESOPHAGITIS AND BARRETT ESOPHAGUS WITH THE BARIUM ESOPHAGRAM

As previously stated, in some centers an emphasis is placed on the detection of abnormalities strongly associated with Barrett esophagus in an attempt to determine which patients should undergo endoscopy.[11] In a group of 309 patients (including 257 reported cases and unpublished data), Barrett esophagus was associated with the following findings on esophagrams: hiatal hernia (87%), esophageal stricture (72%), thickened folds (65%) on the mucosal relief portion of the examination, gastroesophageal reflux (60%), distal esophageal dilation (44%), esophageal ulcer (40%) and a reticular pattern (23%) (see **Fig. 3**; **Fig. 7**).[33] However, this approach has not been rigorously tested and is based on only on relatively small, retrospective, case series investigations. There has never been a large, prospective study comparing the sensitivity of a well-performed barium esophagram with endoscopy in identifying either moderate to severe esophagitis or Barrett esophagus. Furthermore, the most common abnormality associated with Barrett esophagus is a hiatal hernia, a finding that is very common and thus very nonspecific. It is also unlikely that the esophagram would replace endoscopy in the evaluation of these patients. Thus, in the authors' institution the role of the esophagram in the detection of moderate to severe esophagitis is limited. Nevertheless, if an ulcer, stricture, or thickened folds are identified on the barium study, endoscopy is strongly advised.

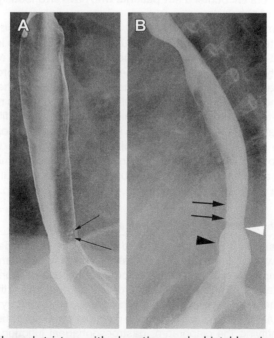

Fig. 7. Distal esophageal stricture with ulcerations and a hiatal hernia. (*A*) Subtle ulcerations (*black arrows*) in the distal esophagus on the upright, air-contrast portion of the examination. (*B*) Diffuse narrowing (nondistensible epiphrenic ampulla) of the distal esophagus (*black arrows*) above the gastroesophageal junction (*white arrowhead*) and a hiatal hernia (*black arrowhead*) on the semiprone, full-column portion of the examination.

THE BARIUM ESOPHAGRAM AFTER ANTIREFLUX PROCEDURES

In the experience of the authors and others, the barium esophagram provides essential information in evaluating symptomatic patients after antireflux procedures.[3,34,35] A careful study best assesses the anatomic problems contributing to these symptoms. At the Cleveland Clinic, all symptomatic post-fundoplication patients have an esophagram as an essential, and usually initial, part of their evaluation.

As with the preoperative examination, eliciting a short history from the patient helps guide the subsequent examination. The authors always ask the patient about the symptoms before the surgery and whether these symptoms were improved or eliminated after the surgery. If the symptoms did not improve after surgery, it is likely that the patient did not have GERD. The patient is also asked about current symptoms, as these often change after the procedure. For instance, a patient may have had severe heartburn before antireflux surgery and developed solid-food dysphagia after the surgery. In such as case the wrap is often too tight.

Initial Upright Phase

If there is any liquid dysphagia, as with the preoperative examination the patient may start by ingesting a small amount of low-density barium to assess for emptying impairment. If there is any delay in emptying, the authors then proceed with a timed barium swallow. Many patients with too tight a wrap have impaired esophageal emptying. This simple test graphically and quantitatively identifies this problem. Furthermore, every year the authors encounter a few patients who have erroneously had a fundoplication in the face of achalasia.

If a timed barium swallow is not performed, the air-contrast phase of the examination begins. An attempt is made to coat the fundoplication so as to identify its length and location vis-à-vis the diaphragm, gastroesophageal junction, and stomach, as well as its integrity. To do so, after the patient ingests the gas-producing crystals and high-density barium and the esophagus is examined upright, the table is rotated to the horizontal position with the patient supine, and the patient is rolled toward the left lateral decubitus position and back again, several times, to fill the posteriorly located fundoplication. Several spot films are taken of the gastroesophageal junction region in multiple planes, even prone. Despite these maneuvers, the best time to examine the wrap is often during the drinking phase of the examination, with the patient in the right anterior oblique position. During this phase, careful attention should be directed to the gastroesophageal junction, diaphragm, and wrap.

Semiprone or Right Anterior Oblique Examination

Motility is then assessed using the standard 5 swallows of low-density barium. In cases where the wrap is too tight, the peristaltic wave may be normal to the level of the epiphrenic ampulla. At this point the epiphrenic ampulla balloons out, and there is retrograde escape of the barium. This process demonstrates that the pressure gradient across the wrap is greater than the pressure of the primary wave.

The distended, full-column or rapid drinking phase of the examination is important in locating and identifying the diaphragm, gastroesophageal junction, gastric fundus, and fundoplication. The authors pay specific attention to this area, attempting to determine: (1) the location of the wrap vis-à-vis the stomach, diaphragm, and esophagus; (2) the integrity and length of the wrap; (3) the lumen the wrap encircles (esophagus, gastroesophageal junction, and/or stomach); and (4) whether there is a recurrent hernia and, if so, its location vis-à-vis the wrap.

Reflux Identification Examination

Next, an attempt is made to identify the presence of reflux using the same maneuvers used in the preoperative patient.

Solid Food Ingestion Examination

The authors then administer the 13-mm barium tablet to determine the tightness of the wrap. The tablet should not obstruct at the level of the fundoplication.

Gastric Motility Assessment

During and at the end of the examination, the motility of the stomach is qualitatively assessed. Unfortunately, the vagus nerve is sometimes damaged during antireflux surgery, which leads to depressed or absent gastric motility, causing bloating, early satiety, and a sense of upper abdominal fullness.

Normal Nissen Fundoplication

A normal Nissen fundoplication should be located below the diaphragm and be no greater than 2 to 3 cm in length (**Fig. 8**).[3,35] The wrap should surround the gastro-esophageal junction and not surround too much of the gastric fundus. There should be no significant narrowing of the lumen at the level of the wrap, and there should not be significant impairment of passage of either a 13-mm tablet or a marshmallow. On single swallows assessing motility, there should be no significant retrograde escape of barium distally, and there should be no significant dilation or ballooning of the esophagus during the rapid drinking phase of the examination. In the upright position, there should be no significant delay in emptying. It may be very difficult to completely opacify a normal fundoplication, as they can be short and small. One will only identify the effect of the wrap on the lumen that is surrounded by the wrap.

Normal Toupet Fundoplication

A Toupet fundoplication is a partial wrap of approximately 270°.[3,35] This uncommon surgery is generally performed in patients with moderate to severe hypomotility. As such, the peristalsis on these patients is often depressed or absent. It may be very difficult to differentiate a Toupet from a Nissen fundoplication on barium examination.

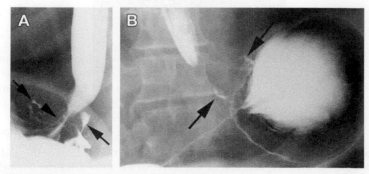

Fig. 8. Normal Nissen fundoplication. (*A*) Small leaves of the fundoplication (*arrows*) encircling the gastroesophageal junction (*arrowhead*) on the semiprone, full-column portion of the examination. (*B*) The leaves of the fundoplication (*arrows*) on a supine view of the fundus.

Collis Gastroplasty–Nissen Fundoplication

A Collis gastroplasty followed by a Nissen fundoplication is performed in patients with foreshortened esophagi.[36,37] In this procedure, lateral stapling of the gastric fundus creates a short neo-esophagus. Thus the distal neo-esophagus is composed of gastric wall and mucosa. A wedge resection of the fundus is often performed to eliminate some of the redundant gastric fundus. The remaining fundus is then used to create the fundoplication. In the authors' experience the fundoplications in patients after a Collis gastroplasty–Nissen procedure are relatively large and "floppy." Knowledge of the presence of a Collis-Nissen procedure is very important to avoid misdiagnosis of a large, long fundoplication or a slipped or malpositioned fundoplication (**Fig. 9**).

After this procedure, in some patients (often with solid-food dysphagia) the 13-mm tablet often obstructs at the level of the gastroplasty or neo-esophagus. In almost all cases, the obstruction is due to a strictured gastroplasty rather than a tight fundoplication (the fundoplications are rarely tight). When the gastroplasty is performed, the blood supply is reduced, often leading to an ischemic stricture.

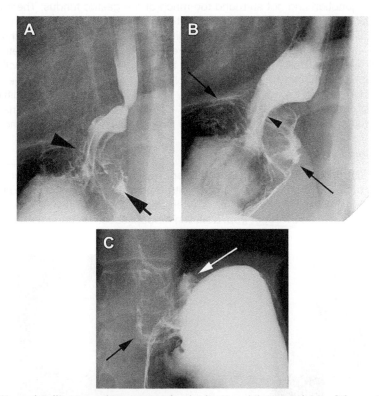

Fig. 9. Normal Collis gastroplasty–Nissen fundoplication. (A) Gastric folds of the gastroplasty (neo-esophagus) (*arrowhead*) and one of the leaves of the fundoplication (*arrow*) on the semiprone, full-column portion of the examination. (B) A cone-down spot film showing both leaves of the fundoplication (*arrows*) encircling the gastroplasty (*arrowhead*) on the semiprone, full-column portion of the examination. (C) The encircling fundoplication (*arrows*) is best shown on a supine view of the fundus.

Abnormal or Failed Fundoplication

As stated previously, it is important for the radiologist to know the preoperative symptoms and whether they resolve after the procedure. It is also important to know whether the postoperative symptoms have recurred or are new. After antireflux surgery, patients may have recurrent heartburn or may have new symptoms of dysphagia, regurgitation, early satiety, or gas-bloat syndrome. It is often easy to predict the radiographic findings based on the patient's postoperative symptoms.

After a Nissen fundoplication patients can present with several findings, a common one being that the fundoplication or wrap is too long and/or too tight and wraps the stomach. This problem often leads to solid-food dysphagia and/or gas bloat (**Fig. 10**). These long, tight wraps surrounding the stomach obstruct the passage of a 13-mm tablet. It is assumed that this failure arises from a poorly formed or malpositioned fundoplication. Another common finding is that the wrap has herniated up into the posterior mediastinum, in a paraesophageal fashion (**Fig. 11**). More often than not, the wrap in these cases is either partially or completely disrupted. In addition, there may be a recurrent hiatal hernia (ie, the gastroesophageal junction is above the diaphragm). The last common finding is that a portion of the stomach is positioned above the wrap, either below or above the diaphragm, with the wrap intact. Some investigators describe this as a slipped Nissen fundoplication. Many surgeons believe that the last 2 findings described are due to failure to recognize a foreshortened esophagus, and/or inadequate mobilization of the esophagus and reduction of the hernia. In some cases the fundoplication may be completely disrupted with recurrence of the hiatal hernia. In unusual cases, incomplete ligation of the short gastric vessels causes rotational tension on the fundoplication, causing a twist at the wrap site.

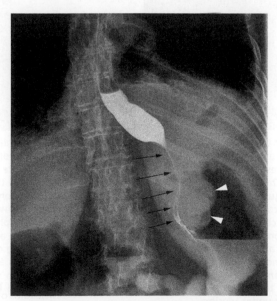

Fig. 10. Long, tight fundoplication, wrapping the stomach in a patient with solid-food dysphagia immediately after surgery. Upright, overhead view of the lower chest and upper abdomen at the end of the examination shows the long fundoplication (*white arrowheads*) wrapping the stomach and causing luminal narrowing (*black arrows*). Note the retained barium in the distal esophagus above the long fundoplication.

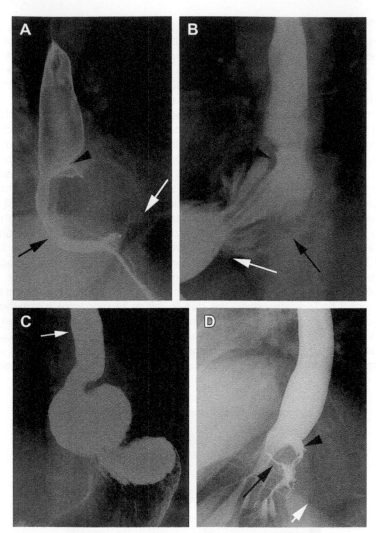

Fig. 11. Status post type III hernia repair with disruption and partial herniation of fundoplication. (*A*) Preoperative fixed, type III hiatal hernia on the upright, air-contrast view (*black arrowhead*, gastroesophageal junction; *black arrow*, hiatal hernia; *white arrow*, diaphragmatic hiatus). (*B*) The same findings on the semiprone, full-column view (*black arrowhead*, gastroesophageal junction; *black arrow*, hiatal hernia; *white arrow*, diaphragmatic hiatus). (*C*) Spontaneous, continuous reflux in the supine position (*white arrow*). (*D, E*) Partially disrupted fundoplication that does not completely encircle the distal esophagus and gastroesophageal junction. A portion of the wrap (*black arrow* in *D* and *E*) is at the level of the diaphragm (*white arrow* in *D*), and a portion of the wrap is above the diaphragm (*black arrowhead* in *D* and *E*). (*F*) A recurrent hiatal hernia with gastric folds above the gastroesophageal junction (*black arrows*). It is likely that either there was too much esophageal foreshortening or there was inadequate esophageal mobilization and hernia reduction, leading to a repair under tension.

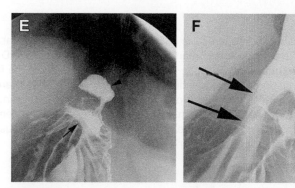

Fig. 11. (*continued*)

OUTCOME OF THE POSTOPERATIVE EXAMINATION

At the end of the examination, gastroenterologists and esophageal surgeons expect that the radiologist has assessed the level of esophageal emptying in patients with liquid dysphagia (**Box 3**),[3] and want a description of: (1) the integrity (intact, partially or completely disrupted) of the wrap; (2) its location vis-à-vis the diaphragm; and (3) which lumen is wrapped. Some investigators have separated the anatomic relationship of the fundoplication vis-à-vis the stomach, esophagus, and diaphragm into various types.[38–40] Because it can be difficult or impossible to easily classify failed fundoplications into neat and tidy types, the authors prefer to describe the individual findings as already described herein. Clinicians also want an assessment of the tightness of the wrap as assessed by the passage of a 13 mm tablet.

In addition to information concerning the fundoplication, the gastroenterologist and, especially, the surgeon expect that a recurrent hiatal hernia is identified. Sometimes the herniated wrap occupies more space in the posterior mediastinum than the recurrent hernia (ie, gastroesophageal junction). An assessment of motility and the presence of recurrent reflux should be reported. Lastly, a qualitative assessment of gastric motility is helpful in identifying the cause of the postoperative bloating or early satiety.

Box 3
What the gastroenterologist and esophageal surgeon want to know from the post-antireflux procedure examination

- Assessment of esophageal emptying
- Fundoplication location vis-à-vis diaphragm
- Fundoplication integrity
- Lumen wrapped by fundoplication
- Fundoplication length
- Fundoplication tightness
- Recurrence of hernia or herniated fundoplication
- Motility
- Gastric emptying

SUMMARY

In their multigroup practice, the authors have found that the barium esophagram forms an integral part of the assessment and management of patients with GERD before and, especially, after antireflux procedures. One could argue that all of the findings revealed by the examination could be identified with endoscopy, a gastric emptying study, and an esophageal motility examination.[41] However, rather than thinking about these examinations as competitors, the authors consider them to be complementary examinations which, when taken as a whole, fully evaluate a patient with suspected GERD as well as symptomatic patients after antireflux procedures.

ACKNOWLEDGMENTS

The authors thank Steven Shay, MD for his helpful and constructive comments and input regarding this article.

REFERENCES

1. Peters JH. Modern imaging for the assessment of gastroesophageal reflux disease begins with the barium esophagram. J Gastrointest Surg 2000;4:346–7.
2. Levine MS, Rubesin SE. Diseases of the esophagus: diagnosis with esophagography. Radiology 2005;237:414–27.
3. Baker ME, Einstein DM, Herts BR, et al. Gastroesophageal reflux disease: integrating the barium esophagram before and after antireflux surgery. Radiology 2007;243:329–39.
4. Levine MS, Rubesin SE, Laufer I. Barium esophagography: a study for all seasons. Clin Gastroenterol Hepatol 2008;6:11–25.
5. deOliveira JM, Birgisson S, Doinoff C, et al. Timed barium swallow: a simple technique for evaluating esophageal emptying in patients with achalasia. AJR Am J Roentgenol 1997;169:473–9.
6. Gastal OL, Hagen JA, Peters JH, et al. Short esophagus. Arch Surg 1999;134:633–8.
7. Mittal SK, Awad ZT, Tasset M, et al. The preoperative predictability of the short esophagus in patients with stricture or paraesophageal hernia. Surg Endosc 2000;14:464–8.
8. Awad ZT, Mittal SK, Roth TA, et al. Esophageal shortening during the era of laparoscopic surgery. World J Surg 2002;25:558–61.
9. Hashemi M, Peters JH, DeMeester TR, et al. Laparoscopic repair of large type III hiatal hernia: objective follow-up reveals high recurrence rate. J Am Coll Surg 2000;190:553–60.
10. Ott DJ. Gastroesophageal reflux disease. Radiol Clin North Am 1994;32:1147–66.
11. Gilchrist AM, Levine MS, Carr RF, et al. Barrett's esophagus: diagnosis by double-contrast esophagography. AJR Am J Roentgenol 1988;150:97–102.
12. Cho YK, Choi MG, Baik CN, et al. Comparison of bolus transit patterns identified by esophageal impedance to barium esophagram in patients with dysphagia. Dis Esophagus 2012;25:17–25.
13. Ott DJ, Chen YM, Hewson EG, et al. Esophageal motility: assessment with synchronous video tape fluoroscopy and manometry. Radiology 1989;173:419–22.
14. Hewson EG, Ott DJ, Dalton CB, et al. Manometry and radiology. Complementary studies in the assessment of esophageal motility disorders. Gastroenterology 1990;98:626–32.
15. Campbell C, Levine MS, Rubesin SE, et al. Association between esophageal dysmotility and gastroesophageal reflux on barium studies. Eur J Radiol 2006;59:88–92.

16. Bulsiewicz WJ, Kahrilas PJ, Kwiatek MA, et al. Esophageal pressure topography criteria indicative of incomplete bolus clearance: a study using high resolution impedance manometry. Am J Gastroenterol 2009;104:2721–8.
17. Zimmerman SL, Levine MS, Rubesin SE, et al. Idiopathic eosinophilic esophagitis in adults: the ringed esophagus. Radiology 2005;236:159–65.
18. Thompson JK, Koehler RE, Richter JE. Detection of gastroesophageal reflux: value of barium studies compared with 24-hr pH monitoring. AJR Am J Roentgenol 1994;162:621–6.
19. Smith DF, Ott DJ, Gelfand DW, et al. Lower esophageal mucosal ring: correlation of referred symptoms with radiographic findings using a marshmallow bolus. AJR Am J Roentgenol 1998;171:1361–5.
20. Samadi F, Levine MS, Rubesin SE, et al. Feline esophagus and gastroesophageal reflux. AJR Am J Roentgenol 2010;194:972–6.
21. Ott DJ, Chen YM, Wu WC, et al. Radiographic and endoscopic sensitivity in detecting lower esophageal mucosal ring. AJR Am J Roentgenol 1986;147:261–5.
22. Jalil S, Castell DO. Schatzki's ring; a benign cause of dysphagia in adults. J Clin Gastroenterol 2002;35:295–8.
23. Kahrilas PJ, Kim HC, Pandolfino JE. Approaches to the diagnosis and grading of hiatal hernia. Best Pract Res Clin Gastroenterol 2008;22:601–16.
24. Ott DJ, Gelfand DW, Chen YM, et al. Predictive relationship of hiatal hernia to reflux esophagitis. Gastrointest Radiol 1985;10:317–20.
25. Ott DJ, Glauser SJ, Ledbetter MS, et al. Association of hiatal hernia and gastroesophageal reflux: correlation between presence and size of hiatal hernia and 24-hour pH monitoring of the esophagus. AJR Am J Roentgenol 1995;165:557–9.
26. Blam ME, Delfyett W, Levine MS, et al. Achalasia: a disease of varied and subtle symptoms that do not correlate with radiographic findings. Am J Gastroenterol 2002;97:1916–23.
27. Amaravadi R, Levine MS, Rubesin SE, et al. Achalasia with complete relaxation of lower esophageal sphincter: radiographic-manometric correlation. Radiology 2005;235:886–91.
28. Richter JE. Achalasia—an update. J Neurogastroenterol Motil 2010;16:232–42.
29. Picus D, Frank PH. Eosinophilic esophagitis. AJR Am J Roentgenol 1981;136:1001–3.
30. Vitellas KM, Bennett WF, Bova JG, et al. Idiopathic eosinophilic esophagitis. Radiology 1993;186:789–93.
31. Levine MS, Saul SH. Idiopathic eosinophilic esophagitis: how common is it? Radiology 1993;186:631–2.
32. White SB, Levine MS, Rubesin SE, et al. The small-caliber esophagus: radiographic sign of idiopathic eosinophilic esophagitis. Radiology 2010;256:127–34.
33. Chen MY, Frederick MG. Barrett esophagus and adenocarcinoma. Radiol Clin North Am 1994;32:1167–81.
34. LeBlanc-Louvry I, Koning E, Zalar A, et al. Severe dysphagia after laparoscopic fundoplication: usefulness of barium meal examination to identify causes other than tight fundoplication – a prospective study. Surgery 2000;128:392–8.
35. Canon CL, Morgan DE, Einstein DM, et al. Surgical approach to gastroesophageal reflux disease: what the radiologist needs to know. Radiographics 2005;25:1485–99.
36. Stirling MC, Orringer MB. Continued assessment of the combined Collis-Nissen operation. Ann Thorac Surg 1989;47:224–30.

37. Pierre AF, Luketich JD, Fernando HC, et al. Results of laparoscopic repair of giant paraesophageal hernias: 200 consecutive patients. Ann Thorac Surg 2002;74: 1909–16.
38. Hainaux B, Sattari A, Coppens E, et al. Intrathoracic migration of the wrap after laparoscopic Nissen fundoplication: radiologic evaluation. AJR Am J Roentgenol 2002;178:859–62.
39. Hatch KF, Daily MF, Christensen BJ, et al. Failed fundoplications. Am J Surg 2004; 188:786–91.
40. Richter JE. Gastroesophageal reflux disease treatment: side effects and complications of fundoplication. Clin Gastroenterol Hepatol 2013;11:465–71.
41. Linke GR, Borovicka J, Schneider P, et al. Is a barium swallow complementary to endoscopy essential in the preoperative assessment of laparoscopic antireflux and hiatal hernia surgery? Surg Endosc 2008;22:96–100.

Ambulatory Esophageal pH Monitoring

Michelle S. Han, MD[a], Jeffrey H. Peters, MD[b],*

KEYWORDS

- Esophageal pH monitoring • Gastroesophageal reflux disease • Catheter-based
- Wireless-based • Impedance

KEY POINTS

- Physicians should have a general knowledge of the diagnostic accuracy of each pH monitoring method.
- Prolonged pH monitoring and the combined impedance function increase the amount of information available for esophageal acid exposure evaluation; however, their effects on gastroesophageal reflux disease (GERD) diagnosis and clinical management are still under ongoing investigation.
- Prolonged pH monitoring increases the reflux detection rate.
- Because of the complexity of GERD diagnosis, routine pH monitoring should be performed for patients who are undergoing evaluation for antireflux surgery.

INTRODUCTION

The first link between gastric acid and gastroesophageal reflux (GER) was reported in 1884 after the retrieval of an acid-contained sponge from the esophagus of a patient with heartburn. The association between esophageal mucosal damage and the presence of acidic juice in the esophagus slowly emerged over the early part of the twentieth century. In 1958, Tuttle and Grossman[1,2] first measured esophageal acid reflux using an existing gastric pH meter with manometry. Johnson and DeMeester[1] established the foundation of esophageal pH monitoring in 1974 after studying GER in normal subjects and patients with reflux symptoms. In this landmark study, not only the methodology of esophageal pH monitoring and the normal reference values were defined but also a composite scoring system, the DeMeester score, was created to quantify acid exposure using 6 pH parameters.[1] This scoring system has been widely validated and is used today. With the advancement of technology, the sponge was replaced by glass

This article originally appeared in Gastrointestinal Endoscopy Clinics, Volume 24, Issue 4, October 2014.

Disclosure: Nothing to disclose.

[a] Department of Surgery, University of Rochester Medical Center, University of Rochester, 601 Elmwood Avenue, Box SURG, Rochester, NY 14642, USA; [b] Department of Surgery, University Hospitals, 11100 Euclid Avenue, Cleveland, OH 44106, USA

* Corresponding author.

E-mail address: jeffrey.peters@UHhospitals.org

and then antimony electrode catheters and in the 1990s to a wireless implantable capsule; but the concept of esophageal pH monitoring for the evaluation of GER disease (GERD) has not changed over the past hundred years. The aims of this article are to review the current methods of ambulatory esophageal pH monitoring, compare the advantage and disadvantage of each test, and to discuss current controversies of each method in an effort to elucidate future directions in the diagnosis of GERD.

ESOPHAGEAL pH MONITORING: WHAT, WHY, AND WHEN

Esophageal pH monitoring is a direct in vivo measurement of esophageal acid exposure over time for the evaluation of GERD. It can be currently performed using either catheter-based or wireless systems (**Fig. 1**). Catheter-based pH monitoring requires transnasal placement of the catheter, with its measuring electrode located 5 cm above the manometrically measured upper border of lower esophageal sphincter (LES). A wireless-based pH capsule is generally placed endoscopically, 6 cm above the squamocolumnar junction (SCJ), or in the setting of Barrett esophagus above the top of the gastric rugal folds. The pH recordings of 24 hours, 48 hours, or 96 hours are currently possible, depending on the choice of device (catheter vs wireless), patient tolerability, and the duration a capsule remains attached. In the case of wireless monitoring, the pH data (sampled at a frequency of once every 6 seconds) are transmitted to an external radiofrequency recorder and then transferred to a computer with commercial software allowing automatic and/or manual analysis. Patients are generally asked to keep a diary recording symptoms, body positions, and meal periods during the time of pH monitoring allowing the analysis of reflux patterns and symptom correlation measures. **Fig. 2** demonstrates the basic steps of the test. Currently available and widely used pH monitoring options are listed in **Box 1**.

Esophageal pH monitoring is a crucial part of GERD evaluation. According to the 2007 American College of Gastroenterology's practice guidelines for esophageal reflux testing, pH monitoring

1. Is useful in documenting abnormal esophageal reflux exposure in endoscopy-negative patients with typical reflux symptoms who failed medical therapy and are being considered for antireflux surgery

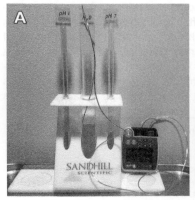
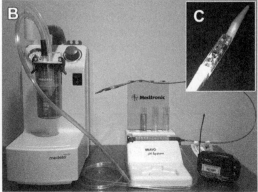

Fig. 1. Ambulatory esophageal pH monitoring: catheter-based (*A*) or wireless-based device (*B*; Bravo, Given Imaging Ltd, Yoqneam, Israel). The Bravo capsule (*C*) is loaded on the delivery system. (Images used with permission from Medtronic, Minneapolis, MN; Sandhill Scientific, Highlands Ranch, CO; Medela Inc, McHenry, IL; and Given Imaging, a Covidien company. The use of any Covidien photo or image does not imply Covidien review or endorsement of any article or publication.)

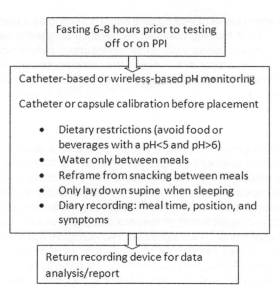

Fig. 2. Basic steps of ambulatory esophageal pH monitoring. PPI, proton pump inhibitor.

2. May be useful in detecting the adequacy of acid control in patients with Barrett esophagus, atypical reflux symptoms, or recurrent symptoms after antireflux surgery[3]
3. May be useful when combined with impedance in detecting nonacid reflux or in evaluating patients whose reflux symptoms are not controlled by a proton pump inhibitor (PPI; PPI nonresponders)[3]

Patients presenting with typical reflux symptoms are given the diagnosis of GERD liberally by health care providers from many specialties. Studies have shown that symptoms, reflux or hiatal hernia detected by barium esophagram, and even findings of mucosal injury on endoscopy are either unreliable or not sensitive in diagnosing GERD; thus, esophageal pH monitoring becomes an integral part of the diagnostic and treatment plan.[4] The Diamond study, a single-blind prospective study of 308 patients published in 2010, concluded that the Reflux Disease Questionnaire, family practitioners, and gastroenterologists all had similar diagnostic accuracy for GERD (sensitivity 62%–67%; specificity 63%–70%). In this study, the 48-hour Bravo (Given Imaging Ltd, Yoqneam, Israel) pH-monitoring result, endoscopic findings of esophagitis, symptom association probability (SAP) of 95% or more, or the borderline pH-monitoring result with response to PPI therapy were used as the gold standard for

---

Box 1
Available pH-monitoring tests

Catheter based (transnasal placement at 5 cm above upper border of LES)

• Conventional 24-hour catheter pH monitoring; dual-channel pH monitoring

• 24-hour multichannel intraluminal impedance pH monitoring

Wireless based (endoscopic placement at 6 cm above SCJ)

• 48-hour Bravo (Given Imaging Ltd, Yoqneam, Israel) pH monitoring

• 96-hour Bravo pH monitoring

diagnosis. A consensus panel of esophageal experts serving as a diagnostic advisory panel concluded in 2012 that the optimal preoperative diagnostic workup for GERD should include pH testing along with upper endoscopy, barium esophagram, and manometry.[5] A diagnostic algorithm outlining the decision making and test selection process when evaluating patients suspected to have abnormal esophageal acid exposure is shown in **Fig. 3**.

TEST SELECTION

A variety of methodologies are available to assess esophageal pH exposure. Single-sensor catheter-based antimony pH probes provide the traditional and heretofore most widely used method. Conventionally, this is a 24-hour study, which detects distal esophageal acid exposure. Dual-channel 24-hour catheter-based pH monitoring provides data on proximal esophageal exposure, although fixed distances between the pH sensors results in misplacement of the proximal probe in as many as 45% of patients, limiting its usefulness.[6] Two significant technological advances were made in the 1990s. First, combined impedance-pH catheters were developed, allowing the assessment of the role of nonacid reflux particularly in patients with atypical and/or refractory reflux symptoms (multichannel intraluminal impedance pH monitoring [MII-pH], **Fig. 4A**). Second, wireless implantable pH sensors were developed, allowing ambulatory recording of 48 hours and now up to 96 hours in the absence of a transnasal catheter (see **Fig. 4B**). The investigators recommend that patients with typical GERD symptoms, such as heartburn and regurgitation, should undergo at least a conventional pH study given the poor sensitivity and specificity of symptom-based diagnosis of GERD.[7] In contrast to common belief, a trial of PPI for symptom response does not improve the diagnostic accuracy.[8] The optimal strategy for test selection

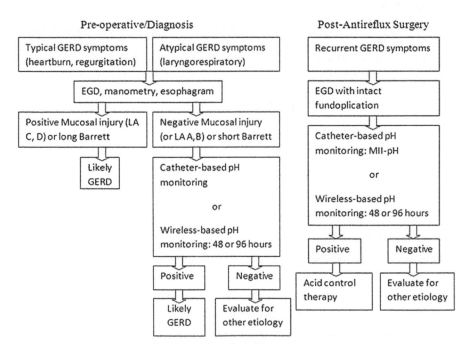

Fig. 3. Diagnostic algorithm for evaluation of GERD symptoms. EGD, esophagogastroduodenoscopy; LA, Los Angeles.

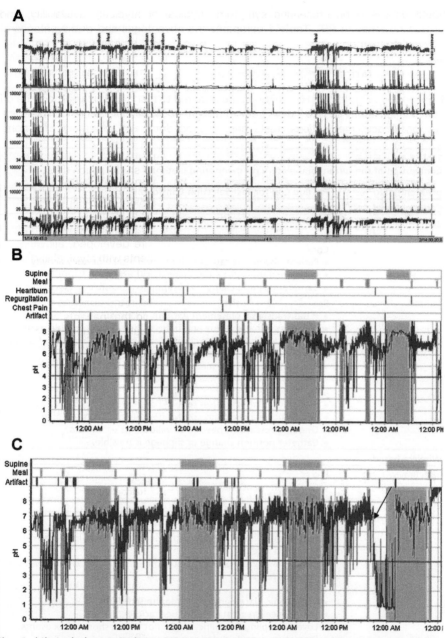

Fig. 4. (*A*) Ambulatory 24-hour MII-pH monitoring: pH tracing. (*B*) pH tracing (96-hour Bravo pH monitoring). Patient positions, meal period, and symptoms are marked along the recording time line. (*C*) The pH tracing showing premature dislodgement of the Bravo capsule on day 4. The pH decreased abruptly to pH less than 1 (*arrow*) and then recovered to pH greater than 8.

should be based on presenting symptoms (typical or atypical), availability, and perhaps response to PPI. **Table 1** compares the advantages and disadvantages of each testing method.

TEST INTERPRETATION

All patients who undergo pH monitoring are required to fast 6 to 8 hours and to be off antacid medications for 5 to 7 days before catheter or capsule placement. On-therapy (stay on antacid medications) tests can also be done and are most commonly

Table 1
Comparison of the current ambulatory pH monitoring methods

pH-Monitoring Test	Pro and Con for Test Selection Consideration
Catheter-based	
24-h conventional	Pro • It has transnasal placement without endoscopy. Con • Patient discomfort causes reduced oral intake or daily activity. • It only measures distal esophageal acid exposure. • Catheter position change and slippage is possible.
MII-pH	Pro • It has transnasal placement without endoscopy. • It detects nonacid reflux and bolus transit. It may provide useful information in patients with atypical symptoms, nonacid reflux, or refractory reflux symptoms. • The multichannel can measure acid and nonacid reflux both distal and proximally. Con • Patient discomfort causes reduced oral intake or daily activity. • Test results may not necessarily alter the management plan. Ongoing research is needed to validate its usefulness. • Catheter position change or slippage is possible.
Wireless-based	
48-h Bravo	Pro • It eliminates patient discomfort. • The capsule is fixed eliminating concerns of movement or slippage. • It is more physiologic and has minimal effects on daily activity or oral intake. • Longer duration of monitoring is possible with an increased reflux detection rate. • Passage with bowel movement eliminates additional clinic visit for catheter removal. Con • Endoscopic placement might require sedation. • it only measures distal esophageal acid exposure. • Lower sampling frequency might not detect short reflux events. • Premature capsule dislodgement could occur. • A rare case with severe discomfort might require endoscopic removal.
96-h Bravo	Pro • They are the same as above. In addition, prolonged duration of monitoring might increase the reflux detection rate further. There is improved sensitivity with high specificity. Con • They are the same as above.

performed on patients who have refractory reflux symptoms.[3] The widely accepted cutoff of a pH less than 4 defining a reflux episode is from Tuttle and colleagues'[9] original work in 1961. It is based on the fact that the onset of pyrosis was induced when the distal esophagus was exposed to acidic fluid perfusion at a pH less than 4[9] and the acidic acid dissociation constant (pKa) of pepsin. Many recommend dietary restrictions, although further studies are needed to evaluate its effect on pH monitoring results.[10] Parameters reported are listed in **Box 2**. Published normal values for the catheter-based and wireless systems are summarized in **Table 2**.

Fig. 5 outlines the brief steps for test interpretation. All pH-monitoring tests provide information on distal esophageal acid exposure, the patterns of reflux, and symptom correlation measures. Monitoring pH with impedance (MII-pH) has the added ability to evaluate bolus transit of gas or liquid and nonacid reflux. A pH less than 4 is the widely accepted cutoff to denote an acid reflux episode. A percent time greater than 5 or DeMeester score greater than 14.72 is used to define a positive study. Wireless tests provide longer duration of monitoring: 48 to 96 hours. The capsule, on average, detaches 5 to 7 days after placement. The success rates (complete data acquisition without premature detachment) for a 48-hour and 96-hour pH recording are 90% and 41% to 90%, respectively.[11–14] Premature capsule dislodgement can be easily identified on the pH tracing with an abrupt decrease of pH to less than 2 (gastric pH) for 3 to 4 hours followed by a recovery of pH to more than 8 (intestinal pH) (see **Fig. 4**C). It is important to recognize premature capsule dislodgement because the software-generated pH parameters, DeMeester scores, and symptom correlation measures would be falsely elevated. The wireless test can be interpreted using the average 48-hour or 96-hour data or the worst-day data. Studies suggest that defining abnormality using the worst-day data is more sensitive,[3] which concurs with the known day-to-day variation in reflux patterns in both health and disease.[15,16]

The 24-hour MII-pH test measures both esophageal impedance and distal esophageal acid exposure (**Fig. 6**). The detection of upward retrograde impedance change (gas or liquid) without a pH decrease to less than 4 is defined as a nonacid reflux event. Nonacid events are further divided into weakly acidic reflux (pH 4.0–6.9) or alkaline reflux (pH≥7). Impedance data of the proximal and distal esophagus can provide information on the height of reflux and the type of refluxate.

Box 2
pH parameters reported by pH-monitoring test

- Total percent time of pH less than 4
- Percent time of pH less than 4 in upright position
- Percent time of pH less than 4 in supine position
- Total number of reflux episodes (pH<4)
- Number of reflux episodes greater than 5 minutes
- Duration of the longest reflux episode
- Calculated DeMeester score
- Total test duration, test duration in upright and supine position, and in postprandial period
- Symptom correlation measures (symptom index, symptom sensitivity index, symptom association probability)
- The complete pH tracing (see **Fig. 4**)
- Impedance data (MII-pH test only)

Table 2
Summary of normal values for each method of pH monitoring (values are 95th percentiles)

Catheter-Based	Johnson & DeMeester[1,a]	Jamieson et al[32]	Richter et al[33]
Total time pH <4 (%)	4.2	4.5	5.78
Upright time pH <4 (%)	6.3	8.4	8.15
Supine time pH <4 (%)	1.2	3.5	3.45
No. of reflux episodes	50.0	46.9	46.0
No. of reflux episodes ≥5 min	3.0	3.5	4.0
Longest episode (min)	9.2	19.8	18.45

MII-pH		Shay et al[34]	Zerbib et al[35]
Total time pH <4 (%)		6.3	5.0
Upright time pH <4 (%)		9.7	6.2
Supine time pH <4 (%)		2.1	5.3
No. of total reflux episodes		73	75
No. of acid reflux episodes		55	50
No. of weakly acid reflux episodes		26	33
No. of non-acid reflux episodes		1	15
Total bolus exposure (%)		1.4	2.0
Upright bolus exposure (%)		9.7	2.7
Supine bolus exposure (%)		2.1	0.9

Wireless-Based[b]	First 24 h	Second 24 h	Combined
Total time pH <4 (%)	6.31	5.87	4.85
Upright time pH <4 (%)	7.99	7.47	7.29
Supine time pH <4 (%)	1.60	1.33	1.39
No. of reflux episodes	58	60	104
No. of reflux episodes ≥5 min	4	3	5
Longest episode (min)	12.24	19.48	16.18
DeMeester score	17.95	15.76	14.98

[a] Values are Mean ± 2 SD.
[b] *Data from* Ayazi S, Lipham JC, Portale G, et al. Bravo catheter-free pH monitoring: normal values, concordance, optimal diagnostic thresholds, and accuracy. Clin Gastroenterol Hepatol 2009;7(1):60–7.

Three clinically distinct patterns of pathologic reflux were described by DeMeester in 1976 and include upright, supine, and combined (bipositional).[17] In this landmark study, the severity of symptoms and physiologic defects were associated with reflux patterns.

Symptom correlation measures provide potentially meaningful associations between symptoms and reflux events. As stated before, pH monitoring only demonstrates distal esophageal acid exposure; judgment is required to conclude that it is the cause of symptoms. Symptom index (SI), symptom sensitivity index (SSI), and symptom association probability (SAP) have been proposed as clinically useful tools to assess how a particular symptom is associated with detected reflux events. Among the 3 measures, it is generally thought that the SAP is most statistically valid[3]; few symptoms other than heartburn have received any meaningful study. Their usefulness in the clinical management of GERD remains an area of investigation. **Box 3** lists the calculation formulas and statistical consideration for each index.

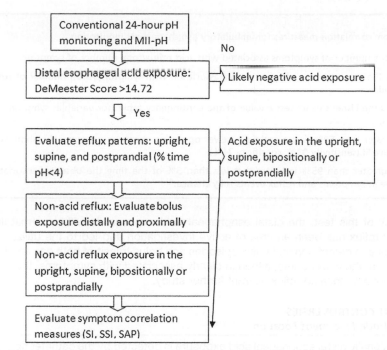

Fig. 5. Test interpretation steps for pH monitoring. SAP, symptom association probability; SI, symptom index; SSI, symptom sensitivity index.

When interpreting test results, it is critically important to know the diagnostic accuracy (sensitivity, specificity, positive predictive value, negative predictive value) of the individual test (**Table 3**). A negative pH-monitoring result does not mean that the patient does not have GERD. It only demonstrates that, with the intrinsic diagnostic

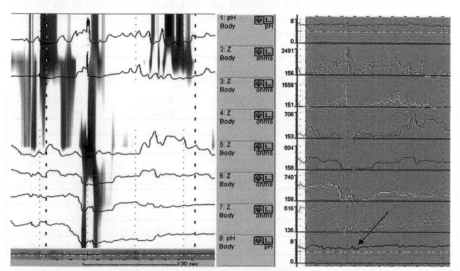

Fig. 6. Twenty-four-hour MII-pH monitoring: the detection of upward impedance change (*left*) without a pH decrease less than 4 (*right, arrow*) is defined as a nonacid reflux event.

> **Box 3**
> **Symptom correlation measures for ambulatory esophageal pH monitoring**
>
> - SI is the number of symptoms associated with acid reflux/total number of symptoms.
> - SSI is the total number of reflux events associated with symptoms/total number of reflux episodes.
> - SAP is the Fisher's exact test *P* value of the contingency table (for variables symptom and reflux).
> - SI greater than 50% is the optimal receiver operating characteristic curve threshold for a positive SI (sensitivity 93%, specificity 71%).
> - SAP greater than 95% indicates that less than 5% of the time the observed association between symptoms and reflux events is by chance.[41]

accuracy of this test, the distal esophageal acid exposure is within normal limits. Nonacid reflux has been an area of active investigation and led to the utilization of impedance to detect nonacid reflux episodes and bolus transit of both gas and liquid; however, at the current time, although clearly associated with symptoms, the clinical implications of nonacid reflux warrant further study.

CURRENT CONTROVERSIES
pH Electrode Placement Location

Conventionally distal esophageal acid exposure is detected by the catheter tip placed at 5 cm above the upper border of the LES or the Bravo capsule located at 6 cm above the SCJ. Both the catheter and capsule position have been areas of investigation. Pandolfino and colleagues[18] compared wireless and catheter-based systems, measuring the tip and the capsule position via fluoroscopy immediately after placement. The mean absolute difference in position between the two systems was 1.0 cm, and the two placement methods resulted in similar tip and capsule positions. More importantly, they showed that the difference in acid exposure between the two systems was not caused by the electrode position. Controversy exists on whether positioning the electrode closer to the gastroesophageal (GE) junction would increase the diagnostic accuracy of pH monitoring.[19,20] Studies have shown that by placing the

Table 3
Summary of sensitivity and specificity for each method of pH monitoring

Catheter-Based[a]	DeMeester et al[37] (%)	Johnsson et al[38] (%)	Mattioli et al[39] (%)	Schindlbeck et al[40,b] (%)
Sensitivity	88.0	87.0	85.0	93.3
Specificity	73.0	97.0	100	92.9

	Pandolfino et al[14]		Ayazi et al[36]	
Wireless-Based	Combined (%)	Worst Day (%)	Combined (%)	Worst Day (%)
Sensitivity	64.9	83.8	82.0	93.0
Specificity	94.8	84.5	100	100
PPV	92.3	83.8	100	100
NPV	74.0	84.6	67.0	83.0

Abbreviations: NPV, negative predictive value; PPV, positive predictive value.
  [a] Ambulatory 24-hour intraesophageal pH monitoring only.
  [b] Only percent time of pH less than 4 is considered.

electrodes closer to the LES than the conventional 5 cm above measures higher acid exposure.[21,22] Wenner and colleagues[19] compared the diagnostic performance between standard electrode placement and a position 1 cm above the SCJ. They reported an increase in test sensitivity from 63% to 86% in patients either with or without esophagitis. A similar study comparing the measurement of acid reflux 1 cm above the gastroesophageal junction to 5 cm showed improved diagnostic accuracy in patients with erosive esophagitis but not in patients with nonerosive reflux disease.[20] Although there is not sufficient evidence to recommend more proximal placement in current clinical practice, the possibility that diagnostic accuracy would be improved by an alternate electrode placement is real and may help explain patients with functional heartburn or those with endoscopic findings of short-segment Barrett esophagus but a negative pH-monitoring result.

Discrepancy Between the Two Systems

Simultaneous catheter-based and Bravo pH monitoring has been conducted over the years to allow comparisons of the two methodologies. In general, studies have reported a higher acid exposure measured by the catheter system comparing with the wireless-based system, although the reasons are largely unclear. Sampling rates may be a cause of discrepancy. Sampling frequency is 4 per second for most catheter-based systems, whereas it is every 6 seconds for the Bravo system, a considerable difference. Des Varannes and colleagues[23] reported significant correlation in acid exposure between the two systems (r = 0.87) and concluded that although the Bravo system under recorded acid exposure, its ability to prolong recording time significantly improved the sensitivity of pH monitoring for the diagnosis of GERD. Pandolfino and colleagues[18] also reported lower acid exposure measurements with the Bravo system. They suggested that electrode thermal calibration and pH drift are potential causes of discrepancy between the two systems. The use of an in vivo pH reference (orange juice) was able to improve the discrepancy between the pH data sets of the two systems. A Swedish study simultaneously comparing the two systems reported similar underestimation of acid exposure by the Bravo system and concluded that the two systems are not interchangeable in practice.[24]

With the added ability to measure bolus transit, reflux height, and nonacid reflux events, MII-pH has been preferentially used to evaluate patients with atypical GERD symptoms, such as laryngo-respiratory symptoms or refractory GERD symptoms (PPI nonresponders). A retrospective review of 66 patients, most with atypical reflux symptoms, who underwent both MII-pH and Bravo pH monitoring at the University of Rochester found that 44% of the patients had discordant results. Of these, 90% had a negative MII-pH but positive Bravo study. The authors concluded that a single 24-hour MII-pH study may be an inadequate test to exclude GERD in this patient population. Prakash and Clouse[25] also reported that the prolonged recording time of the Bravo system increases the reflux detection rate, especially in patients with atypical symptoms. More investigations are needed to study the discrepancies between the two systems in order to make sound clinical recommendations for the clinical utility of each system.

The Influence of Diet on Test Accuracy

Although dietary guidelines are generally not given when pH monitoring is performed, studies have shown that exclusion of the meal period would remove the effects of acidic food ingestion and improve the diagnostic accuracy.[14,26,27] Studies have suggested that 5 minutes of acidic food ingestion has a significant effect on the outcome of pH monitoring.[10] There are no current clinical guidelines on whether or not diet restrictions should be given, and the current preference likely varies among centers and clinics.

On or Off PPI Therapy

A recent diagnostic algorithm for esophageal disorders suggested by Kahrilas and Smout[28] supported the role of a PPI trial as an integral part of the diagnostic workup for GERD. The controversy lies when and if PPIs should be continued during pH monitoring. Most reports have shown that symptomatic PPI nonresponders usually have normal results on pH monitoring.[29] Most experts think that pH monitoring should be performed off PPI therapy to optimize the chance of detecting reflux events.[30,31] Garrean and colleagues[11] combined 48 hours on and off PPI therapy using 96-hour Bravo pH monitoring and reported enhanced test interpretation. According to the American College of Gastroenterology's practice guideline in 2007, testing off therapy is recommended to rule out GERD, whereas on-therapy testing is used to evaluate refractory GERD symptoms.[3] A positive pH-monitoring test of the later scenario suggests that more aggressive therapy or other management plans might be needed.

SUMMARY AND FUTURE DIRECTIONS

- Esophageal pH monitoring is an integral part of the diagnostic workup for GERD.
- There are 2 major systems: the catheter-based or the wireless-based Bravo pH monitoring. All pH monitoring demonstrates distal esophageal acid exposure. MII-pH, in addition, can evaluate bolus transit, reflux height, and nonacid reflux events. Prolonged wireless pH monitoring increases the reflux detection rate and may be the test of choice to evaluate patients with atypical symptoms or PPI nonresponders.
- Test selection should be based on availability, patient symptoms (typical or atypical), and the response to the PPI trial to optimize diagnostic accuracy.
- Test interpretation includes the following: distal esophageal acid exposure, patterns of reflux, inclusion or exclusion of the meal period, impedance (nonacid reflux), and symptom correlation measures (SI, SSI, SAP).
- Monitoring pH, although not perfect, is the single most useful diagnostic test for GERD evaluation. For patients with typical GERD symptoms who are endoscopy-negative, a pH-monitoring test is required for consideration of antireflux surgery. A positive pH study predicts relief of typical symptoms postoperatively.
- Prolonged wireless pH monitoring and possibly a smaller capsule that is placed closer to the GE junction than the conventional position may be useful future advances to improve the diagnosis of GERD.

REFERENCES

1. Johnson LF, Demeester TR. Twenty-four-hour pH monitoring of the distal esophagus. A quantitative measure of gastroesophageal reflux. Am J Gastroenterol 1974;62(4):325–32.
2. Herbella FA, Nipominick I, Patti MG. From sponges to capsules. The history of esophageal pH monitoring. Dis Esophagus 2009;22(2):99–103.
3. Hirano I, Richter JE. ACG practice guidelines: esophageal reflux testing. Am J Gastroenterol 2007;102(3):668–85.
4. Bello B, Zoccali M, Gullo R, et al. Gastroesophageal reflux disease and antireflux surgery-what is the proper preoperative work-up? J Gastrointest Surg 2013;17(1): 14–20 [discussion: p20].

5. Jobe BA, Richter JE, Hoppo T, et al. Preoperative diagnostic workup before anti-reflux surgery: an evidence and experience-based consensus of the Esophageal Diagnostic Advisory Panel. J Am Coll Surg 2013;217(4):586–97.
6. McCollough M, Jabbar A, Cacchione R, et al. Proximal sensor data from routine dual-sensor esophageal pH monitoring is often inaccurate. Dig Dis Sci 2004; 49(10):1607–11.
7. Dent J, Vakil N, Jones R, et al. Accuracy of the diagnosis of GORD by questionnaire, physicians and a trial of proton pump inhibitor treatment: the Diamond Study. Gut 2010;59(6):714–21.
8. Bytzer P, Jones R, Vakil N, et al. Limited ability of the proton-pump inhibitor test to identify patients with gastroesophageal reflux disease. Clin Gastroenterol Hepatol 2012;10(12):1360–6.
9. Tuttle SG, Rufin F, Bettarello A. The physiology of heartburn. Ann Intern Med 1961;55:292–300.
10. Koskenvuo JW, Parkka JP, Hartiala JJ, et al. Ingested acidic food and liquids may lead to misinterpretation of 24-hour ambulatory pH tests: focus on measurement of extra-esophageal reflux. Dig Dis Sci 2007;52(7):1678–84.
11. Garrean CP, Zhang Q, Gonsalves N, et al. Acid reflux detection and symptom-reflux association using 4-day wireless pH recording combining 48-hour periods off and on PPI therapy. Am J Gastroenterol 2008;103(7):1631–7.
12. Grigolon A, Consonni D, Bravi I, et al. Diagnostic yield of 96-h wireless pH monitoring and usefulness in patients' management. Scand J Gastroenterol 2011; 46(5):522–30.
13. Scarpulla G, Camilleri S, Galante P, et al. The impact of prolonged pH measurements on the diagnosis of gastroesophageal reflux disease: 4-day wireless pH studies. Am J Gastroenterol 2007;102(12):2642–7.
14. Pandolfino JE, Richter JE, Ours T, et al. Ambulatory esophageal pH monitoring using a wireless system. Am J Gastroenterol 2003;98(4):740–9.
15. Ayazi S, Hagen JA, Zehetner J, et al. Day-to-day discrepancy in Bravo pH monitoring is related to the degree of deterioration of the lower esophageal sphincter and severity of reflux disease. Surg Endosc 2011;25(7):2219–23.
16. Ahlawat SK, Novak DJ, Williams DC, et al. Day-to-day variability in acid reflux patterns using the BRAVO pH monitoring system. J Clin Gastroenterol 2006;40(1):20–4.
17. Demeester TR, Johnson LF, Joseph GJ, et al. Patterns of gastroesophageal reflux in health and disease. Ann Surg 1976;184(4):459–70.
18. Pandolfino JE, Schreiner MA, Lee TJ, et al. Comparison of the Bravo wireless and Digitrapper catheter-based pH monitoring systems for measuring esophageal acid exposure. Am J Gastroenterol 2005;100(7):1466–76.
19. Wenner J, Hall M, Hoglund P, et al. Wireless pH recording immediately above the squamocolumnar junction improves the diagnostic performance of esophageal pH studies. Am J Gastroenterol 2008;103(12):2977–85.
20. Bansal A, Wani S, Rastogi A, et al. Impact of measurement of esophageal acid exposure close to the gastroesophageal junction on diagnostic accuracy and event-symptom correlation: a prospective study using wireless dual pH monitoring. Am J Gastroenterol 2009;104(12):2918–25.
21. Mekapati J, Knight LC, Maurer AH, et al. Transsphincteric pH profile at the gastroesophageal junction. Clin Gastroenterol Hepatol 2008;6(6):630–4.
22. Wenner J, Johnsson F, Johansson J, et al. Acid reflux immediately above the squamocolumnar junction and in the distal esophagus: simultaneous pH monitoring using the wireless capsule pH system. Am J Gastroenterol 2006;101(8): 1734–41.

23. des Varannes SB, Mion F, Ducrotte P, et al. Simultaneous recordings of oesopha-geal acid exposure with conventional pH monitoring and a wireless system (Bravo). Gut 2005;54(12):1682–6.

24. Hakanson BS, Berggren P, Granqvist S, et al. Comparison of wireless 48-h (Bravo) versus traditional ambulatory 24-h esophageal pH monitoring. Scand J Gastroenterol 2009;44(3):276–83.

25. Prakash C, Clouse RE. Value of extended recording time with wireless pH moni-toring in evaluating gastroesophageal reflux disease. Clin Gastroenterol Hepatol 2005;3(4):329–34.

26. Dhiman RK, Saraswat VA, Naik SR. Ambulatory esophageal pH monitoring: tech-nique, interpretations, and clinical indications. Dig Dis Sci 2002;47(2):241–50.

27. Smout AJ. pH testing: the basics. J Clin Gastroenterol 2008;42(5):564–70.

28. Kahrilas PJ, Smout AJ. Esophageal disorders. Am J Gastroenterol 2010;105(4): 747–56.

29. Charbel S, Khandwala F, Vaezi MF. The role of esophageal pH monitoring in symptomatic patients on PPI therapy. Am J Gastroenterol 2005;100(2):283–9.

30. Hemmink GJ, Bredenoord AJ, Weusten BL, et al. Esophageal pH-impedance monitoring in patients with therapy-resistant reflux symptoms: 'on' or 'off' proton pump inhibitor? Am J Gastroenterol 2008;103(10):2446–53.

31. Kushnir VM, Sayuk GS, Gyawali CP. The effect of antisecretory therapy and study duration on ambulatory esophageal pH monitoring. Dig Dis Sci 2011;56(5): 1412–9.

32. Jamieson JR, Stein HJ, DeMeester TR, et al. Ambulatory 24-h esophageal pH monitoring: normal values, optimal thresholds, specificity, sensitivity, and repro-ducibility. Am J Gastroenterol 1992;87(9):1102–11.

33. Richter JE, Bradley LA, DeMeester TR, et al. Normal 24-hr ambulatory esopha-geal pH values. Influence of study center, pH electrode, age, and gender. Dig Dis Sci 1992;37(6):849–56.

34. Shay S, Tutuian R, Sifrim D, et al. Twenty-four hour ambulatory simultaneous impedance and pH monitoring: a multicenter report of normal values from 60 healthy volunteers. Am J Gastroenterol 2004;99(6):1037–43.

35. Zerbib F, des Varannes SB, Roman S, et al. Normal values and day-to-day vari-ability of 24-h ambulatory oesophageal impedance-pH monitoring in a Belgian-French cohort of healthy subjects. Aliment Pharmacol Ther 2005;22(10):1011–21.

36. Ayazi S, Lipham JC, Portale G, et al. Bravo catheter-free pH monitoring: normal values, concordance, optimal diagnostic thresholds, and accuracy. Clin Gastro-enterol Hepatol 2009;7(1):60–7.

37. DeMeester TR, Wang CI, Wernly JA, et al. Technique, indications, and clinical use of 24 hour esophageal pH monitoring. J Thorac Cardiovasc Surg 1980;79(5): 656–70.

38. Johnsson F, Joelsson B, Isberg PE. Ambulatory 24 hour intraesophageal pH-monitoring in the diagnosis of gastroesophageal reflux disease. Gut 1987; 28(9):1145–50.

39. Mattioli S, Pilotti V, Spangaro M, et al. Reliability of 24-hour home esophageal pH monitoring in diagnosis of gastroesophageal reflux. Dig Dis Sci 1989;34(1):71–8.

40. Schindlbeck NE, Heinrich C, Konig A, et al. Optimal thresholds, sensitivity, and specificity of long-term pH-metry for the detection of gastroesophageal reflux dis-ease. Gastroenterology 1987;93(1):85–90.

41. Singh S, Richter JE, Bradley LA, et al. The symptom index. Differential usefulness in suspected acid-related complaints of heartburn and chest pain. Dig Dis Sci 1993;38(8):1402–8.

Role of Endoscopy in GERD

Virender K. Sharma, MD

KEYWORDS

- Endoscopy • GERD • Barrett • Diagnosis • Therapy • Esophagitis

KEY POINTS

- Endoscopy is the mainstay diagnostic and therapeutic tool in the management of GERD.
- Endoscopy is recommended for the evaluation of medically refractory or atypical GERD, patients with alarm symptoms of dysphagia, anemia or weight loss, for diagnosis and surveillance of Barrett esophagus in patients with chronic GERD, and for application of such therapies as esophageal dilation or ablation.
- Newer imaging techniques in development will further improve the accuracy and use of endoscopy in management of GERD.

INTRODUCTION

Gastroesophageal reflux disease (GERD) is one of the most common conditions encountered in primary care and gastroenterology practices. Almost 40% of the US population suffers from occasional heartburn and up to 20% of patients report bothersome symptoms on at least a weekly basis. Heartburn or indigestion is the commonest symptom of GERD and accounts for nearly 2 million outpatient clinic visits, with dysphagia accounting for additional 1 million visits. GERD is the leading diagnosis for gastrointestinal disorders in outpatient clinic visits in the United States accounting for almost 9 million visits in the year 2009, with Barrett esophagus accounting for an additional 500,000 visits. Endoscopy is commonly performed for the diagnosis and management of GERD, with reflux symptoms (24%) and dysphagia (20%) being the commonest indications.[1]

The prevalence of GERD and use of endoscopy for management of GERD are rising. In a systemic analysis, El-Serag[2] reported an increasing prevalence of GERD over the last two decades. Analysis of CORI and CMMS databases shows an increased use of endoscopy partially accounted for by rising prevalence of GERD.[3]

This article discusses the appropriate indications for endoscopy in patients with GERD and highlights newer imaging technologies that may improve utility and outcomes of endoscopy in management of GERD.

This article originally appeared in Gastroenterology Clinics, Volume 43, Issue 1, March 2014.
Disclosure Statement: Consultant Takeda Pharmaceuticals, Equity/Consultant EndoStim Inc.
Arizona Digestive Health, 2680 South Val Vista, Suite 116, Gilbert, AZ 85295, USA
E-mail address: vksharma@arizonadigestivehealth.com

Clinics Collections 7 (2015) 49–56
http://dx.doi.org/10.1016/j.ccol.2015.06.005

ESOPHAGOGASTRODUODENOSCOPY OR UPPER ENDOSCOPY

High-definition, high-resolution flexible video endoscopy has become the standard of endoscopic care in the United States. Esophagogastroduodenoscopy allows for excellent view of the mucosal details and allows for obtaining photographs, video recordings, and tissue sampling using biopsy and brush cytology. Endoscopy also allows for application of therapies, such as esophageal dilation, Barrett ablation, and endoscopic resection of preneoplastic and early neoplastic lesions. Most esophagogastroduodenoscopy procedures in the United States are performed using conscious sedation or procedural sedations. However, data suggest that unsedated, thin-scope esophagogastroduodenoscopy can be safely and successfully performed in carefully selected patients.[4]

Advances in imaging technology are expanding the accuracy of traditional white light endoscopy. High-definition (>850,000 pixel density), high-magnification (>115×) endoscopes using 1080p technology allow one to see mucosal details with greater resolution improving its diagnostic accuracy. Electronic or virtual chromoendoscopy is replacing traditional chromoendoscopy using dye, which was cumbersome and messy.

Standard white light endoscopy uses blue, green, and red light waves, whereas the NBI technology (Olympus, Center Valley, PA), using electronic light filters, only uses blue (440–460 nm) and green (540–560 nm) wave light, eliminating the use of the red light. The narrower wavelengths highlight the superficial mucosa and blood vessels accentuating the mucosal architecture and microvasculature. The FICE system (Fuji, Wayne, NJ) and I-Scan (Pentax, Montvale, NJ) use postprocessing techniques, such as spectral analysis, or postprocessing enhancements to achieve electronic chromoendoscopy.

Full-spectrum endoscopy (FUSE; EndoChoice, Atlanta, GA) allows for a 245-degree field of view compared with the 160-degree field of view of traditional upper endoscopy and may improve the diagnostic yield of upper endoscopy.

CONFOCAL LASER ENDOMICROSCOPY AND OPTICAL COHERENCE TOMOGRAPHY

Confocal laser endomicroscopy and optical coherence tomography (OCT) use lasers to penetrate to a certain depth below the surface and magnify the images obtained to evaluate deeper structures. Two catheter-based technologies for confocal laser endomicroscopy (Cellvizio; Mauna Kea Technologies, Paris, France) and OCT (NvisionVLE; Ninepoint Medical, Cambridge, MA) have been approved by the Food and Drug Administration for use in the United States.

The Cellvizio probe-based confocal laser endomicroscopy system uses a 7F catheter confocal miniprobe, which is passed down the working channel of the upper endoscope and a low-power blue laser light (wave length 488 nm) passed through a fiberoptic bundle for tissue illumination after application of fluorescence agents (topical Acriflavine hydrochloride and Cresyl Violet, and systemic fluorescein) to obtain confocal images (~1000 × magnification) of the mucosa fixed image plane depth of 55 to 65 μm that are streamed at a frame rate of 12 frames per second.

OCT uses a technique called interferometry that measures the path length of reflected light and processes the information for image generation, a technique similar to an ultrasound that uses sound waves. The NvisionVLE OCT or volumetric laser endomicroscopy uses a balloon catheter that passes through a 2.8-mm or larger scope channel and performs volumetric laser interferometry based on frequency domain OCT to faster, real-time, high-resolution imaging. It provides resolution to 10 mm and imaging depth down to 3 mm, real-time resolution of 7 μm, scanning over a 6-cm length of esophagus for a period of 90 seconds and allowing for the visualization of tissue layers including the esophageal mucosa, submucosa, and muscularis propria.

WIRELESS CAPSULE ENDOSCOPY

Esophageal capsule endoscopy was approved by the Food and Drug Administration in 2004 for the evaluation of the esophagus in patients with GERD and suspected Barrett esophagus. Esophageal capsule endoscopy uses a video capsule endoscope with camera at both ends (height, 11 mm; width, 26 mm; weight, 3.7 g) that takes images of the esophagus at 18 frames per seconds. Esophageal capsule endoscopy allowed for unsedated outpatient evaluation of the esophagus with moderate sensitivity and specificity for the evaluation of Barrett esophagus.[5] However, because of cost and need for mucosal biopsy for the diagnosis of Barrett esophagus, it is not widely used. A tethered multiuse string capsule using the small bowel capsule endoscope was developed to overcome some of the issues of traditional esophageal capsule endoscopy but interest in the technology has waned.[6]

GASTROESOPHAGEAL REFLUX DISEASE

Montreal Consensus Conference defines GERD as a condition that develops when there is reflux of stomach contents into the esophagus causing troublesome symptoms, complications, or both.[7] Presence of mucosal damage and positive endoscopic findings are not a prerequisite for the diagnosis of GERD. GERD can accurately be diagnosed by history of classical symptoms of heartburn and/or regurgitation and a positive response to antisecretory therapy.[7] Almost two-thirds of patients with GERD have nonerosive disease and a normal endoscopy.[8] Los Angeles classification **(Table 1)** is most commonly used to classify the grade of erosive esophagitis in the United States, whereas the Savary-Miller classification is more commonly used in Europe. Los Angeles classification has been shown to have good intraobserver and interobserver agreement among experienced and inexperienced endoscopists and correlates well with the amount of esophageal acid exposure and complications of GERD.[9] However, neither of the classifications accurately predicts symptom severity.

The Clinical Guidelines Committee of the American College of Physicians recommends endoscopy in (1) patients with heartburn and alarm symptoms (dysphagia, bleeding, anemia, weight loss, and recurrent vomiting), (2) typical GERD symptoms that persist despite a therapeutic trial of 4 to 8 weeks of twice-daily proton-pump inhibitor therapy, (3) patients with severe (greater than or equal to Los Angeles grade

Table 1	
Los Angeles classification of endoscopic grades of esophagitis	
Grade	**Endoscopic Description**
A	One or more mucosal break <5 mm that does not extend between the tops of two mucosal folds
B	One or more mucosal break ≥5 mm that does not extend between the tops of two mucosal folds
C	One or more mucosal break that is continuous between the tops of two or more mucosal folds but that involves <75% of the circumference
D	One or more mucosal break that involves ≥75% of the esophageal circumference

C-D) erosive esophagitis after a 2-month course of proton-pump inhibitor therapy to assess healing and rule out Barrett esophagus, and (4) history of esophageal stricture who have recurrent symptoms of dysphagia.[3]

In addition to the above indications, the American Society for Gastrointestinal Endoscopy recommends endoscopy in patients with either extraesophageal symptoms or atypical symptoms of GERD. Endoscopy should also be performed as a part of preoperative evaluation and for the evaluation of patients with recurrent symptoms after endoscopic or surgical antireflux procedures.[10] The American College of Gastroenterology recommends endoscopy to diagnose complications of GERD and identify suspected Barrett esophagus in patients with chronic GERD.[11] Although the American Gastroenterological Association recommends endoscopy for patients with chronic GERD with troublesome dysphagia and nonresponsive to empiric trial of twice-daily proton-pump inhibitor, alarm symptoms other than troublesome dysphagia are classified as "insufficient evidence" to make a recommendation. Biopsies of esophageal abnormalities are recommended; however, routine biopsy of normal squamous mucosa for the diagnosis of GERD is not recommended. Esophageal biopsies (at least five samples) should be performed if the differential diagnosis of eosinophilic esophagitis is being considered (**Box 1**).[12]

ESOPHAGEAL DILATION

Esophageal stricture formation is a well-known complication of GERD. However, the incidence of recurrent stricture has decreased with widespread use of antisecretory therapy with proton-pump inhibitors. Dysphagia is the primary indication for endoscopic dilation and need for dilation in the absence of dysphagia or empiric dilation for dysphagia in the absence of structural abnormality is not routinely recommended.[13]

Three types of dilators are routinely used to perform endoscopic dilation: (1) non–wire-guided mercury or tungsten-filled bougies (Maloney or Hurst), (2) wire-guided polyvinyl dilators (Savary- Gilliard or American), and (3) through-the-scope balloon dilators. Maloney dilators are passed blindly and may have higher risk of perforation compared with wire-guided Savary dilators or through-the-scope balloon dilators. Use of fluoroscopy with Maloney dilators is advised for improved safety and functional results. To avoid complications with dilation, a conservative approach to dilation is the "rule of three," which recommends that after moderate resistance is encountered with

---

Box 1
Indications for endoscopy in GERD

Persistent or progressive GERD symptoms despite appropriate medical therapy

Atypical GERD symptoms

Evaluation of patients with suspected extraesophageal manifestations of GERD

Alarm symptoms

   Dysphagia or odynophagia

   Involuntary weight loss, evidence of gastrointestinal bleeding, or anemia

   Finding of a mass, stricture, or ulcer on imaging studies

Screening for Barrett esophagus in selected patients (as clinically indicated)

Evaluation of patients' before and with recurrent symptoms after endoscopic or surgical antireflux procedures

the bougie dilator, no greater than three consecutive dilators in increments of 1 mm should be used in a single dilation session. In patients with dysphagia caused by Schatzki ring, a larger 16- to 20-mm dilator should be used with the intent of disrupting the stricture.[13] Biopsy of the Schatzki ring before dilation may help in effectively breaking the ring with dilation.

BARRETT ESOPHAGUS

Barrett esophagus is a metaplastic change of the esophageal lining from the normal squamous to specialized columnar epithelium caused by chronic acid damage. Approximately 10% of patients with chronic heartburn symptoms have Barrett esophagus accounting for almost a half million of the visits in 2009.[1] An estimated 3.3 million Americans have a diagnosis of Barrett esophagus. White men have the highest risk for Barrett esophagus, with women, African-Americans, and Asians having lower risks. Hispanics have comparable prevalence of Barrett esophagus as whites.[14] Most (90%) patients with Barrett esophagus have nondysplastic disease and a very low rate of progression to esophageal adenocarcinoma at a rate of 0.3 to 0.4 per patient-year.[15] Guidelines generally recommend that patients with nondysplastic disease undergo endoscopic surveillance every 3 to 5 years to detect progression to dysplasia and/or esophageal adenocarcinoma. Given the large number of subjects with Barrett esophagus, these examinations represent a substantial commitment of resources.

Men older than 50 years with chronic GERD symptoms greater than 5-years duration, nocturnal reflux symptoms, hiatal hernia, elevated body mass index, tobacco use, intra-abdominal distribution of fat, and family history of esophageal cancer are at highest risk for Barrett esophagus and esophageal adenocarcinoma.[3]

The Clinical Guidelines Committee of the American College of Physicians recommends endoscopy in men older than 50 years with chronic (>5 years) GERD symptoms and additional risk factors (nocturnal reflux symptoms, hiatal hernia, elevated body mass index, tobacco use, and intra-abdominal distribution of fat) to detect esophageal adenocarcinoma and Barrett esophagus. In men and women with Barrett esophagus and no dysplasia, surveillance examinations should occur at intervals no more frequently than 3 to 5 years. More frequent intervals are indicated in patients with Barrett esophagus and dysplasia (**Box 2**).[3]

American College of Gastroenterology recommends endoscopy for diagnosis of Barrett esophagus in patients with chronic GERD symptoms. In patients with nondysplastic Barrett esophagus, the recommendation is repeat endoscopy at 1 year and

---

Box 2
Indications for endoscopy for Barrett esophagus

Men older than 50 years with chronic (>5 years) GERD symptoms for detection of Barrett esophagus

Every 3–5 years in patients with nondysplastic Barrett esophagus[a]

In 6 months to confirm the diagnosis of low-grade dysplasia and then annually[b]

Every 3 months in patients with high-grade dysplasia[b]

[a] American College of Gastroenterology guidelines recommend repeat endoscopy in 1 year to exclude incident dysplasia and cancer and then every 3 years; American Gastroenterological Association guidelines recommend endoscopy every 5 years.
[b] Consider endoscopic ablative therapy in select patients.

then 3-year intervals to monitor for progression to dysplasia. Patient with low-grade dysplasia should undergo surveillance at 6- to 12-month intervals and with high-grade dysplasia (HGD) at 3-month intervals. Definitive therapy in the form of ablation or surgery should be considered in patients with HGD.[11]

American Gastroenterological Association guidelines consider the evidence to be insufficient to recommend routine upper endoscopy in the setting of chronic GERD symptoms to diminish the risk of death from esophageal cancer and endoscopic screening for Barrett esophagus and dysplasia in adults 50 years or older with more than 5 to 10 years of heartburn to reduce mortality from esophageal adenocarcinoma.[12]

American Society for Gastrointestinal Endoscopy guidelines recommend endoscopic screening for Barrett esophagus in select patients with multiple risk factors for Barrett esophagus and esophageal adenocarcinoma with the caveat that the patient be informed that there is insufficient evidence to affirm this recommendation. Periodic endoscopic surveillance based on histologic grade and endoscopic ablative therapy in selected patients is recommended.[10]

ADVANCE IMAGING

A recent meta-analysis of electronic or virtual chromoendoscopy showed a 34% increased yield for the diagnosis of dysplasia in patients with Barrett esophagus and the increased yield was comparable with traditional chromoendoscopy without the added hassle or cost of using dyes. The authors recommended targeted biopsies using electronic chromoendoscopy followed by random biopsies using the Seattle protocol as being ideal for dysplasia detection.[16]

Two trials of probe-based confocal endomicroscopy have shown high negative predictive value of this technique, reducing the number of biopsies required and increasing assurance to patients with negative tests, thus overcoming the issue of sampling error and interobserver variability in biopsy interpretation in patients with Barrett esophagus undergoing surveillance.[17–19]

Preliminary results with volumetric laser endomicroscopy reveal a high accuracy in detecting HGD in patients with Barrett esophagus and also buried Barrett glands after ablative therapy.[20] Larger trials are awaited to conclusively establish the accuracy of this technique. However, generalizability of these advanced imaging techniques in accurate diagnosis outside expert academic institutions remains to be established.

EOSINOPHILIC ESOPHAGITIS

Eosinophilic esophagitis is increasingly recognized as a cause of esophageal symptoms, specifically solid food dysphagia and food impactions in the absence of typical GERD symptoms. However, many patients have overlap with both GERD and eosinophilic esophagitis. Additionally, patients with eosinophilic esophagitis can improve on acid suppression with proton-pump inhibitor therapy including patients with proton-pump inhibitor–responsive esophageal eosinophilia making the clinical diagnosis of eosinophilic esophagitis challenging. A high clinical suspicion and endoscopic findings of fixed esophageal rings (feline esophagus, trachealization, or corrugation), white exudates or plaques, longitudinal furrows, edema manifesting as mucosal pallor or decreased vascularity, diffuse esophageal narrowing, and mucosal fragility manifesting as esophageal lacerations induced by scope trauma are suggestive but not pathognomic of this disease. Esophageal biopsies (four to six samples) from mid and distal esophagus showing peak value of greater than or equal to 15 eosinophils per high-power field in the absence of other causes of mucosal eosinophilia are considered diagnostic of this condition.[21]

ENDOSCOPIC THERAPIES FOR GERD

There has been an ongoing attempt at the development of endoscopic therapies for the management of GERD. Most of these therapies were removed from practice because of lack of efficacy or because of safety concerns. There are currently two approved endoscopic GERD therapies available in the United States. Stretta (Mederi Therapeutics Inc, Greenwich, CT) radiofrequency therapy for GERD uses low-energy radiofrequency ablation of the submucosal tissue, resulting in increased lower esophageal sphincter compliance and decreased transient lower esophageal sphincter relaxation. Stretta therapy has been shown to improve esophageal pH and GERD symptoms and decrease medication use. Recently, Stretta therapy received a positive endorsement from the Society of American Gastrointestinal and Endoscopic Surgeons as being "appropriate therapy for patients being treated for GERD who are 18 years of age or older, who have had symptoms of heartburn, regurgitation, or both for 6 months or more, who have been partially or completely responsive to anti-secretory pharmacologic therapy, and who have declined laparoscopic fundoplication."[22]

Transoral fundoplication (EsophyX; EndoGastric Solution, Redwood City, WA) uses polypropylene H fasteners to create a serosa-to-serosa fusion to create a fundoplication. The results from multiple small open label studies reported a modest improvement in esophageal acid exposure, improvement in GERD symptoms, and reduction in medication usage. However, significant complications have been reported with this procedure and the Society of American Gastrointestinal and Endoscopic Surgeons issued a cautionary weak recommendation that transoral fundoplication may be an option for select patients. However, "more studies are needed to define optimal techniques and most appropriate patient selection criteria and to further evaluate device and technique safety."[22]

SUMMARY

Endoscopy is the most important diagnostic tool for evaluation and management of patients with GERD and Barrett esophagus. Newer imaging technologies hold promise in improving diagnostic accuracy. However, their validity and generalizability to routine clinical practice outside select academic institution need to be established.

REFERENCES

1. Peery AF, Dellon ES, LundBurden J, et al. Burden of gastrointestinal disease in the United States: 2012 update. Gastroenterology 2012;143:1179–87.
2. El-Serag HB. Time trends of gastroesophageal reflux disease: a systematic review. Clin Gastroenterol Hepatol 2007;5:17–26.
3. Shaheen NJ, Weinberg DS, Denberg TD, et al. Upper endoscopy for gastroesophageal reflux disease: best practice advice from the clinical guidelines committee of the American College of Physicians. Ann Intern Med 2012;157:808–16.
4. Peery AF, Hoppo T, Garman KS, et al. Feasibility, safety, acceptability, and yield of office-based, screening transnasal esophagoscopy. Gastrointest Endosc 2012; 75:945–53.
5. Eliakim R, Sharma VK, Yassin K, et al. A prospective study of the diagnostic accuracy of PillCam ESO esophageal capsule endoscopy versus conventional upper endoscopy in patients with chronic gastroesophageal reflux diseases. J Clin Gastroenterol 2005;39:572–8.

6. Ramirez FC, Akins R, Shaukat M. Screening of Barrett's esophagus with string-capsule endoscopy: a prospective blinded study of 100 consecutive patients using histology as the criterion standard. Gastrointest Endosc 2008;68:25–31.

7. Vakil N, van Zanten SV, Kahrilas P, et al. Global Consensus Group. The Montreal definition and classification of gastroesophageal reflux disease: a global evidence-based consensus. Am J Gastroenterol 2006;101:1900–20.

8. El-Serag HB. Epidemiology of non-erosive reflux disease. Digestion 2008; 78(Suppl 1):6–10.

9. Rath HC, Timmer A, Kunkel C, et al. Comparison of interobserver agreement for different scoring systems for reflux esophagitis: impact of level of experience. Gastrointest Endosc 2004;60:44–9.

10. Lichtenstein DR, Cash BD, Davila R, et al. Role of endoscopy in the management of GERD. Gastrointest Endosc 2007;66:219–24.

11. Katz PO, Gerson LB, Vela MF. Guidelines for the diagnosis and management of gastroesophageal reflux disease. Am J Gastroenterol 2013;108:308–28.

12. Kahrilas PJ, Shaheen NJ, Vaezi MF, et al. American Gastroenterological Association medical position statement on the management of gastroesophageal reflux disease. Gastroenterology 2008;135:1383–91.

13. Egan JV, Baron TH, Adler DA, et al. Esophageal dilation. Gastrointest Endosc 2006;63:755–60.

14. Balasubramanian G, Singh M, Gupta N, et al. Prevalence and predictors of columnar lined esophagus in gastroesophageal reflux disease (GERD) patients undergoing upper endoscopy. Am J Gastroenterol 2012;107:1655–61.

15. Lenglinger J, Riegler M, Cosentini E, et al. Review on the annual cancer risk of Barrett's esophagus in persons with symptoms of gastroesophageal reflux disease. Anticancer Res 2012;32:5465–73.

16. Qumseya BJ, Wang H, Badie N, et al. Advanced imaging technologies increase detection of dysplasia and neoplasia in patients with Barrett's esophagus: a meta-analysis and systematic review. Clin Gastroenterol Hepatol 2013;11: 1562–70.

17. Nguyen VX, Nguyen CC, De Petris G, et al. Confocal endomicroscopy (CEM) improves efficiency of Barrett surveillance. J Interv Gastroenterol 2012;2:61–5.

18. Sharma P, Meining AR, Coron E, et al. Real-time increased detection of neoplastic tissue in Barrett's esophagus with probe-based confocal laser endomicroscopy: final results of an international multicenter, prospective, randomized, controlled trial. Gastrointest Endosc 2011;74:465–72.

19. Bajbouj M, Vieth M, Rösch T, et al. Probe-based confocal laser endomicroscopy compared with standard four-quadrant biopsy for evaluation of neoplasia in Barrett's esophagus. Endoscopy 2010;42:435–40.

20. Leggett CL, Gorospe EC, Owens VL, et al. Can volumetric LASER endomicroscopy detect dysplasia in Barrett's esophagus? Gastrointest Endosc 2013;77: AB327.

21. Dellon ES, Gonsalves N, Hirano I, et al. ACG Clinical Guideline: evidenced based approach to the diagnosis and management of esophageal eosinophilia and eosinophilic esophagitis (EoE). Am J Gastroenterol 2013;108:679–92.

22. Auyang ED, Carter P, Rauth T, et al. SAGES Guidelines Committee. SAGES clinical spotlight review: endoluminal treatments for gastroesophageal reflux disease (GERD). Surg Endosc 2013;27:2658–72.

Esophageal Strictures and Diverticula

C. Daniel Smith, MD

KEYWORDS

- Esophageal stricture • Esophageal diverticula • Esophageal surgery
- GERD complications • Esophageal stricture management
- Esophageal diverticulectomy

KEY POINTS

- Esophageal disease, and in particular, dysfunction of the lower esophageal sphincter (LES) manifesting as gastroesophageal flux disease, is the most common of all gastrointestinal conditions impacting patients daily.
- Conditions leading impairment of esophageal outflow can be categorized into 2 broad categories, esophageal stricture or narrowing, and disorders of esophageal motility and LES function.
- Management focuses on the diverticulum itself, and relieving the underlying sphincter dysfunction.
- Many conditions can cause esophageal luminal narrowing or stricture; the most common are peptic, malignant, and congenital. Other causes include autoimmune, iatrogenic, medication induced, radiation induced, infectious, caustic, and idiopathic.

INTRODUCTION

The topics of this article can best be understood in the context of impairment of esophageal outflow and its consequences. Conditions that lead to impairment of esophageal outflow can best be categorized into 2 broad categories: esophageal stricture or narrowing and disorders of esophageal motility and lower esophageal sphincter (LES) function. The consequence of esophageal stricture most often involves the immediate mechanical impact of the esophageal narrowing, and treatment focuses on relieving the stricture and control of the underlying process, which lead to the stricture. Esophageal diverticula are most commonly the result of pressurization of the esophagus above a dysfunctional sphincter that fails to open appropriately (lower esophageal and cricopharyngeal), leading to the development of a false diverticulum just proximal to the sphincter. Management focuses on the diverticulum itself, and relieving the underlying sphincter dysfunction. One type of diverticulum not related

This article originally appeared in Surgical Clinics, Volume 95, Issue 3, June 2015.
Piedmont Clinic, 2795 Peachtree Road, Unit 1808, Atlanta, GA 30305, USA
E-mail address: cdanielsmith@icloud.com

Clinics Collections 7 (2015) 57–69
http://dx.doi.org/10.1016/j.ccol.2015.06.006
2352-7986/15/$ – see front matter © 2015 Elsevier Inc. All rights reserved.

to esophageal motor dysfunction, a midesophageal diverticulum is also discussed in this article. In contrast with the false diverticula of the esophagus, a midesophageal diverticulum is a true diverticulum and the result of mediastinal inflammatory processes and the resulting focal traction on the esophageal wall, and is therefore not related to esophageal outflow obstruction.

Many conditions can cause esophageal luminal narrowing or stricture. The most common causes are peptic, malignant, and congenital; other causes include autoimmune, iatrogenic, medication induced, radiation induced, infectious, caustic, and idiopathic.

ESOPHAGEAL STRICTURE

The term 'esophageal stricture' is reserved typically for intrinsic diseases of the esophagus causing luminal narrowing through inflammation, fibrosis, or neoplasia. Strictures are grouped typically into benign and malignant categories, with treatment varying depending on the underlying cause. Other causes of esophageal narrowing sometimes considered under the category of esophageal stricture include extrinsic compromise of the esophageal lumen by direct invasion, lymph node enlargement, or direct compression. This article focuses on the intrinsic causes of esophageal narrowing/stricture.

Presentation

Regardless of the nature of a stricture, the clinical presentation typically involves any or all of the following: dysphagia, food impaction, odynophagia, chest pain, and weight loss. Of these, progressive dysphagia to solids is the most common presenting symptom, with benign strictures following a more slow and insidious progression (eg, months to years), whereas dysphagia of a malignant stricture tends to progress more rapidly (eg, in weeks to months).

The clinical history may help to determine the cause of the dysphagia, although 25% of patient presenting with peptic strictures have no prior heartburn or other symptoms of gastroesophageal reflux disease (GERD). A known history of use of medications known to cause peptic ulcers or irritation, or caustic ingestion, are other examples of clinical history that might suggest the underlying cause.

Diagnosis

Esophagogastroduodenoscopy and contrast swallow are the mainstays of the initial workup and diagnosis for esophageal strictures. Although a contrast swallow is obtained most easily, esophagogastroduodenoscopy can provide more overall information and establish not only the diagnosis of a stricture or esophageal narrowing, but also allow visualization of the esophageal mucosa, including biopsy to establish definitively the underlying cause of the stricture. This becomes especially important in determining whether a stricture is benign or malignant. Contrast swallow may be particularly useful in defining the overall esophageal anatomy and identifying other associated pathology, such as an esophageal diverticulum. Esophageal pH testing, esophageal motility may be needed to confirm a diagnosis of GERD or an underlying esophageal motor abnormality (see Esophageal Diverticula section). Finally, when a stricture is determined to be malignant, or extrinsic pathology is thought to be the cause of esophageal narrowing, CT of the chest and abdomen is indicated to establish the cause of extrinsic narrowing and/or to stage a biopsy-proven malignant stricture. Endoscopic ultrasonography has emerged as a useful diagnostic tool to characterize the nature of a stricture and assess the stage and severity of a malignant or infiltrating process. This has become the mainstay of staging malignant disease of the esophagus.

Benign Esophageal Stricture

Benign strictures are by far the most common, and peptic strictures account for 70% to 80% of all causes of esophageal stricture. Peptic strictures are the result of gastro-esophageal reflux–induced esophagitis and scarring.[1–4] With this, peptic strictures usually occur in the distal esophagus within 4 cm of the squamocolumnar junction. The associated mucosal inflammation and submucosal fibrosis give an appearance of inflammation and smooth narrowing without mass effect (**Fig. 1**).

Another common cause of benign stricture is a Schotski's ring, a ringlike constriction of the distal esophagus, often described as a "bandlike" ring of constriction. The etiology of a Schotski's ring remains elusive. Theories include that (1) the ring is a pleat of redundant mucosa that forms when the esophagus for unknown reasons shortens transiently or permanently, (2) the ring is congenital, (3) the ring is a short peptic stricture related to GERD, and (4) the ring is the result of pill-induced esophagitis.

The treatment of benign stricture is dilation (see details elsewhere in this article) and management of any underlying inflammatory process.[1–4] The treatment of the underlying cause cannot be overemphasized.[5] Patients on maximum medical therapy for GERD have lower redilation rates and better resolution of dysphagia than those who are not on maximal medical GERD therapy. Twice daily dosing of a proton pump inhibitor is more effective than H2 blockers alone and for patients with breakthrough evening GERD symptoms, adding a single evening dose of an H2 blocker is indicated. This regimen is continued for at least 1 month, at which time a repeat esophagogastroduodenoscopy is undertaken to reassess. It may be necessary to repeat the dilation at that time and continue maximum medical therapy until the stricture and inflammatory process has completely resolved. At that time, medication can be tapered to a level for symptom control and an endoscopy planned for 12 months later.[6] For more severe strictures, this plan may be compressed to repeat endoscopy and

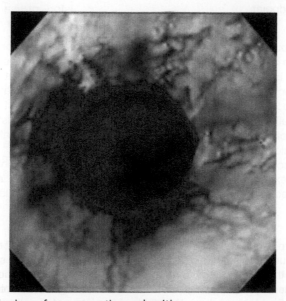

Fig. 1. Endoscopic view of severe peptic esophagitis.

dilation within 1 to 2 weeks of an initial dilation, and more frequent reassessments. Adjuncts such as steroid injections in and around the stricture have been used, especially for more chronic fibrotic strictures. Stenting (see elsewhere in this article) has little role in benign strictures unless the underlying issue with the stricture is anastomotic breakdown and leak from a recent esophageal procedure (which is beyond the scope of this article).

Surgery is indicated for peptic stricture that recurs despite maximal medical therapy, in which case an antireflux procedure is indicated, or for nondilatable fibrotic strictures, which typically requires resection and reconstruction to resolve.[7] One should be cautioned about using a segmental resection of the distal esophagus and esophagogastrostomy to manage a benign stricture because the majority of these patients will have severe GERD after such a procedure, leaving the patient with ongoing issues with peptic injury to the esophagus.[8] If a resection is needed, it is best to use an esophagojejunostomy to avoid severe GERD.

Malignant Esophageal Stricture

The most common cause of malignant esophageal stricture is adenocarcinoma associated with Barrett's esophagus. This is a change from decades ago when most malignant disease of the esophagus was squamous cancer associated with alcohol and tobacco use. The management of malignant stricture centers on tissue diagnosis, staging, and definitive therapy versus palliation. In contrast with benign strictures, dilation plays only a temporizing role, typically to facilitate placement of a stent or prepare for definitive therapy (resection). Stenting (see elsewhere in this article) is much more common in malignant stricture, either as permanent management for advanced disease or temporary management to allow completion of neoadjuvant therapy before undergoing resection.

Management

Dilation
Esophageal dilation[9] for stricture involves selection of technique of dilation, use of adjuncts and endpoint.

Techniques
Mercury-filled bougies (Maloney or Hurst dilators) are reasonable for uncomplicated strictures with an initial diameter of greater than 10 mm. These dilators are inexpensive and fluoroscopy is not needed. This is the technique used for self, at-home dilations.

Wire-guided polyvinyl bougies (Savary-Gilliard dilators) are stiff dilators appropriate for strictures 5 to 20 mm in diameter and are best suited for long, tight strictures. Fluoroscopy is typically needed to assess guidewire placement and to visualize safe passage of the dilator. Use usually requires sedation and is more traumatic on the larynx than other techniques of dilation.[10]

Through-the-scope balloon dilators allow visualized placement and dilation. Although more expensive, balloon dilation seems to result in safe management of more complicated and tighter strictures with fewer sessions and a lower recurrence rate.[11]

Adjuncts
Intralesional steroid injection and endoscopic stricturoplasty are the 2 most commonly talked about adjuncts to stricture dilation. Although few data exist to support a mechanism of action, the first ventures to decrease the inflammatory reaction to the trauma of dilation and thereby limit the degree of restenosis after dilation. Several studies have achieved larger final luminal diameter and lower stricture recurrence with the use of

intralesional steroid.[12] It seems reasonable to use this in a benign stricture where dysphagia persists despite dilations and maximal medical management of GERD.

Four-quadrant stricturoplasty followed by dilation has been described for more fibrotic strictures with limited success.[13] Concern with stricturoplasty relates to perforation making the fibrotic strictures most appealing for this adjunct.

Endpoint of Dilation

How much dilation can be achieved in a single session of dilation, and what luminal diameter should be the goal remain controversial. Most would agree that gaining 1 to 2 mm of luminal diameter through 3 consecutive passes of dilators of increasing size during 1 session is a good general rule. Use of balloon dilators may allow even more increase in luminal diameter during a session. Obviously, perforation remains the concern, and balloon dilation provides real-time, direct visualization of the mechanical effects of the dilation and may allow more aggressive, safe dilation. Most patient experience complete relief of dysphagia when a luminal diameter of 40 to 54F is achieved.

Stenting

Stenting for esophageal structure is used most commonly for malignant strictures, either to provide permanent palliation for advanced disease or temporary palliation while a patient is treated with neoadjuvant therapy in preparation for curative resection.[14,15] Permanent stents are usually self-expanding metal or plastic stents, and temporary stents have the stent itself covered so as to limit tissue ingrowth, allowing the stent to be removed more easily. The details of stent design and placement are beyond the scope of this article.

Surgery

Finally, surgery has a primary role for a malignant stricture where staging reveals a potentially curable cancer. In this case, esophagectomy with either high thoracic or cervical esophageal anastomosis to tubularized stomach or colon interposition is preferred. Distal esophageal segmental resection with esophagogastrectomy should be avoided owing to the severe GERD that often results with the LES gone and an intrathoracic anastomosis to stomach. If it is desirable to preserve as much esophagus as possible, it is better to use jejunum for reestablishing intestinal continuity.

The role of surgery in benign stricture is largely limited to antireflux procedures to manage the GERD that is etiologic in most benign strictures. For a nondilatable benign stricture, segmental resection is reasonable so long as an esophagojejunostomy is performed rather than an esophagogastrostomy (see elsewhere in this article).

ESOPHAGEAL DIVERTICULA

An esophageal diverticulum is an epithelial-lined mucosal pouch that protrudes from the esophageal lumen.[16] Esophageal diverticula are classified according to their location (pharyngoesophageal, midesophageal, or epiphrenic), the layers of the esophagus that accompany them (true diverticulum, which contain all layers, or false diverticulum, containing only mucosa and submucosa), or mechanism of formation (pulsion or traction; Table 1). Most esophageal diverticula are pulsion diverticula and are the consequence of a dysfunctional esophageal sphincter that fails to open appropriately, resulting in pressurization of the esophageal lumen forcing the mucosa and submucosa to herniate through the esophageal musculature (false diverticulum). Pharyngoesophageal and epiphrenic diverticula are pulsion diverticula. Less

Table 1			
Classification of esophageal diverticula			
Diverticulum	Location	Mechanism	Type
Pharyngoesophageal	UES	Pulsion	False
Midesophageal	Tracheal bifurcation	Traction	True
Epiphrenic	Distal esophagus	Pulsion	False

Abbreviation: UES, upper esophageal sphincter.

commonly, a periesophageal inflammatory process adheres to the esophagus and subsequently pulls the esophageal wall focally, resulting in all layers of the esophagus comprising the diverticulum (true diverticulum). Midesophageal diverticula are usually traction diverticula resulting from inflammatory changes in mediastinal lymph nodes.

Pharyngoesophageal Diverticulum (Zenker's)

In 1878, Zenker described 27 cases of pharyngoesophageal diverticulum, and thus his name is associated with this condition. This is the most common of the esophageal diverticula. Pharyngoesophageal diverticula consistently arise within the inferior pharyngeal constrictor, between the oblique fibers of the thyropharyngeus muscle and through or above the more horizontal fibers of the cricopharyngeus muscle (the upper esophageal sphincter; **Fig. 2**). Killian's triangle is the area of weakness through which most pharyngoesophageal diverticula protrude. These diverticula seem to be acquired owing to some degree of incoordination in the swallowing mechanism with

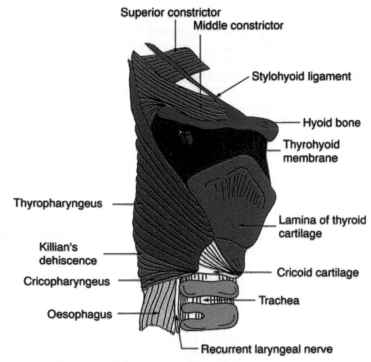

Fig. 2. Anatomy of location of pharyngoesophageal diverticula.

an abnormally high intrapharyngeal pressure leading to protrusion of esophageal mucosa and submucosa through the esophageal wall with subsequent diverticulum formation.

Diagnosis

The presenting symptoms of pharyngoesophageal diverticulum are usually characteristic, and consist of cervical esophageal dysphagia, regurgitation of bland undigested food, frequent aspiration, noisy deglutition (gurgling), halitosis, and voice changes. Dysphagia is present in 98% of patients, and pulmonary aspiration occurs in up to one-third of patients.

The diagnosis of pharyngoesophageal diverticulum is made easily with a barium esophagram (**Fig. 3**). Endoscopy, 24-hour pH monitoring, and esophageal manometry are not indicated unless some features of the symptoms or the esophagram raise suspicion of other conditions (malignancy or GERD). Although these diverticula can reach impressive sizes, it is the degree of upper esophageal sphincter dysfunction that determines the severity of symptoms, not the absolute size of the diverticulum. In most symptomatic cases, treatment is indicated regardless of the size of the diverticulum.

Treatment

As is the case with all pulsion diverticula, proper treatment must be directed at relieving the underlying neuromotor abnormality responsible for the increased intraluminal pressure and then managing the diverticulum.[17] Most techniques described have used division of the cricopharyngeus muscle followed by resection, imbrication, obliteration, or fenestration of the diverticulum (**Table 2**). Most approaches to management agree that relief of the relative obstruction distal to the pouch through cricopharyngeal myotomy is the most important aspect of treatment. Early surgical

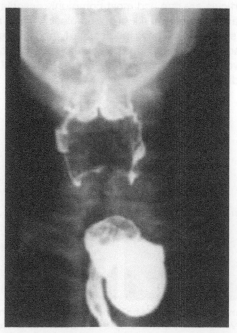

Fig. 3. Barium esophagram showing pharyngoesophageal diverticulum.

Table 2
Treatment options for pharyngoesophageal diverticula

Treatment	Description
Endoscopic diverticulotomy	Endoscopic division of cricopharyngeus and common wall between diverticulum and esophagus (electrocautery, stapler, laser, etc)
Operative myotomy and diverticulectomy	Cricopharyngeal myotomy and excision of diverticulum
Operative myotomy and diverticulopexy	Cricopharyngeal myotomy and mobilization of sac with suture fixation of the sac above the neck of the diverticulum
Operative myotomy alone	Cricopharyngeal myotomy only

strategies using diverticulectomy only, without myotomy, had high failure rates because of esophageal leaks from the suture line, or recurrence. More recently, endoscopic management has emerged as the preferred method of managing these diverticula (ref). Dividing the septum between the esophagus and diverticulum and the cricopharyngeus muscle using either an energy device (eg, cautery, laser; **Fig. 4**) or a stapling device (**Fig. 5**) allows a minimally invasive approach that both addresses the cricopharyngeus muscle and the trapping of content in the diverticulum. The typical advanced age of many who suffer with this condition also makes the endoscopic approach appealing. Success is achieved in more than 90% of patients undergoing endoscopic management with a low morbidity and mortality. Twenty percent of patients may require 2 treatments to achieve these results.[18–21]

Midesophageal Diverticulum

Midesophageal diverticula are rare and most commonly associated with mediastinal granulomatous disease (histoplasmosis or tuberculosis). They are thought to arise because of adhesions between inflamed mediastinal lymph nodes and the esophagus. By contraction, the adhesions exert "traction" on the esophagus with eventual localized diverticulum development. These are true diverticula with all layers of the esophagus present in the diverticulum.

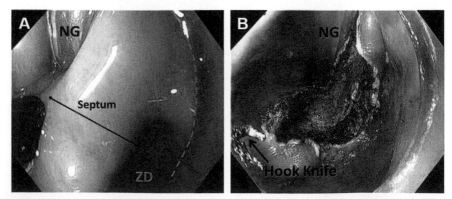

Fig. 4. Endoscopic management of pharyngoesophageal diverticulum. Yellow dashes indicate lateral edge of diverticulum. (*A*) Endoscopic view before diverticulotomy. NG, nasogastric tube in esophagus; ZD, lumen of Zenker's diverticulum. (*B*) Completed diverticulotomy.

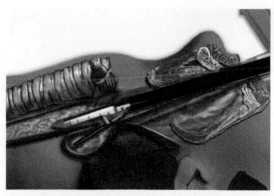

Fig. 5. Stapled endoscopic management of pharyngoesophageal diverticulum.

Diagnosis/treatment

A midesophageal diverticulum is typically asymptomatic and diagnosed incidentally on a barium esophagram undertaken for other reasons. When such an asymptomatic diverticulum is found, no treatment is necessary. In patients with symptoms, esophageal manometry is indicated to ensure that the LES function is normal and that there is not a pulsion diverticulum. Symptomatic diverticula require treatment. Larger diverticula usually require an accompanying resection or diverticulopexy. In the absence of a motor abnormality, diverticulectomy alone may be adequate. Many surgeons will add an esophagogastric myotomy (Heller myotomy) for any esophageal diverticulectomy to minimize the risk of staple line leak that may accompany any early postoperative esophageal lumen pressurization. Data in the literature are mixed related to the requirement of esophagogastric myotomy for true traction diverticula.[22,23] It is this author's preference to add an esophagogastric myotomy (Heller myotomy) myotomy to all cases where esophageal diverticulectomy is indicated (of course, not including pharyngoesophageal diverticula).

Epiphrenic (Pulsion) Diverticulum

An epiphrenic diverticulum typically occurs within the distal 10 cm of the esophagus and is a pulsion type. It is most commonly associated with esophageal motor abnormalities (achalasia, hypertensive LES, diffuse esophageal spasm, nonspecific motor disorders), but may be the result of other causes of increased esophageal pressure (eg, after fundoplication with esophageal outflow obstruction). I have managed several epiphrenic diverticula in patients who have undergone endoluminal fundoplication, in particular transoral incisionless fundoplication, where the esophageal wall has been weakened by the transmural fixation and outflow obstruction has allowed pressurization of the esophagus above and at the fundoplication with subsequent diverticulum formation.

Diagnosis/treatment

Most epiphrenic diverticula are symptomatic because of the underlying esophageal motor disorder. Diagnosis of the diverticulum is made during barium esophagram (**Fig. 6**). Manometry, esophagoscopy, and 24-hour pH testing may be necessary to diagnose associated conditions and direct specific treatments. Most epiphrenic diverticula require esophageal myotomy extending from the neck of the diverticulum

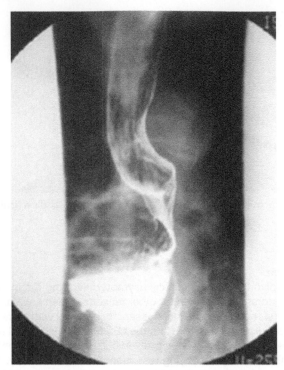

Fig. 6. Barium esophagram showing a large epiphrenic diverticulum.

onto the gastric cardia for a distance of 1.5 to 3.0 cm (see Myotomy for Achalasia). Diverticulectomy, fundoplication, or repair of hiatal hernia may also be necessary, depending on the size of the diverticulum or associated conditions.

Technique of midesophageal and epiphrenic diverticulectomy

In the past, an open thoracic approach has been the preferred approach to these diverticula. Today, a laparoscopic or combined laparoscopic/thoracoscopic approach allows a minimally invasive approach to these diverticula, significantly decreasing the morbidity and mortality of management of these diverticula (ref). If the neck of the diverticulum is above the esophageal hiatus and/or the diverticulum itself is very large and extends up into the chest, the operation commences with a thoracoscopic approach. Prone thoracoscopy[24] significantly facilitates mobilization of the diverticulum (**Figs. 7** and **8**) and stapled transection of the neck (**Figs. 9** and **10**). Once the diverticulum is resected, the patient is flipped into the supine position for laparoscopic esophagogastric myotomy and partial fundoplication. If the neck of the diverticulum is at the level of the esophageal hiatus and the diverticulum does not extend far into the chest, an entirely laparoscopic approach may be adequate. As we have gained experience with prone thoracoscopy, we now approach most epiphrenic diverticula with the combined thoracoscopic/laparoscopic approach.

Several series have documented the feasibility of this approach.[25,26] We have experience in the management of more than 40 cases using laparoscopic/thoracoscopic approach. As stated, we prefer to add an esophagogastric myotomy to all cases to minimize the risk of staple line leak postoperatively.[27]

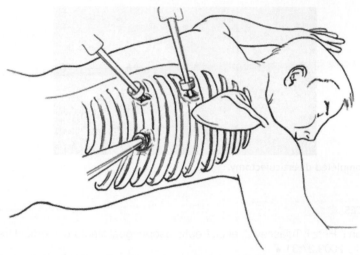

Fig. 7. Illustration of prone thoracoscopy used to approach mid- and large epiphrenic diverticula.

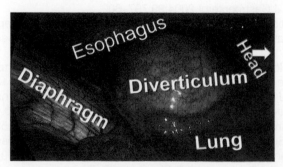

Fig. 8. Prone thoracoscopic view of epiphrenic diverticulum.

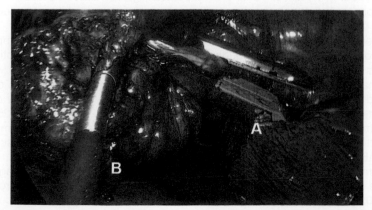

Fig. 9. Prone thoracoscopic view of diverticulum neck being transected with stapler. (A) Stapler across diverticulum neck. (B) Grasper holding diverticulum.

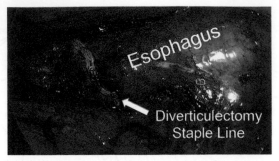

Fig. 10. Completed diverticulectomy.

REFERENCES

1. Pregun I, Hritz I, Tulassay Z, et al. Peptic esophageal stricture: medical treatment. Dig Dis 2009;27:31–7.
2. Pace F, Antinori S, Repici A. What is new in esophageal injury (infection, drug-induced, caustic, stricture, perforation)? Curr Opin Gastroenterol 2009;25:372–9.
3. Guda NM, Vakil N. Proton pump inhibitors and the time trends for esophageal dilation. Am J Gastroenterol 2004;99:797–800.
4. Marks RD, Richter JE, Rizzo J, et al. Omeprazole versus H2-receptor antagonists in treating patients with peptic stricture and esophagitis. Gastroenterology 1994;106:907–15.
5. Dakkak M, Hoare RC, Maslin SC, et al. Oesophagitis is as important as oesophageal stricture diameter in determining dysphagia. Gut 1993;34:152–5.
6. Patterson DJ, Graham DY, Smith JL, et al. Natural history of benign esophageal stricture treated by dilatation. Gastroenterology 1983;85:346–50.
7. Smith CD. Antireflux surgery. Surg Clin North Am 2008;88:943–58.
8. Smith CD. Surgical therapy for gastroesophageal reflux disease: indications, evaluation, and procedures. Gastrointest Endosc Clin N Am 2009;19:35–48, v–vi.
9. de Wijkerslooth LR, Vleggaar FP, Siersema PD. Endoscopic management of difficult or recurrent esophageal strictures. Am J Gastroenterol 2011;106:2080–91 [quiz: 2092].
10. Fan Y, Song HY, Kim JH, et al. Fluoroscopically guided balloon dilation of benign esophageal strictures: incidence of esophageal rupture and its management in 589 patients. AJR Am J Roentgenol 2011;197:1481–6.
11. Saeed ZA, Winchester CB, Ferro PS, et al. Prospective randomized comparison of polyvinyl bougies and through-the-scope balloons for dilation of peptic strictures of the esophagus. Gastrointest Endosc 1995;41:189–95.
12. Ramage JI Jr, Rumalla A, Baron TH, et al. A prospective, randomized, double-blind, placebo-controlled trial of endoscopic steroid injection therapy for recalcitrant esophageal peptic strictures. Am J Gastroenterol 2005;100:2419–25.
13. Raijman I, Siddique I, Rachcal LT. Endoscopic stricturoplasty in the management of recurrent benign esophageal strictures. Gastrointest Endosc 1999;49:AB172.
14. Sharma P, Kozarek R. Practice Parameters Committee of American College of G. Role of esophageal stents in benign and malignant diseases. Am J Gastroenterol 2010;105:258–73 [quiz: 274].
15. Hindy P, Hong J, Lam-Tsai Y, et al. A comprehensive review of esophageal stents. Gastroenterol Hepatol (N Y) 2012;8:526–34.

16. Smith CD. Esophagus. In: Norton JA, Chang AE, Lowry SF, et al, editors. Essential practice of surgery basic science and clinical evidence. New York: Springer - Verlag; 2003. p. 167–84.
17. Zaninotto G, Narne S, Costantini M, et al. Tailored approach to Zenker's diverticula. Surg Endosc 2003;17:129–33.
18. Tang SJ. Flexible endoscopic Zenker's diverticulotomy: approach that involves thinking outside the box (with videos). Surg Endosc 2014;28:1355–9.
19. Parker NP, Misono S. Carbon dioxide laser versus stapler-assisted endoscopic Zenker's diverticulotomy: a systematic review and meta-analysis. Otolaryngol Head Neck Surg 2014;150:750–3.
20. Law R, Baron TH. Transoral flexible endoscopic therapy of Zenker's diverticulum. Dig Surg 2013;30:393.
21. Huberty V, El Bacha S, Blero D, et al. Endoscopic treatment for Zenker's diverticulum: long-term results (with video). Gastrointest Endosc 2013;77:701–7.
22. Isaacs KE, Graham SA, Berney CR. Laparoscopic transhiatal approach for resection of midesophageal diverticula. Ann Thorac Surg 2012;94:e17–9.
23. Galata CL, Bruns CJ, Pratschke S, et al. Thoracoscopic resection of a giant midesophageal diverticulum. Ann Thorac Surg 2012;94:293–5.
24. Goldberg RF, Bowers SP, Parker M, et al. Technical and perioperative outcomes of minimally invasive esophagectomy in the prone position. Surg Endosc 2013;27:553–7.
25. Herbella FA, Patti MG. Modern pathophysiology and treatment of esophageal diverticula. Langenbecks Arch Surg 2012;397:29–35.
26. Soares RV, Montenovo M, Pellegrini CA, et al. Laparoscopy as the initial approach for epiphrenic diverticula. Surg Endosc 2011;25:3740–6.
27. Melman L, Quinlan J, Robertson B, et al. Esophageal manometric characteristics and outcomes for laparoscopic esophageal diverticulectomy, myotomy, and partial fundoplication for epiphrenic diverticula. Surg Endosc 2009;23:1337–41.

Epidemiology of Barrett's Esophagus and Esophageal Adenocarcinoma

Thomas M. Runge, MD, MPH[a], Julian A. Abrams, MD, MS[b],
Nicholas J. Shaheen, MD, MPH[a],*

KEYWORDS

- Barrett's esophagus • Esophageal adenocarcinoma
- Gastroesophageal reflux disease • Epithelium

KEY POINTS

- Barrett's esophagus is a precursor to esophageal adenocarcinoma (EAC).
- The incidence of EAC has increased dramatically and EAC is now the most common form of esophageal cancer in the United States.
- The strongest risk factor for Barrett's esophagus is gastroesophageal reflux (GERD), but central adiposity and tobacco smoking also increase risk.
- Risk factors for EAC include GERD, tobacco smoking, and obesity, whereas *Helicobacter pylori* and nonsteroidal antiinflammatory drugs may be protective.
- Dysplastic changes seen on biopsy predict progression of Barrett's to EAC, but estimates of the incidence of EAC in dysplastic Barrett's epithelium vary.

INTRODUCTION

Barrett's esophagus (BE) is a condition in which the typical squamous epithelium of the esophageal mucosa is replaced with columnar intestinal epithelium.[1,2] BE is a known precursor to the development of esophageal adenocarcinoma (EAC), a

This article originally appeared in Gastroenterology Clinics, Volume 44, Issue 2, June 2015.
Disclosures: Dr N.J. Shaheen receives research funding from Covidien Medical, CSA Medical, NeoGenomics, Takeda Pharmaceuticals, and Oncoscope. He is a consultant for Oncoscope. Dr J.A. Abrams receives research funding from Covidien Medical, CSA Medical, C2 Therapeutics, and Trio Medicines. He is also a consultant for C2 Therapeutics. Dr T.M. Runge has no conflicts to declare.
This research was funded by T32 DK07634 (Robert Sandler) and K24DK100548 (Nicholas Shaheen).
[a] Division of Gastroenterology and Hepatology, Center for Esophageal Diseases and Swallowing, University of North Carolina School of Medicine, University of North Carolina at Chapel Hill, CB#7080, Chapel Hill, NC 27599-7080, USA; [b] Division of Digestive and Liver Diseases, Columbia University Medical Center, 622 West 168th Street, PH 7W-318D, New York, NY 10032, USA
* Corresponding author.
E-mail address: nshaheen@med.unc.edu

malignancy with a dramatically increasing incidence over the past 40 years.[3–5] The risk of EAC among patients with BE is estimated to be 30-fold to 125-fold greater than that of the general population.[6] Endoscopically, the prevalence of BE has been estimated at 1% to 2% in all patients receiving endoscopy for any indication, and from 5% to 15% in patients with symptoms of gastroesophageal reflux disease (GERD).[7] Although uncommon, EAC has a poor prognosis, and is associated with a 5-year survival rate of less than 20%.[8,9]

The incidence of EAC in patients with BE is considerably higher than that in the general population, but only a minority of patients with BE develop EAC, with annual risk estimated at 0.1% to 0.5%.[10,11] Reasons for the rapid increase in the incidence of EAC are not entirely known. However, risk factors for the development of BE and EAC have been identified. Similarly, risk factors for the progression of BE to EAC have also been identified, and are discussed here.

Epidemiology of Barrett's Esophagus

Prevalence and incidence of Barrett's esophagus

BE primarily affects older adults in the developed world. The prevalence in living adults is difficult to ascertain, because individuals with Barrett's are often asymptomatic and do not seek care. One of the earliest estimates of the prevalence of BE was via an autopsy study.[12] Cameron and colleagues[12] estimated a prevalence of long-segment BE (LSBE) of 376 cases per 100,000, or roughly 0.4% of the population, and suggested that only a small minority of cases were detected clinically. Population-based studies have provided estimates of the prevalence of BE in the general public. A Swedish study by Ronkainen and colleagues[13] estimated the prevalence of BE by performing upper endoscopy on 1000 randomly selected adults. These investigators found BE in 16 (1.6%) of the individuals, with 5 subjects (0.5%) in their study showing long-segment disease.[13]

Tertiary care center endoscopy studies have also attempted to estimate the prevalence of BE. Rex and colleagues[14] performed upper endoscopy in 961 individuals presenting for routine screening colonoscopy. These investigators found an overall prevalence of BE of 6.8%, or 65 of 961 individuals, of whom 12 (1.2%) had LSBE. In patients who reported heartburn, the prevalence was slightly higher at 8.3%, but most of the patients (54%) who were found to have BE reported no reflux symptoms. These estimates may be higher than the prevalence in the general population, because this tertiary center population of volunteers may have had more GERD than a random sample of the adult population. Zagari and colleagues[15] analyzed 1033 patients originally identified as part of a large multicenter cross-sectional study on gallstone disease. Of these patients, 1.3% (13) had histologically confirmed BE, whereas 0.2% (2) had LSBE. These estimates suggest that the prevalence of BE is between 0.5% and 2% of unselected individuals. In individuals with reflux symptoms, prevalence estimates are more variable (**Table 1**), ranging from 5% to 15%.[16]

Given that the use of endoscopy depends on the patient's socioeconomic status, access to care, and other nonmedical factors, the incidence of BE has historically been difficult to ascertain. However, the incidence of endoscopically detected BE seems to have increased dramatically over the past 30 years, a finding that is partially attributable to the increasing frequency of endoscopy during the same period.[17] However, data from the United Kingdom[18] and the Netherlands[19] suggest that incidence rates of BE have increased even after controlling for increasing endoscopy rates. These estimates place the increase in BE incidence at near 65% between 1997 and 2002[19] and 159% between 1993 and 2005. Alarmingly, the greatest proportional

Table 1
Studies examining the prevalence of BE

Authors, Year	Country	Setting, Design	Study Sample	Sample Size	% Male	Average Age (y)	Histologic Confirmation	No. with BE (%)	No. with LSBE (%)	No. with SSBE (%)
Gerson et al,[157] 2002	United States	Single VA center, not population based	Individuals without GERD sx receiving sigmoidoscopy for CRC screening	110	92.0	61.0	Yes	27 (24.5)	19 (17.3)	8 (7.3)
Rex et al,[14] 2003	United States	Multicenter, not population based	Individuals receiving colonoscopy, no GI sx other than reflux or regurgitation	961	59.5	59.0	Yes	65 (6.8)[a]	12 (1.2)	53 (5.5)
Ronkainen et al,[13] 2005	United States	Population-based sample from 2 Swedish communities	Random sample of census-based registry	1000	49.0	53.6	Yes	16 (1.6)[b]	5 (0.5)	11 (1.1)
Ward et al,[158] 2006	United States	Single tertiary care center, not population based	Individuals referred for screening colonoscopy	300	53.7	61.0	Yes	50 (16.7)[c]	4 (1.3)	46 (15.3)
Zagari et al,[15] 2008	Italy	Population-based sample from 2 Italian communities	Individuals remaining from original sample who elected to participate	1033	51.1	59.7	Yes	13 (1.3)[d]	2 (0.2)	11 (1.1)
Zou et al,[159] 2011	China	Population-based sample from 2 Chinese areas	Individuals remaining from random sample who elected to participate	1030	42.3	NR	No	19 (1.8)[e]	NR	NR

Abbreviations: CRC, colorectal cancer; GI, gastrointestinal; NR, not reported; SSBE, short-segment BE; sx, symptoms; VA, Veterans' Affairs.
[a] Prevalence among those with GERD symptoms was 8.3%.
[b] Prevalence among those with GERD symptoms was 2.3%.
[c] Prevalence among those with GERD symptoms was 19.8%.
[d] Prevalence among those with GERD symptoms was 1.5%.
[e] Prevalence among those with GERD symptoms was 2.1%.
Data from Refs.[13–15,157–159]

increase in BE diagnosis was in individuals less than 60 years of age, which is in agreement with other work from Europe.[18]

Age, sex, and ethnic variations in Barrett's esophagus
Men, especially white men, have a strong predilection for the development of BE, with a male/female ratio of 2:1 to 3:1 in most studies (**Table 2**).[1,20] Age at diagnosis can vary widely, because many individuals are asymptomatic and undergo diagnostic endoscopy for other reasons.[21] BE on average is diagnosed in the sixth to seventh decade of life, but may develop earlier.[22] In addition to the greater overall prevalence of BE in men, there is evidence that men develop the disease earlier than women. From a British endoscopy center, Van Blankenstein and colleagues[22] reviewed endoscopy records and histology reports of individuals who received upper endoscopy at a single center. Men on average developed BE about 20 years earlier than women in that study. The overall ratio of BE cases was 2:1 favoring men, but in younger adults the ratio of men to women approached 4:1.[22] A similar trend to early development of BE in men was seen in follow-up studies from Europe.[18,19] White people in general are disproportionately affected compared with other races.[23] In a large cross-sectional study, Ford and colleagues,[24] in a sample from the United Kingdom, found that white people had significantly higher prevalence of BE compared with Asians or Afro-Caribbean people. In that population, LSBE was found in 2.9% of white people, compared with 0.31% of Asians and 0.2% of Afro-Caribbean people.

Studies assessing BE prevalence in Latin Americans also show that BE is considerably less prevalent in Latin Americans compared with white people. In a large study by Abrams and colleagues,[25] the prevalence of BE was significantly lower among those of Latin American background than among white people (1.7% vs 6.1%). Other studies have corroborated variations in BE prevalence among ethnic groups living in the same country, possibly suggesting an effect of as-yet unrecognized polygenetic factors across different ethnicities.

Multiple environmental factors are strongly associated with BE. These factors, such as obesity, GERD, and hiatal hernias, are more common in developed countries. However, genetic factors are likely also at play. Work from twin studies suggests that symptoms of GERD, even when adjusted for obesity and other clinical factors, are more concordant in monozygotic twins than in dizygotic twins.[26]

Selected risk factors for Barrett's esophagus development
Gastroesophageal reflux disease GERD is a central risk factor for BE development. Numerous case-control studies have shown that individuals with GERD are 6 to 8 times more likely to have BE, and the propensity to develop BE increases with more severe symptoms (see **Table 1**).[27–29] Longer duration of GERD may create an environment conducive to the development of BE.[30] However, the presence of reflux symptoms is neither sensitive nor specific for pathologic acid reflux,[31,32] and symptom severity does not correlate well with BE risk.[33,34] Some work has suggested that patients with more significant symptoms may be less likely to have BE,[35] perhaps because of impaired acid sensitivity of the columnar metaplasia compared with normal squamous epithelium. However, longer duration of GERD symptoms predicts increased likelihood of BE.[27] A systematic review on the association between symptoms and BE found no association between reflux symptoms and short-segment BE (SSBE) (odds ratio [OR], 1.15; 95% confidence interval [CI], 0.8–1.7) but found increased odds of LSBE in those with reflux symptoms (OR, 4.92; 95% CI, 2.0, 12.0).[36] Because screening programs target both SSBE and LSBE, significant limitations in using symptom severity remain. When patients with Barrett's are compared

Table 2
Reported risk factors for BE, with magnitudes of association represented as odds ratios (ORs)

Risk Factor	Study, Year	Total (n)	Study Type	Comparison Groups	OR (95% CI)
Symptomatic GERD	Anderson et al,[29] 2007	711	Case control	Population controls, asymptomatic	12.0 (7.6, 18.8)
	Johansson et al,[28] 2007	764	Cross sectional	Population controls, asymptomatic	10.7 (3.5, 33.4)
	Conio et al,[27] 2002	457	Case control	Healthy controls	5.8 (4.0, 8.4)
White race	Ford et al,[24] 2005	20,310	Cross sectional	Afro-Caribbean race	12.2[a]
	Ford et al,[24] 2005	20,310	Cross sectional	South Asian race	6.0 (3.6, 10.2)
	Abrams et al,[25] 2008	2100	Cross sectional	Black people	2.9[a]
	Abrams et al,[25] 2008	2100	Cross sectional	Hispanic people	2.6[a]
Male gender	Ford et al,[24] 2005	20,310	Cross sectional	Female gender	2.7 (2.2, 3.4)
	Van Blankenstein et al,[22] 2005	21,899	Cross sectional	Female gender	2.1 (1.8, 2.6)
	Cook et al,[160] 2005	18,765	Meta-analysis	Female gender	2.0 (1.8, 2.2)
	Abrams et al,[25] 2008	2100	Cross sectional	Female gender	1.9 (1.2, 2.9)
Central adiposity[b]	Edelstein et al,[44] 2007	404	Case control	Low WHR	2.4 (1.4, 3.9)
	Corley et al,[161] 2007	636	Nested case control	Abdominal circumference <80 cm	2.2 (1.1, 3.7)
	Kubo et al,[46] 2013	2502	Pooled analysis	Lowest quartile waist circumference, men	2.2 (1.1–4.7)
				Lowest quartile waist circumference, women	3.8 (1.5, 9.6)
Cigarette smoking	Cook et al,[53] 2012	3534	Pooled analysis	Population controls, nonsmokers	1.7 (1.0, 2.7)
	Steevens et al,[49] 2011	120,852	Prospective cohort	Population controls, nonsmokers	1.3 (1.0, 1.8)
	Thrift et al,[51] 2014	1856	Case control	Primary care controls, nonsmokers	0.8 (0.5, 1.3)
				Elective EGD controls, nonsmokers	1.1 (0.8–1.5)
Helicobacter pylori	Corley et al,[56] 2008	617	Case control	Population controls	0.4 (0.3, 0.7)
	Wang et al,[59] 2009	3529	Meta-analysis	Endoscopically normal controls	0.7 (0.4–1.4)
				Healthy blood donors	2.2 (1.1, 4.6)
Low birth weight	Forssell et al,[62] 2013	1183	Case control	Matched controls	8.2 (2.8, 23.9)
Obstructive sleep apnea	Leggett et al,[64] 2014	188	Case control	Randomly matched controls	1.8 (1.1, 3.2)

Abbreviations: CI, confidence interval; EGD, esophagogastroduodenoscopy; WHR, waist/hip ratio.
[a] CI not available.
[b] Reported magnitude of risk of higher group category (high WHR, high abdominal circumference).
Data from Refs.[22,24,25,27–29,44,46,49,51,53,56,59,62,64,160,161]

with those without, the patients with BE have abundant evidence of aberrant acid exposure: longer episodes of acid exposure, lower pH, and also weak peristaltic contractions and decreased baseline lower esophageal sphincter (LES) tone.[37,38]

Although epidemiologic data suggest that gastric acid suppression with proton pump inhibitors (PPIs) may reduce the chance of developing dysplasia and cancer,[39] the impact PPI use has on development of BE is unknown. Among the many adults who have GERD, only a minority develop BE. The prevalence of BE among those with reflux symptoms is higher than that of the general population, but the relationship is not fully explained by GERD. Obesity may be a common mediator of both GERD and BE. Central adiposity is known to predispose to hiatal hernia development[7] and increased GERD symptoms,[40] and even to directly cause LES relaxations.[41]

In summary, reflux is associated with GERD. However, symptoms of reflux cannot reliably distinguish patients with increased acid reflux from those without. It is likely that a genetic milieu predisposing to the development of BE combined with prolonged acid exposure and mutagenic events, including oxidative stress, may act synergistically in patients who develop EAC.

Obesity Obesity, measured by body mass index (BMI) and central adiposity, has been studied extensively as a risk factor for BE. The incidence of BE and EAC have increased dramatically in the past 40 to 50 years in Western societies, concurrent with rapid increases in the rate of obesity. From 1976 to 1991, the prevalence of obesity at all ages increased from 25% to 33%, and it now approaches 35% in adults.[42] Obesity can be assessed in several ways. High BMIs, and especially central adiposity, have been shown to have a significant association with BE. A 2009 meta-analysis that included 11 observational studies showed an increase in the risk of BE (OR, 1.4) in patients with a BMI greater than 30 kg/m^2 compared with those with BMI less than 30 kg/m^2.[43] Patients with BE have been shown to have higher BMIs than either general controls or individuals with GERD but not BE.[44,45]

Because BMI does not take into account the distribution of body fat, the estimated risk increase in the obese may be poorly estimated by BMI measurements. More recent work has shown that central adiposity, rather than BMI, may be the driver of increased BE risk. Edelstein and colleagues,[44] in a case-control study in 2007, found that the overall risk of BE was significantly greater in those with high waist/hip ratios (WHRs) (OR, 2.4); the risk of LSBE in these patients was even higher (OR, 4.3). A pooled analysis by Kubo and colleagues[46] found that waist circumference, as a proxy measure for central adiposity, increased risk for BE for men (OR, 2.24) and women (OR, 3.75). The impact of obesity on BE risk may vary by race as well. In a US case-control study, Kramer and colleagues[23] studied the effect of BMI and WHR on BE prevalence, and the relationship between WHR and BE was strongest and most significant in white people (OR, 2.5), whereas in African Americans and Latin Americans the associations were not significant. Because the strength of the relationship between WHR and BE was strongest in white people, it was suggested that other ethnic groups could potentially carry as-yet unrecognized genes that protect against BE development.[23] It is possible that the overwhelming male predominance among EAC cases could be explained in part by overweight men distributing fat preferentially to their trunks, and this central adiposity drives the risk increase.[47]

Alcohol Alcohol use has been studied extensively as a possible risk factor for BE.[13,27,48–50] Multiple studies have shown no association between the two, but results have been variable.[48,49,51] Some work has suggested an inverse correlation between wine intake and BE risk.[48] The most robust evidence comes from the Barrett's and

Esophageal Adenocarcinoma Consortium (BEACON) consortium, in which the data from 5 studies were pooled to assess risk of alcohol use.[50] Among 1028 cases and 1282 controls, alcohol use was stratified by gender and by number of drinks per day. There was a borderline significant inverse correlation between BE and any degree of alcohol intake (OR, 0.77, 0.60–1.00). Drinking 3 to less than 5 drinks per day was associated with a statistically significant reduction in BE risk (OR, 0.57, 0.38–0.86), but with more or less alcohol consumed no statistically significant results were found (although there was a trend toward an inverse relationship). When assessing beverage-specific data, wine consumption was associated with an inverse risk of BE (OR, 0.71).[46,48]

At this point the preponderance of evidence supports no association between alcohol intake and BE risk. What was once thought to be a minor risk factor for BE now seems to confer no additional risk. Alcohol might be protective, but in order to fully answer this question, more data are needed.

Cigarette smoking Most studies have found an association between cigarette smoking and an increased risk of developing BE.[52,53] A pooled analysis of 5 case-control studies found a consistent increase in risk of BE over several pack-year cut points, with ORs ranging from 1.44 to 1.99 (**Fig. 1**).[53] However, there was significant heterogeneity between studies, and exclusion of a single study yielded pooled ORs with a higher magnitude across all exposure groups, ranging from 1.75 to 2.89, with an average OR of 2.09.[53] To explore a possible synergistic effect between GERD and tobacco use in the genesis of BE, these investigators conducted additional modeling to assess the concurrent effects of smoking and GERD.[53] The OR of Barrett's increased significantly when both GERD and smoking were present, compared with when smokers did not have GERD.

However, not all studies have identified smoking as a risk factor for BE. Thrift and colleagues[51] studied 258 patients with BE in a case-control study from Houston, Texas. These patients were compared with 2 control groups: one group was composed of patients receiving elective esophagogastroduodenoscopy for any indication, and the other was composed of primary care patients undergoing screening colonoscopy. These researchers found no association between smoking and BE in either group, even when stratified by pack-year exposures, length of time smoking, or number of cigarettes per day. In a prospective study design, Steevens and colleagues[49] found ORs of 1.33 in former smokers and 0.93 in current smokers compared with controls. In conclusion, smoking seems to increase risk of BE, but there is wide variability in risk estimates. Further study may clarify the precise role of tobacco in BE pathogenesis.

Helicobacter pylori Helicobacter pylori (H pylori) infection causes chronic gastritis, peptic ulcer disease, and gastric adenocarcinoma. H pylori is known to have a strong association with intestinal metaplasia in the body and antrum of the stomach.[54] Temporal associations have been made between the decreasing prevalence of H pylori infection in developed countries and the increasing prevalence of EAC.[55] Corley and colleagues[56] showed that H pylori was inversely associated with BE (OR, 0.42) in a case-control study design. Although the mechanisms underlying this inverse association are not fully understood, they may relate to decreased acid production in the setting of H pylori infection (especially with associated atrophic gastritis) or via alterations in the microbiome.

Different strains of H pylori may have different abilities to induce risk. The presence of the cytotoxin-associated gene (CagA) identifies H pylori strains more likely to induce gastritis, more extensive gastric inflammation, and gastric cancer.[57] Vaezi and colleagues[58] addressed the role of H pylori in a case-control study, and found that

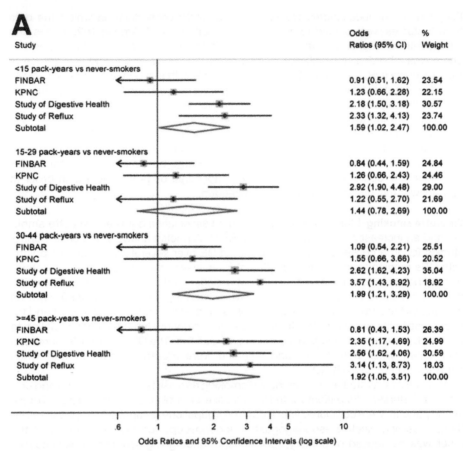

Fig. 1. Forrest plots summarizing the association between smoking and the risk of BE, using population controls. Smoking exposure is grouped by categories. Large unfilled diamonds represent the pooled estimates across all studies within that category. The width of the diamonds represents the 95% CIs. Black squares indicate the point estimate for each individual study. FINBAR, Factors Influencing the Barrett's/Adenocarcinoma Relationship; KPNC, Kaiser Permanente Northern California; UNC, University of North Carolina. (*Adapted from* Cook MB, Shaheen NJ, Anderson LA, et al. Cigarette smoking increases risk of Barrett's esophagus: an analysis of the Barrett's and Esophageal Adenocarcinoma Consortium. Gastroenterology 2012;142:749; with permission.)

patients with BE identified at endoscopy were about 3-fold less likely to be colonized by CagA-positive strains than were controls who did not have BE. However, contradictory findings were noted in a 2009 meta-analysis by Wang and colleagues.[59] Among included studies using endoscopically normal controls, the prevalence of *H pylori* in controls was greater than that in BE, but among those that use healthy blood donors as controls, patients with BE more frequently had *H pylori* infection. The result was a nonsignificant slight trend toward less *H pylori* infection in patients with BE.[59] The investigators cited a need for further study with well-matched cases and controls to make robust conclusions about an association between *H pylori* and BE.

Other possible risk factors Recently, several other possible risk factors for BE have been studied. Low birth weight has been posited as a possible risk factor for BE given the apparent association between preterm birth and systemic inflammation.[60] Forssell and colleagues[61] showed in a Swedish birth cohort that prematurity is associated with the risk of developing esophagitis; a relationship that is most pronounced among those who are small for gestational age (OR, 2.5) or who are born at less than or equal to 32 weeks' gestation (OR, 6.7).[61] Follow-up research by this group suggested that the risk of BE was significantly increased in patients with the lowest birth weights (OR, 8.2).[62] The risk of EAC seems to be increased with reduced gestational time, but the magnitude of effect is smaller (OR, 1.1).[63]

Other factors associated with a proinflammatory state, such as obstructive sleep apnea (OSA) and the metabolic syndrome, seem to increase the risk of BE as well. In a case-control study, Leggett and colleagues[64] found that OSA was associated with an increased risk of BE (OR, 1.8), after controlling for GERD and obesity. Increased levels of adipokines and cytokines have also been found in patients with BE compared with controls.[65] These inflammatory markers may be the intermediaries partially responsible for the increased BE risk seen in individuals with central obesity, OSA, or GERD.

Epidemiology of Esophageal Adenocarcinoma

Prevalence and incidence of esophageal adenocarcinoma
EAC was once a rare form of esophageal malignancy. Surgical series in the early twentieth century showed that EAC made up only 0.8% to 3.7% of all esophageal malignancies.[66] However, by 1990, EAC overtook squamous cell carcinoma of the esophagus, and is now the more common of the two in developed nations.[67] EAC continues to increase in incidence (**Figs. 2** and **3**). In 2014, there are expected to be 18,170 new esophageal cancers diagnosed in the United States.[68] About 15,000 individuals will die from esophageal cancer in 2014, and more than half of these will be from EAC.[68,69]

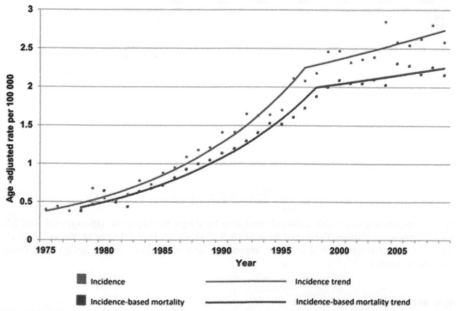

Fig. 2. Incidence and incidence-based mortality from EAC, 1975 to 2009. Produced from SEER 9 data. (*From* Hur C, Miller M, Kong CY, et al. Trends in esophageal adenocarcinoma incidence and mortality. Cancer 2013;119(6):1152; with permission.)

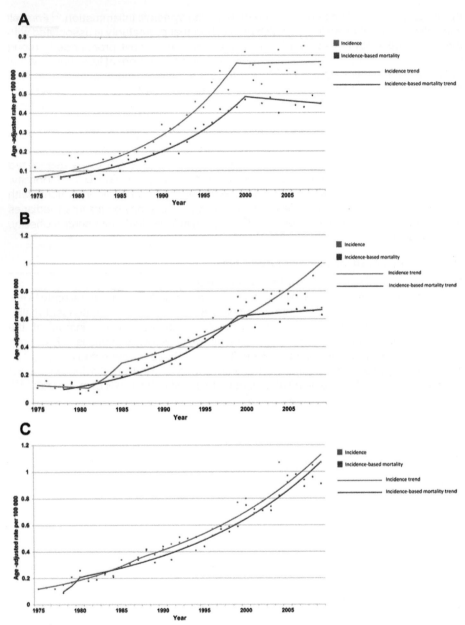

Fig. 3. Incidence and incidence-based mortality by stage, for (A) local, (B) regional, and (C) distant spread of disease. Produced from SEER 9 data. (*From* Hur C, Miller M, Kong CY, et al. Trends in esophageal adenocarcinoma incidence and mortality. Cancer 2013;119(6):1154; with permission.)

Age, sex, and ethnic variations

Esophageal cancer in general affects men in a 4:1 ratio compared with women.[68] With EAC, incidence is highest in white men, with a male/female ratio in white people that approaches 8:1 (See **Table 3**).[70–72] The reported incidence of EAC has risen

Table 3
Reported risk factors for EAC, with magnitudes of association represented as ORs

Risk Factor	Study, Year	Total (n)	Study Type	Comparison Groups	OR (95% CI)
Symptomatic GERD	Lagergren et al,[82] 1999	1271	Case control	Population controls, asymptomatic	43.5[a] (18.3, 103.5)
	Lagergren et al,[82] 1999	1271	Case control	Population controls, asymptomatic	7.7 (5.3, 11.4)
	Whiteman et al,[83] 2008	2373	Case control	Population controls, GERD-once weekly	6.4 (4.5, 9.0)
	Cook et al,[84] 2014	6414	Pooled analysis	Population controls without recurrent heartburn	4.6 (3.3, 6.6)
Male gender	Nordenstedt et al,[70] 2011	9052	Prospective cohort	Women within 13 SEER registries	8.6[b]
	Cook et al,[71] 2009	8783	Prospective cohort	Women within 13 SEER registries	7.7[b]
	Hur et al,[72] 2013	NA	Prospective cohort	Women within SEER registries	7.2[b]
White race	Cook et al,[71] 2009	8783	Prospective cohort	African Americans	4.6[c]
	Nordenstedt et al,[70] 2011	9052	Prospective cohort	African Americans	5.4[c]
	Nordenstedt et al,[70] 2011	9052	Prospective cohort	Hispanics	2.2[c]
Obesity (BMI)	Chow et al,[87] 1998	1284	Case control	Lowest quartile of BMI	3.0[d] (1.7, 5.0)
	Hoyo et al,[90] 2012	12,378	Pooled analysis	Lowest category of BMI	2.8 (1.9, 4.1)
	Steffen et al,[92] 2009	346, 354	Prospective cohort	Lowest quintile of BMI	2.8 (1.3, 5.9)
Obesity (central adiposity)	Steffen et al,[92] 2009	346, 354	Prospective cohort	Lowest quintile of waist circumference	3.4 (1.5, 7.7)
	Singh et al,[93] 2013	841	Meta-analysis	Lowest category of waist circumference	2.0 (1.5, 2.6)
Tobacco use	Cook et al,[94] 2010	10,993	Pooled analysis	Never smokers	2.0 (1.6, 2.3)
	Lagergren et al,[95] 2000	1009	Case control	Never smokers	1.6 (0.9, 2.7)
H pylori	Chow et al,[57] 1998	353	Case control	Population controls	0.4 (0.2, 0.8)
	De Martel et al,[101] 2005	200	Nested case control	Ambulatory patients	0.4 (0.2, 0.9)
NSAIDs	Corley et al,[104] 2003	442	Meta-analysis	Varied[e]	0.7 (0.5, 0.9)
	Abnet et al,[162] 2009	NA	Meta-analysis	Nonusers of NSAIDs[f]	0.65 (0.5, 0.9)

Abbreviations: BMI, body mass index; NA, not available; NSAID, nonsteroidal antiinflammatory drug; SEER, Surveillance, Epidemiology, and End Results.
[a] Severe GERD symptoms.
[b] White women; no CIs available.
[c] IRRs; no CIs available.
[d] Men only.
[e] Included studies compared with no NSAID use, no acetylsalicylic acid (ASA) use, no ASA use for 1 month, or no daily ASA use for greater than 1 month.
[f] Precise comparison groups not available.
Data from Refs.[57,70–72,82–84,87,90,92–95,101,104,162]

dramatically over the past 30 to 40 years.[3] By some estimates the incidence has increased from 300% to 500% over this time,[2] or by a 10% annual increase in men, and between 5% and 7% annually in women.[73] In the United States from 1975 to 2006, the incidence of EAC increased 7-fold, an increase greater than that of any other major malignancy.[74] Among women, rates of EAC increased from 0.17 per 100,000 in 1975 to 1979 to 0.74 per 100,000 from 2000 to 2004.[73] With EAC similar increases have been seen in the Latin American population of the United States[73] Fewer analyses have been done on African American men or women, often because of significantly lower numbers of reported cases of disease, yielding unstable estimates of risk.[75] In the last quarter of the twentieth century, men more than 65 years of age saw the greatest increase in incidence of EAC (about 600%).[76] Similar increases have been seen in European and some Asian populations as well.[75,77] More recent data suggest that, when separated by stage of disease at diagnosis, incidences of localized EAC have slowed, whereas distant and regional cases have continued a rapid increase (see **Fig. 3**).[72,76]

Multiple studies assessing Surveillance, Epidemiology, and End Results (SEER) data have suggested a ratio of EAC cases in white people to African Americans of approximately 5:1.[71] These results parallel data on the prevalence of both erosive esophagitis and BE in white people versus African Americans, in which rates are significantly higher in white people.[25,78] The increased incidence in EAC among white people is counterintuitive, in that African Americans, white people, and Asians report a similar prevalence of heartburn.[71,78] Similarly, across multiple races, women in general often have fewer complications of GERD, whereas men are more likely to have erosive disease, BE, or EAC.[70]

The greatest gender disparity in EAC cases is seen in white people, with an 8:1 ratio. In African Americans, a 3:1 ratio is seen, and, in Latin Americans, there is a 7:1 predominance of men compared with women.[71] Other work has placed male/female ratios for Latin Americans even higher than those of white people in some age groups.[70]

Recent research suggests that age-related incidence rates show similar patterns in different ethnic groups, and that older individuals are disproportionately affected. Nordenstedt and colleagues,[70] in an analysis of SEER data, showed that incidence of EAC peaks in the 70-year-old and older category in white people, African Americans, and Latin Americans. The reasons for the great gender disparity in EAC incidence are not known. A greater proportion of abdominal fat, or possibly unknown influences of estrogen or testosterone on disease activity and severity, are possible explanations.[70,79]

In the immediate future, the incidence of EAC is expected to continue its increase. Kong and colleagues[80] conducted an analysis of 3 models assessing projections of EAC incidence, progression, and mortality. According to recent predictions, the incidence of EAC is expected to increase until at least 2030 in men. At that point, the estimates place the incidence of EAC at 8.4 to 10.1 per 100,000 person-years.[81]

Selected risk factors for esophageal adenocarcinoma

Gastroesophageal reflux disease The association between GERD symptoms and EAC risk has been shown to be strong, with risk estimates in individuals with frequent GERD symptoms ranging from 3-fold to 5-fold higher or more compared with asymptomatic controls (See **Table 3**).[40,82–84] In a pivotal case-control study in Sweden in 1999, Lagergren and colleagues[82] found that, compared with individuals without GERD symptoms, those with recurrent symptoms had a risk of EAC more than 7 times higher. Among those with severe and long-standing symptoms, the risk was increased dramatically, by a factor of 43, compared with controls (OR, 43.5). This association was also seen in several other studies,[40,83] with estimates of the risk of EAC ranging from 3-fold to 5-fold higher in individuals with GERD. ORs increased with more severe or more frequent symptoms.[40,83] Pooled data from the BEACON consortium, analyzed by Cook and colleagues,[84] found similar effects. Individuals with longer duration of GERD symptoms had an approximately 5-fold increase in risk, and this increased to a 6-fold increase with symptoms longer than 20 years.[84]

What can be concluded from this information? The relationship between GERD symptoms and risk of EAC is predictable and robust. Data supporting this relationship are more robust than those supporting the relationship between GERD and BE, in which an inconsistent relationship between symptom severity and risk of disease is seen.[21] The association between GERD and EAC has been less rigorously studied in minority populations and in women, and estimates of risk may differ when these patient populations are considered.

Obesity Obesity is a risk factor for development of EAC, and some authorities have suggested that obesity is the central driver of BE and EAC rates in the developed world.[30,85] However, the initial increase in EAC incidence predated the obesity epidemic, and thus obesity does not fully explain observed EAC incidence trends.[86] The risk of EAC in patients in the highest categories of BMI has consistently been shown to be 3-fold to 7-fold higher than in those with normal body weight.[74,87,88] This relationship has been reliably shown in other population-based studies as well, and, remarkably, occurs whether or not reflux is present. Other studies have suggested a linear risk increase with increasing BMI (**Fig. 4**).[40,89] A pooled analysis of 10 case-control studies assessed the relationship between BMI and EAC. Compared with the referent group (BMI<25), increasing BMI was associated with increased risk at cut points of 30 to 34.9 (OR, 2.39), 35.0 to 39.9 (OR, 2.79), and greater than 40.0 (OR, 4.76).[90] Prospective studies have shown similar trends. In a prospective cohort study design, Abnet and colleagues[91] compared individuals with BMIs of 18.5 to 25 (normal body weight) with those with obesity (BMI >30.0) and found that the risk of EAC was increased by more than a factor of 2 (hazard ratio [HR], 2.1). The risk of EAC increased further in those with BMIs greater than 35 (HR, 2.64).

As in BE, the obesity risk in EAC may lie primarily in patients with truncal obesity. In a prospective cohort study, Steffen and colleagues[92] found a rate ratio (RR) for EAC of 2.6 compared with those in the highest quartile of waist circumference versus those in the lower quartile. This finding has been corroborated in other recent studies.[93]

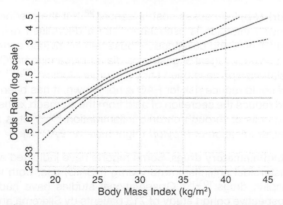

Fig. 4. Restricted cubic regression splines depicting the relationship between BMI and adenocarcinomas of the esophagus and esophageal junction. (*From* Hoyo C, Cook MB, Kamangar F, et al. Body mass index in relation to esophageal and oesophagogastric junction adenocarcinomas: a pooled analysis from the international BEACON consortium. Int J Epidemiol 2012;41:1706–18; with permission.)

Tobacco use Smokers are reported to have at least twice the risk of EAC as non-smokers.[52,94] However, evidence of a possible dose-response relationship has been inconsistent.[94,95] In 2000, Lagergren and colleagues[95] performed a case-control study of possible dose-dependent effects among nearly 200 patients with EAC and 820 controls. In their study, no dose-response trend was seen for either cigarette smokers or pipe smokers, despite such a relationship being seen with esophagogastric junction (EGJ) adenocarcinomas. More recently, in 2010, Cook and colleagues[94] pooled data on tobacco use and EAC risk in both EAC and EGJ adenocarcinoma from the BEACON consortium. An association between smoking and cancer was observed for both EAC (OR, 1.96) and EGJ adenocarcinoma (OR, 2.18). Risks for EAC by gender differed slightly but were not statistically significantly different; there was a trend toward higher risk in men (OR, 2.10 vs 1.74 in women) and a dose-response relationship was seen. Heavy smokers had the highest risk, with ORs of 2.7 (male) and 3.6 (female).[94] These data provide compelling evidence that EAC risk increases with increasing levels of exposure to tobacco. The investigators did not find any modulating effects of GERD or BMI on the effect of smoking and EAC risk.

In summary, smoking for any duration seems to increase risk, and smoking most likely leads to more risk. After quitting, risk likely decreases, but this effect is not immediate.[94] Much of these observed associations may be caused in part by the effects of smoking on both GERD and BE risk. Whether smoking increases the risk of EAC in patients with BE is less clear.

Alcohol Alcohol is strongly associated with squamous cell carcinoma of the esophagus. However, as is seen with BE, alcohol has been shown to have little correlation with development of EAC. In an analysis comparing 260 controls with 227 EAC cases, Anderson and colleagues[96] found no association between any beverage type or amount of alcohol with development of EAC. In a pooled analysis across 11 studies, Freedman and colleagues[97] found no increased risk of EAC in individuals who use alcohol, irrespective of duration or intensity of use. The summary ORs indicated slightly reduced risk in low-alcohol-use and moderate-alcohol-use groups (ORs, 0.78 and 0.77) but there was no association between alcohol and EAC in very-low or high-alcohol-use groups.[97]

Helicobacter pylori H pylori causes gastric cancer,[98] but the predominance of data suggest that H pylori infection is associated with a decreased risk of EAC.[99] In a case-control study, Chow and colleagues[57] observed an inverse correlation between H pylori infection and esophageal or gastric cardia adenocarcinoma (OR, 0.4, 0.2–0.8). Similar inverse relationships have been shown in other studies.[100,101] The mechanism by which H pylori could reduce risk for EAC is not known. It has been suggested that the bacteria could reduce the secretion of acid from the stomach, either through direct action on parietal cells or through chronic inflammation.[101,102] It is also not known what effect, if any, eradication of H pylori might have on EAC risk.

Nonsteroidal antiinflammatory drugs Some reports have indicated a decreased risk of EAC with nonsteroidal antiinflammatory drug (NSAID) use, both with aspirin and with other nonaspirin drugs.[103,104] Observational studies have had conflicting results.[105,106] A prospective cohort study of 713 patients by Sikkema and colleagues[105] found no association between NSAIDs and cancer risk, whereas Nguyen and colleagues[106] found a reduced risk of EAC (OR, 0.64) in a nested case-control study in 2010. However, systematic reviews have shown a decreased risk of EAC in patients taking NSAIDs. Corley and colleagues[104] found a decreased risk among those using

NSAIDs or aspirin (OR, 0.57; 95% CI, 0.47–0.71). A more recent meta-analysis by Abnet and colleagues in 2009 also found an inverse correlation between NSAID use and EAC (OR, 0.64; 95% CI, 0.52–0.79). In summary, EAC risk may be slightly reduced by taking NSAIDs, but the magnitude of risk reduction is small. A clearer pattern in individual studies would make this conclusion more robust.

Progression of Barrett's Esophagus to Esophageal Adenocarcinoma

Earlier estimates placed the annual rate of progression from BE to EAC at 0.5%.[2,107] However, more recent large cohort studies have reported lower rates of progression, ranging from 0.1% to 0.3%.[10,11,108] Clinical guidelines have recommended periodic endoscopic surveillance for the detection of dysplasia and early cancer in patients with BE. However, surveillance becomes less cost-effective at lower EAC risks, and therefore understanding factors associated with progression are key to guiding management.

Dysplasia in Barrett's esophagus

Dysplasia in BE is a histologic diagnosis suggesting that epithelial cells have acquired genetic or epigenetic alterations that predispose them to the development of malignancy.[1] When identified in a patient with BE, dysplasia predicts a higher risk of EAC, but several issues have limited its utility. For example, sampling error during surveillance endoscopy is an obstacle that has hindered the effectiveness of dysplasia as an accurate marker of cancer risk. Because dysplasia is not readily distinguished endoscopically from typical BE, an area of dysplastic epithelium can easily be missed.[109] Thus, even with extensive sampling, by the time histology shows dysplasia, cancer may be present.[110] Surgical series have shown that cancer was often present at referral for esophagectomy when the referral was for endoscopically diagnosed high-grade dysplasia (HGD).[11,109] Because of sampling error, guidelines recommend use of the Seattle biopsy protocol, an aggressive biopsy technique that seeks to minimize sampling error and improve reliability of cancer and dysplasia detection.[111] Studies have shown that strict adherence to the Seattle protocol improves detection of HGD and cancer.[45] After implementing the strict guidelines, a hospital system in the United Kingdom improved detection of HGD or cancer by more than 4-fold.[112] Despite the benefits of aggressive biopsy protocol, in practice adherence is suboptimal. In a 2009 study by Abrams and colleagues[113] of a national pathology database, these biopsy guidelines were followed in slightly more than half (51.2%) of more than 2200 BE surveillance cases. Furthermore, nonadherence was associated with a significant reduction in dysplasia detection (summary OR, 0.53).

Another issue is the rate of progression. Rates of EAC development in low-grade dysplasia (LGD) were once thought to be as high as 7% to 8% or more per year, or higher.[110,114–117] More recent estimates place the annual risk of progression in BE with LGD closer to 0.5% to 3%, with some newer estimates even lower.[118] However, these estimates are heterogeneous (**Table 4**). Numerous issues confound the accurate interpretation of the presence and severity of dysplasia in BE. Even among experienced pathologists, the extent of interobserver agreement when diagnosing LGD can be less than 50%.[117,119] Other work has shown difficulty in reproducing the diagnosis of BE,[120] in part because inflammation can cause cytologic atypia in the bases of crypts that mimics dysplasia. Regression of LGD, or the failure to detect dysplastic changes on subsequent endoscopies, also occurs in half or more of patients with LGD.[121,122] Because of uncertainties regarding LGD-associated cancer risk, there remains debate over the optimal management strategy in these patients. Incidence of EAC or HGD is estimated at 1.1% to 6% annually but some estimates are as high as 13.4% per year.[10,11,108,123,124] With HGD, interobserver agreement is better but is still less than

Table 4
Prospective and registry-based cohort studies reporting progression risk in LGD, because 2000

Authors, Year	Setting	Study Design	Patients With BE Followed	Male	Incidence of EAC in NDBE (% per y)	Incidence of EAC or HGD in NDBE (% per y)	Incidence of EAC in LGD (% per y)	Incidence of EAC or HGD in LGD (% per y)
Thota et al,[142] 2015	United States	Prospective cohort	299	79.0	NR	NR	0.80	3.10
Picardo et al,[133] 2014	United Kingdom	Prospective cohort	1093	67.1	0.13	0.72	1.98	6.49
Duits et al,[141] 2014	Netherlands	Retrospective cohort	293	76.0	NR	0.60	NR	9.10
Rugge et al,[132] 2012	Italy	Prospective cohort	841	77.0	NR	0.53	NR	3.17
Hvid-Jensen et al,[10] 2011	Netherlands	Prospective cohort	11,028	66.8	0.09	0.25	0.55	1.67
Bhat et al,[11] 2011	United Kingdom	Retrospective cohort	8522	57.9	0.10	0.15	0.92	1.31
Wani et al,[108] 2011	United States	Prospective cohort	1755	85.0	NR	NR	0.44	1.83
Schouten et al,[140] 2011	Netherlands	Retrospective cohort	605	54.0	0.30	NR	0.41	NR
den Hoed et al,[131] 2011	Netherlands	Prospective cohort	133	54.9	NR	0.35	NR	1.62
Jung et al,[139] 2011	United States	Retrospective cohort	355	72.0	0.25$	0.66	0.23	0.71
De Jonge et al,[123] 2010	Netherlands	Retrospective cohort	42,207	62.5	0.39	0.51	0.77	1.06

Study	Country	Design	N					
Curvers et al,[138] 2010	Netherlands	Retrospective cohort	1198	67.0	NR	0.49	0.34	13.40
Wong et al,[137] 2010	United States	Retrospective cohort	248	NR	0.51	0.61	1.51	1.51
Gatenby et al,[122] 2009	United Kingdom	Retrospective cohort	146	NR	NR	NR	2.70	4.60
Alcedo et al,[136] 2009	Spain	Retrospective cohort	386	79.0	0.52	0.95	0.00	0.00
Swizer-Taylor et al,[130] 2008	United Kingdom	Retrospective cohort	212	69.0	0.68	0.85	0.75	3.16
Lim et al,[129] 2007	United Kingdom	Retrospective cohort	357	57.7	NR	0.62	NR	3.30
Vieth et al,[135] 2006	Germany	Retrospective cohort	748	67.8	0.23	0.23	4.67	4.67
Dulai et al,[128] 2005	United States	Retrospective cohort	575	99.0	0.09	0.36	36.00	1.28
Conio et al,[127] 2003	Italy	Prospective cohort	166	81.3	0.36	0.61	2.27	3.44
Schnell et al,[134] 2001	United States	Retrospective cohort	1099	NR	NR	NR	0.19	NR
Weston et al,[115] 2001	United States	Prospective cohort	48	100.0	NR	NR	0.61	2.43
Reid et al,[109] 2000	United States	Prospective cohort	327	NR	1.05	NR	1.50	NR
Skacel et al,[114] 2000	United States	Retrospective cohort	25	84.0	NR	NR	0.15	0.52

Abbreviation: NDBE, nondysplastic BE.
Data from Refs. [10,11,108,109,114,115,122,123,127–142].

90%.[109] Given the high cumulative incidence of progression from HGD to EAC, current guidelines recommend endoscopic intervention for such patients.[125,126]

Factors that increase risk for dysplasia progression

The strongest predictor of progression to HGD or EAC is baseline LGD. Sikkema and colleagues[105] followed 713 patients with BE with or without LGD for a mean of 4 years, and found that the strongest predictor of incident EAC was the presence of LGD (with OR, 9.6). In longitudinal studies, progression rates are significantly higher in those with LGD, but estimates of increased risk vary widely (see **Table 2**). Most studies following both patients with nondysplastic BE (NDBE) and patients with LGD have found increased risk in the 4-fold to 9-fold range if LGD is present[11,127–133] but estimates have ranged from 2-fold to 27-fold increases in progression rates.[10,11,108,109,114,115,122,123,127,128,130–142]

When patients' slides are reviewed by an expert panel of pathologists, the risk of cancer progression increases because of many patients with LGD being downstaged to NDBE.[138,141] Curvers and colleagues[138] found an annual progression rate of 9.4% in those with LGD confirmed by expert review, compared with an annual risk of 0.53% in those who were downstaged to NDBE after review. This finding was corroborated by Duits and colleagues[141] in 2014. These investigators found that approximately 75% of patients deemed to have LGD by community pathologists were subsequently downgraded to nondysplastic reads by expert pathologists. Among the quarter of patients who had their LGD readings confirmed, progression rates were extremely high: 9.1% of these patients progressed to either HGD or EAC on an annual basis.

Duration of BE is also a risk factor for disease progression. Sikkema and colleagues[105] found that the cumulative incidence of HGD or EAC was 9.6% over 4 years in patients with BE duration greater than 10 years. In those with BE duration less than 10 years, the cumulative incidence was 3.1%. Incidence was 13.3% in those with esophagitis compared with 3.0% in those without.

Among patients with HGD, the risk of cancer is substantially higher. Reid and colleagues[109] reported a cancer risk of 59% over 5 years (or 11.8% annually) in patients with HGD at index endoscopy, compared with 1.5% annual cancer risk in patients with LGD. A meta-analysis published in 2008 yielded a crude incidence rate of 5.6% across 4 studies, with point estimates of annual incidence rates ranging from 2.3% per year to 10.3% per year.[143] Endoscopic therapy is highly effective for the eradication of BE and associated dysplasia, and is now considered the preferred management strategy for patients with HGD.[125]

In summary, LGD represents a marker of increased risk of progression to cancer in patients with BE. However, the magnitude of risk increase is unclear, because reported progression rates to EAC in LGD have been widely variable. This variability is caused in part by the poor reproducibility of this diagnosis. Patients with HGD are at very high risk of progression to cancer, prompting recommendations for therapeutic intervention when it is found. More robust data on progression risk may help better tailor surveillance strategies to each patient in the future.

Barrett's esophagus segment length

Other risk factors have been identified that increase the risk of developing EAC in the setting of BE. Several studies have found that the risk of EAC is greater in longer segments of BE compared with shorter segments.[113,144,145] A study by Weston and colleagues[145] found that the risk increased by a factor of 6 in longer segments. Sikkema and colleagues,[105] in a prospective study design, found that for every additional centimeter of BE the cumulative risk of HGD or EAC increased by 11% over 4 years. The relationship between segment length and increased risk of EAC is not always linear,[146] but the preponderance of evidence suggests that greater surface area of columnar-lined mucosa correlates with increased cancer risk.

Extent of dysplasia

Studies have attempted to determine whether greater extent of dysplasia within a Barrett's segment confers increased risk of neoplastic progression. Studies have had conflicting results as to whether or not more extensive LGD or HGD increases the risk of subsequent EAC.[108,140,147–149] A study by Srivastava and colleagues[147] suggested that, when looking at crypts showing dysplasia (as a criteria for LGD diagnosis), increased fractions of dysplastic crypts correlated with increased EAC risk. Buttar and colleagues[148] also found a 4-fold higher risk of cancer progression in patients with extensive HGD compared with those with unifocal HGD. However, this result could not be duplicated in a follow-up study.[149] Intuitively, it seems that the presence of greater numbers of dysplastic crypts would confer an increased risk of future cancer. However, in part because of sampling error limitations of endoscopic surveillance, the utility of focal versus multifocal dysplasia as a risk stratification tool is unclear.

Molecular/biological markers for progression from Barrett's esophagus to dysplasia/cancer

Numerous studies have attempted to assess the utility of molecular biomarkers to predict progression and assist with risk stratification. If low-risk patients can be accurately identified, then little or no follow-up may be warranted. Alternatively, chemopreventive or endoscopic interventions could be targeted to high-risk patients. However, to date none of the candidate biomarkers has been prospectively validated.

P53 may have the most promise of any of the biomarkers for predicting neoplastic progression in patients with Barrett's. Kastelein and colleagues[150] studied the effect of aberrant p53 expression in a nested case-control study and found striking results. P53 overexpression assessed by immunohistochemistry was associated with significantly increased risk of progression to either HGD or EAC (RR, 5.6; 95% CI, 3.1, 10.3). Among patients with loss of p53 expression, the risk of progression was even higher (RR, 14.0; 95% CI, 5.3, 37.2). LGD alone was far less predictive of progression (RR, 2.4; 95% CI, 0.9, 6.0), and the positive predictive value of progression was 15% with LGD alone compared with 33% in patients with both LGD and aberrant p53 expression.[150] P53 has been found to increase the risk of progression in other studies as well. In a prospective cohort study, Reid and colleagues[151] found that loss of heterozygosity of the chromosome harboring p53 was associated with a 7-fold increase in progression risk.[152]

In a prospective study design, Reid and colleagues[109] analyzed abnormalities in genetic content by flow cytometry and found that, among patients with HGD, incidence of esophageal cancer varied from 58% over 3 years in patients with baseline cytologic abnormalities, to 7.7% in those without baseline cytometric changes. In such lower risk patients, a less invasive management strategy might be warranted. Bird-Lieberman and colleagues[153] performed a retrospective, nested case-control study from a large cohort of patients in Northern Ireland. In that study, LGD, abnormal DNA ploidy, and Aspergillus oryzae lectin (AOL) were all risk factors for progression. Expert LGD contributed significantly, but AOL (OR, 3.7) and ploidy (OR, 2.8) were also independent predictors of advancement to EAC.[153]

Another retrospective study found that, among 322 patients with BE, aneuploidy and/or tetraploidy, when assessed by flow cytometry, was associated with an RR of 11.7 for neoplastic progression to cancer.[154]

Fluorescence in situ hybridization (FISH) is a method by which a tissue sample can be tested for a panel of genetic abnormalities.[155] A prospective study by Davelaar and colleagues[156] tested a protocol comparing p53 staining by immunohistochemistry and FISH on brush cytology specimens. They found that p53 abnormalities detected by immunohistochemistry (OR, 17; 95% CI, 3.2, 96) and FISH (OR, 7.3; 95% CI, 1.3, 41) were both independent predictors of progression. In addition, when both p53 and FISH were used, detection of LGD, HGD, and EAC was 100% accurate, both p53 and FISH improved the risk stratification capability of p53 alone, and because flow cytometry requires frozen sections of tissue (something rarely done in clinical practice)[45] the potential for clinical use of FISH may be greater.

Despite the significant advances in biomarker development, significant barriers remain. Of all the biomarkers currently identified, the greatest potential for clinical application may lie with assays using p53. P53 can easily be tested, and in multiple studies has been documented to improve the reproducibility of the diagnosis of dysplasia and to predict neoplastic progression.[155] Because of the imperfect nature of dysplasia alone as a predictor of neoplastic progressions, work on molecular biomarkers continues at a rapid pace. However, to date, no biomarkers are approved for diagnosis or risk stratification, and the most recent guidelines from the American Gastroenterological Association recommend against use of molecular biomarkers for risk stratification.[45] Recent British Society of Gastroenterology guidelines propose that p53 immunostaining should be considered, in addition to routine clinical diagnosis, for BE diagnosis.[126] However, pathology societies have yet to develop guidelines for the interpretation and reporting of p53 staining by immunohistochemistry in BE.

SUMMARY

There has been a remarkable increase in the incidence of EAC. In addition, the spectrum of BE and EAC presents multiple challenges to the medical system. Rapidly increasing incidence, high mortality from EAC, and difficulties with risk stratification are all issues to be overcome for effective intervention in this disease state. Some risk factors for BE and EAC are modifiable, such as tobacco use and obesity. In addition to these clinical factors, continued rigorous study of appropriate methods for risk stratification continues. Molecular and genetic biomarkers have considerable promise in risk prediction models, and may in the future be used as part of a prognostic panel, designed to help clinicians focus attention on the patients most at risk.

REFERENCES

1. Spechler SJ. Barrett's esophagus and esophageal adenocarcinoma: pathogenesis, diagnosis, and therapy. Med Clin North Am 2002;86(6):1423–45, vii.
2. Shaheen N, Ransohoff DF. Gastroesophageal reflux, Barrett esophagus, and esophageal cancer: scientific review. JAMA 2002;287(15):1972–81.
3. Blot WJ. Esophageal cancer trends and risk factors. Semin Oncol 1994;21(4): 403–10.
4. Daly JM, Karnell LH, Menck HR. National Cancer Data Base report on esophageal carcinoma. Cancer 1996;78(8):1820–8.
5. Hesketh PJ, Clapp RW, Doos WG, et al. The increasing frequency of adenocarcinoma of the esophagus. Cancer 1989;64(2):526–30.
6. Cameron AJ, Ott BJ, Payne WS. The incidence of adenocarcinoma in columnar-lined (Barrett's) esophagus. N Engl J Med 1985;313(14):857–9.
7. Shaheen NJ, Richter JE. Barrett's oesophagus. Lancet 2009;373(9666):850–61.

8. Lund O, Kimose HH, Aagaard MT, et al. Risk stratification and long-term results after surgical treatment of carcinomas of the thoracic esophagus and cardia. A 25-year retrospective study. J Thorac Cardiovasc Surg 1990;99(2):200–9.
9. Siegel R, Naishadham D, Jemal A. Cancer statistics, 2013. CA Cancer J Clin 2013;63(1):11–30.
10. Hvid-Jensen F, Pedersen L, Drewes AM, et al. Incidence of adenocarcinoma among patients with Barrett's esophagus. N Engl J Med 2011;365(15):1375–83.
11. Bhat S, Coleman HG, Yousef F, et al. Risk of malignant progression in Barrett's esophagus patients: results from a large population-based study. J Natl Cancer Inst 2011;103(13):1049–57.
12. Cameron AJ, Zinsmeister AR, Ballard DJ, et al. Prevalence of columnar-lined (Barrett's) esophagus. Gastroenterology 1990;99(4):918–22.
13. Ronkainen J, Aro P, Storskrubb T, et al. Prevalence of Barrett's esophagus in the general population: an endoscopic study. Gastroenterology 2005;129(6):1825–31.
14. Rex DK, Cummings OW, Shaw M, et al. Screening for Barrett's esophagus in colonoscopy patients with and without heartburn. Gastroenterology 2003;125(6):1670–7.
15. Zagari RM, Fuccio L, Wallander MA, et al. Gastro-oesophageal reflux symptoms, oesophagitis and Barrett's oesophagus in the general population: the Loiano–Monghidoro study. Gut 2008;57(10):1354–9.
16. Westhoff B, Brotze S, Weston A, et al. The frequency of Barrett's esophagus in high-risk patients with chronic GERD. Gastrointest Endosc 2005;61(2):226–31.
17. Conio M, Cameron AJ, Romero Y, et al. Secular trends in the epidemiology and outcome of Barrett's oesophagus in Olmsted County, Minnesota. Gut 2001;48(3):304–9.
18. Coleman HG, Bhat S, Murray LJ, et al. Increasing incidence of Barrett's oesophagus: a population-based study. Eur J Epidemiol 2011;26(9):739–45.
19. van Soest EM, Dieleman JP, Siersema PD, et al. Increasing incidence of Barrett's oesophagus in the general population. Gut 2005;54(8):1062–6.
20. Cameron AJ, Lomboy CT. Barrett's esophagus: age, prevalence, and extent of columnar epithelium. Gastroenterology 1992;103:1241–5.
21. Wong A, Fitzgerald RC. Epidemiologic risk factors for Barrett's esophagus and associated adenocarcinoma. Clin Gastroenterol Hepatol 2005;3(1):1–10.
22. van Blankenstein M, Looman CW, Johnston BJ, et al. Age and sex distribution of the prevalence of Barrett's esophagus found in a primary referral endoscopy center. Am J Gastroenterol 2005;100(3):568–76.
23. Kramer JR, Fischbach LA, Richardson P, et al. Waist-to-hip ratio, but not body mass index, is associated with an increased risk of Barrett's esophagus in white men. Clin Gastroenterol Hepatol 2013;11(4):373–81.e1.
24. Ford AC, Forman D, Reynolds PD, et al. Ethnicity, gender, and socioeconomic status as risk factors for esophagitis and Barrett's esophagus. Am J Epidemiol 2005;162(5):454–60.
25. Abrams JA, Fields S, Lightdale CJ, et al. Racial and ethnic disparities in the prevalence of Barrett's esophagus among patients who undergo upper endoscopy. Clin Gastroenterol Hepatol 2008;6(1):30–4.
26. Cameron AJ, Lagergren J, Henriksson C, et al. Gastroesophageal reflux disease in monozygotic and dizygotic twins. Gastroenterology 2002;122(1):55–9.
27. Conio M, Filiberti R, Blanchi S, et al. Risk factors for Barrett's esophagus: a case-control study. Int J Cancer 2002;97(2):225–9.

28. Johansson J, Håkansson HO, Mellblom L, et al. Risk factors for Barrett's oesophagus: a population-based approach. Scand J Gastroenterol 2007; 42(2):148–56.
29. Anderson LA, Watson RG, Murphy SJ, et al. Risk factors for Barrett's oesophagus and oesophageal adenocarcinoma: results from the FINBAR study. World J Gastroenterol 2007;13(10):1585.
30. de Jonge PJ, van Blankenstein M, Grady WM, et al. Barrett's oesophagus: epidemiology, cancer risk and implications for management. Gut 2013;63(1): 191–202.
31. Bansal A, Wani S, Rastogi A, et al. Impact of measurement of esophageal acid exposure close to the gastroesophageal junction on diagnostic accuracy and event-symptom correlation: a prospective study using wireless dual pH monitoring. Am J Gastroenterol 2009;104(12):2918–25.
32. Lacy BE, Chehade R, Crowell MD. A prospective study to compare a symptom-based reflux disease questionnaire to 48-h wireless pH monitoring for the identification of gastroesophageal reflux (revised 2-26-11). Am J Gastroenterol 2011; 106(9):1604–11.
33. Avidan B, Sonnenberg A, Schnell TG, et al. Hiatal hernia size, Barrett's length, and severity of acid reflux are all risk factors for esophageal adenocarcinoma. Am J Gastroenterol 2002;97(8):1930–6.
34. Cameron AJ. Barrett's esophagus: prevalence and size of hiatal hernia. Am J Gastroenterol 1999;94(8):2054–9.
35. Eloubeidi MA, Provenzale D. Clinical and demographic predictors of Barrett's esophagus among patients with gastroesophageal reflux disease: a multivariable analysis in veterans. J Clin Gastroenterol 2001;33(4):306–9.
36. Taylor JB, Rubenstein JH. Meta-analyses of the effect of symptoms of gastroesophageal reflux on the risk of Barrett's esophagus. Am J Gastroenterol 2010;105(8):1730–7.
37. Brandt MG, Darling GE, Miller L. Symptoms, acid exposure and motility in patients with Barrett's esophagus. Can J Surg 2004;47(1):47.
38. Singh P, Taylor RH, Colin-Jones DG. Esophageal motor dysfunction and acid exposure in reflux esophagitis are more severe if Barrett's metaplasia is present. Am J Gastroenterol 1994;89(3):349–56.
39. El-Serag HB, Aguirre TV, Davis S, et al. Proton pump inhibitors are associated with reduced incidence of dysplasia in Barrett's esophagus. Am J Gastroenterol 2004;99(10):1877–83.
40. Wu AH, Tseng CC, Bernstein L. Hiatal hernia, reflux symptoms, body size, and risk of esophageal and gastric adenocarcinoma. Cancer 2003;98(5): 940–8.
41. Lagergren J. Influence of obesity on the risk of esophageal disorders. Nat Rev Gastroenterol Hepatol 2011;8(6):340–7.
42. Ogden CL, Carroll MD, Kit BK, et al. Prevalence of childhood and adult obesity in the United States, 2011-2012. JAMA 2014;311(8):806–14.
43. Kamat P, Wen S, Morris J, et al. Exploring the association between elevated body mass index and Barrett's esophagus: a systematic review and meta-analysis. Ann Thorac Surg 2009;87(2):655–62.
44. Edelstein ZR, Farrow DC, Bronner MP, et al. Central adiposity and risk of Barrett's esophagus. Gastroenterology 2007;133(2):403–11.
45. Spechler SJ, Sharma P, Souza RF, et al. American Gastroenterological Association technical review on the management of Barrett's esophagus. Gastroenterology 2011;140(3):e18.

46. Kubo A, Cook MB, Shaheen NJ, et al. Sex-specific associations between body mass index, waist circumference and the risk of Barrett's oesophagus: a pooled analysis from the international BEACON consortium. Gut 2013; 62(12):1684–91.
47. Berger NA, Dannenberg AJ, editors. Obesity, inflammation and cancer. New York (NY): Springer; 2013.
48. Kubo A, Levin TR, Block G, et al. Alcohol types and sociodemographic characteristics as risk factors for Barrett's esophagus. Gastroenterology 2009;136(3): 806–15.
49. Steevens J, Schouten LJ, Driessen AL, et al. A prospective cohort study on overweight, smoking, alcohol consumption, and risk of Barrett's esophagus. Cancer Epidemiol Biomarkers Prev 2011;20(2):345–58.
50. Thrift AP, Cook MB, Vaughan TL, et al. Alcohol and the risk of Barrett's esophagus: a pooled analysis from the International BEACON Consortium. Am J Gastroenterol 2014;109(10):1586–94.
51. Thrift AP, Kramer JR, Richardson PA, et al. No significant effects of smoking or alcohol consumption on risk of Barrett's esophagus. Dig Dis Sci 2014;59(1): 108–16.
52. Lepage C, Drouillard A, Jouve JL, et al. Epidemiology and risk factors for oesophageal adenocarcinoma. Dig Liver Dis 2013;45(8):625–9.
53. Cook MB, Shaheen NJ, Anderson LA, et al. Cigarette smoking increases risk of Barrett's esophagus: an analysis of the Barrett's and Esophageal Adenocarcinoma Consortium. Gastroenterology 2012;142(4):744–53.
54. Stemmermann GN. Intestinal metaplasia of the stomach. A status report. Cancer 1994;74(2):556–64.
55. El-Serag HB, Sonnenberg A. Opposing time trends of peptic ulcer and reflux disease. Gut 1998;43(3):327–33.
56. Corley DA, Kubo A, Levin TR, et al. Helicobacter pylori infection and the risk of Barrett's oesophagus: a community-based study. Gut 2008;57(6):727–33.
57. Chow WH, Blaser MJ, Blot WJ, et al. An inverse relation between cagA+ strains of Helicobacter pylori infection and risk of esophageal and gastric cardia adenocarcinoma. Cancer Res 1998;58(4):588–90.
58. Vaezi MF, Falk GW, Peek RM, et al. CagA-positive strains of Helicobacter pylori may protect against Barrett's esophagus. Am J Gastroenterol 2000;95(9):2206–11.
59. Wang C, Yuan Y, Hunt RH. Helicobacter pylori infection and Barrett's esophagus: a systematic review and meta-analysis. Am J Gastroenterol 2009; 104(2):492–500.
60. Goldenberg RL, Culhane JF, Iams JD, et al. Epidemiology and causes of preterm birth. Lancet 2008;371(9606):75–84.
61. Forssell L, Cnattingius S, Bottai M, et al. Risk of esophagitis among individuals born preterm or small for gestational age. Clin Gastroenterol Hepatol 2012; 10(12):1369–75.
62. Forssell L, Cnattingius S, Bottai M, et al. Increased risk of Barrett's esophagus among individuals born preterm or small for gestational age. Clin Gastroenterol Hepatol 2013;11(7):790–4.
63. Forssell L, Cnattingius S, Bottai M, et al. Risk of oesophageal adenocarcinoma among individuals born preterm or small for gestational age. Eur J Cancer 2013; 49(9):2207–13.
64. Leggett CL, Gorospe EC, Calvin AD, et al. Obstructive sleep apnea is a risk factor for Barrett's esophagus. Clin Gastroenterol Hepatol 2014;12(4): 583–8.e1.

65. Garcia JM, Splenser AE, Kramer J, et al. Circulating inflammatory cytokines and adipokines are associated with increased risk of Barrett's esophagus: a case-control study. Clin Gastroenterol Hepatol 2014;12(2):229–38.e3.

66. Bosch A, Frias Z, Caldwell WL. Adenocarcinoma of the esophagus. Cancer 1979;43(4):1557–61.

67. Devesa SS, Blot WJ, Fraumeni JF. Changing patterns in the incidence of esophageal and gastric carcinoma in the United States. Cancer 1998;83(10):2049–53.

68. American Cancer Society. Cancer facts and figures. Atlanta (GA): American Cancer Society; 2014.

69. Eloubeidi MA, Mason AC, Desmond RA, et al. Temporal trends (1973–1997) in survival of patients with esophageal adenocarcinoma in the United States: a glimmer of hope? Am J Gastroenterol 2003;98(7):1627–33.

70. Nordenstedt H, El-Serag H. The influence of age, sex, and race on the incidence of esophageal cancer in the United States (1992-2006). Scand J Gastroenterol 2011;46(5):597–602.

71. Cook M, Chow W, Devesa S. Oesophageal cancer incidence in the United States by race, sex, and histologic type, 1977–2005. Br J Cancer 2009; 101(5):855–9.

72. Hur C, Miller M, Kong CY, et al. Trends in esophageal adenocarcinoma incidence and mortality. Cancer 2013;119(6):1149–58.

73. Younes M, Henson DE, Ertan A, et al. Incidence and survival trends of esophageal carcinoma in the United States: racial and gender differences by histological type. Scand J Gastroenterol 2002;37(12):1359–65.

74. Pera M, Manterola C, Vidal O, et al. Epidemiology of esophageal adenocarcinoma. J Surg Oncol 2005;92(3):151–9.

75. Reid BJ, Li X, Galipeau PC, et al. Barrett's oesophagus and oesophageal adenocarcinoma: time for a new synthesis. Nat Rev Cancer 2010;10(2):87–101.

76. Brown LM, Devesa SS, Chow WH. Incidence of adenocarcinoma of the esophagus among white Americans by sex, stage, and age. J Natl Cancer Inst 2008; 100(16):1184–7.

77. Vizcaino AP, Moreno V, Lambert R, et al. Time trends incidence of both major histologic types of esophageal carcinomas in selected countries, 1973–1995. Int J Cancer 2002;99(6):860–8.

78. El-Serag HB, Petersen NJ, Carter J, et al. Gastroesophageal reflux among different racial groups in the United States. Gastroenterology 2004;126(7): 1692–9.

79. Lagergren J, Nyrén O. Do sex hormones play a role in the etiology of esophageal adenocarcinoma? A new hypothesis tested in a population-based cohort of prostate cancer patients. Cancer Epidemiol Biomarkers Prev 1998;7(10):913–5.

80. Kong CY, Kroep S, Curtius K, et al. Exploring the recent trend in esophageal adenocarcinoma incidence and mortality using comparative simulation modeling. Cancer Epidemiol Biomarkers Prev 2013;23:997–1006.

81. Thrift AP, Whiteman D. The incidence of esophageal adenocarcinoma continues to rise: analysis of period and birth cohort effects on recent trends. Ann Oncol 2012;23(12):3155–62.

82. Lagergren J, Bergström R, Lindgren A, et al. Symptomatic gastroesophageal reflux as a risk factor for esophageal adenocarcinoma. N Engl J Med 1999; 340(11):825–31.

83. Whiteman DC, Sadeghi S, Pandeya N, et al. Combined effects of obesity, acid reflux and smoking on the risk of adenocarcinomas of the oesophagus. Gut 2008;57(2):173–80.

84. Cook MB, Corley DA, Murray LJ, et al. Gastroesophageal reflux in relation to adenocarcinomas of the esophagus: a pooled analysis from the Barrett's and Esophageal Adenocarcinoma Consortium (BEACON). PLoS one 2014;9(7): e103508.

85. Ryan AM, Duong M, Healy L, et al. Obesity, metabolic syndrome and esophageal adenocarcinoma: epidemiology, etiology and new targets. Cancer Epidemiol 2011;35(4):309–19.

86. Abrams JA, Sharaiha RZ, Gonsalves L, et al. Dating the rise of esophageal adenocarcinoma: analysis of Connecticut Tumor Registry data, 1940–2007. Cancer Epidemiol Biomarkers Prev 2011;20(1):183–6.

87. Chow WH, Blot WJ, Vaughan TL, et al. Body mass index and risk of adenocarcinomas of the esophagus and gastric cardia. J Natl Cancer Inst 1998;90(2):150–5.

88. Lagergren J. Adenocarcinoma of oesophagus: what exactly is the size of the problem and who is at risk? Gut 2005;54(suppl 1):i1–5.

89. Lagergren J, Bergström R, Nyrén O. Association between body mass and adenocarcinoma of the esophagus and gastric cardia. Ann Intern Med 1999; 130(11):883–90.

90. Hoyo C, Cook MB, Kamangar F, et al. Body mass index in relation to oesophageal and oesophagogastric junction adenocarcinomas: a pooled analysis from the International BEACON Consortium. Int J Epidemiol 2012;41(6):1706–18.

91. Abnet CC, Freedman ND, Hollenbeck AR, et al. A prospective study of BMI and risk of oesophageal and gastric adenocarcinoma. Eur J Cancer 2008;44(3): 465–71.

92. Steffen A, Schulze MB, Pischon T, et al. Anthropometry and esophageal cancer risk in the European prospective investigation into cancer and nutrition. Cancer Epidemiol Biomarkers Prev 2009;18(7):2079–89.

93. Singh S, Sharma AN, Murad MH, et al. Central adiposity is associated with increased risk of esophageal inflammation, metaplasia, and adenocarcinoma: a systematic review and meta-analysis. Clin Gastroenterol Hepatol 2013; 11(11):1399–412.e7.

94. Cook MB, Kamangar F, Whiteman DC, et al. Cigarette smoking and adenocarcinomas of the esophagus and esophagogastric junction: a pooled analysis from the international BEACON consortium. J Natl Cancer Inst 2010;102(17):1344–53.

95. Lagergren J, Bergström R, Lindgren A, et al. The role of tobacco, snuff and alcohol use in the aetiology of cancer of the oesophagus and gastric cardia. Int J Cancer 2000;85(3):340–6.

96. Anderson LA, Cantwell MM, Watson RG, et al. The association between alcohol and reflux esophagitis, Barrett's esophagus, and esophageal adenocarcinoma. Gastroenterology 2009;136(3):799–805.

97. Freedman ND, Murray LJ, Kamangar F, et al. Alcohol intake and risk of oesophageal adenocarcinoma: a pooled analysis from the BEACON Consortium. Gut 2011;60(8):1029–37.

98. Parsonnet J, Friedman GD, Vandersteen DP, et al. *Helicobacter pylori* infection and the risk of gastric carcinoma. N Engl J Med 1991;325(16):1127–31.

99. Islami F, Kamangar F. *Helicobacter pylori* and esophageal cancer risk: a meta-analysis. Cancer Prev Res 2008;1(5):329–38.

100. Wu AH, Crabtree JE, Bernstein L, et al. Role of *Helicobacter pylori* CagA+ strains and risk of adenocarcinoma of the stomach and esophagus. Int J Cancer 2003;103(6):815–21.

101. de Martel C, Llosa AE, Farr SM, et al. *Helicobacter pylori* infection and the risk of development of esophageal adenocarcinoma. J Infect Dis 2005;191(5):761–7.

102. Engel LS, Chow WH, Vaughan TL, et al. Population attributable risks of esophageal and gastric cancers. J Natl Cancer Inst 2003;95(18):1404–13.
103. Farrow DC, Vaughan TL, Hansten PD, et al. Use of aspirin and other nonsteroidal anti-inflammatory drugs and risk of esophageal and gastric cancer. Cancer Epidemiol Biomarkers Prev 1998;7(2):97–102.
104. Corley DA, Kerlikowske K, Verma R, et al. Protective association of aspirin/NSAIDs and esophageal cancer: a systematic review and meta-analysis. Gastroenterology 2003;124(1):47–56.
105. Sikkema M, Looman CW, Steyerberg EW, et al. Predictors for neoplastic progression in patients with Barrett's esophagus: a prospective cohort study. Am J Gastroenterol 2011;106(7):1231–8.
106. Nguyen DM, Richardson P, El-Serag HB. Medications (NSAIDs, statins, proton pump inhibitors) and the risk of esophageal adenocarcinoma in patients with Barrett's esophagus. Gastroenterology 2010;138(7):2260–6.
107. Shaheen NJ, Crosby MA, Bozymski EM, et al. Is there publication bias in the reporting of cancer risk in Barrett's esophagus? Gastroenterology 2000;119(2):333–8.
108. Wani S, Falk GW, Post J, et al. Risk factors for progression of low-grade dysplasia in patients with Barrett's esophagus. Gastroenterology 2011;141(4):1179–86.e1.
109. Reid BJ, Levine DS, Longton G, et al. Predictors of progression to cancer in Barrett's esophagus: baseline histology and flow cytometry identify low-and high-risk patient subsets. Am J Gastroenterol 2000;95(7):1669–76.
110. Levine DS, Haggitt RC, Blount PL, et al. An endoscopic biopsy protocol can differentiate high-grade dysplasia from early adenocarcinoma in Barrett's esophagus. Gastroenterology 1993;105:40–50.
111. Wang KK, Sampliner RE, Practice Parameters Committee of the American College of Gastroenterology. Updated guidelines 2008 for the diagnosis, surveillance and therapy of Barrett's esophagus. Am J Gastroenterol 2008;103(3):788–97.
112. Fitzgerald RC, Saeed IT, Khoo D, et al. Rigorous surveillance protocol increases detection of curable cancers associated with Barrett's esophagus. Dig Dis Sci 2001;46(9):1892–8.
113. Abrams JA, Kapel RC, Lindberg GM, et al. Adherence to biopsy guidelines for Barrett's esophagus surveillance in the community setting in the United States. Clin Gastroenterol Hepatol 2009;7(7):736.
114. Skacel M, Petras RE, Gramlich TL, et al. The diagnosis of low-grade dysplasia in Barrett's esophagus and its implications for disease progression. Am J Gastroenterol 2000;95(12):3383–7.
115. Weston AP, Banerjee SK, Sharma P, et al. p53 protein overexpression in low grade dysplasia (LGD) in Barrett's esophagus: immunohistochemical marker predictive of progression. Am J Gastroenterol 2001;96(5):1355–62.
116. Hameeteman W, Tytgat GN, Houthoff HJ, et al. Barrett's esophagus: development of dysplasia and adenocarcinoma. Gastroenterology 1989;96(5 Pt 1):1249–56.
117. Montgomery E, Goldblum JR, Greenson JK, et al. Dysplasia as a predictive marker for invasive carcinoma in Barrett esophagus: a follow-up study based on 138 cases from a diagnostic variability study. Hum Pathol 2001;32(4):379–88.
118. Singh S, Manickam P, Amin AV, et al. Incidence of esophageal adenocarcinoma in Barrett's esophagus with low-grade dysplasia: a systematic review and meta-analysis. Gastrointest Endosc 2014;79(6):897–909.e4.
119. Reid B, Haggitt RC, Rubin CE, et al. Observer variation in the diagnosis of dysplasia in Barrett's esophagus. Hum Pathol 1988;19(2):166–78.

120. Meining A, Ott R, Becker I, et al. The Munich Barrett follow up study: suspicion of Barrett's oesophagus based on either endoscopy or histology only—what is the clinical significance? Gut 2004;53(10):1402–7.
121. Sharma P, Falk GW, Weston A, et al. Dysplasia and cancer in a large multicenter cohort of patients with Barrett's esophagus. Clin Gastroenterol Hepatol 2006; 4(5):566–72.
122. Gatenby P, Ramus J, Caygill C, et al. Routinely diagnosed low-grade dysplasia in Barrett's oesophagus: a population-based study of natural history. Histopathology 2009;54(7):814–9.
123. de Jonge PJ, van Blankenstein M, Looman CW, et al. Risk of malignant progression in patients with Barrett's oesophagus: a Dutch nationwide cohort study. Gut 2010;59(8):1030–6.
124. Gaddam S, Singh M, Balasubramanian G, et al. Persistence of nondysplastic Barrett's esophagus identifies patients at lower risk for esophageal adenocarcinoma: results from a large multicenter cohort. Gastroenterology 2013;145(3): 548–53.e1.
125. Spechler SJ, Sharma P, Souza RF, et al. American Gastroenterological Association medical position statement on the management of Barrett's esophagus. Gastroenterology 2011;140(3):1084–91.
126. Fitzgerald RC, di Pietro M, Ragunath K, et al. British Society of Gastroenterology guidelines on the diagnosis and management of Barrett's oesophagus. Gut 2014;63(1):7–42.
127. Conio M, Blanchi S, Lapertosa G, et al. Long-term endoscopic surveillance of patients with Barrett's esophagus. Incidence of dysplasia and adenocarcinoma: a prospective study. Am J Gastroenterol 2003;98(9):1931–9.
128. Dulai GS, Shekelle PG, Jensen DM, et al. Dysplasia and risk of further neoplastic progression in a regional Veterans Administration Barrett's cohort. Am J Gastroenterol 2005;100(4):775–83.
129. Lim C, Treanor D, Dixon MF, et al. Low-grade dysplasia in Barrett's esophagus has a high risk of progression. Endoscopy 2007;39(07):581–7.
130. Switzer-Taylor V, Schlup M, Lübcke R, et al. Barrett's esophagus: a retrospective analysis of 13 years surveillance. J Gastroenterol Hepatol 2008;23(9):1362–7.
131. den Hoed C, van Blankenstein M, Dees J, et al. The minimal incubation period from the onset of Barrett's oesophagus to symptomatic adenocarcinoma. Br J Cancer 2011;105(2):200–5.
132. Rugge M, Zaninotto G, Parente P, et al. Barrett's esophagus and adenocarcinoma risk: the experience of the North-Eastern Italian Registry (EBRA). Ann Surg 2012;256(5):788–95.
133. Picardo S, O'Brien MP, Feighery R, et al. A Barrett's esophagus registry of over 1000 patients from a specialist center highlights greater risk of progression than population-based registries and high risk of low grade dysplasia. Dis Esophagus 2014;28(2):121–6.
134. Schnell TG, Sontag SJ, Chejfec G, et al. Long-term nonsurgical management of Barrett's esophagus with high-grade dysplasia. Gastroenterology 2001;120(7): 1607–19.
135. Vieth M, Schubert B, Lang-Schwarz K, et al. Frequency of Barrett's neoplasia after initial negative endoscopy with biopsy: a long-term histopathological follow-up study. Endoscopy 2006;38(12):1201–5.
136. Alcedo J, Ferrández A, Arenas J, et al. Trends in Barrett's esophagus diagnosis in Southern Europe: implications for surveillance. Dis Esophagus 2009;22(3): 239–48.

137. Wong T, Tian J, Nagar AB. Barrett's surveillance identifies patients with early esophageal adenocarcinoma. Am J Med 2010;123(5):462–7.
138. Curvers WL, ten Kate FJ, Krishnadath KK, et al. Low-grade dysplasia in Barrett's esophagus: overdiagnosed and underestimated. Am J Gastroenterol 2010; 105(7):1523–30.
139. Jung KW, Talley NJ, Romero Y, et al. Epidemiology and natural history of intestinal metaplasia of the gastroesophageal junction and Barrett's esophagus: a population-based study. Am J Gastroenterol 2011;106(8):1447–55.
140. Schouten LJ, Steevens J, Huysentruyt CJ, et al. Total cancer incidence and overall mortality are not increased among patients with Barrett's esophagus. Clin Gastroenterol Hepatol 2011;9(9):754–61.
141. Duits LC, Phoa KN, Curvers WL, et al. Barrett's oesophagus patients with low-grade dysplasia can be accurately risk-stratified after histological review by an expert pathology panel. Gut 2014. [Epub ahead of print].
142. Thota PN, Lee HJ, Goldblum JR, et al. Risk stratification of patients with Barrett's esophagus and low-grade dysplasia or indefinite for dysplasia. Clin Gastroenterol Hepatol 2015;13(3):459–65.e1.
143. Rastogi A, Puli S, El-Serag HB, et al. Incidence of esophageal adenocarcinoma in patients with Barrett's esophagus and high-grade dysplasia: a meta-analysis. Gastrointest Endosc 2008;67(3):394–8.
144. Wani S, Falk G, Hall M, et al. Patients with nondysplastic Barrett's esophagus have low risks for developing dysplasia or esophageal adenocarcinoma. Clin Gastroenterol Hepatol 2011;9(3):220–7.e1.
145. Weston AP, Badr AS, Hassanein RS. Prospective multivariate analysis of clinical, endoscopic, and histological factors predictive of the development of Barrett's multifocal high-grade dysplasia or adenocarcinoma. Am J Gastroenterol 1999; 94(12):3413–9.
146. Gatenby PA, Caygill CP, Ramus JR, et al. Short segment columnar-lined oesophagus: an underestimated cancer risk? A large cohort study of the relationship between Barrett's columnar-lined oesophagus segment length and adenocarcinoma risk. Eur J Gastroenterol Hepatol 2007;19(11):969–75.
147. Srivastava A, Hornick JL, Li X, et al. Extent of low-grade dysplasia is a risk factor for the development of esophageal adenocarcinoma in Barrett's esophagus. Am J Gastroenterol 2007;102(3):483–93.
148. Buttar NS, Wang KK, Sebo TJ, et al. Extent of high-grade dysplasia in Barrett's esophagus correlates with risk of adenocarcinoma. Gastroenterology 2001; 120(7):1630–9.
149. Dar M, Goldblum JR, Rice TW, et al. Can extent of high grade dysplasia in Barrett's oesophagus predict the presence of adenocarcinoma at oesophagectomy? Gut 2003;52(4):486–9.
150. Kastelein F, Biermann K, Steyerberg EW, et al. Aberrant p53 protein expression is associated with an increased risk of neoplastic progression in patients with Barrett's oesophagus. Gut 2013;62(12):1676–83.
151. Reid BJ, Prevo LJ, Galipeau PC, et al. Predictors of progression in Barrett's esophagus II: baseline 17p (p53) loss of heterozygosity identifies a patient subset at increased risk for neoplastic progression. Am J Gastroenterol 2001; 96(10):2839–48.
152. Allison RK, Skipper HE, Reid MR, et al. Studies on the photosynthetic reaction. I. The assimilation of acetate by Nostoc muscorum. J Biol Chem 1953;204(1): 197–205.

153. Bird-Lieberman EL, Dunn JM, Coleman HG, et al. Population-based study reveals new risk-stratification biomarker panel for Barrett's esophagus. Gastroenterology 2012;143(4):927–35.e3.
154. Rabinovitch PS, Longton G, Blount PL, et al. Predictors of progression in Barrett's esophagus III: baseline flow cytometrio variables. Am J Gastroenterol 2001;96(11):3071–83.
155. Timmer M, Sun G, Gorospe EC, et al. Predictive biomarkers for Barrett's esophagus: so near and yet so far. Dis Esophagus 2013;26(6):574–81.
156. Davelaar AL, Calpe S, Lau L, et al. Aberrant TP53 detected by combining immunohistochemistry and DNA-FISH improves Barrett's esophagus progression prediction: a prospective follow-up study. Genes Chromosomes Cancer 2015; 54(2):82–90.
157. Gerson LB, Shetler K, Triadafilopoulos G. Prevalence of Barrett's esophagus in asymptomatic individuals. Gastroenterology 2002;123(2):461–7.
158. Ward EM, Wolfsen HC, Achem SR, et al. Barrett's esophagus is common in older men and women undergoing screening colonoscopy regardless of reflux symptoms. Am J Gastroenterol 2006;101(1):12–7.
159. Zou D, He J, Ma X, et al. Epidemiology of symptom-defined gastroesophageal reflux disease and reflux esophagitis: the systematic investigation of gastrointestinal diseases in China (SILC). Scand J Gastroenterol 2011;46(2):133–41.
160. Cook M, Wild C, Forman D. A systematic review and meta-analysis of the sex ratio for Barrett's esophagus, erosive reflux disease, and nonerosive reflux disease. Am J Epidemiol 2005;162(11):1050–61.
161. Corley DA, Kubo A, Levin TR, et al. Abdominal obesity and body mass index as risk factors for Barrett's esophagus. Gastroenterology 2007;133(1):34–41.
162. Abnet C, Freedman ND, Kamangar F, et al. Non-steroidal anti-inflammatory drugs and risk of gastric and oesophageal adenocarcinomas: results from a cohort study and a meta-analysis. Br J Cancer 2009;100(3):551–7.

Predictors of Progression to High-Grade Dysplasia or Adenocarcinoma in Barrett's Esophagus

Matthew J. Whitson, MD, Gary W. Falk, MD, MS*

KEYWORDS

- Barrett's esophagus • Esophageal adenocarcinoma • Dysplasia • Risk factors
- Neoplastic progression

KEY POINTS

- Barrett's esophagus is the most well-established risk factor for the development of esophageal adenocarcinoma.
- Risk factors for neoplastic progression in patients with Barrett's esophagus include endoscopic findings (ie, erosive esophagitis), pathologic findings (ie, dysplasia), and clinical aspects (ie, male sex, older age, tobacco).
- Protective factors against neoplastic progression include medication use (ie statins, aspirin) and dietary considerations.

INTRODUCTION

The incidence of esophageal adenocarcinoma, a disease characterized by high mortality and an estimated 5-year survival rate of 20%, has increased dramatically in recent decades.[1,2] Barrett's esophagus is the most well-established risk factor for the development of esophageal adenocarcinoma.[3] The annual risk of progression from Barrett's esophagus to adenocarcinoma is approximately 0.33% per year.[4] When including both esophageal adenocarcinoma and high-grade dysplasia as a combined end point of progression, the incidence rate is approximately 0.9% to 1.0% per year.[5,6] Despite this neoplastic risk, the vast majority of patients with Barrett's esophagus die of causes other than esophageal adenocarcinoma.[7] At present, it remains unclear which patients

This article originally appeared in Gastroenterology Clinics, Volume 44, Issue 2, June 2015.
This work was supported in part by the NIH/NCI U54-CA163004, NIH/NIDDK P30-DK050306 (and its Molecular Pathology and Imaging and Molecular Biology Cores), NIH/NCI P01-CA098101 and institutional funds.
Division of Gastroenterology, Hospital of the University of Pennsylvania, University of Pennsylvania Perelman School of Medicine, 7th floor, South Pavillion, 3400 Civic Center Boulevard, Philadelphia, PA 19104, USA
* Corresponding author.
E-mail address: gary.falk@uphs.upenn.edu

Clinics Collections 7 (2015) 101–117
http://dx.doi.org/10.1016/j.ccol.2015.06.008
2352-7986/15/$ – see front matter © 2015 Elsevier Inc. All rights reserved.

with Barrett's esophagus progress on to neoplasia, a fact that makes current surveillance programs problematic. This article examines the endoscopic, pathologic, and epidemiologic risk factors for neoplastic progression in Barrett's esophagus (**Table 1**).

ENDOSCOPIC RISK FACTORS
Segment Length

While esophageal adenocarcinoma can develop in both short and long segments of Barrett's esophagus (traditionally defined as >3 cm), the understanding of the relationship between segment length and the risk of progression has evolved in recent years.[8] A 2012 meta-analysis found a lower annual incidence of esophageal adenocarcinoma in patients with short-segment Barrett's esophagus (<3 cm) than in the overall Barrett's esophagus population (0.19% vs 0.33% per year).[4] Work from the Northern Ireland Barrett's Esophagus Registry demonstrated an increased risk for progression to adenocarcinoma or high-grade dysplasia in long-segment Barrett's esophagus (hazard ratio [HR], 7.1; 95% confidence interval [CI], 1.74–29.04).[9] A recent case-control study from Berlin also found an association of segment length with progression to adenocarcinoma or high-grade dysplasia.[10] Patients with long-segment Barrett's esophagus had an increased risk of progression when compared with those with short-segment Barrett's esophagus (odds ratio [OR], 2.69; 95% CI, 1.48–4.88).

Newer studies have examined the relationship of segment length and risk of progression not only as a binary variable of long versus short but also as a continuous variable. In a large multicenter study, increasing segment length was an independent risk factor for neoplastic progression in patients with nondysplastic Barrett's esophagus.[11] Patients who progressed to adenocarcinoma or high-grade dysplasia had a longer Barrett's segment (6.1 cm vs 3.5 cm). Perhaps more importantly, the risk for neoplastic progression increased by 28% for every 1-cm increase in length of the Barrett's segment. Similarly, a Netherlands cohort study of more than 700 patients with nondysplastic Barrett's esophagus or low-grade dysplasia confirmed the concept of increasing risk with increasing segment length.[12] The relative risk of neoplastic progression to adenocarcinoma or high-grade dysplasia was 1.11 (95% CI, 1.01–1.2) per 1-cm increase in segment length. The recently completed SURF (Surveillance vs Radiofrequency Ablation) trial of radiofrequency ablation in patients with Barrett's esophagus with low-grade dysplasia also found segment length to be an independent predictor of neoplastic progression in the surveillance arm of the study (OR, 1.35 per cm; 95% CI, 1.04–1.76).[13]

Table 1 Risk factors for neoplastic progression to esophageal adenocarcinoma	
Clinical	Older age
	White race
	Male sex
	Family history
	Tobacco
	Obesity
Endoscopic	Long-segment Barrett's esophagus
	Hiatal hernia
	Mucosal abnormalities
	Right hemisphere position
Pathologic	Intestinal metaplasia
	Dysplasia
	p53 Overexpression

However, progression does occur in shorter segments of Barrett's esophagus, and a population-based study of over 8000 patients in Ireland found no relationship between segment length and risk of progression.[14] Taken together, it would seem that longer segments of Barrett's esophagus are associated with an increased risk of progression to adenocarcinoma or high-grade dysplasia.

Hiatal Hernia

Hiatal hernia is a well-documented risk factor for the development of Barrett's esophagus.[15] In addition, some data suggest that a larger hiatal hernia size may increase the risk of neoplastic progression in Barrett's esophagus (OR, 1.20 per cm hiatal hernia; 95% CI, 1.04–1.39).[16] In a cohort study of 550 patients from the Veterans Affairs Medical Center, Kansas City, a large hiatal hernia (>6 cm) was associated with an increased risk of neoplastic progression to adenocarcinoma or high-grade dysplasia when compared with patients with no hiatal hernia.[17] However, other studies find contrary results. A 2013 case-control study of approximately 600 patients demonstrated that although the presence of hiatal hernia increased the risk for Barrett's esophagus, it did not increase the risk of neoplastic progression to adenocarcinoma or high-grade dysplasia.[10] Overall, it is unclear if hiatal hernia size is an independent risk factor for neoplastic progression in Barrett's esophagus.

Mucosal Abnormalities

Several mucosal changes within the Barrett's segment are associated with an increased risk of progression to adenocarcinoma or high-grade dysplasia. Erosive esophagitis has emerged as a potential risk factor for esophageal adenocarcinoma. A Dutch multicenter cohort study found an increased risk of progression to adenocarcinoma or high-grade dysplasia in patients with Barrett's esophagus with esophagitis at baseline endoscopy (risk ratio [RR], 3.5; 95% CI, 1.3–9.5).[12] A Danish cohort study also found an increased standardized incidence ratio for esophageal adenocarcinoma among patients with Barrett's esophagus with erosive esophagitis when compared with the general population (standardized incidence ratio, 5.2; 95% CI, 4.6–5.8).[18]

Ulceration within a Barrett's segment is also associated with an increased risk of neoplastic progression to adenocarcinoma or high-grade dysplasia. The above-mentioned population-based case-control study from Northern Ireland also found that patients with ulceration in the Barrett's segment at diagnosis, but not elsewhere in the esophagus, were more likely to progress to cancer or high-grade dysplasia than those without (HR, 1.72; 95% CI, 1.08–2.76).[9]

It is unclear if mucosal abnormalities such as erosive esophagitis or ulceration are in fact risk factors for progression or rather are markers of prevalent adenocarcinoma or high-grade dysplasia, as shown by current endoscopic eradication studies. Overall, it seems that mucosal abnormalities are associated with an increased risk of neoplastic progression in patients with Barrett's esophagus.

Circumferential Position

Early adenocarcinoma and high-grade dysplasia seem to have a predilection to develop in the right hemisphere of the esophagus.[19–22] The author's group found that 85% of patients with adenocarcinoma or high-grade dysplasia referred for endoscopic management had these abnormalities located in the right hemisphere of the esophagus, predominantly in the area between 12-o'clock and 3-o'clock positions.[20] Similar findings were described in an Australian study, where more than 50% of advanced lesions were found between 2-o'clock and 5-o'clock positions.[19] Both of these studies are in line with previous data demonstrating greater chances for esophagitis to be found on the right hemisphere of the esophagus, suggesting a potential inflammatory mechanism to explain this observation.[23]

PATHOLOGIC RISK FACTORS
Intestinal Metaplasia Versus Columnar Metaplasia

At present, there is some disagreement among gastrointestinal (GI) societies as to the definition of Barrett's esophagus. The major difference is whether or not the presence of intestinal metaplasia within the columnar lined esophagus is required for the diagnosis. Early data from Scandinavia suggested that the risk of progression to adenocarcinoma or high-grade dysplasia in the columnar lined esophagus was equivalent in patients with and without intestinal metaplasia.[24] However, multiple subsequent studies have demonstrated an increased risk of neoplastic progression in patients with intestinal metaplasia.

Work from the population-based Northern Ireland Barrett's Esophagus Registry examined the risk of progression to high-grade dysplasia and esophageal adenocarcinoma in 8522 patients diagnosed with Barrett's esophagus defined as a columnar lined esophagus both with and without intestinal metaplasia.[6] The risk of cancer for patients with intestinal metaplasia at index endoscopy was increased compared with that of those without intestinal metaplasia at index endoscopy (0.38% per year vs 0.07% per year; HR, 3.54; 95% CI, 2.09–6.0).

An observational study from the University of Chicago demonstrated that among 379 patients with a columnar lined esophagus without goblet cells on pathologic findings, none progressed to adenocarcinoma or high-grade dysplasia during an average follow-up of 5 years.[25] In contrast, 8.9% of patients with a columnar lined esophagus with goblet cells progressed to adenocarcinoma or high-grade dysplasia.

Although there are not yet enough data to definitively state that intestinal metaplasia is a necessary component to the neoplastic risk of Barrett's esophagus, it does seem that there is an increased risk of neoplastic progression in patients with intestinal metaplasia compared with that in those without intestinal metaplasia.

Dysplasia

Dysplasia remains the single best marker for risk of progression in Barrett's esophagus. For patients with nondysplastic Barrett's esophagus, the risk of neoplastic progression remains low. A 2012 meta-analysis found an incidence of esophageal adenocarcinoma of 1 case per 300 patient-years in patients with nondysplastic Barrett's epithelium.[4] Two large, population-based studies not included in this meta-analysis also support these findings. A cohort study from Denmark evaluated the incidence of adenocarcinoma in more than 11,000 patients with Barrett's esophagus.[26] The incidence rate was 1 case per 1000 person-years in patients with nondysplastic Barrett's esophagus over a median follow-up of 5.2 years. A cohort study from Ireland also had similar low rates of progression in patients with nondysplastic Barrett's esophagus, 0.17% per year.[14]

Recent work of a large US multicenter consortium evaluated the importance of repeated biopsy-proven nondysplastic Barrett's esophagus during surveillance endoscopy.[27] Patients were found to have a lower annual risk of progressing to either adenocarcinoma or high-grade dysplasia if they had multiple endoscopies documenting persistent nondysplastic Barrett's esophagus (0.34% in patients with 5 endoscopies vs 0.75% In patients with 1 endoscopy). Overall, the neoplastic progression risk in nondysplastic Barrett's esophagus seems to be very low.

Low-Grade Dysplasia

Low-grade dysplasia has been extensively studied as a risk factor for progression with highly variable results. Probably due to the interobserver variability in the diagnosis of this lesion, the diagnosis becomes problematic.[28] A large, multicenter outcomes study from the United States investigated 210 patients with low-grade dysplasia to determine the rate of neoplastic progression.[29] There was a 1.83% per year incidence of progression to adenocarcinoma or high-grade dysplasia in this cohort. While the progression to esophageal adenocarcinoma was 0.18% per year if only 1 of 3 pathologists confirmed the diagnosis of low-grade dysplasia, the incidence rate increased to 0.39% per year if all 3 pathologists agreed. Critics of the study point out that there was a low interobserver agreement among the 2 expert pathologists (κ, 0.14).[30] In addition, approximately 1 in 4 of the original low-grade dysplasia samples were subsequently upgraded to high-grade dysplasia in this study, further calling into question the results. In a landmark study from the Netherlands, 293 patients with low-grade dysplasia were assessed.[31] Biopsy samples were confirmed by 2 independent pathologists with extensive experience with dysplasia within Barrett's esophagus from a panel of 6 pathologists. Upon expert review, almost three-quarters of patients were downstaged to either nondysplastic Barrett's esophagus or indefinite for dysplasia. In the patients who were confirmed to have low-grade dysplasia on expert review, the risk of neoplastic progression was 9.1% per patient-year with a median follow-up of over 3 years. The patients with nondysplastic Barrett's esophagus or those who were indefinite for dysplasia had a significantly lower risk of neoplastic progression (0.6%–0.9% per patient-year).

These results are similar to previous reports from the Academic Medical Center group in the Netherlands, which put the risk of progression to adenocarcinoma or high-grade dysplasia at 13.4% per year in patients with confirmed low-grade dysplasia.[32] In the surveillance arm of the SURF study examining radiofrequency ablation for patients with confirmed low-grade dysplasia, 26.5% of patients progressed to adenocarcinoma or high-grade dysplasia during a median follow-up of 30 months.[13] Similarly, a high progression rate was seen in the original clinical trial of radiofrequency ablation for low-grade dysplasia where expert gastrointestinal pathologist confirmation was required: 14% of patients in the sham treatment arm developed high-grade dysplasia at 1 year of follow-up.[33] Finally, in a population-based cohort study from Denmark, the standardized incidence ratio for esophageal adenocarcinoma in patients with low-grade dysplasia was 5.1 per 1000 patient-years (95% CI, 3.0–8.6).[26]

These rates are considerably higher than those described in the most recent meta-analysis, which found a rate of progression from low-grade dysplasia to adenocarcinoma of 0.54% per year (95% CI, 0.32%–0.76%) and to adenocarcinoma or high-grade dysplasia of 1.73% per year (95% CI, 0.99%–2.47%).[34] However, the investigators reported significant heterogeneity between the studies and acknowledged that rates of neoplastic progression were higher in the studies when expert pathologists confirmed low-grade dysplasia.

In summary, low-grade dysplasia is a challenging lesion to diagnose but seems to be a risk factor for neoplastic progression when confirmed by multiple pathologists with expertise in GI pathology.

Biomarkers of Increased Risk

Given the low rate of neoplastic progression in Barrett's esophagus and the inherent limitations of current endoscopic surveillance programs, there has long been interest in identifying biomarkers of increased risk in patients with Barrett's esophagus. Although multiple biomarkers have been studied, a select few are discussed here.

One of the best studied biomarkers is the tumor suppressor gene p53. In patients with Barrett's esophagus, loss of heterozygosity (LOH) for p53 (RR, 16; CI, 6.2–39.0) as well as overexpression of p53 (OR, 8.42; 95% CI, 2.37–30.0) are associated with progression to adenocarcinoma or high-grade dysplasia.[35,36] A nested case-control study demonstrated similar results; loss of p53 (RR, 14.0; 95% CI, 5.3–37.2) and over-expression of p53 (RR, 5.6; 95% CI, 3.1–10.3) were associated with a higher risk of progression to adenocarcinoma or high-grade dysplasia.[37] In addition, biopsies with both low-grade dysplasia and aberrant p53 expression seem to have higher rates of neoplastic progression.[37,38]

Other tumor suppressor genes (ie, p16), cell-cycle-related proteins (ie, cyclin A, cyclin D1), growth factor receptors (ie, epidermal growth factor receptor), and flow cytometry for DNA abnormalities (ie, aneuploidy and tetraploidy) have been studied at length. Despite some promising results, none of these potential biomarkers are appropriate for clinical practice at this time.

Considerable efforts have also gone into developing panels of these biomarkers that may assist in the identification of patients at increased risk for progression. A combination of 17p LOH, 9p LOH, and aneuploidy/tetraploidy was found to have a relative risk of 38.7 (95% CI, 10.8–138.5) for neoplastic progression and a 10-year cumulative incidence of adenocarcinoma of nearly 80%.[39] In patients with none of these biomarkers, only 12% progressed to adenocarcinoma. A panel of methylation biomarkers for 8 different genes (including p16, RUNX3, HPP1) had sensitivity for detection of progression of less than 50%.[40] The panel of just p16, RUNX3, and HPP1 has also been studied.[41,42] Finally, a nested case-control study from the Northern Ireland Barrett's Esophagus Registry evaluated a combination of biomarkers and anatomic pathology.[43] The panel of low-grade dysplasia, DNA aneuploidy/tetraploidy detected by image cytometry, and *Aspergillus oryzae* lectin demonstrated an increasing OR for each component of the panel that was present (OR, 3.73 per biomarker; 95% CI, 2.43–5.79).

Biomarkers and biomarker panels may in the future assist in determining who is likely to progress to adenocarcinoma or high-grade dysplasia. At the present time, there are multiple limitations that need to be addressed before these biomarkers are incorporated into daily clinical practice.

EPIDEMIOLOGIC RISK FACTORS
Age

The incidence of esophageal adenocarcinoma increases with age, regardless of sex or race.[44,45] Between the ages of 50 and 59 years, white males have an esophageal adenocarcinoma incidence rate of 8.44 per 100,000 person-years (95% CI, 8.05–8.85), which increases to 26.31 per 100,000 person-years (95% CI, 25.27–27.38) between ages 70 and 79 years.[44] The most recent publication of the Surveillance, Epidemiology, and End Results (SEER) registry reaffirms the increase in esophageal adenocarcinoma with age.[45] Starting at age 40 years and continuing until 79 years, the incidence rates of esophageal adenocarcinoma continue to rise. Beyond the age of 80 years, the incidence rate seems to level off in most groups.

In patients with Barrett's esophagus, most studies suggest an increase in the risk of neoplastic progression with increasing age. A Dutch population-based study found that the risk of progression increased with increasing age at diagnosis, with a marked increase in risk after the age of 75 years (HR, 12; 95% CI, 8.0–18).[46] Similarly, in the

Danish Barrett's esophagus population-based study, the incidence of adenocarcinoma or high-grade dysplasia increased progressively with age and was greatest in patients older than 70 years.[26]

Race

White race is a known risk factor for esophageal adenocarcinoma.[47–49] There is a fourfold increase in the incidence rate of esophageal adenocarcinoma in white males compared with black males and twofold increase compared with that of Hispanic males.[50] Similar patterns are also seen in women, although with lower incidence rates in all races. While the cause of this difference is unclear, a recent study of patients with Barrett's esophagus found a higher rate of dysplasia (7% vs 0%) and of long-segment Barrett's esophagus (26% vs 12%) at the time of endoscopy in Caucasians compared with black patients.[51] As both dysplasia and long-segment Barrett's esophagus are independent risk factors for esophageal adenocarcinoma, this may be an avenue worthy of further study.

Sex

Male gender is another well-documented risk factor for esophageal adenocarcinoma with a 6- to 10-fold risk increase compared with that of women.[45,52] However, both genders have seen a dramatic increase in the number of esophageal cancers. Newer data from the SEER registry have demonstrated the largest gender difference exists largely in the earlier-age cancers (ie, younger than 65 years).[45] Furthermore, the age-adjusted incidence rate in women older than 80 years continues to increase, whereas the rate in men plateaus. This difference may relate to estrogen exposure. Previously, estrogen exposure was suggested as a protective mechanism against both gastric and colon cancers and was demonstrated to reduce apoptosis and cell growth in esophageal adenocarcinoma.[53–55] As women age, there is a significant decrease in estrogen, which may explain the delayed increase in esophageal adenocarcinoma incidence, as seen in the SEER database data. Studies examining how risk factors with possible male predominance, including gastroesophageal reflux disease (GERD), obesity, and tobacco, may affect neoplastic progression risk have not yet provided a clear mechanistic answer to this epidemiologic difference.[56] Among patients with Barrett's esophagus, male gender is also a clearly recognized risk factor for progression to esophageal adenocarcinoma.[4,10,46]

Family History/Genetic Risk

Familial aggregation of Barrett's esophagus and esophageal adenocarcinoma has suggested a potential genetic component to these disease entities. Much of the work in this area has come from Chak and colleagues[57] who initially found that a positive family history (first- or second-degree relative with Barrett's esophagus, esophageal adenocarcinoma, or esophagogastric junction carcinoma) was higher among case subjects than among GERD controls (24% vs 5%). On multivariate analysis, a positive family history for Barrett's esophagus, adenocarcinoma of the esophagus, or esophagogastric junction was associated with an increased risk of developing these lesions when compared with patients with GERD alone (OR, 12.23; 95% CI, 3.34–44.76).

A subsequent segregation analysis by the same group found an incomplete autosomal dominant inheritance pattern for familial aggregations of Barrett's esophagus, esophageal adenocarcinoma, and gastroesophageal junction carcinoma.[58] Finally, in multiplex aggregations characterized by 3 or more members of a family with Barrett's esophagus and/or esophageal adenocarcinoma, the median age for the diagnosis of adenocarcinoma was approximately 5 years less than that in duplex families or sporadic cases.[59] Others have found an increased prevalence of Barrett's esophagus in first-degree relatives of patients with adenocarcinoma.[60]

Last, examination of germline mutations in patients with Barrett's esophagus and esophageal adenocarcinoma has yielded interesting results. In a model-free linkage analysis comparing both concordant sibling pairs with Barrett's and esophageal adenocarcinoma and discordant sibling pairs, 3 genes were identified with significant mutations (MSR1, ASCC1, and CTHRC1).[61] MSR1 was associated with the presence of both Barrett's esophagus and esophageal adenocarcinoma. A genome-wide association study from the BEACON (Barrett's and Esophageal Adenocarcinoma Consortium) group of more than 1500 cases of esophageal adenocarcinoma and 2300 cases of Barrett's esophagus found a high genetic correlation between Barrett's esophagus and adenocarcinoma as well as between multiple shared genes underlying the development of both.[62]

Taken together, these data suggest that there is a genetic component to neoplastic progression in some patients with Barrett's esophagus. More data are still needed to fully characterize this risk.

Tobacco

Tobacco use is a clear risk factor for the development of both Barrett's esophagus and esophageal adenocarcinoma.[63,64] A pooled analysis evaluating approximately 3000 cases of either esophageal adenocarcinoma or esophagogastric junctional adenocarcinoma found an OR of 1.67 (95% CI, 1.04–2.67) for developing esophageal adenocarcinoma in patients with tobacco use, with a significant increase with increased number of pack-years smoking.[65] Current or prior tobacco use also increases the risk of neoplastic progression in patients with Barrett's esophagus.[66,67] A population-based cohort study from the Northern Ireland Barrett's Esophagus Registry demonstrated an increased risk of neoplastic progression to adenocarcinoma or high-grade dysplasia in current smokers when compared with nonsmokers (HR, 2.03; 95% CI, 1.29–3.17).[66] Overall, tobacco is an established risk factor for progression to esophageal adenocarcinoma.

Obesity

Obesity is a well-described risk factor for esophageal adenocarcinoma.[68,69] A 2013 meta-analysis of more than 8000 cancers examined the relationship between body mass index (BMI), calculated as the weight in kilograms divided by the height in meters squared, and esophageal and gastric cardia adenocarcinoma.[69] The relative risk for developing esophageal adenocarcinoma increased with an increasing BMI; the relative risk was 1.71 (95% CI, 1.50–1.96) for a BMI in the range 25 to 30 and 2.34 (95% CI, 1.95–2.81) for a BMI greater than 30. An observational study from England showed a significant increase in esophageal adenocarcinoma with a BMI greater than 35 (HR, 4.95), but only an upward trend at lower BMIs.[70] This finding corresponds to earlier data suggesting that the largest risk was in patients with BMI greater than 35.[68] It would seem that male pattern central obesity is the key component of this risk, with a 2013 meta-analysis reporting an OR of 2.51 (95% CI, 1.56–4.04) for developing esophageal adenocarcinoma in patients with central adiposity.[71]

The impact of obesity and abdominal adiposity specifically on neoplastic progression of Barrett's esophagus to adenocarcinoma is a bit more unclear. A small cross-sectional analysis from Seattle Barrett's Esophagus Project demonstrated an increasing risk of histologic and genetic abnormalities associated with a high likelihood of neoplastic progression in patients with a predominantly abdominal fat distribution.[72] However, a recent cohort study of more than 400 patients with Barrett's esophagus found no relation between higher waist-hip ratios and neoplastic progression to adeno-carcinoma.[67] Although the role of neoplastic progression in Barrett's esophagus is not fully known, it is clear that obesity and specifically abdominal adiposity are associated with an increased overall risk of esophageal adenocarcinoma.

The exact mechanism underlying this risk is not fully known but may involve increased levels of insulinlike growth factor 1, insulin resistance, and adipokines such as leptin.[73–75] These relationships are explored at length by Chandar and Iyer, elsewhere in the issue.

PROTECTIVE FACTORS
Medications

There is emerging evidence that statins may have a protective effect for multiple cancers, including esophageal adenocarcinoma (**Table 2**). In vitro studies of statins have demonstrated multiple potential mechanisms for chemoprevention including antiproliferation, antiangiogenesis, and proapoptotic effects.[76–78] Two studies have demonstrated that regular statin use results in decreased malignant transformation from Barrett's esophagus to esophageal adenocarcinoma or high-grade dysplasia.[79,80] A cohort study from the United Kingdom found an inverse relationship between regular statin use of any dose (10+ months) and developing esophageal adenocarcinoma (OR, 0.58; 95% CI, 0.39–0.87).[81] The protective effect of statins seems to become more apparent with longer-term use. Overall, it seems that statins are protective against neoplastic progression.

Nonsteroidal antiinflammatory drugs (NSAIDs) have also been investigated as potential protective agents against neoplastic progression in Barrett's esophagus. In Barrett's esophagus, there is an increase in cyclooxygenase-2 (COX-2) expression as disease progresses from nondysplastic Barrett's esophagus to adenocarcinoma or high-grade dysplasia.[82] As such, the effect of NSAIDs, including aspirin, on prostaglandin E_2 production via the COX-2 pathways may serve as a potential protective mechanism against neoplastic progression. A pooled analysis by the BEACON group of 6 studies totaling 1226 patients with esophageal adenocarcinoma and 1140 patients with esophagogastric junctional adenocarcinoma examined the impact of aspirin and/or NSAID use on the development of these cancers.[83] "Anytime users" of NSAIDs or aspirin had reduced risk of esophageal adenocarcinoma compared with nonusers (OR, 0.68; 95% CI, 0.56–0.83). The OR improved further with daily use for 10 or more years (OR, 0.56; 95% CI, 0.43–0.73) in patients. For aspirin, the overall OR for developing esophageal adenocarcinoma in anytime users was 0.77 (95% CI, 0.60–0.97).

Table 2	
Protective factors against neoplastic progression to esophageal adenocarcinoma	
Dietary	Significant fruits and vegetables
	Fiber
Medications	Statins
	NSAIDs
	Aspirin
Acid suppression	PPIs
H pylori infection	

Abbreviations: NSAIDs, nonsteroidal antiinflammatory drugs; PPIs, proton pump inhibitors.

Multiple studies have examined the impact of NSAID and/or aspirin use on neoplastic progression of Barrett's esophagus. Work from the Seattle Barrett's Esophagus Project found a decreased HR for progression to adenocarcinoma in current NSAID users (HR, 0.32; 95% CI, 0.14–0.70) over an average follow-up of 65 months.[84] In addition, a multicenter, prospective cohort from the Netherlands showed a reduced risk of progression to cancer in patients with Barrett's esophagus taking NSAIDs (HR, 0.47; 95% CI, 0.24–0.93).[85] This study showed an additive benefit when both NSAIDs and statins were used (HR, 0.22; 95% CI, 0.06–0.85). Finally, a meta-analysis found an overall reduced risk of adenocarcinoma or high-grade dysplasia among patients with Barrett's esophagus taking COX inhibitors (RR, 0.64; 95% CI, 0.53–0.77) or aspirin (RR, 0.63; 95% CI, 0.43–0.94) reaffirming the protective effects of NSAIDs and aspirin against neoplastic progression.[86]

The seminal work by Lagergren and colleagues[87] demonstrated a striking association between more frequent, more severe, and more persistent reflux symptoms and esophageal adenocarcinoma. Thus it makes sense that the effect of acid suppression on neoplastic progression in Barrett's esophagus has been studied. Multiple small studies have suggested a reduced risk of neoplastic progression in patients with Barrett's esophagus who use proton pump inhibitors (PPIs).[79,88] Furthermore, a 2014 meta-analysis demonstrated an adjusted OR of 0.29 (95% CI, 0.12–0.79) for neoplastic progression in patients with Barrett's esophagus taking PPIs.[89] There was no benefit noted from histamine2 antagonists. However, a recent Danish case-control study of 140 patients with Barrett's esophagus found no benefit for PPI long-term users.[90] As such, it is still unclear if PPIs themselves reduce the risk of neoplastic progression in patients with Barrett's esophagus, although there seems to be no role for histamine2 antagonists.

Helicobacter pylori

As treatment and eradication rates of *H pylori* have increased, the rates of esophageal adenocarcinoma have also increased, prompting investigators to examine the potential relationship between the 2 observations. Multiple studies have demonstrated an inverse relationship between *H pylori* infection and development of Barrett's esophagus.[91,92] These observations have also suggested a possible protective effect of *H pylori* infection against the development of esophageal adenocarcinoma. A recent meta-analysis of 13 studies, pooling 1145 esophageal cases with 3453 controls, demonstrated a protective benefit of *H pylori* against developing adenocarcinoma (OR, 0.57; 95% CI, 0.44–0.73).[93] This study did not specifically address patients with Barrett's esophagus.

Overall, it does seem that *H pylori* infection has some protective benefit against developing both Barrett's esophagus and esophageal adenocarcinoma. However, the effect of neoplastic progression in patients with Barrett's esophagus has yet to be studied.

Diet

High consumption of fruits and vegetables seems to decrease the risk of adenocarcinoma in patients with Barrett's esophagus.[10,94] A National Institutes of Health study examined dietary patterns in the general population, finding a decreased risk for developing esophageal adenocarcinoma in patients reporting a positive Healthy Eating Index, which puts a premium on vegetables and fruits (HR, 0.75; 95% CI, 0.57–0.98).[95] On the other hand, increased meat consumption, particularly processed red meats, seems to increase the risk of esophageal adenocarcinoma.[96–98] These studies did not address neoplastic progression in patients with Barrett's esophagus.

Multiple different vitamins and supplements have also been studied. The most consistent data, although limited, suggest that fiber may play a protective role against adenocarcinoma.[99,100] Mixed data exist regarding the potential benefit of using a daily multivitamin, folate, or vitamin B_{12}.[100–104] Overall, a healthy diet including significant consumption of fruits and vegetables likely decreases the risk of developing esophageal adenocarcinoma.

SUMMARY

As the prevalence of esophageal adenocarcinoma increases, research has discovered epidemiologic, endoscopic, and pathologic factors that may help determine the risk for neoplastic progression. It is hoped that algorithms can be developed to risk stratify patients in the future to tailor optimal therapy and intervention to prevent the development of adenocarcinoma.

REFERENCES

1. Lepage C, Drouillard A, Jouve JL, et al. Epidemiology and risk factors for oesophageal adenocarcinoma. Dig Liver Dis 2013;45:625–9.
2. Pennathur A, Gibson MK, Jobe BA, et al. Oesophageal carcinoma. Lancet 2013; 381:400–12.
3. Verbeek RE, Leender M, Ten Kate FJ, et al. Surveillance of Barrett's esophagus and mortality from esophageal adenocarcinoma: a population-based cohort study. Am J Gastroenterol 2014;109:1215–22.
4. Desai TK, Krishnan K, Samala N, et al. The incidence of oesophageal adenocarcinoma in non-dysplastic Barrett's oesophagus: a meta-analysis. Gut 2012;61: 970–6.
5. Yousef F, Cardwell C, Cantwell MM, et al. The incidence of esophageal cancer and high-grade dysplasia in Barrett's esophagus: a systematic review and meta-analysis. Am J Epidemiol 2008;168:237–49.
6. Sikkema M, de Jonge PJ, Steyerberg EW, et al. Risk of esophageal adenocarcinoma and mortality in patients with Barrett's esophagus; a systematic review and meta-analysis. Clin Gastroenterol Hepatol 2010;8:235–44.
7. Milind R, Attwood SE. Natural history of Barrett's esophagus. World J Gastroenterol 2012;18(27):3483–91.
8. Gatenby P, Caygill C, Wall C, et al. Lifetime risk of esophageal adenocarcinoma in patients with Barrett's esophagus. World J Gastroenterol 2014;20(28):9611–7.
9. Coleman HG, Bhat SK, Murray LJ, et al. Symptoms and endoscopic features at Barrett's esophagus diagnosis: implications for neoplastic progression risk. Am J Gastroenterol 2014;109:527–34.
10. Pohl H, Wrobel K, Bojarski C, et al. Risk factors in the development of esophageal adenocarcinoma. Am J Gastroenterol 2013;108:200–7.
11. Anaparthy R, Gaddam S, Kanakadandi V, et al. Association between length of Barrett's esophagus and risk of high-grade dysplasia or adenocarcinoma in patients without dysplasia. Clin Gastroenterol Hepatol 2013;11:1430–6.
12. Sikkema M, Looman CW, Steyerberg EW, et al. Predictors of neoplastic progression in patients with Barrett's esophagus: a prospective cohort study. Am J Gastroenterol 2011;106:1231–8.
13. Phoa KN, van Vilsteren FGI, Weusten BL, et al. Radiofrequency ablation vs endoscopic surveillance for patients with Barrett esophagus and low-grade dysplasia. JAMA 2014;311(12):1209–17.

14. Bhat S, Coleman HG, Yousef F, et al. Risk of malignant progression in Barrett's esophagus patients: Results form a large population based study. J Natl Cancer Inst 2011;103:1049–57.

15. Andrici J, Tio M, Cox MR, et al. Hiatal hernia and the risk of Barrett's esophagus. J Gastroenterol Hepatol 2013;28:415–31.

16. Avidan B, Sonnenberg A, Schnell TG, et al. Hiatal hernia size, Barrett's length, and severity of acid reflux are all risk factors for esophageal adenocarcinoma. Am J Gastroenterol 2002;97:1930–6.

17. Weston AP, Sharma P, Mathur S, et al. Risk stratification of Barrett's esophagus: Updated prospective multivariate analysis. Am J Gastroenterol 2004;99: 1657–66.

18. Erichsen R, Robertson D, Farkas DK, et al. Erosive reflux disease increases risk for esophageal adenocarcinoma, compared with nonerosive reflux. Clin Gastroenterol Hepatol 2012;10:475–80.

19. Kariyawasam VC, Bourke MJ, Hourigan LF, et al. Circumferential location predicts the risk of high-grade dysplasia and early adenocarcinoma in short-segment Barrett's esophagus. Gastrointest Endosc 2012;75:938–44.

20. Enestvedt BK, Lugo R, Guarner-Argente C, et al. Location, location, location: does early cancer in Barrett's esophagus have a preference. Gastrointest Endosc 2013;78:462–7.

21. Pech O, Gossner L, Manner H, et al. Prospective evaluation of the macroscopic types and location of early Barrett's neoplasia in 380 lesions. Endoscopy 2007; 39:588–93.

22. Cassani L, Sumner E, Slaughter JC, et al. Directional distribution of neoplasia in Barrett's esophagus is not influenced by distance from the gastroesophageal junction. Gastrointest Endosc 2013;77:877–82.

23. Edebo A, Vieth M, Tam W, et al. Circumferential and axial distribution of esophageal mucosal damage in reflux disease. Dis Esophagus 2007;20:232–8.

24. Gatenby PA, Ramus JR, Caygill CP, et al. Relevance of the detection of intestinal metaplasia in non-dysplastic columnar-lined oesophagus. Scand J Gastroenterol 2008;43:524–30.

25. Westerhoff M, Hovan L, Lee C, et al. Effects of dropping the requirement for goblet cells from the diagnosis of Barrett's esophagus. Clin Gastroenterol Hepatol 2012;10:1232–6.

26. Hvid-Jensen F, Pedersen L, Drewes AM, et al. Incidence of adenocarcinoma among patients with Barrett's esophagus. N Engl J Med 2011;365:1375–83.

27. Gaddam S, Singh M, Gokulakrishnan B, et al. Persistence of nondysplastic Barrett's esophagus identifies patients at lower risk for esophageal adenocarcinoma: results from a large multicenter cohort. Gastroenterology 2013;145:548–53.

28. Montgomery E, Broner MP, Goldblum JR, et al. Reproducibility of the diagnosis of dysplasia in Barrett esophagus: a reaffirmation. Hum Pathol 2001;32:368–78.

29. Wani S, Falk GW, Post J, et al. Risk Factors for progression of low-grade dysplasia in patients with Barrett's esophagus. Gastroenterology 2011;141:1179–86.

30. Bergman J, Vieth M. Let's not jump to conclusions regarding low-grade dysplasia in Barrett's esophagus. Gastroenterology 2012;142(5):e18–9.

31. Duits L, Phoa KN, Curvers WL, et al. Barrett's oesophagus patients with low-grade dysplasia can be accurately risk-stratified after histological review by an expert pathology panel. Gut 2014. [Epub ahead of print].

32. Curvers WL, ten Kate FJ, Krishnadath KK, et al. Low-grade dysplasia in Barrett's esophagus: overdiagnosed and underused. Am J Gastroenterol 2010;15: 1523–30.

33. Shaheen NJ, Sharma P, Overholt BF, et al. Radiofrequency ablation in Barrett's esophagus with dysplasia. N Engl J Med 2009;360:2277–88.

34. Singh S, Manickmam P, Amin AV, et al. Incidence of esophageal adenocarcinoma in Barrett's esophagus with low-grade dysplasia: a systematic review and meta-analysis. Gastrointest Endosc 2014;79:897–909.

35. Reid BJ, Prevo LJ, Galipeau PC, et al. Predictors of progression in Barrett's esophagus II: baseline 17p (p53) loss of heterozygosity identifies a patient subset at increased risk for neoplastic progression. Am J Gastroenterol 2001;96: 2839–48.

36. Murray L, Sedo A, Scott M, et al. TP53 and progression from Barrett's metaplasia to oesophageal adenocarcinoma in a UK population cohort. Gut 2006;55: 1390–7.

37. Kastelein F, Biermann K, Steyerberg EW, et al. Aberrant p53 protein expression is associated with an increased risk of neoplastic progression in patients with Barrett's oesophagus. Gut 2013;62:1676–83.

38. Kaye PV, Haider SA, Ilyas M, et al. Barrett's dysplasia and the Vienna classification: reproducibility, prediction of progression and impact of consensus reporting and p53 immunohistochemistry. Histopathology 2009;54(6):699–712.

39. Galipeau PC, Li X, Blount PL, et al. NSAIDs modulate cdkn2a, tp53, and DNA content risk for progression to esophageal adenocarcinoma. PLoS Med 2007; 4(2):e67.

40. Jin Z, Cheng Y, Gu W, et al. A multi-center, double-blinded validation study of methylation biomarkers for progression prediction in Barrett's esophagus. Cancer Res 2009;69:4112–5.

41. Sato F, Jin Z, Schulmann K, et al. Three-tiered risk stratification model to predict progression in Barrett's esophagus using epigenetic and clinical features. PLoS One 2008;101:1193–9.

42. Schulmann K, Sterian A, Berki A, et al. Inactivation of p16, RUNX3, and HPP1 occurs early in Barrett's associated neoplastic progression and predicts progression risk. Oncogene 2005;24:4138–48.

43. Bird-Lieberman EL, Dunn JM, Coleman HG, et al. Population-based study reveals new risk-stratification biomarker panel for Barrett's esophagus. Gastroenterology 2012;143:927–35.

44. Nordenstedt H, El-Serag H. The influence of age, sex, and race on the incidence of esophageal cancer in the United States (1992–2006). Scand J Gastroenterol 2011;46:597–602.

45. Mathieu LN, Kanark NF, Tsai HL, et al. Age and sex differences in the incidence of esophageal adenocarcinoma: results from the Surveillance, Epidemiology, and End Results (SEER) registry (1973–2008). Dis Esophagus 2014;27:757–63.

46. de Jonge PJ, van Blankenstein M, Looman CW, et al. Risk of malignant progression in patients with Barrett's oesophagus: a Dutch nationwide cohort study. Gut 2010;59:1030–6.

47. Coupland VH, Lagergren J, Konfortion J, et al. Ethnicity in relation to incidence of oesophageal and gastric cancer in England. Br J Cancer 2012;107:1908–14.

48. Ashktorab H, Nouri Z, Nouraie M, et al. Esophageal carcinoma in African Americans: a five-decade experience. Dig Dis Sci 2011;56:3577–82.

49. Sadler GJ, Jothiamni D, Zanetta U, et al. The effect of ethnicity on the presentation and management of oesophageal and gastric cancers: a UK perspective. Eur J Gastroenterol Hepatol 2009;21:996–1000.

50. Kubo A, Corley DA. Marked multi-ethnic variation of esophageal and gastric cardia carcinomas within the United States. Am J Gastroenterol 2004;99:582–8.

51. Khoury JE, Chisholm S, Jamal MM, et al. African Americans with Barrett's esophagus are less likely to have dysplasia at biopsy. Dig Dis Sci 2012;57: 419–23.

52. El-Serag HB, Mason AC, Petersen N, et al. Epidemiological differences between adenocarcinoma of the oesophagus and adenocarcinoma of the gastric cardia in the USA. Gut 2002;50:368–72.

53. Camargo MC, Goto Y, Zabaleta J, et al. Sex hormones, hormonal interventions, and gastric cancer risk: a meta-analysis. Cancer Epidemiol Biomarkers Prev 2012;21:20–38.

54. Chlebowski RT, Wactawski-Wende J, Ritenbaugh C, et al. Estrogen plus progestin and colorectal cancer in postmenopausal women. N Engl J Med 2004;350: 991–1004.

55. Sukocheva OA, Wee C, Ansar A, et al. Effect of estrogen on growth and apoptosis in esophageal adenocarcinoma cells. Dis Esophagus 2012;26(6): 628–35.

56. Rutegard M, Nordenstedt H, Lu Y, et al. Sex-specific exposure prevalence of established risk factors for oesophageal adenocarcinoma. Br J Cancer 2010;103: 735–40.

57. Chak A, Lee T, Kinnard MF, et al. Familial aggregation of Barrett's oesophagus, oesophageal adenocarcinoma, and oesophagogastric junctional adenocarcinoma in Caucasian adults. Gut 2002;51:323–8.

58. Sun X, Elston R, Barnholtz-Sloan J, et al. A segregation analysis of Barrett's esophagus and associated adenocarcinomas. Cancer Epidemiol Biomarkers Prev 2010;19:666–74.

59. Chak A, Chen Y, Vengoechea J, et al. Variation in age at cancer diagnosis in familial versus nonfamilial Barrett's esophagus. Cancer Epidemiol Biomarkers Prev 2012;21:376–83.

60. Juhasz A, Mittal SK, Lee TH, et al. Prevalence of Barrett esophagus in first-degree relatives of patients with esophageal adenocarcinoma. J Clin Gastroenterol 2011;45(10):867–71.

61. Orloff M, Peterson C, He X, et al. Germline mutations in MSR1, ASCC1, and CTHRC1 in patients with Barrett esophagus and esophageal adenocarcinoma. JAMA 2011;206(4):410–9.

62. Weronica E, Levine DM, D'Amato M, et al. Germline genetic contributions to risk for esophageal adenocarcinoma, Barrett's esophagus, and gastroesophageal reflux. J Natl Cancer Inst 2013;105:1711–8.

63. Cook MB, Shaheen NJ, Anderson LA, et al. Cigarette smoking increases risk of Barrett's Esophagus: an analysis of the Barrett's and Esophageal Adenocarcinoma Consortium. Gastroenterology 2012;142(4):744–53.

64. Tramacere I, La Vecchia C, Negri E. Tobacco smoking and esophageal and gastric cardia adenocarcinoma. Epidemiology 2011;22(3):344–9.

65. Cook MB, Kamangar F, Whiteman DC, et al. Cigarette smoking and adenocarcinomas of the esophagus and esophagogastric junction: a pooled analysis from the International BEACON Consortium. J Natl Cancer Inst 2010;102: 1344–53.

66. Coleman HG, Bhat S, Johnston BT, et al. Tobacco smoking increases the risk of high-grade dysplasia and cancer among patients with Barrett's esophagus. Gastroenterology 2012;142:233–40.

67. Hardikar S, Onstatd L, Blount PL, et al. The role of tobacco, alcohol, and obesity in neoplastic progression to esophageal adenocarcinoma: a prospective study of Barrett's Esophagus. PLoS One 2013;8(1):e52192.

68. Abnet CC, Freedman ND, Hollenbeck AR, et al. A prospective study of BMI and risk of oesophageal and gastric adenocarcinoma. Eur J Cancer 2008;44:465–71.
69. Turati F, Tramacere I, La Vecchia C, et al. A meta-analysis of body mass index and esophageal and gastric cardia adenocarcinoma. Ann Oncol 2013;24:609–17.
70. Yates M, Cheong E, Luben R, et al. Body mass index, smoking, and alcohol and risks of Barrett's esophagus and esophageal adenocarcinoma: a UK prospective cohort study. Dig Dis Sci 2014;59:1552–9.
71. Singh S, Sharma AN, Murad MH, et al. Central adiposity is associated with increased risk of esophageal inflammation, metaplasia, and adenocarcinoma: a systematic review and meta-analysis. Clin Gastroenterol Hepatol 2013;11: 1399–412.
72. Vaughan TL, Kristal AR, Blount PL, et al. Nonsteroidal anti-inflammatory drug use, body mass index, and anthropometry in relation to genetic and flow cytometric abnormalities in Barrett's esophagus. Cancer Epidemiol Biomarkers Prev 2002;11:745–52.
73. Doyle SL, Donohoe CL, Finn SP, et al. IGF-1 and its receptor in esophageal cancer: association with adenocarcinoma and visceral obesity. Am J Gastroenterol 2012;107:196–204.
74. Alexandre L, Long E, Beales IL. Pathophysiological mechanism linking obesity and esophageal adenocarcinoma. World J Gastrointest Pathophysiol 2014; 5(4):534–49.
75. Ogunwobi O, Mutungi G, Beales IL. Leptin stimulates proliferation and inhibits apoptosis in Barrett's esophageal adenocarcinoma cells by cycloxygenase-2-dependent, prostatglandin-E2-mediated transactivation of the epidermal growth factor receptor and c-Jun NH2-terminal kinase activation. Endocrinology 2006; 147:4505–16.
76. Ogunwobi OO, Beales IL. Statins inhibit proliferation and induce apoptosis in Barrett's esophageal adenocarcinoma cells. Am J Gastroenterol 2008;103:825–37.
77. Sadaria MR, Reppert AE, Yu JA, et al. Statin therapy attenuates growth and malignant potential of human esophageal adenocarcinoma cells. J Thorac Cardiovasc Surg 2011;142:1152–60.
78. Konturek PC, Burnat G, Hahn EG. Inhibition of Barrett's adenocarcinoma cell growth by simvastatin: involvement of COX-2 and apoptosis-related proteins. J Physiol Pharmacol 2007;58(Suppl 3):141–8.
79. Nguyen DM, Richardson P, El-Serag HB. Medications (NSAIDs, statins, proton pump inhibitors) and the risk of esophageal adenocarcinoma in patients with Barrett's esophagus. Gastroenterology 2010;138:2260–6.
80. Beales IL, Vardi I, Dearman L. Regular statin and aspirin use in patients with Barrett's oesophageal adenocarcinoma. Eur J Gastroenterol Hepatol 2012;24:917–23.
81. Alexandre L, Clark AB, Bhutta HY, et al. Statin use is associated with reduced risk of histologic subtypes of esophageal cancer: a nested case-control analysis. Gastroenterology 2014;146:661–8.
82. Morris CD, Armstrong GR, Bigley G, et al. Cyclooxygenase-2 expression in the Barrett's metaplasia-dysplasia-adenocarcinoma sequence. Am J Gastroenterol 2001;96:990–6.
83. Liao LM, Vaughan TL, Corley DA, et al. Nonsteroidal anti-inflammatory drug use reduces risk of adenocarcinomas of the esophagus and esophagogastric junction in a pooled analysis. Gastroenterology 2012;142:442–52.
84. Vaughan TL, Dong LM, Blount PL, et al. Non-steroidal anti-inflammatory drugs and risk of neoplastic progression in Barrett's oesophagus: a prospective study. Lancet Oncol 2005;6:945–52.

85. Kastelein F, Spaander MC, Biermann K, et al. Nonsteroidal anti-inflammatory drugs and statins have chemopreventative effects in patients with Barrett's esophagus. Gastroenterology 2011;141:2000–8.

86. Zhang S, Zhang XQ, Ding XW, et al. Cyclooxygenase inhibitors use is associated with reduced risk of esophageal adenocarcinoma in patients with Barrett's esophagus: a meta-analysis. Br J Cancer 2014;110:2378–88.

87. Lagergren J, Bergstrom R, Lindren A, et al. Symptomatic Gastroesophageal reflux as a risk factor for esophageal adenocarcinoma. N Engl J Med 1999; 340(11):825–31.

88. Kastelein F, Spaander MC, Steyerberg EW, et al. Proton pump inhibitors reduce the risk of neoplastic progression in patients with Barrett's esophagus. Clin Gastroenterol Hepatol 2013;11:382–8.

89. Singh S, Garg SK, Singh PP, et al. Acid-suppressive medications and risk of oesophageal adenocarcinoma in patients with Barrett's oesophagus: a systematic review and meta-analysis. Gut 2014;63(8):1229–37.

90. Hvid-Jensen F, Pedersen L, Funch-Jensen P, et al. Proton pump inhibitor use may not prevent high-grade dysplasia and oesophageal adenocarcinoma in Barrett's oesophagus: a nationwide study of 9883 patients. Aliment Pharmacol Ther 2014;39:984–91.

91. Rubenstein JH, Inadomi JM, Scheiman J, et al. Association between Helicobacter pylori and Barrett's esophagus, erosive esophagitis, and gastroesophageal reflux symptoms. Clin Gastroenterol Hepatol 2014;12:239–45.

92. Corley DA, Kubo A, Levin TR, et al. Helicobacter pylori infection and the risk of Barrett's oesophagus: a community-based study. Gut 2007;57:727–33.

93. Nie S, Chen T, Yang X, et al. Association of Helicobacter pylori infection with esophageal adenocarcinoma and squamous cell carcinoma: a meta-analysis. Dis Esophagus 2014;27:645–53.

94. Steevens J, Schouten LJ, Goldbohm RA, et al. Vegetables and fruits consumption and risk of esophageal and gastric cancer subtypes in the Netherlands cohort study. Int J Cancer 2011;129:2681–93.

95. Li WQ, Park Y, Wu JW, et al. Index-based dietary patterns and risk of esophageal and gastric cancer in a large cohort study. Clin Gastroenterol Hepatol 2013;11:1130–6.

96. Zhu HC, Yang X, Xu LP, et al. Meat consumption in associated with esophageal cancer risk in a meat- and cancer-histological-type dependent manner. Dig Dis Sci 2014;59:664–73.

97. Salehi M, Moradi-Lakeh M, Salehi MH, et al. Meat, fish, and esophageal cancer risk: a systematic review and dose-response meta analysis. Nutr Rev 2013; 71(5):257–67.

98. O'Doherty MG, Cantwell MM, Murray LJ, et al. Dietary fat and meat intakes and risk of reflux esophagitis, Barrett's esophagus, and esophageal adenocarcinoma. Int J Cancer 2011;129:1493–502.

99. Coleman HG, Murray LJ, Hicks B, et al. Dietary Fiber and the risk of precancerous lesions and cancer of the esophagus: a systematic review and meta-analysis. Nutr Rev 2013;71(7):474–82.

100. Mayne ST, Risch HA, Dubrow R, et al. Nutrient Intake and risk of subtypes of esophageal and gastric cancer. Cancer Epidemiol Biomarkers Prev 2001;10: 1055–62.

101. Dong LM, Sanchez CA, Rabinovitch PS, et al. Dietary supplement use and risk of neoplastic progression in esophageal adenocarcinoma: a prospective study. Nutr Cancer 2008;60(1):39–48.

102. Dawsey SP, Hollenbeck A, Schatzkin A, et al. A prospective study of vitamin and mineral supplement use and the risk of upper gastrointestinal cancers. PLoS One 2014;9(2):e88774.
103. Sharp L, Carsin AE, Cantwell MM, et al. Intakes of dietary folate and other B vitamins are associated with risks of esophageal adenocarcinoma, Barrett's esophagus, and reflux esophagitis. J Nutr 2013;143:1966–73.
104. Xiao Q, Freedman ND, Ren J, et al. Intakes of folate methionine, vitamin b6, and vitamin b12 with a risk of esophageal and gastric cancer in a large cohort study. Br J Cancer 2014;110:1328–33.

Surveillance in Barrett's Esophagus
Utility and Current Recommendations

Joel H. Rubenstein, MD, MSc[a,b],*

KEYWORDS

- Esophageal neoplasms • Surveillance • Endoscopy

KEY POINTS

- Empirical evidence supporting the efficacy of surveillance of Barrett's esophagus is limited to observational studies with important limitations.
- Guidelines provide weak recommendations in favor of surveillance of Barrett's esophagus.
- In nondysplastic Barrett's esophagus, it is recommended to not perform surveillance more frequently than every 3 years.
- Adequate biopsies should be performed during surveillance endoscopies (4 quadrant every 2 cm plus of any mucosal irregularities).

INTRODUCTION

The notion of endoscopic surveillance of Barrett's esophagus with the aim of decreasing the burden of esophageal adenocarcinoma (EAC) is very attractive for several reasons. The incidence of EAC has risen dramatically over the past 4 decades in many Western nations. The mortality rate from the cancer is high. There exists a relatively easily identifiable precursor lesion in Barrett's esophagus, and tissue can be acquired from the lesion for histology with relative ease and safety (when compared with sampling, for instance, lesions of the pancreas, kidney, liver, or lung). Although survival from even most early-stage esophageal cancers is still poor,[1] a growing body of evidence has demonstrated the efficacy of endoscopic therapy directed at dysplasia and even adenocarcinoma confined to the mucosa (invading the lamina propria or muscularis mucosae, T1a cancers).[2,3] Therefore, it would seem reasonable that an effort should be made to reduce the burden of EAC by performing periodic

This article originally appeared in Gastroenterology Clinics, Volume 44, Issue 2, June 2015.
Conflict of Interest: J.H. Rubenstein has been a paid consultant for ORC International.
[a] Veterans Affairs Center for Clinical Management Research, VA Medical Center 111-D, 2215 Fuller Road, Ann Arbor, MI 48105, USA; [b] Barrett's Esophagus Program, Division of Gastroenterology, University of Michigan Medical School, 3912 Taubman Center, SPC 5362, Ann Arbor, MI 48109, USA
* VA Medical Center, 111-D, 2215 Fuller Road, Ann Arbor, MI 48105.
E-mail address: jhr@umich.edu

endoscopic surveillance in patients with Barrett's esophagus in order to identify and intervene on patients who develop dysplasia or intramucosal cancer. Herein, the author reviews the evidence regarding the effectiveness and efficiency of surveillance, caveats in interpreting that evidence, recommendations from published guidelines, details regarding the logistics of how surveillance should be conducted, and potential future directions.

INCIDENCE OF CANCER IN BARRETT'S ESOPHAGUS

Whether surveillance of Barrett's esophagus is rational depends heavily on the incidence of EAC in that setting. Some relatively small cohorts have published estimates of the incidence of EAC in nondysplastic Barrett's esophagus exceeding 2% per year.[4] However, there was likely a bias for disseminating the studies with the greatest observed risk. A recent meta-analysis of cohort studies has estimated the incidence at 0.33% per year.[5] Some large cohort studies have estimated the incidence as low as 0.12% per year.[6,7] When the risk of cancer is as low as 2% per decade, it is not clear that any intervention, even if it is efficacious for preventing cancer mortality, is worth the expected expense and complications. In low-grade dysplasia, the incidence of cancer may be higher, but it still ranges between 0.2% and 0.4% per year.[8–10] The incidence is clearly greater when high-grade dysplasia is present, but in that case, the standard of care has become endoscopic therapy rather than surveillance.[11]

LEAD-TIME AND LENGTH-TIME BIASES

In order to interpret the results of surveillance in Barrett's esophagus, an understanding of lead-time and length-time biases is necessary. Studies of the effects of screening or surveillance on cancer mortality are inherently fraught with the potential for bias by lead-time and length-time effects. Lead-time effects are best understood through a thought experiment (**Fig. 1**). A hypothetical set of twin brothers is imagined who were born on the same day, destined to develop EAC on the same day, and destined to die from EAC on the same day. Twin A does not undergo any screening or surveillance and instead is diagnosed with EAC when he presents with dysphagia, say at the age of 68 years. Assuming he dies at the age of 70 years, his survival time with EAC is 2 years. Twin B decided to undergo screening, was found to have Barrett's esophagus, and underwent surveillance; he was diagnosed with EAC while asymptomatic, say at the age of 63 years. He undergoes esophagectomy but still ends up dying from recurrent metastatic EAC at the age of 70 years. His survival time with EAC is observed to be 7 years. In practice, it is not known when someone is destined to develop cancer or when one is destined to die (even among twins), so this difference of 5 years between the 2 patients would be mistakenly attributed as an extension of the duration of life by 5 years, when in fact all that was accomplished with screening and surveillance was increasing the proportion of life with a known diagnosis of EAC in twin B and not delaying the date of his death at all. Even if there is a true effect of screening and surveillance on survival, it can be expected that lead-time effects will bias the observation of survival toward a stronger effect.

Length-time effects refer to the predilection of screening and surveillance examinations to identify indolent disease. Cancers are heterogeneous, with some progressing quickly and others slowly (**Fig. 2**). Any screening or surveillance examination is more likely to identify a slow-growing tumor than a fast-growing one because there is more time available to detect the cancer between onset and death. A reasonable assumption is that a slow-growing tumor is also less likely to be fatal than a fast-growing tumor; so any screening or surveillance examination is more likely to detect cancers

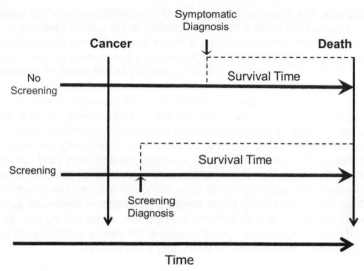

Fig. 1. Lead-time bias. Each of a pair of twins is destined to develop cancer on the same day and die from cancer on the same day. One twin does not undergo screening and is diagnosed with cancer because of symptoms. The other twin is diagnosed with cancer when he undergoes screening. If it is not known that they are destined to live the exact same number of days in their entire life, it would be observed that the second twin survives longer with his cancer than the first twin. But in fact, screening did not extend his life; it only increased the proportion of his life with a diagnosis of cancer.

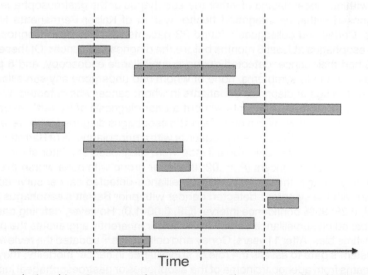

Fig. 2. Length-time bias. Cancers are heterogeneous. Slow-growing (less-fatal) cancers are represented by long bars (duration of time a patient is alive with the cancer). Fast-growing (more fatal) cancers are represented by short bars. In this example, the prevalence of slow-growing and fast-growing cancers is equal (there are 6 of each type). Surveillance is performed at the 4 times represented by the dashed lines. Because the slow-growing cancers are present for a longer period, surveillance is inherently more likely to identify slow-growing tumors (all 6 in this example), but miss fast-growing tumors (only 2 of 6 are detected in this example).

that are less fatal. The observed longer survival in surveillance-detected cases could be entirely because of the differences in the biology of the tumors detected by surveillance versus symptom-detected tumors and not a causal effect of surveillance. The potential for length-time bias can be aggravated by the manner in which cases and controls are classified. For instance, in one analysis of the effect of surveillance of Barrett's esophagus, the cases were defined as cancers detected by surveillance and controls as cancers detected by symptoms in the interval between surveillance. Such a design inherently compares slow-growing to fast-growing cancers; the investigators found a strong inverse association between surveillance (and likely preferential detection of slow-growing cancers) and mortality.[12] Analyzing the data from the same population in a different manner wherein patients with fatal cancer were compared with those with Barrett's esophagus for the presence of a prior endoscopy, the same investigators strikingly found no evidence of a protective effect of endoscopy.[13] The only way to entirely avoid length-time effects in studies of surveillance (even in randomized trials) is to perform surveillance so frequently that all tumors are detected by surveillance and not in the interval between surveillance (for instance, in an absurd scenario, with weekly or even daily endoscopies).

EMPIRICAL STUDIES OF THE EFFECTIVENESS OF SURVEILLANCE ENDOSCOPY

There have not been any published randomized trials of surveillance in Barrett's esophagus. Several retrospective studies have suggested that prior upper endoscopy among patients with EAC is associated with earlier stage of cancer at the time of initial diagnosis and improved survival. One must pay careful attention to the design of those studies in order to interpret the results. For instance, in a retrospective review of 589 patients with adenocarcinoma of either the esophagus or the gastroesophageal junction diagnosed within an integrated health system of Kaiser Permanente Northern California, Corley and colleagues[12] found 23 patients who had been diagnosed with Barrett's esophagus at least 6 months before the diagnosis of cancer. Of these 23 patients, 15 had their cancer detected during a surveillance endoscopy, and 8 patients were detected due to symptoms, none of whom had undergone any surveillance endoscopies. The age at diagnosis of patients in whom cancer was detected by surveillance was similar to that of patients without a prior diagnosis of Barrett's esophagus, but less than that of those with a prior Barrett's esophagus diagnosis who were not undergoing surveillance. The cancers in patients with a prior diagnosis of Barrett's esophagus who were not undergoing surveillance were diagnosed at a later stage than the surveillance-detected cancers ($P = .02$; the latter group with none worse than stage IIA). Adjusting for age, the patients with surveillance-detected cancer survived longer than those with the symptom-detected cancer with prior Barrett's esophagus (hazard ratio [HR], 0.25; 95% confidence interval [CI], 0.06–1.0). However, defining cases and controls based on surveillance detection of cancer inherently aggravates the potential for length-time bias. After 11 years, Corley and colleagues[13] updated the review of their health system's data to assess the role of surveillance in cancer mortality; they identified 38 deaths from adenocarcinoma of the esophagus or gastroesophageal junction in patients with a diagnosis of Barrett's esophagus at least 6 months before their cancer diagnosis and compared these to 101 patients with Barrett's esophagus matched for age, sex, and year of Barrett's esophagus diagnosis. In this analysis, they did not find any association between cancer mortality and receipt of surveillance endoscopy within 3 years prior (odds ratio [OR], 0.99, 95% CI, 0.36–2.75).

In a case-control study within the US Veterans Health Administration, Kearney and colleagues[14] identified 245 cases of death from adenocarcinoma of the esophagus or gastric cardia in patients diagnosed with gastroesophageal reflux disease (GERD) using International Classification of Diseases diagnostic billing codes, and compared them to 980 controls with GERD, matched for age, sex, and race. Receipt of a prior upper endoscopy at least 1 year prior was associated with a decreased odds of death from cancer (OR, 0.66; 95% CI, 0.45–0.96), but the investigators noted that none of the controls had been diagnosed with EAC and none had undergone esophagectomy, raising the likelihood that the results were biased in some way. For instance, those who underwent upper endoscopy may have been more conscious of their health and may have had other health-conscious habits such as avoidance of tobacco, healthy diet, and exercise, which were not measured. The author's group also examined the effect of prior upper endoscopy on patients with EAC with GERD using the same database.[15] Differences in the analysis were that data from 4 additional years were included, all subjects were required to have at least 1 encounter with the Veterans Health Administration in each of the 5 years preceding the diagnosis of cancer, and electronic medical records were reviewed to verify case status, dates of endoscopies, stage at diagnosis, and follow-up. From 311 potential subjects using administrative data, 155 subjects with EAC and a prior diagnosis of GERD were verified. Of the 155 subjects with EAC, 25 cases had undergone upper endoscopy between 1 and 5 years before the diagnosis of cancer. Those undergoing prior upper endoscopy were diagnosed at an earlier stage ($P = .03$), but there was no survival benefit (HR, 0.93; 95% CI, 0.58–1.50, adjusting for age, comorbidities, and year of diagnosis). Adherence with the recommended interval of surveillance (eg, 3 years for nondysplastic Barrett's esophagus), trended toward an association with improved survival (adjusted HR, 0.52; 95% CI, 0.24–1.12), but even among patients who did not undergo cancer resection, there seemed to be an association between adherence and survival (adjusted HR, 0.42; 95% CI, 0.16–1.09). This observation suggests that even if there had been a statistically significant association between surveillance and survival from EAC, it may not be a causal relation, but instead the result of bias such as selection of health-conscious patients for endoscopy and other biases described below.

In an analysis of the US Surveillance, Epidemiology, and End Results (SEER) cancer registry linked to Medicare data, Cooper and colleagues[16] identified 777 patients with EAC who were at least 70 years old at diagnosis. An upper endoscopy was performed at least 1 year before cancer diagnosis in 13%, but Barrett's esophagus was coded in only 7%. The stage of cancer was earlier in those with a prior upper endoscopy (62% vs 35% local cancer or dysplasia; notably, approximately 12% of the patients with a prior upper endoscopy and classified as having cancer by the study actually only had dysplasia). Patients classified with EAC with a prior upper endoscopy had longer median survival time (7 months vs 5 months, $P<.01$). Adjusting for age, sex, race, and comorbidities, prior upper endoscopy was associated with improved survival (HR, 0.73; 95% CI, 0.57–0.93). Results were similar for patients who not only underwent a prior upper endoscopy but also were diagnosed with Barrett's esophagus.

Cooper and colleagues[17] updated their analysis of the SEER-Medicare linked database 7 years later but limited the newer analysis to the receipt of an upper endoscopy between 6 months and 3 years before the diagnosis of EAC and lowered the minimum age to 68 years. A total of 2754 patients with EAC were identified, 11.5% of whom had undergone upper endoscopy within the defined time, and Barrett's esophagus was coded in 8.1%. Among those who had undergone prior upper endoscopy, the median number of prior endoscopies was 4. A prior diagnosis of Barrett's esophagus was more strongly associated with both earlier stage and improved survival than merely a prior upper endoscopy (for survival: prior Barrett's esophagus HR, 0.45; 95% CI, 0.25–0.80 vs prior endoscopy HR, 0.66; 95% CI, 0.47–0.93).

Verbeek and colleagues[18] analyzed data from the Netherlands National Cancer Registry linked to a nationwide pathology registry. The investigators identified 9780 cases of EAC, 791 (8%) of whom had a diagnosis of Barrett's esophagus at least 1 year before the cancer diagnosis, including 452 undergoing adequate surveillance (defined as at least 1 additional set of biopsies performed within 1.5 times the recommended interval; eg, 4.5 years for nondysplastic Barrett's esophagus). Those classified as undergoing adequate surveillance were more likely to be detected at stage I (47% vs 18% for inadequate surveillance, 17% for no surveillance but prior diagnosis of Barrett's esophagus, and 6% for no known prior Barrett's esophagus). Adequate surveillance was associated with improved 5-year survival compared with those without a prior diagnosis of Barrett's esophagus (OR, 0.74; 95% CI, 0.58–0.94, adjusting for sex, age, year of diagnosis, academic vs community hospital, location of tumor, stage, differentiation, and type of treatment). Although Barrett's esophagus with inadequate surveillance or without surveillance were both associated with improved survival in univariate analysis, there were no associations in the adjusted analyses. The definition for adequate surveillance used in this study aggravates the potential for length-time bias because patients with only 1 endoscopy before the diagnosis of EAC would be classified as no surveillance, even if that procedure had been performed within 4.5 years of the cancer diagnosis. This fact likely explains why patients classified as not undergoing surveillance had a shorter interval between diagnosis of Barrett's esophagus and EAC than those classified as adequate surveillance (median 5.2 years vs 7.5 years). Patients with inadequate surveillance were older at the time of diagnosis than those with adequate surveillance but had longer interval between diagnosis of Barrett's esophagus and EAC (median 12.6 years), suggesting that their age at diagnosis of Barrett's esophagus may have been similar. As the survival analyses were conducted starting at the age of diagnosis of cancer, this suggests that at least some of the observed association between adequate surveillance and survival is likely because of lead-time bias. Strangely, the association of adequate surveillance with survival persisted after adjusting for stage and treatment modality; if the effect of surveillance is mediated through earlier stage at diagnosis and greater likelihood of surgical resection, then it should be expected that association with adequate surveillance should no longer be evident after adjusting for those factors. This suggests that at least some of the observed association between surveillance and survival is biased by length-time effects and/or confounded by other unmeasured factors such as comorbidities or health-conscious behaviors.

Recently, Bhat and colleagues[19] reported results from a population-based study in Northern Ireland. The investigators identified 716 cases of EAC, 52 (7.3%) of whom had a diagnosis of Barrett's esophagus at least 6 months prior. Those with a prior diagnosis of Barrett's esophagus were more likely to be diagnosed at stage I or II (44.2% vs 11.1%) and more likely to undergo surgical resection (50.0% vs 25.5%). Patients with EAC with a prior diagnosis of Barrett's esophagus seemed to survive longer (HR, 0.44; 95% CI, 0.30–0.64; adjusted for age, sex, and tumor grade). However, there was a survival benefit of prior Barrett's esophagus even in patients who did not undergo esophagectomy (HR, 0.50; 95% CI, 0.32–0.79), suggesting that the estimate of the effect was likely biased. The investigators attempted to adjust for the potential of lead-time bias by estimating the duration of asymptomatic, but clinically detectable cancer (the sojourn time) by comparing the average age at cancer diagnosis between those with and without prior Barrett's esophagus diagnosis (67.4 vs 69.9 years, a difference of 2.5 years). In the analysis adjusting for lead-time bias, the effect of a prior diagnosis of Barrett's esophagus on survival was attenuated (HR, 0.65; 95% CI, 0.45–0.95). The investigators also attempted to adjust for the potential of length-time bias by accounting for the relative proportions of low-grade differentiated tumors in both groups, and the expected survival difference between grades of differentiation, finding that it only slightly altered the estimate for the effect of prior diagnosis of Barrett's esophagus on survival.

In summary, several retrospective studies have observed apparent associations between surveillance and improved survival from EAC, but the results have not been consistent and the studies are prone to several important potential biases.

WHAT IS THE TRUE EFFECTIVENESS OF SURVEILLANCE?

Given the inherent predilection of studies of surveillance to be biased by lead-time and length-time effects, and the likely selection effects for health-conscious patients to undergo surveillance in the observational studies, the available empirical data on surveillance almost certainly overestimate the magnitude of the effect of surveillance of Barrett's esophagus on improving survival from EAC. Of the studies described above, there was no evidence of an effect of surveillance in the Kaiser Permanente Northern California system or in the US Veterans Health Administration, but both effect estimates had fairly wide CIs, which could allow for some substantial undetected effect. In the larger SEER-Medicare linked data set and in the much larger Dutch national study, the effect estimates for mortality ranged from 0.45 to 0.74. These effects should be interpreted as the best-case scenario; the true effect is likely weaker, and it is conceivable that there is no true effect. In the Northern Ireland study, which formally attempted to account for the potential for lead-time and length-time effects, a prior diagnosis of Barrett's esophagus was associated with an HR of approximately 0.65.

Notably, all the studies described estimated the effect of surveillance on survival from EAC. In the current era of endoscopic therapy, there is the potential for an additional effect of surveillance on preventing EAC. Endoscopic therapy in dysplastic Barrett's esophagus prevents progression to EAC, at least in the short term.[2,20] However, 60% to 67% of patients with Barrett's esophagus who have been adherent with surveillance and yet progressed to invasive cancer were never found to have high-grade dysplasia on any surveillance endoscopy and 30% to 54% were never found to have low-grade dysplasia either.[18,21] So even if endoscopic therapy could prevent progression to EAC in 100% of patients with dysplastic Barrett's esophagus, a substantial proportion of patients undergoing surveillance would still develop EAC. A randomized controlled trial of surveillance plus endoscopic therapy for dysplasia compared with no surveillance would be needed to better estimate the efficacy and effectiveness of surveillance.

COST-EFFECTIVENESS OF SURVEILLANCE

Several investigators have sought to estimate the cost-effectiveness of surveillance. These estimates depend on the effectiveness of surveillance, which is not known with much precision. For the purposes of their analyses, the investigators have all assumed that surveillance is indeed effective. Before the widespread advent of endoscopic therapy, Inadomi and colleagues[22] published a cost-effectiveness analysis, which found that screening for Barrett's esophagus and surveillance in patients with dysplasia was cost-effective, but that additionally performing surveillance in patients with nondysplastic Barrett's esophagus even as infrequently as every 5 years cost $596,000 per quality-adjusted life-year (QALY) gained; the typically accepted willingness-to-pay thresholds of society ranges from $50,000 to $250,000 per QALY. In a model incorporating endoscopic therapy for high-grade dysplasia and surveillance every 2 years for nondysplastic Barrett's esophagus, Gordon and colleagues[23] estimated that surveillance would prevent 28% of EAC and cost $60,858 per QALY. In a European model of long-segment Barrett's esophagus incorporating endoscopic therapy for high-grade dysplasia, Kastelein and colleagues[24] estimated that surveillance every 5 years cost €5283 per QALY compared with no surveillance. Surveillance every 4 years cost an additional €62,619 per QALY compared with every 5 years and surveillance every 3 years cost an additional €105,755 per QALY compared with every 4 years. Similar to the study by Inadomi and colleagues,[22] they found that a strategy of surveillance every 5 years without endoscopic therapy would cost €413,500 per QALY compared with no surveillance. The investigators concluded that the optimal strategy was surveillance every 5 years with endoscopic therapy for high-grade dysplasia. Although these studies do not prove that surveillance is effective, they demonstrate that if surveillance is indeed effective, then surveillance followed by endoscopic therapy for high-grade dysplasia is likely cost effective. However, surveillance of nondysplastic Barrett's esophagus without endoscopic therapy for high-grade dysplasia (as had been practiced for many years before the advent of endoscopic resection and radiofrequency ablation) was likely a very inefficient practice.

GUIDELINE RECOMMENDATIONS

The published guidelines regarding surveillance of Barrett's esophagus have evolved over time (**Table 1**). The 1998 guidelines from the American College of Gastroenterology recommended surveillance with biopsies every 2 to 3 years in patients without dysplasia

Table 1
A history of guideline recommendations regarding surveillance of Barrett's esophagus

Year	Society	Recommendation	Grade
1998	ACG[25]	Surveillance every 2–3 y after 2 sets of biopsies without dysplasia	N/A
2002	ACG[23]	Surveillance every 3 y after 2 sets of biopsies without dysplasia	N/A
2005	BSG[41]	Surveillance every 2 y	C (weakest)
2005	AGA[42]	Surveillance at 1 y, then every 5 y	N/A
2006	ASGE[43]	Surveillance at 1 y, then every 3 y	N/A
2007	FSDE[27]	Surveillance every 2 y for >6 cm, 3 y for 3–6 cm, and 5 y for <3 cm	N/A
2008	ACG[30]	Surveillance every 3 y after 2 sets of biopsies without dysplasia	N/A
2011	AGA[11]	Surveillance every 3–5 y	Weak
2012	DSGH[44]	Surveillance every 3 y	IIIB (on scale of IA to IV with IA being best-quality evidence)
2012	ACP[45]	Surveillance every 3–5 y	May be indicated
2012	ASGE[26]	Surveillance every 3–5 y	Low-quality evidence
2014	BSG[28]	Surveillance should be offered: • For ≥3 cm, every 2–3 y • For <3 cm with intestinal metaplasia, every 3–5 y	B C (weakest) C (weakest)

Abbreviations: ACG, American College of Gastroenterology; ACP, American College of Physicians; AGA, American Gastroenterology Association; ASGE, American Society for Gastrointestinal Endoscopy; BSG, British Society of Gastroenterology; DSGH, Danish Society of Gastroenterology and Hepatology; FSDE, French Society of Digestive Endoscopy; N/A, not applicable.
    Data from Refs.[11,23,25–28,30,41–45]

on at least 2 prior endoscopies (because of concern of sampling error for missing dysplasia on the first endoscopy).[25] The 2011 guidelines from the American Gastroenterology Association dropped the recommendation for a repeat endoscopy within 1 year after the initial diagnosis of Barrett's esophagus and gave a weak recommendation for surveillance every 3 to 5 years in nondysplastic Barrett's esophagus.[11] Similarly, the 2012 guidelines from the American Society for Gastrointestinal Endoscopy specifically recommended against surveillance at 1 year from the initial diagnosis and recommended surveillance every 3 to 5 years in nondysplastic Barrett's esophagus.[26] In 2007, the French Society of Digestive Endoscopy introduced the recommendation of surveillance interval stratified by the length of Barrett's esophagus.[27] The most recent guidelines from the British Society of Gastroenterology endorsed a similar framework.[28] All these recommendations have been characterized as weak and based on low-quality evidence. The general theme over time has been a prolongation of the recommended interval between surveillance, such that current US guidelines recommend surveillance every 3 to 5 years. The Choosing Wisely campaign of the American Board of Internal Medicine and Consumer Reports is aimed at decreasing overutilization of testing and therapy. In 2012, the American Gastroenterology Association included in its list for Choosing Wisely of Five Things Physicians and Patients Should Question surveillance endoscopy in Barrett's esophagus more frequently than every 3 years.

EMPIRICAL EVIDENCE FOR THE FREQUENCY OF SURVEILLANCE

Despite the trend toward recommendations for less-frequent surveillance intervals, there is very little empirical data to guide the decision about the correct interval. The initial recommendation of surveillance every 2 to 3 years was justified by the expectation that the incidence of EAC in nondysplastic Barrett's esophagus is likely low and more frequent surveillance would not be justified.[25] Some guidelines have cited the earlier case-control study within the US Veterans Health Administration described above, which found that an endoscopy performed between 2 and 4 years prior was the only interval studied that was statistically significantly associated with a decreased odds of death from EAC.[14] However, as described above, the investigators themselves noted that the results of the study were suspect because none of the controls were ever diagnosed with EAC or underwent esophagectomy, suggesting that the association of endoscopy (at any interval) with protection from EAC mortality was likely biased by selection effects. The trend toward recommendations of less-frequent intervals seems to be driven primarily by the emerging data that the true incidence of EAC in nondysplastic Barrett's esophagus is lower than it was believed when the initial guidelines were published. The cost-effectiveness analysis by Kastelein and colleagues[24] found that surveillance more frequently than every 5 years was expensive but did not examine surveillance intervals less frequent than every 5 years. Given the rarity of incident EAC in nondysplastic Barrett's esophagus, a surveillance interval as long as every 10 years might even be reasonable. On the other hand, if the transition from dysplasia to cancer is a rapid event, lengthening the interval of surveillance might substantially reduce the effectiveness of surveillance because most patients would develop their cancer in the interval between surveillances. For instance, in the Seattle Barrett's Esophagus Study cohort of patients with high-grade dysplasia under surveillance every 3 months, those who ultimately progressed to cancer had somatic chromosomal alterations present at the earliest 2 to 4 years before their cancer.[29] So it is unclear what the correct interval of surveillance should be. In light of the uncertainty, the very low incidence of EAC in Barrett's esophagus argues in favor of infrequent surveillance, if surveillance is performed at all.

BIOPSY PROTOCOL IN SURVEILLANCE

Guidelines have recommended biopsies of visible mucosal abnormalities in addition to random biopsies in 4 quadrants every 2 cm in nondysplastic Barrett's esophagus and every 1 cm in dysplastic Barrett's esophagus.[11,26,28,30] Unfortunately, adherence to the protocol has been demonstrated to be inversely associated with the length of Barrett's esophagus; patients with longer Barrett's esophagus and thus at highest risk of progression are the least likely to undergo an adequate biopsy regimen.[31,32] The observation of nonadherence in longer segments of Barrett's esophagus suggests that endoscopist fatigue, time pressures, and financial incentives may be responsible. Adherence to the biopsy protocol has been associated with an increased detection of dysplasia and cancer.[31,33] If one is going to undertake the risks and costs of surveillance, one ought to make certain that the surveillance endoscopy is as effective as possible, even if that requires a few more minutes for the procedure.

FUTURE DIRECTIONS

Although surveillance of Barrett's esophagus has been recommended, it is not clear if it is effective. A randomized trial of surveillance would provide higher-quality evidence regarding whether time is being wasted with surveillance. Such a trial would have to be very large, but the cost would be a very small proportion of the money currently spent on screening and surveillance in Barrett's esophagus. The efficiency of surveillance might be improved by developing and implementing risk-stratified strategies of surveillance. For instance, the French Society of Digestive Endoscopy and the British Society of Gastroenterology have recommended surveillance intervals stratified by the length of Barrett's esophagus.[27,28] Other potential clinical markers that could be leveraged for risk stratification include age, sex, obesity, tobacco use, and family history.[34–36] Aside from clinical markers, the use of molecular biomarkers might improve the efficiency of surveillance. Promising examples include loss of heterozygosity in the p53 gene, abnormally increased tetraploidy, aneuploidy, hypermethylated genes, and specific lectins.[37–39] Use of such markers to guide surveillance decisions could improve the cost-effectiveness of surveillance.[23] In addition, strategies that use adjunctive imaging technologies during endoscopy could improve the accuracy of detection of neoplasia, thereby decreasing the number of biopsies required and potentially lengthening the duration required between surveillance procedures. Finally, nonendoscopic technologies for performing surveillance, such as the cytosponge device, if both accurate and inexpensive could improve the effectiveness of surveillance, possibly at a lower cost than endoscopic surveillance.[40]

SUMMARY

Surveillance of Barrett's esophagus for incident dysplasia or EAC has become an accepted practice, receiving weak recommendations in favor from multiple specialty societies. Although the strategy makes good sense intuitively, the body of evidence supporting the practice is relatively weak and there are legitimate concerns that the practice may not be particularly effective. As such, there has been momentum toward at least decreasing the frequency of surveillance. In addition, if surveillance is undertaken, then evidence does demonstrate that an adequate biopsy protocol should be performed. Otherwise, endoscopists squander much of whatever chance they have for effectively reducing the burden of EAC.

REFERENCES

1. Hur C, Miller M, Kong CY, et al. Trends in esophageal adenocarcinoma incidence and mortality. Cancer 2013;119:1149–58.
2. Shaheen NJ, Sharma P, Overholt BF, et al. Radiofrequency ablation in Barrett's esophagus with dysplasia. N Engl J Med 2009;360:2277–88.
3. Pech O, May A, Manner H, et al. Long-term efficacy and safety of endoscopic resection for patients with mucosal adenocarcinoma of the esophagus. Gastroenterology 2014;146:652–60.e1.
4. Shaheen N, Crosby M, Bozymski E, et al. Is there publication bias in the reporting of cancer risk in Barrett's esophagus? Gastroenterology 2000;119:333–8.
5. Desai TK, Krishnan K, Samala N, et al. The incidence of oesophageal adenocarcinoma in non-dysplastic Barrett's oesophagus: a meta-analysis. Gut 2012;61:970–6.
6. Hvid-Jensen F, Pedersen L, Drewes AM, et al. Incidence of adenocarcinoma among patients with Barrett's esophagus. N Engl J Med 2011;365:1375–83.
7. Wani S, Falk G, Hall M, et al. Patients with nondysplastic Barrett's esophagus have low risks for developing dysplasia or esophageal adenocarcinoma. Clin Gastroenterol Hepatol 2011;9:220–7 [quiz: e26].
8. Wani S, Falk GW, Post J, et al. Risk factors for progression of low-grade dysplasia in patients with Barrett's esophagus. Gastroenterology 2011;141:1179–86.
9. Bhat S, Coleman HG, Yousef F, et al. Risk of malignant progression in Barrett's esophagus patients: results from a large population-based study. J Natl Cancer Inst 2011;103:1049–57.
10. de Jonge PJ, van Blankenstein M, Looman CW, et al. Risk of malignant progression in patients with Barrett's oesophagus: a Dutch nationwide cohort study. Gut 2010;59:1030–6.
11. Spechler SJ, Sharma P, Souza RF, et al. American gastroenterological association medical position statement on the management of Barrett's esophagus. Gastroenterology 2011;140:1084–91.
12. Corley DA, Levin TR, Habel LA, et al. Surveillance and survival in Barrett's adenocarcinomas: a population-based study. Gastroenterology 2002;122:633–40.
13. Corley DA, Mehtani K, Quesenberry C, et al. Impact of endoscopic surveillance on mortality from Barrett's esophagus–associated esophageal adenocarcinomas. Gastroenterology 2013;145:312–9.
14. Kearney DJ, Crump C, Maynard C, et al. A case-control study of endoscopy and mortality from adenocarcinoma of the esophagus or gastric cardia in persons with GERD. Gastrointest Endosc 2003;57:823–9.
15. Rubenstein JH, Sonnenberg A, Davis J, et al. Prior endoscopy does not improve long-term survival from esophageal adenocarcinoma among United States veterans. Am J Gastroenterol 2006;101:S46 [Abstract].
16. Cooper GS, Yuan Z, Chak A, et al. Association of prediagnosis endoscopy with stage and survival in adenocarcinoma of the esophagus and gastric cardia. Cancer 2002;95:32–8.
17. Cooper GS, Kou TD, Chak A. Receipt of previous diagnoses and endoscopy and outcome from esophageal adenocarcinoma: a population-based study with temporal trends. Am J Gastroenterol 2009;104:1356.
18. Verbeek RE, Leenders M, Ten Kate FJ, et al. Surveillance of Barrett's esophagus and mortality from esophageal adenocarcinoma: a population-based cohort study. Am J Gastroenterol 2014;109:1215–22.
19. Bhat SK, McManus DT, Coleman HG, et al. Oesophageal adenocarcinoma and prior diagnosis of Barrett's oesophagus: a population-based study. Gut 2015;64:20–5.

20. Phoa KN, van Vilsteren FG, Weusten BL, et al. Radiofrequency ablation vs endoscopic surveillance for patients with Barrett esophagus and low-grade dysplasia: a randomized clinical trial. JAMA 2014;311:1209–17.
21. Rubenstein JH, Sonnenberg A, Davis J, et al. Effect of a prior endoscopy on outcomes of esophageal adenocarcinoma among United States veterans. Gastrointest Endosc 2008;68:849–55.
22. Inadomi JM, Sampliner R, Lagergren J, et al. Screening and surveillance for Barrett esophagus in high-risk groups: a cost-utility analysis. Ann Intern Med 2003;138:176–86.
23. Gordon LG, Mayne GC, Hirst NG, et al. Cost-effectiveness of endoscopic surveillance of non-dysplastic Barrett's esophagus. Gastrointest Endosc 2014;79: 242–56.e6.
24. Kastelein F, van Olphen S, Steyerberg EW, et al. Surveillance in patients with long-segment Barrett's oesophagus: a cost-effectiveness analysis. Gut 2014. [Epub ahead of print].
25. Sampliner RE. Practice guidelines on the diagnosis, surveillance, and therapy of Barrett's esophagus. The Practice Parameters Committee of the American College of Gastroenterology. Am J Gastroenterol 1998;93:1028–32.
26. Evans JA, Early DS, Fukami N, et al. The role of endoscopy in Barrett's esophagus and other premalignant conditions of the esophagus. Gastrointest Endosc 2012; 76:1087–94.
27. Boyer J, Laugier R, Chemali M, et al. French Society of Digestive Endoscopy SFED guideline: monitoring of patients with Barrett's esophagus. Endoscopy 2007;39:840–2.
28. Fitzgerald RC, di Pietro M, Ragunath K, et al. British Society of Gastroenterology guidelines on the diagnosis and management of Barrett's oesophagus. Gut 2014; 63:7–42.
29. Li X, Galipeau PC, Paulson TG, et al. Temporal and spatial evolution of somatic chromosomal alterations: a case-cohort study of Barrett's esophagus. Cancer Prev Res (Phila) 2014;7:114–27.
30. Wang KK, Sampliner RE. Practice parameters committee of the American college of G. Updated guidelines 2008 for the diagnosis, surveillance and therapy of Barrett's esophagus. Am J Gastroenterol 2008;103:788–97.
31. Abrams JA, Kapel RC, Lindberg GM, et al. Adherence to biopsy guidelines for Barrett's esophagus surveillance in the community setting in the United States. Clin Gastroenterol Hepatol 2009;7:736–42 [quiz: 710].
32. Curvers WL, Peters FP, Elzer B, et al. Quality of Barrett's surveillance in the Netherlands: a standardized review of endoscopy and pathology reports. Eur J Gastroenterol Hepatol 2008;20:601–7.
33. Fitzgerald RC, Saeed IT, Khoo D, et al. Rigorous surveillance protocol increases detection of curable cancers associated with Barrett's esophagus. Dig Dis Sci 2001;46:1892–8.
34. Hardikar S, Onstad L, Blount PL, et al. The role of tobacco, alcohol, and obesity in neoplastic progression to esophageal adenocarcinoma: a prospective study of Barrett's esophagus. PLoS One 2013;8:e52192.
35. Coleman HG, Bhat S, Johnston BT, et al. Tobacco smoking increases the risk of high-grade dysplasia and cancer among patients with Barrett's esophagus. Gastroenterology 2012;142:233–40.
36. Prasad GA, Bansal A, Sharma P, et al. Predictors of progression in Barrett's esophagus: current knowledge and future directions. Am J Gastroenterol 2010; 105:1490–502.

37. Jin Z, Cheng Y, Gu W, et al. A multicenter, double-blinded validation study of methylation biomarkers for progression prediction in Barrett's esophagus. Cancer Res 2009;69:4112–5.
38. Bird-Lieberman E, Dunn J, Coleman H, et al. Population-based study reveals new risk-stratification biomarker panel for Barrett's esophagus. Gastroenterology 2012;143:927–35.e3.
39. Reid BJ, Levine DS, Longton G, et al. Predictors of progression to cancer in Barrett's esophagus: baseline histology and flow cytometry identify low- and high-risk patient subsets. Am J Gastroenterol 2000;95:1669–76.
40. Kadri SR, Lao-Sirieix P, O'Donovan M, et al. Acceptability and accuracy of a non-endoscopic screening test for Barrett's oesophagus in primary care: cohort study. BMJ 2010;341:c4372.
41. Watson A, Heading RC, Shepherd NA. Guidelines for the diagnosis and management of Barrett's columnar-lined oesophagus. 2005. Available at: http://www.bsg.org.uk/bsgdisp1.php?id=3f4a76385e42599499e9&h=1&sh=1&i=1&b=1&m=00023. Accessed January 22, 2007.
42. Wang KK, Wongkeesong M, Buttar NS. American Gastroenterological Association medical position statement: role of the gastroenterologist in the management of esophageal carcinoma. Gastroenterology 2005;128:1468–70.
43. Hirota W, Zuckerman M, Adler D, et al. ASGE guideline: the role of endoscopy in the surveillance of premalignant conditions of the upper GI tract. Gastrointest Endosc 2006;63:570–80.
44. Bremholm L, Funch-Jensen P, Eriksen J, et al. Barrett's esophagus. Diagnosis, follow-up and treatment. Dan Med J 2012;59:C4499.
45. Shaheen NJ, Weinberg DS, Denberg TD, et al. Upper endoscopy for gastro-esophageal reflux disease: best practice advice from the clinical guidelines committee of the American College of Physicians. Ann Intern Med 2012;157:808–16.

Epidemiology and Diagnosis of Acute Nonvariceal Upper Gastrointestinal Bleeding

Gianluca Rotondano, MD

KEYWORDS

- Nonvariceal bleeding • Epidemiology • Diagnosis • Risk factors • Peptic ulcer
- Endoscopy • Timing

KEY POINTS

- There is a trend toward a decrease in the overall incidence and hospitalization for nonvariceal upper gastrointestinal bleeding (UGIB) worldwide. Peptic ulcer is still the most common cause of hemorrhage.
- The changing epidemiology is characterized by an aging population, with multiple comorbidities and increased use of aspirin, nonsteroidal antiinflammatory drugs (NSAIDs), or other antiplatelets/anticoagulants.
- Mortality for UGIB is still approximately 5% and is usually related to multiorgan failure, cardiopulmonary conditions, and end-stage malignancy.
- Endoscopy is the mainstay in the management of UGIB, allowing for proper diagnosis, risk stratification, and treatment of the bleeding lesion.
- Unless contraindicated, endoscopy should be performed within 24 hours of patient presentation to maximize benefits and improve economic outcomes.

EPIDEMIOLOGY OF ACUTE NONVARICEAL UPPER GASTROINTESTINAL BLEEDING

UGIB is predominantly nonvariceal in origin and remains one of the most common challenges faced by gastroenterologists and endoscopists in daily clinical practice. Despite major advances in the approach to the management of nonvariceal UGIB over the past 2 decades, including prevention of peptic ulcer bleeding, optimal use of endoscopic therapy, and adjuvant high-dose proton pump inhibitors (PPIs), it still carries considerable morbidity, mortality, and health economic burden.

This article originally appeared in Gastroenterology Clinics, Volume 43, Issue 4, December 2014.
The author has no conflict of interest to disclose.
Division of Gastroenterology & Digestive Endoscopy, Hospital Maresca, ASLNA3sud, Via Montedoro, Torre del Greco 80059, Italy
E-mail address: gianluca.rotondano@virgilio.it

Incidence of Acute Upper Gastrointestinal Bleeding

With more than 300,000 hospital admissions annually in the United States,[1,2] UGIB is one of the most common gastrointestinal (GI) emergencies. A 2012 update on the burden of GI disease in the United States reports that GI hemorrhage still ranked 7th among the principal GI discharge diagnoses from hospital admissions in 2009, with a 22% increase compared with year 2000, and 10th among causes of death from GI and liver diseases.[3]

The incidence rates of UGIB demonstrate a large geographic variation, ranging from 48 to 160 cases per 100,000 population per year, with consistent reports of higher incidences among men and the elderly.[4–10] Possible explanations for the reported geographic variations in incidence are differences in definition of UGIB in various studies, population characteristics, prevalence of gastroerosive medications, in particular aspirin and NSAIDs, and *Helicobacter pylori* prevalence.

Some but not all time-trend studies have reported a significant decline in incidence of all-cause acute UGIB, especially peptic ulcer bleeding, in recent years. In the Netherlands, the incidence of UGIB decreased from 61.7/100,000 in 1993/1994 to 47.7/100,000 persons annually in 2000, corresponding to a 23% decrease in incidence after age adjustment.[6,7] This was confirmed in a population-based study carried out in Northern Italy in which the overall incidence of UGIB decreased from 112.5 to 89.8/100,000 per year, which corresponds to a 35.5% decrease after adjustment for age.[8] Trends for incidence of hospitalization due to GI complications in the United States from 2001 to 2009 confirm decreases in UGIB (78.4–60.6/100,000) and peptic ulcer bleeding (48.7–32.1/100,000).[11] The reasons for the observed decrease in hospitalizations due to nonvariceal UGIB are not well defined, but it is reasonable to assume that the use of eradication therapy in patients with ulcer disease and the progressive increase in the implementation of preventive strategies in patients taking aspirin and NSAIDs may have played a role.[12–14]

Outcome data from multicenter observational registries of UGIB, originating from Italy,[15] Canada,[16] and the United Kingdom,[17] reported a mean age of bleeders over 60 years and a prevalence of UGIB in men. In-hospital bleeding (ie, GI hemorrhage that occurs in patients already hospitalized for another medical-surgical condition) occurs in 10% to 25%.[7,18–20]

Causes of Acute Upper Gastrointestinal Bleeding

Peptic ulcer bleeding is still the most common cause of nonvariceal UGIB, responsible for approximately 31% to 67% of all cases, followed by erosive disease, esophagitis, malignancy, and Mallory-Weiss tears. In 2% to 8% of cases, uncommon causes, such as Dieulafoy lesion, hemobilia, angiodysplasia, vascular-enteric fistula, and gastric antral vascular ectasia are found (**Table 1**).[6–9,15–17,21–26]

In recent years, there has been an overall decrease in the incidence of UGIB related to bleeding peptic ulcers, at least in subjects under 70 years of age,[8] whereas its incidence is stable or even higher among patients of more advanced age.[27] A study from Australia on bleeding ulcers over a 10-year period (1997–2007) confirmed that the number of bleeding ulcers remained unchanged despite a decreased incidence of uncomplicated peptic ulcer.[28] Gastric ulcers increased significantly in both bleeding and nonbleeding patients whereas the proportion of duodenal ulcers fell significantly. The proportion of bleeding ulcers related to NSAIDs or aspirin increased significantly over 10 years, from 51% to 71%. Gastroduodenal ulcers are also the most frequent causes of nonvariceal bleeding in cirrhotic patients (48%–51%).[29,30]

Table 1	
Causes of upper gastrointestinal bleeding according to recent epidemiologic studies	
	%
Peptic ulcer	31–67
Erosive disease	7–31
Variceal bleeding	4–20
Esophagitis	3–12
Mallory-Weiss tears	4–8
Malignancy	2–8
Vascular lesions	2–8
None (no lesion identified)	3–19

Data from Refs.[8,15–17,24,33]

Nonvariceal UGIB is not just about peptic ulcers. According to different registries, nonvariceal nonulcer bleeding accounts for 34% to 64% of all presenting cases of nonvariceal UGIB.[15–17] Recent data from Italy[31] show that patients with Dieulafoy lesions have high rebleeding rates (19.1%); although rare causes of nonvariceal UGIB, they can cause torrential bleeding and can be difficult to locate. Patients with Dieulafoy lesions were more likely to present with hematemesis, shock, syncope, and a lower hemoglobin concentration and require blood transfusion compared with patients presenting with other endoscopic diagnoses. Of greater concern was the reported rebleeding rate for Mallory-Weiss tears (6.3%), traditionally considered benign, low-risk, and self-limiting lesions. It is possible that this may represent endoscopic undertreatment because of the perceived low-risk nature of Mallory-Weiss tears but also raises questions regarding uniform diagnostic criteria.

The source and outcomes of UGIB in oncologic patients are poorly investigated. The causes of UGIB in oncologic patients seem to be different from those in the general population. Retrospective data on 324 patients with cancer referred for endoscopy due to UGIB[32] showed that tumor was the most common cause of bleeding (23.8%), followed by varices (19.7%), peptic ulcer (16.3%), and gastroduodenal erosions (10.9%). If considering only patients with tumors outside the GI tract, however, the most common causes of UGIB are similar to those in the general population, that is, peptic ulcer, gastroduodenal erosions, and varices. On the other hand, even in patients with tumors outside the GI tract, metastases were the source of bleeding in a significant number of patients (11%).

Risk Factors for Acute Nonvariceal Upper Gastrointestinal Bleeding

Risk factors for peptic ulcer bleeding are H pylori infection, use of NSAIDs, use of low-dose aspirin, and other antiplatelet medications or oral anticoagulants.

Helicobacter pylori infection
H pylori infection is found in 43% to 56% of peptic ulcer bleeding patients.[15–17,23,33] The true H pylori prevalence in bleeding peptic ulcer is probably underestimated: in a recent meta-regression on 71 studies, including 8496 patients, the mean prevalence of H pylori infection in peptic ulcer bleeding was 72%.[34] The most significant variables associated with a high prevalence of H pylori infection were the use of a diagnostic test delayed until at least 4 weeks after the bleeding episode (odds ratio [OR] 2.08; 95% CI, 1.10–3.93) and a lower mean age of patients (OR 0.95 per

additional year; 95% CI, 0.92–0.99). The low prevalence of *H pylori* infection reported in peptic ulcer bleeding may be due to the methodology of the studies and to patient characteristics. These data also support the recent recommendations of an international consensus on nonvariceal UGIB[35] regarding the performance of a delayed diagnostic test when *H pylori* tests carried out during the acute bleeding episode are negative.

The incidence of *H pylori*–negative idiopathic bleeding ulcers (ie, those not related to NSAIDs or other gastroerosive medications) is rising. These bleeding ulcers account for 16.1% of patients admitted for UGIB and 42.4% of patients who bled while in the hospital.[36] These ulcers are also prone to recurrent complications at 12 months: 13.4% (95% CI, 7.3%–19.5%) versus 2.5% (95% CI, 0.4%–4.6%) in patients with *H pylori*–positive ulcers who received eradication therapy.[36]

H pylori–negative bleeding ulcers are also associated with poorer outcomes regardless of use of NSAIDs. In a study from the University of Texas, patients without *H pylori* infection had significantly more comorbid medical conditions and higher Charlson index comorbidity scores than those with *H pylori*. Recurrent bleeding within 30 days was more frequent (11% vs 5%, $P = .009$) and hospital length of stay was significantly longer compared with *H pylori*–positive patients.[37] Such outcome data confirm previous findings of significantly higher incident rates of rebleeding and death in patients with *H pylori*-negative idiopathic ulcers than in controls with *H pylori*–positive bleeding ulcers. Moreover, gastroprotective agents, such as PPIs or H_2-receptor antagonists, did not reduce the risk of recurrent bleeding or mortality for patients with *H pylori*–negative idiopathic bleeding ulcers.[38]

Current guidelines recommend testing for *H pylori* infection among users of low-dose aspirin who are at high risk for developing ulcers, because the long-term incidence of rebleeding with aspirin use is reduced after *H pylori* is eradicated.[35] This was confirmed by a recent prospective study from Hong Kong,[39] in which the incidence of ulcer bleeding (per 100 patient-years) in the *H pylori*–eradicated cohort did not differ significantly from that of the average-risk cohort (no history of ulcers). Aspirin users without current or past *H pylori* infections who develop ulcer bleeding have a 5-fold incidence of recurrent bleeding.

Low-dose aspirin, antiplatelets, and nonsteroidal antiinflammatory drugs

Long-term use of aspirin is recommended for prevention of cardiovascular events among patients with prior cardiovascular disease or multiple risk factors.[40] Regular aspirin use is associated with an increased risk of major GI bleeding. A recent meta-analysis found an approximately 2-fold higher risk of GI bleeding among individuals regularly using aspirin compared with placebo, with no difference between 75 to 162.5 mg/d and greater than 162.5 to 325 mg/d.[41] Such a magnitude of risk is confirmed by a large prospective study of 87,680 women in which the relative risk (RR) of major UGIB requiring hospitalization or blood transfusion was 1.43 (95% CI, 1.29–1.59) over a 24-year follow-up period.[42] Furthermore, when used for primary prevention of cardiovascular disease, the absolute harms of aspirin seem to exceed its benefits: a meta-analysis of 27 studies showed that 60 to 84 major cardiovascular events per 100,000 person-years were averted, whereas 68 to 117 GI bleeds were incurred. There was a nonsignificant change in total cardiovascular disease, whereas risks were increased by 37% for GI bleeds.[43] Risk factors for UGIB among low-dose aspirin users include (1) a history of peptic ulcer disease or GI bleeding; (2) older age; (3) concomitant use of NSAIDs, including cyclooxygenase (COX)-2 inhibitors; (4) concomitant use of anticoagulants or other platelet aggregation inhibitors; (5) the presence of severe medical comorbidities; and (6) high aspirin dose. *H pylori* and aspirin seem to be independent risk factors for peptic ulcer bleeding, so that in patients with a history of peptic ulcer disease, *H pylori* infection should be assessed and treated if present.[44]

At-risk low-dose aspirin users are recommended to take gastroprotective agents. PPIs seem superior to eradication only to prevent recurrent ulcer bleeding in patients using low-dose aspirin.[35] Moreover, in patients with acute coronary syndrome or myocardial infarction receiving aspirin, clopidogrel, enoxaparin, or thrombolytics, PPIs are superior to H_2-receptor antagonists.[45]

Population-based epidemiologic data confirm that the use of low-dose aspirin, NSAIDs, warfarin, and the combination thereof are significantly more common among UGI bleeders than nonbleeders.[8,15–17,21,22,25] An increasing proportion of patients are nowadays hospitalized due to medication-related UGIB. Comparing data from Italy and the United Kingdom, the proportion of UGIB patients taking NSAIDs or antiplatelet agents and that of patients on anticoagulants was almost identical (46.4% vs 44.2% and 11.7% vs 13.2%, respectively).[8,17] The increased risk of UGIB associated with NSAIDs seems lower than previously reported: in a Spanish primary care research database study of more than 660,000 subjects,[46] increased risks were found with current use of NSAIDs (RR 1.72; 95% CI, 1.41–2.09), low-dose aspirin (RR 1.74; 95% CI, 1.37–2.21), other antiplatelet drugs (RR 1.73; 95% CI, 1.27–2.36), and oral anticoagulants (RR 2.00; 95% CI, 1.44–2.77). The use of oral corticosteroids, selective serotonin reuptake inhibitors, or acetaminophen was not associated with an increased risk.

In patients at risk for GI bleeding and using NSAIDs, a protective drug is recommended.[35] Acid-suppressing drugs reduce the risk among users of NSAIDs (OR 0.58; 0.39–0.85), particularly in users with antecedent peptic ulcer (OR 0.16; 0.05–0.58).[47] Unfortunately, despite several society and national guidelines that have been formulated, these are poorly followed in clinical practice and gastroprotection is largely underused. Data from Europe show that although approximately one-half of all patients with peptic ulcer bleeding were using NSAIDs or aspirin, an effective gastroprotective agent was only used in 10% to 15% of at-risk patients.[7,23,47,48] A multinational study from the United Kingdom, Italy, and the Netherlands confirmed that the risk of UGIB is significantly higher in nonselective NSAID users with gastroprotective nonadherence. Among 618,684 nonselective NSAID users, nonadherers to gastroprotection had a 2-fold risk of UGIB (OR 1.89; 95% CI, 1.09–3.28).[49] Selective cyclooxygenase (COX)-2 inhibitors are associated with a lower risk of clinically significant UGIB than nonselective NSAIDs[7,48]; however, concerns over the possible cardiovascular adverse effects of some of these agents should be taken into account. Moreover, switching to selective COX-2 inhibitors in patients with previous bleeding is not completely risk-free, and concomitant PPI therapy may also be needed. The combination of COX-2 inhibitors with PPIs promotes the greatest risk reduction for NSAID-related UGIB.[48]

A retrospective study among general practitioners in France[50] documented that within 2 years after prescribing a PPI, physicians did not renew this prescription for approximately 33% of those patients at risk for GI events (>65 years, past history of GI ulcer, or receiving antiplatelet agents) receiving continuous NSAIDs. Predictors for no longer receiving a prescription for a PPI included switching to a COX-2 selective inhibitor or to a nonselective NSAID and female gender. The risk for upper GI injury was higher among patients with discontinued PPI prescriptions (OR 1.45; 95% CI, 1.06–2.09).

UGIB is a rare but serious potential side effect of bisphosphonate therapy. In a population-based nested cohort study in Canada within an exposure cohort of 26,223 subjects,[51] 117 individuals suffered a serious UGIB within 120 days of starting a bisphosphonate (0.4%). Age greater than 80 (adjusted OR 2.03; 95% CI, 1.40–2.94) and a past history of serious UGIB (adjusted OR 2.28; 95% CI, 1.29–4.03) were the strongest predictors. Men were 70% more likely to suffer an UGIB compared with women (adjusted OR 1.69; 95% CI, 1.05–2.72).

Patients with UGIB have increasing non-GI comorbidities. Results of a matched case-control study on 16,355 patients with nonvariceal UGIB and 81,636 controls showed that non-GI comorbidity had a strong association with UGIB; the adjusted OR for a single comorbidity was 1.43 (95% CI, 1.35–1.52) and for multiple or severe comorbidity was 2.26 (95% CI, 2.14–2.38). The additional population attributable fraction for comorbidity (19.8%; 95% CI, 18.4–21.2) was considerably larger than that for any other measured risk factor, including aspirin or NSAIDs use (3.0% and 3.1%, respectively).[52] Non-GI comorbidity is an independent risk factor for UGIB and contributes to a greater proportion of patients with bleeding in the population than other recognized risk factors. These findings could explain why the incidence of nonvariceal bleeding remains high in older populations.

Mortality from Acute Upper Gastrointestinal Bleeding

Despite advances in endoscopic hemostasis and adjuvant pharmacologic treatment, the overall mortality from UGIB remains 5% to 14%, although most studies from the United States, Europe, and Asia place that figure closer to 5%.[15–17,22,25] A systematic review of 18 studies (10 using administrative databases and 8 using bleeding registries) showed mortality rates from acute UGIB ranging from 1.1% in Japan to 11% in Denmark.[53] The 28-day mortality after nonvariceal UGIB in England decreased from 14.7% in 1999 to 13.1% in 2007.[54] A recent analysis of the trends for incidence of hospitalization and death due to UGIB in the United States from 2001 to 2009 confirmed that age/gender-adjusted case fatality owing to bleeding is low (2.5%) and increases with age but remains less than 5% even in elderly patients.[11] These discrepancies in reported mortality rates of nonvariceal UGIB are attributable to differences in study methodologies and populations studied (heterogeneous definitions of case ascertainment, differing patient populations with regard to severity of presentation and associated comorbidities, varying durations of follow-up, and different health care system-related practices). More uniform standards in reporting would enable a better understanding of causes of death and the apparent discrepant outcome in endoscopic end points versus clinical end points. Nonvariceal UGIB is now predominantly a disease of the elderly, with more than 60% of patients over the age of 60 years and approximately 20% over the age of 80 years.[8,15] Because elderly patients have more comorbid illness, are more likely users of aspirin and NSAIDs, and are less tolerant of hemodynamic insult, the management of this high-risk population is a major challenge.[55] Current evidence indicates that most peptic ulcer bleeding–linked deaths are not a direct sequela of the bleeding ulcer itself. Instead, mortality derives from multiorgan failure, cardiopulmonary conditions, or end-stage malignancy, suggesting that improving further current treatments for the bleeding ulcer may have a limited impact on mortality unless supportive therapies are developed for the global management of these patients.[18] In a prospective cohort study enrolling more than 10,000 cases of peptic ulcer bleeding at the Prince of Wales Hospital in Hong Kong,[22] one of the most reputed bleeding centers worldwide, overall mortality was 6.2%. The study reported that approximately 80% of deceased patients died of non–bleeding-related causes.

Risk factors for mortality after nonvariceal UGIB[6,15–17,22,24,25,55–57] are

- Increasing age
- Hemodynamic instability on admission
- Presence of severe and life-threatening comorbid medical conditions

Recent data from Italy also identified an American Society of Anesthesiologists (ASA) score of 3 or 4 versus 1 or 2 as the variable with the greatest OR for predicting mortality (OR 3.92; 95% CI, 2.37–6.50).[31] One or more comorbidities are present in almost two-thirds of UGIB patients.[15–17,21] Underlying comorbidity is consistently associated with an increased short-term mortality in patients with peptic ulcer bleeding. A systematic review and meta-analysis of 16 studies[58] showed that the risk of 30-day or in-hospital mortality was significantly greater in patients with comorbidity than in those without (RR 4.44; 95% CI, 2.45–8.04). Patients with 3 or more comorbidities had a greater risk of dying than those with 1 or 2 (RR 3.46; 95% CI, 1.34–8.89). Among individual comorbidities that significantly increased the risk of death, RRs were higher for hepatic, renal, and malignant disease (RR range, 4.04–6.33) than for cardiovascular and respiratory disease and diabetes (2.39, 2.45, and 1.63, respectively). Coagulation disorders are also independently associated with more than a 5-fold increase in the odds of in-hospital mortality.[59]

Cirrhotic patients suffering a nonvariceal bleed have significantly greater in-hospital mortality than noncirrhotic patients.[29,30,60] The presence of cirrhosis independently increased mortality (adjusted OR 3.3; 95% CI, 2.2–4.9). Decompensated cirrhosis had higher mortality than compensated cirrhosis.[60] Cryptogenic etiology of cirrhosis, renal dysfunction, actively bleeding ulcers on hospital admission, concurrent presence of duodenal ulcer and erosive disease, and bleeding from vascular lesions are all independent predictors of mortality.[29,30]

Impaired renal function is an independent risk factor for UGIB. Crude rates of acute nonvariceal UGIB among patients undergoing dialysis have not decreased in the past 10 years.[61] Although 30-day mortality related to UGIB declined, the burden on the end-stage renal disease population remains substantial. Overall 30-day mortality is 4.8% to 13.7%, with a 2-fold risk of death in peptic ulcer bleeding patients with end-stage renal disease compared with those without.[62,63] Such a high mortality in patients undergoing dialysis was significantly correlated with older age, female gender, infection during hospitalization, single episodic UGIB, abnormal white blood cell count, and albumin level less than or equal to 3 g/dL.[62]

Mortality is also increased in patients who are already admitted in hospital for another medical problem. In-hospital bleeding accounts for 10% to 25% of the overall nonvariceal bleeding population[7,19,20,33] and is associated with poorer outcome, with mortality rates as high as 26%.[8,15–17,19,21] Nonetheless, the reasons for increased mortality in this subgroup of patients have not been consistently identified. Guidelines on optimal management of inpatients who develop nonvariceal UGIB[35,64–66] have been derived essentially from studies on outpatient bleeding, whereas few data are available that focus on in-hospital bleeding and its management. Recent data from Italy shed some light on the issue, showing that the mortality rate for in-hospital bleeding was significantly higher than that of outpatient bleeding (8.9% vs 3.8%; OR 2.44; 95% CI, 1.57–3.79). Hemodynamic instability on presentation and the presence of severe comorbidity were the strongest predictors of mortality for in-hospital bleeders.[20]

The risk of mortality increases with rebleeding, which is thus another major outcome parameter. Rebleeding rates, using a combination of endoscopic hemostasis and adjuvant acid-suppressing therapy, have been shown to be reduced to less than 10%[21,22,25] and it would be difficult, if not impossible, to reduce this further. Because a majority of nonvariceal UGIB patients today are of advanced age, users of NSAIDs and aspirin, and with multiple comorbid illnesses, the "endeavor to further reduce this rebleeding rate is an uphill battle."[22]

Little is known about mortality associated with nonulcer, nonvariceal UGIB. This may stem from a perception among clinicians that, other than those patients with a GI malignancy as the causative bleeding lesion, outcomes of patients with nonulcer bleeding are favorable. Therefore, it is possible that the usual algorithms of postendoscopy care, pharmacotherapy, and monitoring that are applied to patients in whom endoscopic hemostasis has been achieved after peptic ulcer bleeding may not be applied with the same rigor to those with nonulcer bleeding. A large prospective, multicenter study of 3207 patients with documented nonulcer UGIB have a risk of death similar to bleeding peptic ulcers.[20] Mortality was 9.8% for neoplasia, 4.8% for Mallory-Weiss tears, 4.8% for vascular lesions, 4.4% for gastroduodenal erosions, 4.4% for duodenal ulcer, and 3.1% for gastric ulcer. Frequency of death was not different among benign endoscopic diagnoses. The strongest predictor of mortality was the overall ASA score. After adjusting for ASA score, the endoscopic diagnosis had no impact on mortality, suggesting that nonulcer causes of bleeding carry a risk of mortality similar to that of peptic ulcers. Therefore, even a bleed from what is perceived to be a minor lesion in a high-risk patient can be a sufficient precipitant to initiate a downward cascade of clinical events, resulting in multiorgan failure and death. The message could not be clearer: treat the patient and not just the source of GI bleeding.

DIAGNOSIS OF ACUTE NONVARICEAL UPPER GASTROINTESTINAL BLEEDING

Upper GI endoscopy is an essential part of UGIB management and is the mainstay of diagnosis and treatment of most causes of UGIB.[26]

Endoscopy seems to reduce mortality among patients hospitalized for UGIB and specialty care in a gastroenterology ward offers additional protective effects. In a prospective study on 13,427 hospitalizations for UGIB in Italy, the 30-day mortality was 6.9%. Significantly lower rates were observed among hospitalizations that included endoscopy (OR 0.30; 95% CI, 0.26–0.34), specialist care (OR 0.55; 95% CI, 0.37–0.82), or both (OR 0.12; 95% CI, 0.07–0.22). The protective effects of endoscopy and specialist care remained strong after adjustment for potential confounders.[67]

Endoscopy provides crucial prognostic data as to the risk for recurrent bleeding through the assessment of the stigmata of recent hemorrhage (ie, endoscopic appearance of the ulcer crater). These are categorized according to the Forrest classification, developed 4 decades ago and first published by Forrest and colleagues in *The Lancet* in 1974.[68] The purpose of the classification was initially to uniformly describe lesions that are or have been bleeding. The Forrest classification, however, has since been mostly used to stratify patients with ulcer bleeding into high- and low-risk categories for rebleeding and mortality (**Table 2**).[69] Several endoscopic findings portend a higher risk for recurrent bleeding and their recognition is essential for proper therapeutic planning. Endoscopic treatment is indicated for patients found to have active spurting (Forrest Ia) or oozing bleeding (Forrest Ib) (**Fig. 1**) and for those with a nonbleeding visible vessel (Forrest IIa, NBVV) (**Fig. 2**) in an ulcer. Overlying adherent clots (Forrest IIb) (**Fig. 3**) should be vigorously irrigated to evaluate and potentially treat any underlying lesion. The management of peptic ulcers with adherent clots that are resistant to removal by vigorous irrigation remains, however, controversial.[35] Ulcers with low-risk stigmata (ie, those with flat pigmented spots [Forrest IIc] of hematin or fibrin-covered clean base [Forrest III] [**Fig. 4**]) do not warrant any endoscopic intervention.[26,35,64–66]

A recent prospective reassessment of the predictive value of Forrest classification documented that it still has predictive value for rebleeding of peptic ulcers, especially

Table 2	
The Forrest classification of peptic ulcer hemorrhage	
Active hemorrhage	
Forrest Ia	Active spurting hemorrhage
Forrest Ib	Oozing hemorrhage
Signs of recent hemorrhage	
Forrest IIa	NBVV
Forrest IIb	Adherent clot
Forrest IIc	Flat pigmented spot on ulcer base
Lesions without active bleeding	
Forrest III	Clean-base ulcer

Data from Forrest JA, Finlayson ND, Shearman DJ. Endoscopy in gastrointestinal bleeding. Lancet 1974;2:394–7.

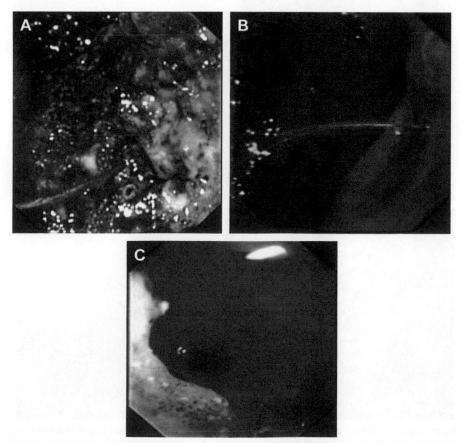

Fig. 1. Actively bleeding lesions: (*A*) malignant ulcerated lesion of the gastric angulus with a spurting arterial vessel; (*B*) an NSAID-related gastric ulcer in the upper portion of the gastric body with a brisk flow of arterial blood; and (*C*) oozing bleeding from an exposed vessel in a duodenal ulcer.

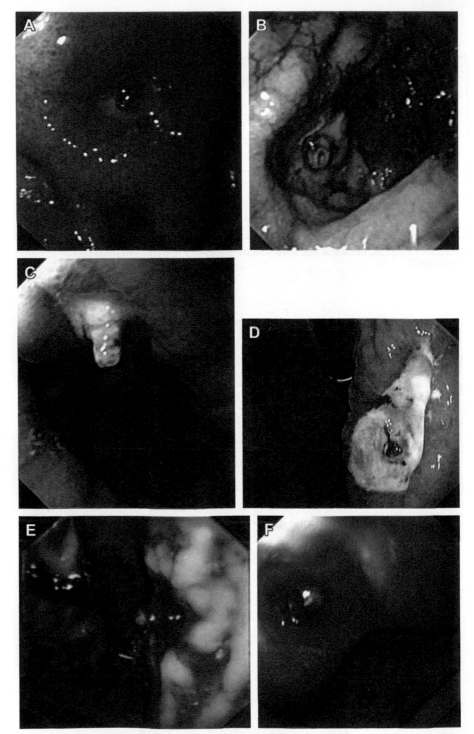

Fig. 2. Examples of NBVVs: (*A*) central pink-reddish slightly protuberant vessel in a duodenal ulcer; (*B*) ulcer of the pyloric channel with a white translucent eccentric vessel; (*C*) ulcer of the lesser curvature of the stomach with a protuberant white vessel; (*D*) retroflexed view of a gastric ulcer in the corpus with a brownish consolidated flattened vessel (sentinel clot); (*E*) ulcer of the gastric body showing a large protuberant aneurysmic dark red vessel seen in retroflexion; and (*F*) ulcer of the duodenal bulb with a red protuberant vessel.

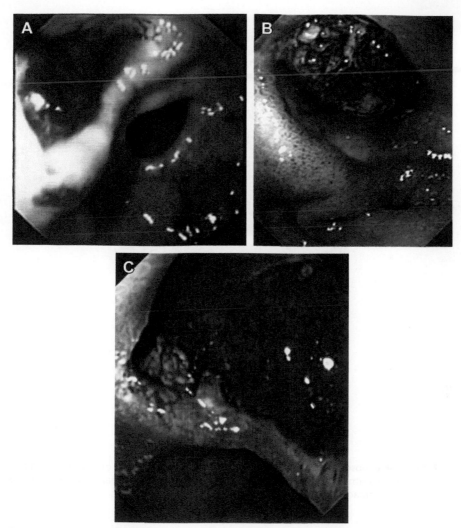

Fig. 3. Various types of adherent clots: (*A*) gastric ulcer with a freshly formed clot; (*B*) ulcer of the anterosuperior duodenal wall with an organized clot covering the ulcer base; and (*C*) a black hardened clot overlying the base of a duodenal bulb ulcer.

for gastric ulcers; however, it does not predict mortality.[70] Another study finding was that a proposed simplified classification into high risk (Forrest Ia), increased risk (Forrest Ib–IIc), and low risk (Forrest III) had similar test characteristics to the original Forrest classification.

The finding of an NBVV has been touted as a reliable predictor of the risk of recurrent bleeding and poor outcome.[69,71–73] Not all exposed vessels carry the same risk of recurrent bleeding, however, with pale, protuberant vessels shown much more risky than dark, flattened ones.[74] The distinction between NBVV and clots can be difficult[75,76]; hence the presence of an NBVV may not be in itself a sufficiently reliable indicator to select patients for invasive therapy. Enhanced endoscopic imaging of bleeding ulcers to identify and characterize an involved buried vessel may allow for more cost-effective management. Although the endoscopic Doppler ultrasound

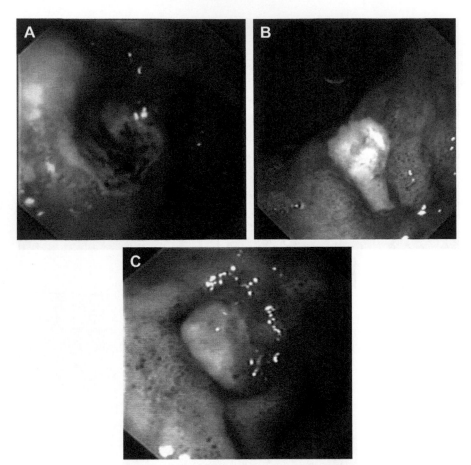

Fig. 4. Low-risk endoscopic stigmata: (*A*) flat gray sloughs of hematin on the base of an ulcer in the gastric antrum; (*B*) endoscopic view in retroflexion of a clean-base ulcer on the angulus of the stomach; and (*C*) clean-base duodenal bulb ulceration.

probes[77] have been proposed to evaluate the size and patency of underlying vessels, these systems have not gained widespread popularity. A pilot study from Italy investigated the role of magnification endoscopy in improving the characterization of exposed vessels in ulcer hemorrhage.[78] Zoom endoscopy after methylene blue staining provided clear images of the vessel and allowed visualization of the artery, the site of rupture, and the presence of a clot plugging the hole. A diagnostic gain (ie, an upgrading from low-to high-risk category of the vessel) was achieved in 33% of cases. No lesion was downstaged, possibly because frankly protruding reddish or pale vessels are already very clear under standard endoscopic visualization. The vessels that appear only slightly protuberant or that resemble clots or pigment spots were the ones most likely to be upgraded by magnification endoscopy.

Upper GI endoscopy in a bleeding patient should be carried out in an adequately equipped setting—the endoscopy suite or operating theater—by qualified endoscopists. A therapeutic endoscope with 3.7-mm operative working channel should be used. Scopes with 6-mm jumbo channels or double-channel scopes may occasionally be required. All devices for endoscopic hemostasis (injection needles and solutions, monopolar or bipolar thermal probes, and mechanical devices, such as hemoclips) should be available and ready to be used by skilled personnel. The use of modern high-frequency generators with built-in argon plasma coagulation modules is advisable. Patients should ideally be hemodynamically stable at the time of upper endoscopy. The assistance of an anesthesiologist is required in patients with severe hematemesis and endotracheal intubation should be considered in such selected cases to prevent aspiration.

The quality of endoscopy can be adversely affected by poor visibility in patients requiring urgent endoscopy with UGIB due to obscuring blood in the gastric lumen. In 3% to 19% of cases, no apparent cause of UGIB can be identified.[15,17,21,23,33] This may be related either to the aforementioned presence of food or blood debris hampering proper endoscopic visualization (in particular for awkwardly positioned lesions) or to the presence of faint lesions that are difficult to identify if not actively bleeding, specifically vascular lesions (**Fig. 5**). Apart from the routine use of

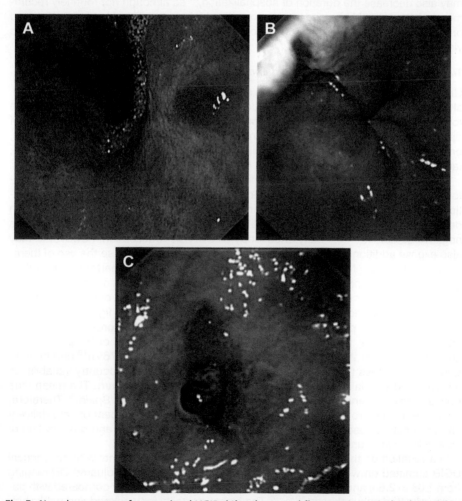

Fig. 5. Nonulcer causes of nonvariceal UGIB: (*A*) a cherry-red flat gastric angiodysplasia; (*B*) a Mallory-Weiss tear covered with hematin; and (*C*) a Dieulafoy lesion of the gastric fundus with an overlying clot.

water-jet irrigation and adequate suction applied to the endoscope, a patient may need to be rolled over in different positions to improve visibility. In cases of large fundic blood clots, a large-bore nasogastric or orogastric tube should be considered for inserting to empty the stomach and repeat the examination shortly thereafter. The systematic use of a nasogastric tube before endoscopy is not recommended,[35] but in selected patients it may offer important prognostic information. The presence of blood in the nasogastric aspirate is a significant predictor of high-risk stigmata at index upper endoscopy.[79]

Pre-endoscopic administration of intravenous erythromycin or metoclopramide (20–120 minutes before endoscopy) has been shown to reduce the need for repeat endoscopy to determine the site and cause of bleeding in patients with UGIB (OR 0.55; 95% CI, 0.32–0.94).[80] This is an important adjunct to treatment with regard to the ability to make a diagnosis, apply definitive treatment, and avoid unnecessary exposure of patients to repeat procedures; additional data show that the use of prokinetic agents may also decrease the duration of hospitalization,[81] so although not routinely recommended, they should be used in patients with a high probability of having fresh blood or a clot in the stomach when undergoing upper endoscopy to improve diagnostic yield.

Timing of Endoscopy: When Should Endoscopy Be Performed?

Urgent EGD has been proposed as the standard of care in patients with acute UGIB, although the optimal timing for early endoscopy is still uncertain. A 24-hour time frame for endoscopic examination is internationally recommended as the optimal window of opportunity,[35,64,66] especially for patients with a history of malignancy or cirrhosis, presentation with hematemesis, and signs of hypovolemia, including hypotension, tachycardia, hemodynamic shock, and hemoglobin less than 8 g/dL.[26]

Although no study has been able to show a direct reduction in mortality through performance of early endoscopy, available data from observational studies favor a reduction in length of hospital stay, recurrent bleeding, and need for surgery,[82–85] with decreased mortality in a subgroup analysis of patients at particularly high risk of a negative outcome.[57,85,86] Early endoscopy aids in risk stratification; however, it may also expose additional cases of active bleeding and hence increase the use of therapeutic intervention. No evidence exists that earlier endoscopy, performed less than 12 hours of patient presentation, can reduce the risk of rebleeding or improve survival compared with later (>24 hours) endoscopy.[87,88] In the UK audit, only 50% of all patients underwent endoscopy within 24 hours of presentation (a figure that had not improved from the previous audit performed 14 years earlier), probably related to the lack of 24-hour provision of emergency endoscopy in 48% of hospitals at the time of the audit in 2007.[17] These figures are better in Canada (76%)[16] and in other European countries (78%–81%),[15,21,24] despite a wide between-country variability in the area and speciality of the nonvariceal UGIB management team. The mean time from admission to endoscopy was less than 1 day only in Italy and Spain.[89] Therefore, there seems to be room for considerable improvement in this aspect of care delivery and this could be used as a key parameter to monitor standards and organization of care delivery in future studies of UGIB.

In a variation on this theme, several studies indicate that patients with nonvariceal UGIB admitted on weekends have higher in-hospital mortality (adjusted OR ranging from 1.08 to 2.68) and significantly lower rates of early endoscopy compared with patients admitted on weekdays.[10,90–92] The higher mortality for weekend and public holiday admissions could not be explained by measures of case mix and may indicate a possible impact of reduced staffing levels and delays to endoscopy on weekends in some hospitals. Also, when the quality of care did not seem to differ between weekday/weekend admissions, UGIB patients admitted during the weekend were at higher risk of an adverse outcome,[93] possibly because this subgroup is more likely to present with hemodynamic shock and hematemesis and receive red blood cell transfusion,[94] Nonetheless, in the UK audit there was no evidence of increased mortality for weekend versus weekday presentation despite patients being more critically ill and having greater delays to endoscopy on the weekends. The absence of a weekend effect on mortality from peptic ulcer bleeding was confirmed in a large Asian cohort of 8222 patients.[95] An overall 19.1% of patients were admitted on holidays and there was no difference in mortality between holiday versus weekday admissions (4.1% vs 4.0%). The waiting time for endoscopy was correlated with the risk of 30-day mortality. When therapeutic endoscopy can be offered within 1 day of hospital admission, holiday admission does not adversely affect bleeding mortality.[95]

In theory, the availability both of on-call physicians proficient in endoscopic hemostasis and on-call support staff with technical expertise in usage of endoscopic devices enables performance of endoscopy on a 24/7 basis. This is especially important to achieve in those countries that have demonstrated evidence of a weekend effect for UGIB mortality, including the United States[90–92] and Wales.[10] In contrast, no evidence of a weekend effect for mortality was found in Hong Kong[95] or in the United Kingdom.[94] In the latter case, there was even no difference in the risk of death for weekend compared with weekday presentation between patients presenting to hospitals with an out-of-hours endoscopy rota compared with those presenting to hospitals without such a facility, questioning the need for provision of 24/7 access to emergency endoscopy.

In appropriate settings, endoscopy can be used to assess the need for inpatient admission. Hemodynamically stable patients who are evaluated for UGIB with upper endoscopy and subsequently found to have low-risk stigmata for recurrent bleeding can be safely discharged and followed as outpatients, reducing the need for hospitalization and consequently hospital costs.[96,97]

In conclusion, upper GI endoscopy is the cornerstone of diagnosis and management of patients with UGIB. Early endoscopy (within 24 hours of patient presentation) ensures a correct identification of the bleeding source and allows risk stratification, valuable in allocating the patient to the adequate level of care. High-risk patients should be treated endoscopically and followed in monitored or high-dependency units. Low-risk patients can be safely discharged home or even be treated as outpatients.

REFERENCES

1. Yavorski RT, Wong RK, Maydonovitch C, et al. Analysis of 3,294 cases of upper gastrointestinal bleeding in military medical facilities. Am J Gastroenterol 1995; 90:568–73.
2. Longstreth GF. Epidemiology of hospitalization for acute upper gastrointestinal hemorrhage: a population-based study. Am J Gastroenterol 1995;90:206–10.
3. Peery AF, Dellon ES, Lund J, et al. Burden of gastrointestinal disease in the United States: 2012 update. Gastroenterology 2012;143:1179–87.
4. Targownik LE, Nabalamba A. Trends in management and outcomes of acute nonvariceal upper gastrointestinal bleeding: 1993-2003. Clin Gastroenterol Hepatol 2006;4:1459–66.
5. Theocharis GJ, Thomopoulos KC, Sakellaropoulos G, et al. Changing trends in the epidemiology and clinical outcome of acute upper gastrointestinal bleeding in a defined geographical area in Greece. J Clin Gastroenterol 2008;42:128–33.

6. van Leerdam ME, Vreeburg EM, Rauws EA, et al. Acute upper GI bleeding: did anything change? Time trend analysis of incidence and outcome of acute upper GI bleeding between 1993/1994 and 2000. Am J Gastroenterol 2003;98:1494–9.

7. van Leerdam ME. Epidemiology of acute upper gastrointestinal bleeding. Best Pract Res Clin Gastroenterol 2008;22:209–24.

8. Loperfido S, Baldo V, Piovesana E, et al. Changing trends in acute upper-GI bleeding: a population-based study. Gastrointest Endosc 2009;70:212–24.

9. Hreinsson JP, Kalaitzakis E, Gudmundsson S, et al. Upper gastrointestinal bleeding: incidence, etiology and outcomes in a population-based setting. Scand J Gastroenterol 2013;48:439–47.

10. Button LA, Roberts SE, Evans PA, et al. Hospitalized incidence and case fatality for upper gastrointestinal bleeding from 1999 to 2007: a record linkage study. Aliment Pharmacol Ther 2011;33:64–76.

11. Laine L, Yang H, Chang SC, et al. Trends for incidence of hospitalization and death due to GI complications in the United States from 2001 to 2009. Am J Gastroenterol 2012;107:1190–5.

12. Lanas A, García-Rodríguez LA, Polo-Tomás M, et al. Time trends and impact of upper and lower gastrointestinal bleeding and perforation in clinical practice. Am J Gastroenterol 2009;104:1633–41.

13. Sonnenberg A. Time trends of ulcer mortality in Europe. Gastroenterology 2007; 132:2320–7.

14. Chan FK, Abraham NS, Scheiman JM, et al. Management of patients on nonsteroidal anti-inflammatory drugs: a clinical practice recommendation from the First International Working Party on Gastrointestinal and Cardiovascular Effects of Nonsteroidal Anti-inflammatory Drugs and Anti-platelet Agents. Am J Gastroenterol 2008;103:2908–18.

15. Marmo R, Koch M, Cipolletta L, et al, PNED Investigators. Predictive factors of mortality from nonvariceal upper gastrointestinal hemorrhage: a multicenter study. Am J Gastroenterol 2008;103:1639–47.

16. Barkun A, Sabbah S, Enns R, et al. The Canadian Registry on Nonvariceal Upper Gastrointestinal Bleeding and Endoscopy (RUGBE): endoscopic hemostasis and proton pump inhibition are associated with improved outcomes in a real-life setting. Am J Gastroenterol 2004;99:1238–46.

17. Hearnshaw SA, Logan RF, Lowe D, et al. Acute upper gastrointestinal bleeding in the UK: patient characteristics, diagnoses and outcomes in the 2007 UK audit. Gut 2011;60:1327–35.

18. Sostres C, Lanas A. Epidemiology and demographics of upper gastrointestinal bleeding: prevalence, incidence, and mortality. Gastrointest Endosc Clin N Am 2011;21:567–81.

19. Müller T, Barkun AN, Martel M. Non-variceal upper GI bleeding in patients already hospitalized for another condition. Am J Gastroenterol 2009;104:330–9.

20. Marmo R, Koch M, Cipolletta L, et al. Predicting mortality in patients with in-hospital nonvariceal upper GI bleeding: a prospective, multicenter database study. Gastrointest Endosc 2014;79(5):741–9.e1.

21. Marmo R, Koch M, Cipolletta L, et al, Italian Registry on Upper Gastrointestinal Bleeding (PNED2). Predicting mortality in non-variceal upper gastrointestinal bleeders: validation of the Italian PNED score and prospective comparison with the Rockall Score. Am J Gastroenterol 2010;105:1284–91.

22. Sung JJ, Tsoi KK, Ma TK, et al. Causes of mortality in patients with peptic ulcer bleeding: a prospective cohort study of 10,428 cases. Am J Gastroenterol 2010; 105:84–9.

23. Enestvedt BK, Gralnek IM, Mattek N, et al. An evaluation of endoscopic indications and findings related to nonvariceal upper-GI hemorrhage in a large multicenter consortium. Gastrointest Endosc 2008;67:422–9.

24. Nahon S, Hagège H, Latrive JP, et al, Groupe des Hémorragies Digestives Hautes de l'ANGH. Epidemiological and prognostic factors involved in upper gastrointestinal bleeding: results of a French prospective multicenter study. Endoscopy 2012;44:998–1008.

25. Del Piano M, Bianco MA, Cipolletta L, et al, Prometeo Study Group of the Italian Society of Digestive Endoscopy (SIED). The "Prometeo" study: online collection of clinical data and outcome of Italian patients with acute nonvariceal upper gastrointestinal bleeding. J Clin Gastroenterol 2013;47:33–7.

26. Hwang JH, Fisher DA, Ben-Menachem T, et al, Standards of Practice Committee of the American Society for Gastrointestinal Endoscopy. The role of endoscopy in the management of acute non-variceal upper GI bleeding. Gastrointest Endosc 2012;75:1132–8.

27. Yachimski PS, Friedman LS. Gastrointestinal bleeding in the elderly. Nat Clin Pract Gastroenterol Hepatol 2008;5:80–93.

28. Gururatsakul M, Ching KJ, Talley NJ, et al. Incidence and risk factors of uncomplicated peptic ulcer and bleeding peptic ulcer over a 10-year period. Gastrointest Endosc 2009;69:AB607.

29. González-González JA, García-Compean D, Vázquez-Elizondo G, et al. Nonvariceal upper gastrointestinal bleeding in patients with liver cirrhosis. Clinical features, outcomes and predictors of in-hospital mortality. A prospective study. Ann Hepatol 2011;10:287–95.

30. Marmo R, del Piano M, Cipolletta L, et al. Mortality from non variceal upper gastrointestinal bleeding in patients with liver cirrhosis: an individual patient data meta-analysis. Gastrointest Endosc 2013;77:AB180.

31. Marmo R, Del Piano M, Rotondano G, et al. Mortality from nonulcer bleeding is similar to that of ulcer bleeding in high-risk patients with nonvariceal hemorrhage: a prospective database study in Italy. Gastrointest Endosc 2012;75:263–72.

32. Maluf-Filho F, da Costa Martins B, Simas de Lima M, et al. Etiology, endoscopic management and mortality of upper gastrointestinal bleeding in patients with cancer. United European Gastroenterol J 2013;1:60–7.

33. Holster IL, Kuipers EJ. Management of acute nonvariceal upper gastrointestinal bleeding: current policies and future perspectives. World J Gastroenterol 2012;18:1202–7.

34. Sánchez-Delgado J, Gené E, Suárez D, et al. Has H. pylori prevalence in bleeding peptic ulcer been underestimated? A meta-regression. Am J Gastroenterol 2011;106:398–405.

35. Barkun AN, Bardou M, Kuipers EJ, et al. International consensus recommendations on the management of patients with nonvariceal upper gastrointestinal bleeding. Ann Intern Med 2010;152:101–13.

36. Hung LC, Ching JY, Sung JJ, et al. Long-term outcome of Helicobacter pylori-negative idiopathic bleeding ulcers: a prospective cohort study. Gastroenterology 2005;128:1845–50.

37. Chason RD, Reisch JS, Rockey DC. More favorable outcomes with peptic ulcer bleeding due to Helicobacter pylori. Am J Med 2013;126:811–8.

38. Wong GL, Au KW, Lo AO, et al. Gastroprotective therapy does not improve outcomes of patients with Helicobacter pylori-negative idiopathic bleeding ulcers. Clin Gastroenterol Hepatol 2012;10:1124–9.

39. Chan FK, Ching JY, Suen BY, et al. Effects of Helicobacter pylori infection on long-term risk of peptic ulcer bleeding in low-dose aspirin users. Gastroenterology 2013;144:528–35.

40. US Preventive Services Task Force. Aspirin for the prevention of cardiovascular disease: U.S. Preventive Services Task Force recommendation statement. Ann Intern Med 2009;150:396–404.

41. McQuaid KR, Laine L. Systematic review and meta-analysis of adverse events of low-dose aspirin and clopidogrel in randomized controlled trials. Am J Med 2006;119:624–38.

42. Huang ES, Strate LL, Ho WW, et al. Long-term use of aspirin and the risk of gastrointestinal bleeding. Am J Med 2011;124:426–33.

43. Sutcliffe P, Connock M, Gurung T, et al. Aspirin in primary prevention of cardiovascular disease and cancer: a systematic review of the balance of evidence from reviews of randomized trials. PLoS One 2013;8:e81970.

44. Valkhoff VE, Sturkenboom MC, Kuipers EJ. Risk factors for gastrointestinal bleeding associated with low-dose aspirin. Best Pract Res Clin Gastroenterol 2012;26:125–40.

45. Ng FH, Tunggal P, Chu WM, et al. Esomeprazole compared with famotidine in the prevention of upper gastrointestinal bleeding in patients with acute coronary syndrome or myocardial infarction. Am J Gastroenterol 2012;107:389–96.

46. de Abajo FJ, Gil MJ, Bryant V, et al. Upper gastrointestinal bleeding associated with NSAIDs, other drugs and interactions: a nested case-control study in a new general practice database. Eur J Clin Pharmacol 2013;69:691–701.

47. Ramsoekh D, van Leerdam ME, Rauws EA, et al. Outcome of peptic ulcer bleeding, nonsteroidal anti-inflammatory drug use, and *Helicobacter pylori* infection. Clin Gastroenterol Hepatol 2005;3:859–64.

48. Targownik LE, Metge CJ, Leung S, et al. The relative efficacies of gastroprotective strategies in chronic users of nonsteroidal anti-inflammatory drugs. Gastroenterology 2008;134:937–44.

49. van Soest EM, Valkhoff VE, Mazzaglia G, et al. Suboptimal gastroprotective coverage of NSAID use and the risk of upper gastrointestinal bleeding and ulcers: an observational study using three European databases. Gut 2011;60:1650–9.

50. Le Ray I, Barkun AN, Vauzelle-Kervroëdan F, et al. Failure to renew prescriptions for gastroprotective agents to patients on continuous nonsteroidal anti-inflammatory drugs increases rate of upper gastrointestinal injury. Clin Gastroenterol Hepatol 2013;11:499–504.

51. Knopp-Sihota JA, Cummings GG, Homik J, et al. The association between serious upper gastrointestinal bleeding and incident bisphosphonate use: a population-based nested cohort study. BMC Geriatr 2013;13:36.

52. Crooks CJ, West J, Card TR. Comorbidities affect risk of non variceal upper gastrointestinal bleeding. Gastroenterology 2013;144:1384–93.

53. Jairath V, Martel M, Logan RF, et al. Why do mortality rates for nonvariceal upper gastrointestinal bleeding differ around the world? A systematic review of cohort studies. Can J Gastroenterol 2012;26:537–43.

54. Crooks C, Card T, West J. Reductions in 28-day mortality following hospital admission for upper gastrointestinal hemorrhage. Gastroenterology 2011;141:62–70.

55. Lau JY, Barkun A, Fan DM, et al. Challenges in the management of acute peptic ulcer bleeding. Lancet 2013;381:2033–43.

56. Rosenstock SJ, Møller MH, Larsson H, et al. Improving quality of care in peptic ulcer bleeding: nationwide cohort study of 13,498 consecutive patients in the

Danish Clinical Register of Emergency Surgery. Am J Gastroenterol 2013;108: 1449–57.

57. Wysocki JD, Srivastav S, Winstead NS. A nationwide analysis of risk factors for mortality and time to endoscopy in upper gastrointestinal haemorrhage. Aliment Pharmacol Ther 2012;36:30–6.

58. Leontiadis GI, Molloy-Bland M, Moayyedi P, et al. Effect of comorbidity on mortality in patients with peptic ulcer bleeding: systematic review and meta-analysis. Am J Gastroenterol 2013;108:331–45.

59. Jairath V, Kahan BC, Stanworth SJ, et al. Prevalence, management, and outcomes of patients with coagulopathy after acute nonvariceal uppergastrointestinal bleeding in the United Kingdom. Transfusion 2013;53:1069–76.

60. Venkatesh PG, Parasa S, Njei B, et al. Increased mortality with peptic ulcer bleeding in patients with both compensated and decompensated cirrhosis. Gastrointest Endosc 2014;79(4):605–14.

61. Yang JY, Lee TC, Montez-Rath ME, et al. Trends in acute nonvariceal upper gastrointestinal bleeding in dialysis patients. J Am Soc Nephrol 2012;23: 495–506.

62. Weng SC, Shu KH, Tarng DC, et al. In-hospital mortality risk estimation in patients with acute nonvariceal upper gastrointestinal bleeding undergoing hemodialysis: a retrospective cohort study. Ren Fail 2013;35:243–8.

63. Parasa S, Navaneethan U, Sridhar AR, et al. End-stage renal disease is associated with worse outcomes in hospitalized patients with peptic ulcer bleeding. Gastrointest Endosc 2013;77:609–16.

64. Gralnek IM, Barkun AN, Bardou M. Management of acute bleeding from a peptic ulcer. N Engl J Med 2008;359:928–37.

65. Sung JJ, Chan FK, Chen M, et al. Asia-Pacific Working Group consensus on non-variceal upper gastrointestinal bleeding. Gut 2011;60:1170–7.

66. Laine L, Jensen DM. Management of patients with ulcer bleeding. Am J Gastroenterol 2012;107:345–60.

67. Kohn A, Ancona C, Belleudi V, et al. The impact of endoscopy and specialist care on 30-day mortality among patients with acute non-variceal upper gastrointestinal hemorrhage: an Italian population-based study. Dig Liver Dis 2010;42: 629–34.

68. Forrest JA, Finlayson ND, Shearman DJ. Endoscopy in gastrointestinal bleeding. Lancet 1974;2:394–7.

69. Laine L, Peterson WL. Bleeding peptic ulcer. N Engl J Med 1994;331:717–27.

70. de Groot NL, van Oijen MG, Kessels K, et al. Reassessment of the predictive value of the Forrest classification for peptic ulcer rebleeding and mortality: can classification be simplified? Endoscopy 2014;46:46–52.

71. Griffiths WJ, Neumann DA, Welsh JD. The visible vessel as an indicator of uncontrolled or recurrent gastrointestinal hemorrhage. N Engl J Med 1979;300: 1411–3.

72. Wara P. Endoscopic prediction of major rebleeding - a prospective study of stigmata of hemorrhage in bleeding ulcer. Gastroenterology 1985;88(5 Pt 1):1209–14.

73. Freeman ML. Stigmata of hemorrhage in bleeding ulcers. Gastrointest Endosc Clin N Am 1997;7:559–74.

74. Freeman ML, Cass OW, Peine CJ, et al. The non-bleeding visible vessel versus the sentinel clot: natural history and risk of rebleeding. Gastrointest Endosc 1993;39:359–66.

75. Laine L, Freeman M, Cohen H. Lack of uniformity in evaluation of endoscopic prognostic features of bleeding ulcers. Gastrointest Endosc 1994;40:411–7.

76. Lau JY, Sung JJ, Chan AC, et al. Stigmata of hemorrhage in bleeding peptic ulcers: an interobserver agreement study among international experts. Gastrointest Endosc 1997;46:33–6.

77. Wong RC. Endoscopic Doppler US probe for acute peptic ulcer hemorrhage. Gastrointest Endosc 2004;60:804–12.

78. Cipolletta L, Bianco MA, Salerno R, et al. Improved characterization of visible vessels in bleeding ulcers by using magnification endoscopy: results of a pilot study. Gastrointest Endosc 2010;72:413–8.

79. Wyse JM, Barkun AN, Bardou M, et al. Can the presence of endoscopic high-risk stigmata be confidently predicted before gastroscopy? Gastrointest Endosc 2009;69:AB181.

80. Barkun AN, Bardou M, Martel M, et al. Prokinetics in acute upper GI bleeding: a meta-analysis. Gastrointest Endosc 2010;72:1138–45.

81. Altraif I, Handoo FA, Aljumah A, et al. Effect of erythromycin before endoscopy in patients presenting with variceal bleeding: a prospective, randomized, double-blind, placebo-controlled trial. Gastrointest Endosc 2011;73:245–50.

82. Cooper GS, Chak A, Way LE, et al. Early endoscopy in upper gastrointestinal hemorrhage: associations with recurrent bleeding, surgery, and length of hospital stay. Gastrointest Endosc 1999;49:145–52.

83. Chak A, Cooper GS, Lloyd LE, et al. Effectiveness of endoscopy in patients admitted to the intensive care unit with upper GI hemorrhage. Gastrointest Endosc 2001;53:6–13.

84. Cooper GS, Kou TD, Wong RC. Use and impact of early endoscopy in elderly patients with peptic ulcer hemorrhage: a population-based analysis. Gastrointest Endosc 2009;70:229–35.

85. Lim LG, Ho KY, Chan YH, et al. Urgent endoscopy is associated with lower mortality in high-risk but not low-risk nonvariceal upper gastrointestinal bleeding. Endoscopy 2011;43:300–6.

86. Karsan SS, Kanwal F, Huang ES, et al. Early endoscopy predicts lower mortality in acute gastrointestinal haemorrhage. Gastroenterology 2009;136(5 Suppl 1): A606.

87. Tsoi KK, Ma TK, Sung JJ. Endoscopy for upper gastrointestinal bleeding: how urgent is it? Nat Rev Gastroenterol Hepatol 2009;6:463–9.

88. Jairath V, Kahan BC, Logan RF, et al. Outcomes following acute nonvariceal upper gastrointestinal bleeding in relation to time to endoscopy: results from a nationwide study. Endoscopy 2012;44:723–30.

89. Lanas A, Aabakken L, Fonseca J, et al. Variability in the management of nonvariceal upper gastrointestinal bleeding in Europe: an observational study. Adv Ther 2012;29:1026–36.

90. Ananthakrishnan AN, McGinley EL, Saeian K. Outcomes of weekend admissions for upper gastrointestinal hemorrhage: a nationwide analysis. Clin Gastroenterol Hepatol 2009;7:296–302.

91. Shaheen AA, Kaplan GG, Myers RP. Weekend versus weekday admission and mortality from gastrointestinal hemorrhage caused by peptic ulcer disease. Clin Gastroenterol Hepatol 2009;7:303–10.

92. Dorn SD, Shah ND, Berg BP, et al. Effect of weekend hospital admission on gastrointestinal hemorrhage outcomes. Dig Dis Sci 2010;55:1658–66.

93. de Groot NL, Bosman JH, Siersema PD, et al, RASTA Study Group. Admission time is associated with outcome of upper gastrointestinal bleeding: results of a multicentre prospective cohort study. Aliment Pharmacol Ther 2012;36:477–84.

94. Jairath V, Kahan BC, Logan RF, et al. Mortality from acute upper gastrointestinal bleeding in the United Kingdom: does it display a "weekend effect"? Am J Gastroenterol 2011;106:1621–8.

95. Tsoi KK, Chiu PW, Chan FK, et al. The risk of peptic ulcer bleeding mortality in relation to hospital admission on holidays: a cohort study on 8,222 cases of peptic ulcer bleeding. Am J Gastroenterol 2012;107:405–10.

96. Lee JG, Turnipseed S, Romano PS, et al. Endoscopy-based triage significantly reduces hospitalization rates and costs of treating upper GI bleeding: a randomized controlled trial. Gastrointest Endosc 1999;50:755–61.

97. Cipolletta L, Bianco MA, Rotondano G, et al. Outpatient management for low-risk nonvariceal upper GI bleeding: a randomized controlled trial. Gastrointest Endosc 2002;55:1–5.

Gastroduodenal Perforation

Raminder Nirula, MD, MPH

KEYWORDS

- Gastroduodenal • Perforation • Ulcer-reducing surgery

KEY POINTS

- The most common cause of gastroduodenal perforation is peptic ulcer disease.
- Nonoperative management can be considered in patients with minimal symptoms who are younger than 70 years.
- Abdominal washout, ulcer biopsy, and omental patch are appropriate in most circumstances.
- Acid-reducing surgery is indicated in patients who have a history of failed medical therapy.

The cause and management of gastroduodenal perforation has changed as a result of increasing use of nonsteroidal antiinflammatories and improved pharmacologic treatment of acid hypersecretion, as well as the recognition and treatment of *Helicobacter pylori* (**Fig. 1**). As a result of the reduction in ulcer recurrence with medical therapy, the surgical approach to patients with gastroduodenal perforation has also changed over the last 3 decades, with ulcer-reducing surgery being performed infrequently.[1,2]

CAUSE

- The most common cause of gastroduodenal perforation is ulcer disease
  - Ulcer disease may be secondary to acid hypersecretion, *H pylori* infection, or from medications (steroids, nonsteroidal antiinflammatories)
- Other causes include trauma, neoplasm, foreign body ingestion, or iatrogenic (endoscopic procedures).
  - Blunt trauma resulting in gastroduodenal perforation is rare, comprising only 5% of blunt hollow viscous injuries.
  - Malignant perforations may be secondary to necrotic tumor in the stomach or duodenum that perforates or from an obstructing tumor, leading to proximal dilation and perforation.
  - Foreign bodies may cause perforation from direct injury to the stomach or duodenum or as a result of luminal obstruction.[1]

This article originally appeared in Surgical Clinics, Volume 94, Issue 1, February 2014.
Department of Surgery, University of Utah, 50 North Medical Drive, Salt Lake City, UT 84132, USA
E-mail address: r.nirula@hsc.utah.edu

Clinics Collections 7 (2015) 155–158
http://dx.doi.org/10.1016/j.ccol.2015.06.011

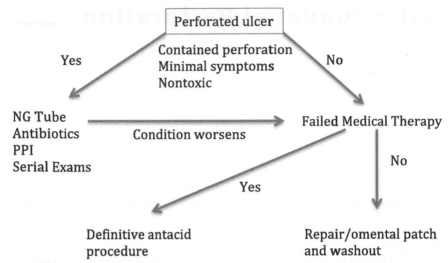

Fig. 1. Treatment of perforated gastroduodenal ulcer. Exams, examinations; NG, nasogastric; PPI, proton pump inhibitor.

PRESENTATION

- Sudden onset of severe epigastric and right upper quadrant abdominal pain in patients with a history of gastroesophageal reflux is common among those with peptic ulcer disease perforations.
- Peritonitis may be minimal in the case of contained leaks.
- Mental status changes and septic shock (fever, hypotension, tachycardia) may be observed in diffuse leakage of the perforation.

DIAGNOSIS

- Leukocytosis, metabolic acidosis, and hyperamylasemia may be present but are not sensitive.
- Upright chest radiograph may show free air.
- Computed tomography (CT) with enteral contrast shows free air, free fluid, mesenteric fat stranding, and bowel wall thickening and may localize the site of perforation. Early CT scans after traumatic injury may be falsely negative in up to 12% of cases.[3]

MANAGEMENT
Nonoperative Management

Approximately half of the perforations spontaneously seal, which raises the question as to whether these patients can be managed nonoperatively. The difficulty is identifying those patients who have sealed without compromising the outcomes for those who have not sealed while one observes them for signs of clinical deterioration.[4] Factors mandating surgical management include shock and generalized peritonitis. Risk factors that have been associated with failure of nonoperative management include age greater than 70 years, symptoms of greater than 24 hours, and lack of improvement after 12 hours of conservative therapy. Conservative therapy includes showing that there is no free extravasation of contrast and that the leak is confined either by CT or gastroduodenography. Once this information is verified, a nasogastric tube for decompression is required. The patient should receive antimicrobial therapy directed at aerobic gram-positive cocci such as ampicillin/sulbactam, as well as a proton pump inhibitor.[5] Should the patient fail to improve or worsen (fever, shock, worsening peritonitis), prompt surgical intervention is required.

Operative Management

Patients who have free perforation, shock, generalized peritonitis, or progressive symptoms should undergo surgery. The decision to perform an acid-reducing operation is made based on the patient's history. Those patients who have perforated despite antacid therapy and H pylori eradication or who require ulcerogenic medications such as steroids should undergo an acid-reducing operation. For those who have not received adequate medical therapy, ulcer biopsy for gastric ulcers, omental patch, and abdominal washout followed by medical therapy provide acceptably low ulcer recurrence rates, of less then 10%.[6–8]

In patients who have failed medical therapy and are hemodynamically stable, there are several antacid operations, each with its merits: truncal vagotomy with pyloroplasty, truncal vagotomy with antrectomy, and either a Bilroth I or Bilroth II reconstruction, or highly selective vagotomy. These operations should generally be reserved for ulcers that are related to acid hypersecretion, which include prepyloric ulcers or gastric ulcers within the body that occur in conjunction with duodenal ulcers. The choice of which operation to perform needs to take into account the location of the perforation and the ability to achieve closure along with the risk for ulcer recurrence balanced by the risk of complications related to the operation. Vagotomy and antrectomy carries the lowest risk for ulcer recurrence, at approximately 2%, whereas vagotomy and pyloroplasty carries a recurrence rate of 5%, and 10% to 20% for highly selective vagotomy.[9,10]

Closure of gastric perforations can typically be easily performed, because of the mobility and redundancy of the stomach, which can then be reinforced with an omental patch. Duodenal perforations frequently cannot be primarily closed unless they are small without causing duodenal narrowing. Therefore, an omental or jejunal serosal patch may be necessary. If the integrity of the repair is in question, the right upper quadrant should be drained in anticipation of a duodenal fistula and a gastrostomy tube for drainage, and a jejunal feeding tube should be placed. In patients who are hemodynamically normal, this procedure may be performed laparoscopically. If the perforation is proximal and an antacid operation is being performed, then, the ulcer may be resected if the remaining duodenal stump is not indurated, and the resection can be performed without injury to the ampulla.

REFERENCES

1. Lui FY, Davis KA. Gastroduodenal perforation: maximal or minimal intervention? Scand J Surg 2010;99(2):73–7.
2. Meissner K. H2-receptor antagonists and the incidence of gastroduodenal ulcer perforation and hemorrhage. An epidemiological study. Chirurg 1990;61(6): 449–52 [discussion: 453]. [in German].
3. Fakhry SM, Watts DD, Luchette FA. Current diagnostic approaches lack sensitivity in the diagnosis of perforated blunt small bowel injury: analysis from 275,557 trauma admissions from the EAST multi-institutional HVI trial. J Trauma 2003;54(2):295–306.
4. Crofts TJ, Park KG, Steele RJ, et al. A randomized trial of nonoperative treatment for perforated peptic ulcer. N Engl J Med 1989;320(15):970–3.

5. Solomkin JS, Mazuski JE, Bradley JS, et al. Diagnosis and management of complicated intra-abdominal infection in adults and children: guidelines by the Surgical Infection Society and the Infectious Diseases Society of America. Clin Infect Dis 2010;50(2):133–64.
6. Wong BC, Lam SK, Lai KC, et al. Triple therapy for *Helicobacter pylori* eradication is more effective than long-term maintenance antisecretory treatment in the prevention of recurrence of duodenal ulcer: a prospective long-term follow-up study. Aliment Pharmacol Ther 1999;13(3):303–9.
7. Axon AT, O'Morain CA, Bardhan KD, et al. Randomised double blind controlled study of recurrence of gastric ulcer after treatment for eradication of *Helicobacter pylori* infection. BMJ 1997;314(7080):565–8.
8. Graham DY, Lew GM, Klein PD, et al. Effect of treatment of *Helicobacter pylori* infection on the long-term recurrence of gastric or duodenal ulcer. A randomized, controlled study. Ann Intern Med 1992;116(9):705–8.
9. Busman DC, Volovics A, Munting JD. Recurrence rate after highly selective vagotomy. World J Surg 1988;12(2):217–23.
10. Sawyer JL, Scott HW Jr. Selective gastric vagotomy with antrectomy or pyloroplasty. Ann Surg 1971;174(4):541–7.

Endoscopic Management of Nonvariceal, Nonulcer Upper Gastrointestinal Bleeding

Eric T.T.L. Tjwa, MD, PhD*, I. Lisanne Holster, MD, PhD,
Ernst J. Kuipers, MD, PhD

KEYWORDS

• UGIB • Angiodysplasia • Dieulafoy • GAVE • Gastric cancer • Hemospray • OTSC

KEY POINTS

- Although peptic ulcer and esophagogastric varices remain the most common causes of upper gastrointestinal bleeding, a quarter to half of these events is due to a range of other conditions.
- Endoscopy is the mainstay for diagnosis of these bleeds, as well as the management of the largest proportion of them.
- Endoscopic treatment makes use of the same modalities as used for peptic ulcer and varices.
- Evidence for specific endoscopic therapy per specific cause is mounting.
- The use of novel modalities such as hemostatic powder, self-expandable metal stents, and over-the-scope-clips have expanded and may replace other treatment methods.

INTRODUCTION

The endoscopic management of gastrointestinal (GI) hemorrhage consists of injection therapy (with epinephrine or cyanoacrylate and other sclerosing agents), endoscopic thermal therapy, mechanical modalities such as hemoclips and over-the-scope-clips, and more recently, topical hemostatic sprays.[1,2] Solid evidence exists on how these modalities can be used in peptic ulcer and variceal bleeds, but it is less clear for other causes. This article deals with the endoscopic management of nonvariceal, nonulcer upper gastrointestinal bleeding (UGIB).[3–6]

This article originally appeared in Gastroenterology Clinics, Volume 43, Issue 4, December 2014.
Financial disclosures: E.T.T.L. Tjwa has received an unrestricted educational grant from Cook Medical Ireland.
Department of Gastroenterology and Hepatology, Erasmus MC University Medical Centre, PO box 2040, 3000 CA, Rotterdam, The Netherlands
* Corresponding author. Erasmus MC University Medical Centre, Room Hs-312, 's Gravendijkwal 230, Rotterdam 3015 CE, The Netherlands.
E-mail address: E.tjwa@erasmusmc.nl

Clinics Collections 7 (2015) 159–171
http://dx.doi.org/10.1016/j.ccol.2015.06.012
2352-7986/15/$ – see front matter © 2015 Elsevier Inc. All rights reserved.

EROSIVE CAUSES OF UGIB

Nonsteroidal antiinflammatory drugs are the principal cause for drug-induced erosions. They can be responsible for intramucosal petechial hemorrhage, superficial hemorrhagic erosions, gastroduodenitis, and ulceration.[7] In an endoscopic study of 187 patients using low-dose aspirin for at least 3 months with and without gastroprotective agents, erosions were observed in 34% and 63% of subjects, respectively.[8,9]

Other classes of drugs that can lead to erosions and ulceration are selective serotonin reuptake inhibitors, corticosteroids, nitrogen-containing bisphosphonates, potassium tablets, some antibiotics (eg, erythromycin, nalidixic acid, sulfonamides, and derivatives), and various chemotherapeutic agents.[7]

Larger hiatal hernia can result in linear erosions and ulcers or so-called *Cameron lesions* within the stomach at the impression of the diaphragm.[10] They predominantly occur along the lesser curvature. They most likely occur as a result of the combination of chronic mechanical trauma (eg, rubbing of the mucosal folds at the level of the diaphragm during respiratory excursions) and acid injury. Local ischemia may also play a role. Cameron lesions are found in about 5% of patients with hiatal hernia undergoing upper endoscopy; two-thirds of these patients have multiple lesions.[11] They may occur in 10% to 20% of patients with a hernia greater than or equal to 5 cm.[12]

Erosive esophago-gastro-duodenitis has many possible causes such as excessive alcohol consumption, use of mucosal erosion–causing drugs (see earlier discussion),[13] gastroesophageal reflux, and *Helicobacter pylori* infection.[14–16] Gastroduodenal erosions infrequently cause clinically significant blood loss.[3,5,14,17–20]

Endoscopic Management of Erosive Causes of UGIB

Endoscopy has only a marginal role in the treatment of hemorrhage caused by erosions. The treatment of choice is acid suppression, leading to healing of erosions and normalization of hemoglobin levels. The outcome is generally excellent. Acute bleeds sometimes require endoscopic treatment such as of a visible vessel, for which the treatment is similar to the approach of gastroduodenal ulcers. A different approach may be the control of bleeding by a topical hemostatic spray. Hemospray (Cook Medical, Winston Salem, NC, USA) is a novel proprietary powder specifically developed for the treatment of UGIB.[21,22] It is a nonorganic mineral blended powder that is thought to work via absorption of liquids at the bleeding site, forming an adhesive and cohesive mechanical barrier over the bleeding site. In a large European observational study in 63 patients with UGIB due to various causes, the application of Hemospray as primary monotreatment led to immediate hemostasis in 85% of patients with a 7-day rebleeding rate of 15%. When used as salvage therapy, after failure of conventional endoscopic treatment modalities, initial hemostasis was 100% and rebleeding 25%, reflecting the refractory nature of these lesions. Causes of nonvariceal, nonulcer UGIB included erosive esophagitis, gastritis, and/or duodenitis (n = 7), as well as Dieulafoy lesions, gastric antral vascular ectasia (GAVE), and Mallory-Weiss lesions.[23] Concomitant use of antithrombotics, mostly causative for erosive UGIB, do not appear to influence the success rates of Hemospray.[22]

UGIB CAUSED BY VASCULAR ANOMALIES

Vascular anomalies that most commonly cause UGIB include angiodysplasia, Dieulafoy lesions, and GAVE. Although not a true anomaly, but rather the result of congestion, portal hypertensive gastropathy is also ranked in this same category of vascular lesions.

Angiodysplasia

Angiodysplasia is defined as a sharply delineated vascular lesion within the mucosa, with a typical red appearance, with flat or slightly raised surface. Angiodysplasia is generally believed to be acquired, but the exact causes are unknown.[24–26] These lesions are often multiple and frequently seen in the colon, but may also involve the stomach and small bowel, including the duodenum. Patients with angiodysplasia can present with chronic iron-deficiency anemia, as well as with acute GI bleeding with melena and seldom hematemesis.[27]

Dieulafoy Lesion

Dieulafoy lesions most commonly occur in the proximal stomach along the lesser curve, but they are incidentally seen in the esophagus,[28] small intestine, and colon.[29] A Dieulafoy lesion consists of a dilated tortuous artery with a diameter up to 3 mm that protrudes through the mucosa and may cause massive GI hemorrhage by erosion of the artery. It is thought that this is due to a combination of factors such as straining of the vascular wall during peristalsis and peptic digestion.[30,31] Bleeding due to Dieulafoy lesions account for 1% to 6% of cases of acute nonvariceal UGIB.[30]

Gastric Antral Vascular Ectasia

GAVE is endoscopically recognized as a pattern of linear red stripes in the antrum separated by normal mucosa. GAVE has been associated with several autoimmune conditions, renal failure, and bone marrow transplantation.[32–35]

GAVE or so-called *watermelon stomach* is often confused with portal hypertensive gastropathy. Although GAVE is closely related to portal hypertension, it can also appear in the absence of portal hypertension, and GAVE generally does not respond to treatments that reduce portal pressure.

Portal Hypertensive Gastropathy

Portal hypertensive gastropathy or congestive gastropathy corresponds to dilated gastric mucosal capillaries without inflammation.[36] It is exclusively observed in patients with portal hypertension. When present in the small intestine or colon, it is termed portal hypertensive enteropathy[37] and portal hypertensive colopathy.[38] The degree of portal hypertension needed for development of portal hypertensive gastropathy remains controversial.[39] Bleeding from these conditions usually occurs as slow, diffusely oozing, but it may also be acute (and even) massive.

Endoscopic Management of Vascular Anomalies and Portal Hypertensive Gastropathy

The current standard of endoscopic treatment of bleeding angiodysplasia consists of coagulation therapy. Although high success rates are achieved for treatment of individual lesions, patients may experience recurrent anemia or overt bleeding. Banding of angiodysplasia has also been demonstrated in a small study of 11 subjects.[40] In case of bleeding angiodysplasia in the small intestines, (repeated) argon plasma coagulation (APC) via enteroscopy has been proved feasible and successful.[41]

Endoscopic treatment is also the first choice in bleeding Dieulafoy lesions[42] and is able to achieve hemostasis in more than 90% of cases.[30] Treatment is usually performed with clipping or band ligation of the lesion.

The first-line treatment of actively bleeding GAVE as well as recurrent bleeding from GAVE has for a long time consisted of repetitive sessions of APC.[43] In case of recurrence, patients have been successfully retreated with APC.[44] More recent publications show that band ligation of bleeding GAVE resulted in fewer treatment sessions for control of bleeding and higher rates of cessation of further bleeding than APC treatment.[45–48] Whether this also pertains to persistently decreased recurrence rates remains to be demonstrated (**Fig. 1**).

Endoscopic management has no place in treating portal hypertensive gastropathy.[43] Successful treatment should aim at reducing portal venous pressure by means of nonselective β-blockers, vasoactive drugs, and/or transjugular intrahepatic portosystemic shunts.

NEOPLASTIC BLEEDING LESIONS

Neoplastic lesions (both primary and metastatic) of the upper GI tract account for 2% to 8% of the cases of UGIB.[3,5,17–19] Gastric adenocarcinoma is the most prevalent among patients presenting with UGIB.

Endoscopic Management of Neoplastic Bleeding

Conventional endoscopic therapy for bleeding GI tumors is generally not very successful, because most tumors are beyond the reach of thermal or mechanical modalities due to their complex neoangiogenesis.[49] Endoscopic management was assessed in a study of 42 patients with primary upper GI cancer. In approximately half of these patients, severe UGIB was the first presentation of their malignancy, most of which were at an advanced stage with larger ulcerating tumor masses. Endoscopic hemostasis was only achieved in the lesser advanced, nondiffusely bleeding cancers. Severe bleeding correlated with a poor 1-year survival irrespective of initial hemostasis.[50] Against this background, radiotherapy and/or transarterial embolization (TAE) were for a long time the only alternative treatments for management of bleeding. Radiotherapy has a delayed effect, and the effect of both radiotherapy and embolization may be transient. In a retrospective study of 30 patients with UGIB from gastric cancer, almost 75% responded to radiotherapy, but rebled within 3 months. Patients who received concurrent chemoradiotherapy had a significant lower rebleeding rate (18%).[51] In a retrospective study of 23 patients with neoplastic UGIB treated with TAE, the overall treatment success was only 50%.[52]

Hemostatic powders are increasingly advocated as an endoscopic treatment of neoplastic bleeding because of its ability to stop diffuse bleeding. Two case series from Canada and France, including a total of 10 patients, showed promising short-term results in the use of Hemospray in bleeding esophageal, gastric, and pancreatic

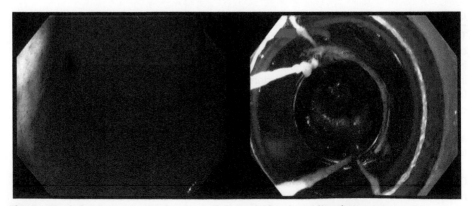

Fig. 1. Dieulafoy lesion in the fundus before and after band ligation.

cancers. In both reports, immediate hemostasis was reached in 100% of the patients and the rebleeding rate after 3 days was 20%.[53,54] Because powder can be endoscopically delivered during the index endoscopy, it provides a rapid and effective treatment modality in the bleeding oncology patient in the acute setting (**Fig. 2**).

UGIB CAUSED BY TRAUMA
Mallory-Weiss Tear

A Mallory-Weiss tear is a common cause of UGIB and typically presents as hematemesis after an initial episode of vomiting without blood. It is defined as a mucosal laceration at the gastroesophageal junction or gastric cardia, usually caused by retching or forceful vomiting.[55] Many factors have been associated with the development of Mallory-Weiss lesions, including alcohol use, use of aspirin and coumarins, paroxysms of coughing, pregnancy, heavy lifting, straining, seizure, blunt abdominal trauma, colonic lavage, and cardiopulmonary resuscitation.[56,57] The amount of blood loss is usually mild. Several epidemiologic studies reported these lesions as the bleeding source in 2% to 8% of patients presenting with acute UGIB.[3,17,18,58,59] In a large UK audit of 5004 patients who underwent endoscopy for UGIB, Mallory-Weiss lesions were the only bleeding source identified in 2.1% of cases and were present in a total 4.3% of cases.[59]

Boerhaave Syndrome and Other Causes of Transmural Perforation

Boerhaave syndrome is a rupture of the esophagus caused by a rapid increase in intraluminal pressure in the distal esophagus combined with negative intrathoracic pressure caused by straining or vomiting. Other causes of benign esophageal perforation include endoscopic and surgical handling and foreign body impaction.[60] In some cases, bleeding may be an accompanying symptom.

Caustic Injury and Foreign Body Ingestion

Ingestion of foreign bodies and toxic substances can be accidental or intentional. The ingestion of strong alkali results in liquefactive necrosis, which is associated with deep tissue penetration and may result in perforation accompanied by bleeding.[61] Acidic agents cause more superficial coagulation necrosis with scarring that may limit the

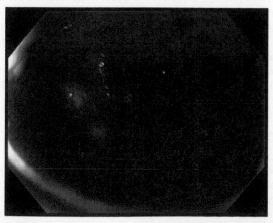

Fig. 2. Hemorrhagic gastric adenocarcinoma of the corpus after hemostasis with Hemospray.

extent of the injury.[62] Bleeding may occur as a result of widespread ulceration. More severe bleeding is however rare.

UGIB is also seen after foreign body ingestion. Most noteworthy in this respect is the ingestion of batteries and magnets leading to leakage and pressure adhesion, which can lead to local ulceration and perforation.[63] Hemorrhage is a frequent complication after foreign body ingestion[64] and results from local pressure or puncture of the mucosa with sometimes fistula formation to an underlying vessel.[65]

Endoscopic Management for Traumatic Bleeding

Most of the Mallory-Weiss lesions stop bleeding spontaneously.[58,66] A minority of cases require endoscopic treatment. In a French series of 218 patients with Mallory-Weiss bleeding, 56 (26%) had active bleeding on endoscopy. In other series, this prevalence ranged from 5% to 44%.[58,67] Various studies have looked at optimal endoscopic treatment. In a trial that randomized 63 patients to either supportive treatment or endoscopic therapy, rebleeding rates after only supportive therapy were higher than that after endoscopic epinephrine injection (25% vs 6%).[67] Endoscopic epinephrine injection, hemoclip placement, and band ligation were equivalent for primary hemostasis, all achieving 100% primary hemostasis.[67–71] Rebleeding rates after band ligation and hemoclip placement were similar in a randomized Korean trial (6%–10%),[70] but significantly lower after band ligation in a French trial (0% vs 18%).[71] It is unknown whether prescription of a proton pump inhibitor accelerates healing.

The "bear-claw" or over-the-scope-clip system (Ovesco Endoscopy, Tübingen, Germany) is a new clipping device developed for closure of large luminal GI defects.[72] These defects may be spontaneous like Boerhaave syndrome or iatrogenic (post-endoscopic submucosal dissection[73] or dehiscence after surgical anastomosis[74]) and include both perforated and bleeding lesions. Until now, evidence regarding the effectiveness of the device only came from case series,[75] but it is expected that over-the-scope-clip system may become an alternative to conventional surgical therapy for traumatic lesions. Endoscopic placement of a self-expandable metal stent (SEMS) can also be considered for Boerhaave syndrome.[60] The authors reported a series of 33 patients with nonmalignant esophageal perforation treated with SEMS placement. Initial sealing of the perforation was achieved in 97% of patients, long-term success without the need for surgical repair in 88%. Treatment was complicated in one-third of patients by stent migration, managed by SEMS repositioning or restenting. In their center, this has now become the initial endoscopic treatment of choice for esophageal perforations that require intervention. Stents need to be removed within 6 weeks after placement, because a longer time in situ often impairs the ease of removal. When a persistent perforation is observed after stent removal, placement of another stent should be considered.

Endoscopy often has little to offer in terms of treatment of bleeding caused by caustic injury. Early prophylactic esophageal stenting preventing stricture formation is currently under investigation.[76]

BLEEDING FROM THE HEPATOPANCREATICOBILIARY TRACT
Hemobilia

Hemobilia or bleeding from the hepatobiliary tract is a rare cause of UGIB. The causes include liver biopsy,[77] percutaneous transhepatic cholangiography, cholecystectomy, endoscopic biliary biopsies/stenting, and hepatic or bile duct tumors. In a review of 222 cases of hemobilia, 65% were iatrogenic, whereas accidental trauma accounted for only 6%.[78,79] In rare cases, bleeding may occur due to a fistula to the portal system or the hepatic vein, which can also lead to rapid onset of extreme jaundice.[80] In most cases, these bleeds are self-limiting and do not require intervention other than preventing biliary obstruction due to clots.

Symptoms of hemobilia can be variable. The classic triad of jaundice, biliary colic, and overt UGIB was in the most recent series only observed in 22% of the patients.[79] Endoscopic retrograde cholangiography is helpful to confirm diagnosis and establish the underlying cause. It can also be of help in clearance of the biliary tree, with stenting if necessary to reduce the risk of renewed obstruction. In rare cases, a lesion of the hepatic vein can establish a connection between the hepatic vein and the biliary tract and instead of hemobilia give rise to opposite flow of bile into the vein. Such bilhemia may lead to marked, acute onset of jaundice. In such a case, biliary stenting can reverse the flow, by rapidly reducing jaundice and allow closure of the leak.[80]

Hemosuccus Pancreaticus

Hemosuccus pancreaticus is caused by a bleeding source in the pancreas, pancreatic duct, or adjacent structures, such as the splenic artery connecting to the pancreatic duct.[81] Hemosuccus is most often due to pancreatic pseudoaneurysms resulting from acute or chronic pancreatitis.[82–84] Usually this involves erosion of the splenic artery leading to hemorrhage into the pancreatic duct. It has been estimated to occur in about 1 in 500 to 1500 cases of UGIB.[82,84] In 2 retrospective studies (n = 40 total), the most frequent complaints at presentation were melena, hematochezia, hematemesis, and epigastric pain.[82,84] Patients may also develop symptoms of nausea and vomiting, weight loss, and jaundice (when the bleed also leads to obstruction of the common bile duct). In an observational report including 31 patients with hemosuccus pancreaticus, the presence of duodenal blood was observed during upper GI endoscopy in only half of the patients.[84]

Endoscopic Management of Hemobilia and Hemosuccus Pancreaticus

Because hemobilia is mostly self-limiting, the role of endoscopic treatment is limited to clearance of the biliary system if needed, with occasional stenting to maintain an open biliary tract. Also for hemosuccus pancreaticus, there is no major role for endoscopic treatment. Selective arterial embolization is successful in 50% of the patients, whereas surgery is often necessary in emergency situations or after failure to control the bleeding by TAE.[84]

MISCELLANEOUS CAUSES OF BLEEDING

In rare cases, UGIB is caused by large- or small-vessel vasculitis,[85–89] which may occur throughout the GI tract.[89] Lesions may typically be very topical, affecting sharply demarcated areas, yet arising at multiple sites. Endoscopic biopsy specimens of the affected area may reveal ulceration and inflammation, but are often insufficient to demonstrate the underlying vasculitis. Diagnosis of the underlying disease is nevertheless mandatory. Treatment mostly starts with corticosteroids and immunosuppressive therapy, together with proton pump inhibitors in patients with upper GI lesions.

Acute gastric ischemia is uncommon because of the stomach's rich vascular supply. Nevertheless it is important to recognize, because progression to necrosis can lead to ulceration, including complications such as bleeding, perforation, and sepsis.[90,91] It may also occur if there is stenosis of the celiac trunk with insufficient collateral circulation.[92] UGIB due to ischemia has been described in a few case reports.[93,94]

Table 1
Causes of nonvariceal, nonulcer UGIB and their specific endoscopic management

Type of Bleeding	Subtype	Endoscopic Management
Erosive		None, possible role for hemostatic powder
Vascular	Angiodysplasia	Coagulation
	Dieulafoy lesion	Hemoclips, band ligation
	GAVE	Coagulation, band ligation
	Portal hypertensive gastropathy	None
Traumatic	Mallory-Weiss lesion	Band ligation, hemoclips, epinephrine injection
	Associated with perforation	Over-the-scope-clips, SEMS
	Caustic	None
Neoplastic		Possible role for hemostatic powder
Hepatopancreaticobiliary	Hemobilia, hemosuccus pancreaticus	None, ERCP to prevent obstruction or to treat bilhemia
Miscellaneous	Vasculitis, ischemic	Possible role for hemostatic powder

Endoscopic Management

Bleeding from these miscellaneous causes usually prohibit successful endoscopic therapy because bleeding is often diffuse and/or nonpulsatile hampering targeted therapy such as hemoclips, band ligation, or thermal therapy. Even though some data are available on the successful use of liberally deployed hemostatic powder,[23] the generalizability of this method is under further investigation. Treating the cause of vasculitis, systemic disease of ischemia will remain cornerstone in the treatment of associated bleeding.

SUMMARY

Although peptic ulcer and esophagogastric varices remain the most common causes of UGIB, a quarter to half of these events is due to a range of other conditions.[3,5,17–19] Endoscopy is the mainstay for diagnosis of these bleeds, as well as the management of the largest proportion of them. Endoscopic treatment makes use of the same modalities as used for peptic ulcer and varices. Evidence for specific endoscopic therapy per specific cause is mounting (**Table 1**). The use of novel modalities such as hemostatic powder, SEMS, and over-the-scope-clips have expanded and often replaced other treatment methods.

REFERENCES

1. Committee ASoP, Early DS, Ben-Menachem T, et al. Appropriate use of GI endoscopy. Gastrointest Endosc 2012;75:1127–31.
2. Barkun AN, Moosavi S, Martel M. Topical hemostatic agents: a systematic review with particular emphasis on endoscopic application in GI bleeding. Gastrointest Endosc 2013;77:692–700.
3. Czernichow P, Hochain P, Nousbaum JB, et al. Epidemiology and course of acute upper gastro-intestinal haemorrhage in four French geographical areas. Eur J Gastroenterol Hepatol 2000;12:175–81.

4. Enestvedt BK, Gralnek IM, Mattek N, et al. An evaluation of endoscopic indi-cations and findings related to nonvariceal upper-GI hemorrhage in a large multicenter consortium. Gastrointest Endosc 2008;67:422–9.
5. van Leerdam ME, Vreeburg EM, Rauws EA, et al. Acute upper GI bleeding: did anything change? Time trend analysis of incidence and outcome of acute upper GI bleeding between 1993/1994 and 2000. Am J Gastroenterol 2003; 98:1494–9.
6. Holster IL, Kuipers EJ. Other causes of upper gastrointestinal bleeding. In: Sung JJ, Kuipers EJ, Barkun AN, editors. Gastrointestinal bleeding. 2nd edition. London: Blackwell Publishing Ltd; 2012. p. 135–76.
7. Gore RM, Levine MS, Ghahremani GG. Drug-induced disorders of the stomach and duodenum. Abdom Imaging 1999;24:9–16.
8. Yeomans ND, Lanas AI, Talley NJ, et al. Prevalence and incidence of gastrodu-odenal ulcers during treatment with vascular protective doses of aspirin. Aliment Pharmacol Ther 2005;22:795–801.
9. Tamura A, Murakami K, Kadota J, Investigators O-GS. Prevalence and indepen-dent factors for gastroduodenal ulcers/erosions in asymptomatic patients taking low-dose aspirin and gastroprotective agents: the OITA-GF study. QJM 2011; 104(2):133–9.
10. Cameron AJ, Higgins JA. Linear gastric erosion. A lesion associated with large diaphragmatic hernia and chronic blood loss anemia. Gastroenterology 1986; 91:338–42.
11. Weston AP. Hiatal hernia with cameron ulcers and erosions. Gastrointest Endosc Clin N Am 1996;6:671–9.
12. Maganty K, Smith RL. Cameron lesions: unusual cause of gastrointestinal bleeding and anemia. Digestion 2008;77:214–7.
13. Sugawa C, Lucas CE, Rosenberg BF, et al. Differential topography of acute erosive gastritis due to trauma or sepsis, ethanol and aspirin. Gastrointest Endosc 1973;19:127–30.
14. Toljamo KT, Niemela SE, Karttunen TJ, et al. Clinical significance and outcome of gastric mucosal erosions: a long-term follow-up study. Dig Dis Sci 2006;51:543–7.
15. Morris A, Nicholson G. Ingestion of campylobacter pyloridis causes gastritis and raised fasting gastric pH. Am J Gastroenterol 1987;82:192–9.
16. Kuipers EJ. Review article: exploring the link between Helicobacter pylori and gastric cancer. Aliment Pharmacol Ther 1999;13(Suppl 1):3–11.
17. Di Fiore F, Lecleire S, Merle V, et al. Changes in characteristics and outcome of acute upper gastrointestinal haemorrhage: a comparison of epidemiology and practices between 1996 and 2000 in a multicentre French study. Eur J Gastroenterol Hepatol 2005;17:641–7.
18. Theocharis GJ, Thomopoulos KC, Sakellaropoulos G, et al. Changing trends in the epidemiology and clinical outcome of acute upper gastrointestinal bleeding in a defined geographical area in Greece. J Clin Gastroenterol 2008;42:128–33.
19. Paspatis GA, Matrella E, Kapsoritakis A, et al. An epidemiological study of acute upper gastrointestinal bleeding in Crete, Greece. Eur J Gastroenterol Hepatol 2000;12:1215–20.
20. McQuaid KR, Laine L. Systematic review and meta-analysis of adverse events of low-dose aspirin and clopidogrel in randomized controlled trials. Am J Med 2006;119:624–38.
21. Sung JJ, Luo D, Wu JC, et al. Early clinical experience of the safety and effec-tiveness of Hemospray in achieving hemostasis in patients with acute peptic ulcer bleeding. Endoscopy 2011;43:291–5.

22. Holster IL, Kuipers EJ, Tjwa ET. Hemospray in the treatment of upper gastrointestinal hemorrhage in patients on antithrombotic therapy. Endoscopy 2013;45: 63–6.
23. Smith LA, Stanley AJ, Bergman JJ, et al. Hemospray application in nonvariceal upper gastrointestinal bleeding: results of the survey to evaluate the application of hemospray in the luminal tract. J Clin Gastroenterol 2013. [Epub ahead of print].
24. Gilmore PR. Angiodysplasia of the upper gastrointestinal tract. J Clin Gastroenterol 1988;10:386–94.
25. Kaaroud H, Fatma LB, Beji S, et al. Gastrointestinal angiodysplasia in chronic renal failure. Saudi J Kidney Dis Transpl 2008;19:809–12.
26. Mishra PK, Kovac J, de Caestecker J, et al. Intestinal angiodysplasia and aortic valve stenosis: let's not close the book on this association. Eur J Cardiothorac Surg 2009;35:628–34.
27. Chalasani N, Cotsonis G, Wilcox CM. Upper gastrointestinal bleeding in patients with chronic renal failure: role of vascular ectasia. Am J Gastroenterol 1996;91: 2329–32.
28. Ertekin C, Barbaros U, Taviloglu K, et al. Dieulafoy's lesion of esophagus. Surg Endosc 2002;16:219.
29. Moreira-Pinto J, Raposo C, Teixeira da Silva V, et al. Jejunal Dieulafoy's lesion: case report and literature review. Pediatr Surg Int 2009;25:641–2.
30. Lee YT, Walmsley RS, Leong RW, et al. Dieulafoy's lesion. Gastrointest Endosc 2003;58:236–43.
31. Lara LF, Sreenarasimhaiah J, Tang SJ, et al. Dieulafoy lesions of the GI tract: localization and therapeutic outcomes. Dig Dis Sci 2010;55:3436–41.
32. Goel A, Christian CL. Gastric antral vascular ectasia (watermelon stomach) in a patient with Sjogren's syndrome. J Rheumatol 2003;30:1090–2.
33. Viiala CH, Kaye JM, Hurley DM, et al. Watermelon stomach arising in association with Addison's disease. J Clin Gastroenterol 2001;33:173.
34. Ingraham KM, O'Brien MS, Shenin M, et al. Gastric antral vascular ectasia in systemic sclerosis: demographics and disease predictors. J Rheumatol 2010; 37:603–7.
35. Burak KW, Lee SS, Beck PL. Portal hypertensive gastropathy and gastric antral vascular ectasia (GAVE) syndrome. Gut 2001;49:866–72.
36. Thuluvath PJ, Yoo HY. Portal hypertensive gastropathy. Am J Gastroenterol 2002;97:2973–8.
37. Higaki N, Matsui H, Imaoka H, et al. Characteristic endoscopic features of portal hypertensive enteropathy. J Gastroenterol 2008;43:327–31.
38. Bini EJ, Lascarides CE, Micale PL, et al. Mucosal abnormalities of the colon in patients with portal hypertension: an endoscopic study. Gastrointest Endosc 2000;52:511–6.
39. Cubillas R, Rockey DC. Portal hypertensive gastropathy: a review. Liver Int 2010;30:1094–102.
40. Ljubicic N. Endoscopic detachable mini-loop ligation for treatment of gastroduodenal angiodysplasia: case study of 11 patients with long-term follow-up. Gastrointest Endosc 2004;59:420–3.
41. Godeschalk MF, Mensink PB, van Buuren HR, et al. Primary balloon-assisted enteroscopy in patients with obscure gastrointestinal bleeding: findings and outcome of therapy. J Clin Gastroenterol 2010;44:e195–200.
42. Yanar H, Dolay K, Ertekin C, et al. An infrequent cause of upper gastrointestinal tract bleeding: "Dieulafoy's lesion". Hepatogastroenterology 2007;54:1013–7.

43. Garcia N, Sanyal AJ. Portal hypertensive gastropathy and gastric antral vascular ectasia. Curr Treat Options Gastroenterol 2001;4:163–71.
44. Fuccio L, Zagari RM, Serrani M, et al. Endoscopic argon plasma coagulation for the treatment of gastric antral vascular ectasia-related bleeding in patients with liver cirrhosis. Digestion 2009;79:143–50.
45. Sato T, Yamazaki K, Akaike J. Endoscopic band ligation versus argon plasma coagulation for gastric antral vascular ectasia associated with liver diseases. Dig Endosc 2012;24:237–42.
46. Chiu YC, Lu LS, Wu KL, et al. Comparison of argon plasma coagulation in management of upper gastrointestinal angiodysplasia and gastric antral vascular ectasia hemorrhage. BMC Gastroenterol 2012;12:67.
47. Wells CD, Harrison ME, Gurudu SR, et al. Treatment of gastric antral vascular ectasia (watermelon stomach) with endoscopic band ligation. Gastrointest Endosc 2008;68:231–6.
48. Kumar R, Mohindra S, Pruthi HS. Endoscopic band ligation: a novel therapy for bleeding gastric antral vascular ectasia. Endoscopy 2007;39(Suppl 1):E56–7.
49. Heller SJ, Tokar JL, Nguyen MT, et al. Management of bleeding GI tumors. Gastrointest Endosc 2010;72:817–24.
50. Savides TJ, Jensen DM, Cohen J, et al. Severe upper gastrointestinal tumor bleeding: endoscopic findings, treatment, and outcome. Endoscopy 1996;28: 244–8.
51. Asakura H, Hashimoto T, Harada H, et al. Palliative radiotherapy for bleeding from advanced gastric cancer: is a schedule of 30 Gy in 10 fractions adequate? J Cancer Res Clin Oncol 2010;137:125–30.
52. Lee HJ, Shin JH, Yoon HK, et al. Transcatheter arterial embolization in gastric cancer patients with acute bleeding. Eur Radiol 2009;19:960–5.
53. Chen YI, Barkun AN, Soulellis C, et al. Use of the endoscopically applied hemostatic powder TC-325 in cancer-related upper GI hemorrhage: preliminary experience (with video). Gastrointest Endosc 2012;75:1278–81.
54. Leblanc S, Vienne A, Dhooge M, et al. Early experience with a novel hemostatic powder used to treat upper GI bleeding related to malignancies or after therapeutic interventions (with videos). Gastrointest Endosc 2013;78:169–75.
55. Mallory GK, Weiss SW. Hemorrhages from lacerations of the cardiac orifice of the stomach due to vomiting. Am J Med Sci 1929;178:506–12.
56. Younes Z, Johnson DA. The spectrum of spontaneous and iatrogenic esophageal injury: perforations, Mallory-Weiss tears, and hematomas. J Clin Gastroenterol 1999;29:306–17.
57. Eisen GM, Baron TH, Dominitz JA, et al. Complications of upper GI endoscopy. Gastrointest Endosc 2002;55:784–93.
58. Kim JW, Kim HS, Byun JW, et al. Predictive factors of recurrent bleeding in Mallory-Weiss syndrome. Korean J Gastroenterol 2005;46:447–54.
59. Hearnshaw SA, Logan RF, Lowe D, et al. Use of endoscopy for management of acute upper gastrointestinal bleeding in the UK: results of a nationwide audit. Gut 2010;59:1022–9.
60. van Heel NC, Haringsma J, Spaander MC, et al. Short-term esophageal stenting in the management of benign perforations. Am J Gastroenterol 2010;105: 1515–20.
61. Poley JW, Steyerberg EW, Kuipers EJ, et al. Ingestion of acid and alkaline agents: outcome and prognostic value of early upper endoscopy. Gastrointest Endosc 2004;60:372–7.
62. Kay M, Wyllie R. Caustic ingestions in children. Curr Opin Pediatr 2009;21:651–4.

63. Sahin C, Alver D, Gulcin N, et al. A rare cause of intestinal perforation: ingestion of magnet. World J Pediatr 2010;6:369–71.
64. Syrakos T, Zacharakis E, Antonitsis P, et al. Surgical intervention for gastrointestinal foreign bodies in adults: a case series. Med Princ Pract 2008;17:276–9.
65. Huiping Y, Jian Z, Shixi L. Esophageal foreign body as a cause of upper gastrointestinal hemorrhage: case report and review of the literature. Eur Arch Otorhinolaryngol 2008;265:247–9.
66. Kortas DY, Haas LS, Simpson WG, et al. Mallory-Weiss tear: predisposing factors and predictors of a complicated course. Am J Gastroenterol 2001;96: 2863–5.
67. Llach J, Elizalde JI, Guevara MC, et al. Endoscopic injection therapy in bleeding Mallory-Weiss syndrome: a randomized controlled trial. Gastrointest Endosc 2001;54:679–81.
68. Huang SP, Wang HP, Lee YC, et al. Endoscopic hemoclip placement and epinephrine injection for Mallory-Weiss syndrome with active bleeding. Gastrointest Endosc 2002;55:842–6.
69. Park CH, Min SW, Sohn YH, et al. A prospective, randomized trial of endoscopic band ligation vs. epinephrine injection for actively bleeding Mallory-Weiss syndrome. Gastrointest Endosc 2004;60:22–7.
70. Cho YS, Chae HS, Kim HK, et al. Endoscopic band ligation and endoscopic hemoclip placement for patients with Mallory-Weiss syndrome and active bleeding. World J Gastroenterol 2008;14:2080–4.
71. Lecleire S, Antonietti M, Iwanicki-Caron I, et al. Endoscopic band ligation could decrease recurrent bleeding in Mallory-Weiss syndrome as compared to haemostasis by hemoclips plus epinephrine. Aliment Pharmacol Ther 2009;30:399–405.
72. Monkemuller K, Peter S, Toshniwal J, et al. Multipurpose use of the 'bear claw' (over-the-scope-clip system) to treat endoluminal gastrointestinal disorders. Dig Endosc 2014;26(3):350–7.
73. Nishiyama N, Mori H, Kobara H, et al. Efficacy and safety of over-the-scope clip: including complications after endoscopic submucosal dissection. World J Gastroenterol 2013;19:2752–60.
74. Weiland T, Fehlker M, Gottwald T, et al. Performance of the OTSC system in the endoscopic closure of iatrogenic gastrointestinal perforations: a systematic review. Surg Endosc 2013;27:2258–74.
75. Singhal S, Changela K, Papafragkakis H, et al. Over the scope clip: technique and expanding clinical applications. J Clin Gastroenterol 2013;47:749–56.
76. Lee M. Caustic ingestion and upper digestive tract injury. Dig Dis Sci 2010;55: 1547–9.
77. Prata Martins F, Bonilha DR, Correia LP, et al. Obstructive jaundice caused by hemobilia after liver biopsy. Endoscopy 2008;40(Suppl 2):E265–6.
78. Sandblom P. Hemobilia (biliary tract hemorrhage). History, pathology, diagnosis, treatment. Springfield (IL): Charles C Thomas; 1972.
79. Green MH, Duell RM, Johnson CD, et al. Haemobilia. Br J Surg 2001;88:773–86.
80. Hommes M, Kazemier G, van Dijk LC, et al. Complex liver trauma with bilhemia treated with perihepatic packing and endovascular stent in the vena cava. J Trauma 2009;67:E51–3.
81. Sandblom P. Gastrointestinal hemorrhage through the pancreatic duct. Ann Surg 1970;171:61–6.
82. Etienne S, Pessaux P, Tuech JJ, et al. Hemosuccus pancreaticus: a rare cause of gastrointestinal bleeding. Gastroenterol Clin Biol 2005;29:237–42.

83. Kuganeswaran E, Smith OJ, Goldman ML, et al. Hemosuccus pancreaticus: rare complication of chronic pancreatitis. Gastrointest Endosc 2000;51:464–5.
84. Vimalraj V, Kannan DG, Sukumar R, et al. Haemosuccus pancreaticus: diagnostic and therapeutic challenges. HPB (Oxford) 2009;11:345–50.
85. Pore G. GI lesions in Henoch-Schonlein purpura. Gastrointest Endosc 2002;55: 283–6.
86. Chae EJ, Do KH, Seo JB, et al. Radiologic and clinical findings of Behcet disease: comprehensive review of multisystemic involvement. Radiographics 2008;28:e31.
87. Perez RA, Silver D, Banerjee B. Polyarteritis nodosa presenting as massive upper gastrointestinal hemorrhage. Surg Endosc 2000;14:87.
88. Pagnoux C, Mahr A, Cohen P, et al. Presentation and outcome of gastrointestinal involvement in systemic necrotizing vasculitides: analysis of 62 patients with polyarteritis nodosa, microscopic polyangiitis, Wegener granulomatosis, Churg-Strauss syndrome, or rheumatoid arthritis-associated vasculitis. Medicine (Baltimore) 2005;84:115–28.
89. Kuipers EJ, van Leeuwen MA, Nikkels PG, et al. Hemobilia due to vasculitis of the gall bladder in a patient with mixed connective tissue disease. J Rheumatol 1991;18:617–8.
90. Steen S, Lamont J, Petrey L. Acute gastric dilation and ischemia secondary to small bowel obstruction. Proc (Bayl Univ Med Cent) 2008;21:15–7.
91. Lewis S, Holbrook A, Hersch P. An unusual case of massive gastric distension with catastrophic sequelae. Acta Anaesthesiol Scand 2005;49:95–7.
92. Mensink PB, Moons LM, Kuipers EJ. Chronic gastrointestinal ischaemia: shifting paradigms. Gut 2010;60:722–37.
93. Fiddian-Green RG, Stanley JC, Nostrant T, et al. Chronic gastric ischemia. A cause of abdominal pain or bleeding identified from the presence of gastric mucosal acidosis. J Cardiovasc Surg (Torino) 1989;30:852–9.
94. Sharlow JW, Cone JB, Schaefer RF. Acute gastric necrosis in the postoperative period. South Med J 1989;82:529–30.

Endoscopic Management of Acute Peptic Ulcer Bleeding

Yidan Lu, MD[a], Yen-I Chen, MD[a], Alan N. Barkun, MD, MSc[a,b],*

KEYWORDS

- Peptic ulcer bleeding • Upper gastrointestinal bleeding • Endoscopy • Gastric ulcer
- Duodenal ulcer • Nonvariceal upper gastrointestinal hemorrhage

KEY POINTS

- Endoscopy should be performed within 24 hours of presentation in patients with upper gastrointestinal bleeding.
- Pre-endoscopic prokinetics should be considered in patients who are suspected of having a significant amount of blood in the upper gastrointestinal tract, such as those with positive nasogastric aspirate or active hematemesis, to improve the endoscopic view and decrease the need for repeat endoscopy.
- Endoscopic therapy should be performed in lesions with high-risk stigmata (Forrest classification I–IIB) with combination therapy or monotherapy using current endoscopic hemostatic agents except for epinephrine, which should not be used alone as definitive therapy.
- Postendoscopic care includes testing and eradication of *Helicobacter pylori*, avoidance of nonsteroidal anti-inflammatory drugs whenever possible, and the use of proper gastroprotective strategies in patients requiring ongoing antiplatelet and anticoagulant therapy.

INTRODUCTION

Peptic ulcers are the most frequently encountered cause of upper gastrointestinal bleeding (UGIB), with an annual incidence of 19.4 to 57.0 per 100,000 individuals.[1] Ulcers account for one-third to half of all presentations of acute UGIB.[1–3] A large United States inpatient database reveals declining trends in the incidence of both UGIB and peptic ulcer bleeding.[1] Similarly, the mortality from UGIB has also

This article originally appeared in Gastroenterology Clinics, Volume 43, Issue 4, December 2014.
Disclosure: No conflicts of interest to disclose.
Yidan Lu and Yen-I Chen are co-authors.
[a] Division of Gastroenterology, McGill University Health Center, McGill University, 1650 Cedar Avenue, Montréal H3G 1A4, Canada; [b] Division of Clinical Epidemiology, McGill University Health Center, McGill University, 687 Pine Avenue West, Montréal H3A 1A1, Canada
* Corresponding author. Division of Gastroenterology, McGill University Health Center, Montreal General Hospital Site, 1650 Cedar Avenue, Room D7-185, Montréal H3G 1A4, Canada.
E-mail address: alan.barkun@muhc.mcgill.ca

decreased from 2.95% to 2.45%.[1] In the management of UGIB, the use of endoscopy plays a fundamental role in the diagnosis, treatment, and prognostication of UGIB. Pre-endoscopic considerations such as the use of prokinetics and timing of endoscopy are reviewed, with a focus on the endoscopic management of peptic ulcer bleeding. Such management includes the use of the available hemostatic modalities, including emerging therapies, which will be reviewed along with their comparative effectiveness. Proton-pump inhibitors (PPIs) after endoscopy, indications for second-look endoscopy, and the use of secondary pharmacologic prophylaxis are also discussed. Issues of risk stratification and initial resuscitation are discussed in an article elsewhere in this issue by Meltzer and Klein.

PROKINETICS

Prokinetic agents such as erythromycin and metoclopramide can be administered before endoscopy to improve endoscopic yield and reduce the need for a repeat endoscopy. Erythromycin, a motilin agonist, can be given at a dose of 250 mg intravenously, and metoclopramide 10 mg intravenously 30 to 60 minutes before endoscopy. The use of erythromycin is favored based on current data. Doses used in the literature range from 3 to 4 mg/kg of erythromycin administered 20 to 90 minutes before endoscopy. Furthermore, the QT-interval–prolonging effect of erythromycin should be taken into consideration, and an electrocardiogram first performed.

The use of prokinetics should be considered in acute UGIB, particularly when targeting patients with active bleeding and/or evidence of blood in the stomach.[4] A meta-analysis comprising 3 randomized controlled trials (RCTs) with erythromycin and 2 abstracts with metoclopramide included a total of 162 patients, all showing evidence of active bleeding with blood in the stomach,[5] showed that a prokinetic agent, in comparison with placebo or no treatment, led to a significant reduction in the need for repeat endoscopy (odds ratio [OR] 0.55; 95% confidence interval [CI] 0.32–0.94). This effect was not preserved when analyzing metoclopramide alone (OR 1.22; 95% CI 0.35–4.25).[5] No differences were noted for blood transfusions or need for surgery, while mortality was not analyzed. A more recent meta-analysis solely looking at erythromycin showed similar results, with improvement in the visualization of the gastric mucosa (OR 3.43; 95% CI 1.81–6.50), and a decrease in the need for a second-look endoscopy (OR 0.47; 95% CI 0.26–0.83).[6] Of note, the effect of erythromycin in decreasing units of blood transfused and length of stay in hospital reached significance[7] when an additional trial that only included patients with variceal bleeding[8] was added to the meta-analysis.[7,9]

Pre-endoscopic intravenous PPI administration and nasogastric lavage can also be considered before endoscopy; these details are discussed elsewhere.

TIMING OF ENDOSCOPY

The performance of early endoscopy within 24 hours of patient presentation is warranted for most patients.[4,10] This practice has been shown to be safe for all patients at risk, allows for earlier discharge of low-risk patients,[11] and improves outcomes in those at high risk.[4] Lower costs are also associated with early discharge after endoscopy of low-risk patients.[12]

Several RCTs and retrospective cohort studies have examined very early endoscopy at less than 2 to 3, less than 6, less than 8, and less than 12 hours, compared with less than 24 to 48 hours.[13] Faster time to endoscopy yielded higher rates of finding high-risk stigmata of bleeding at endoscopy,[14–16] and similarly higher rates of hemostasis being performed[16,17] without demonstrable effects on outcomes of rebleeding, need for surgery, or duration of hospitalization. This finding contrasts with those of studies looking at early endoscopy (<24 hours) showing a significant decreased length of stay in hospital.[18] Moreover, decreased rebleeding and need for surgery[19] were also observed, particularly among high-risk patients (ulcer with active bleeding or visible vessel, or varices).[18]

In higher-risk patients, one study randomizing patients to endoscopy at less than 12 hours versus greater than 12 hours from patient presentation detected a significantly reduced need for blood transfusions, and shorter hospitalization (4 vs 14.5 days) in the subgroup of patients with coffee grounds or bloody nasogastric aspirate.[20] In parallel, one observational study demonstrated, using a receiver-operating curve analysis, that a longer time to endoscopy (>13 hours) predicted all-cause in-hospital mortality in patients with a Blatchford score of 12 or higher.[21] The robustness of the results is limited by the lack of randomization and adjustment for possible confounders that can influence mortality. As a result, the American College of Gastroenterology guidelines on ulcer bleeding suggest that endoscopy within 12 hours may be considered in high-risk patients. Similarly, the United Kingdom UGIB toolkit produced by the Academy of Royal Medical Colleges recommends endoscopy at less than 6 to 12 hours in "urgent-risk" patients,[22] a practice that is currently not supported by high-quality evidence for nonvariceal UGIB (NVUGIB),[23] though appropriate in the context of suspected variceal bleeding, in which case endoscopy within 12 hours is suggested.[24]

Data from bleeding registries show that a significant proportion of patients have a delay greater than 24 hours before undergoing upper endoscopy. Though variable, rates of early endoscopy range from 50% in a United Kingdom bleeding audit[25] up to 82% in a large Danish registry.[26] Reasons behind such delays are likely multifactorial; however, several reports from administrative databases relay a "weekend effect" whereby patients presenting on weekends are less likely to undergo early endoscopy, and have higher mortality, which may[27-29] or may not result from longer endoscopy delays.[30] Nevertheless, endoscopy within 24 hours of patient presentation should be targeted as a stand-alone quality indicator when managing patients with acute UGIB.[31]

ENDOSCOPIC DIAGNOSIS AND RISK STRATIFICATION

The endoscopic findings of a bleeding ulcer have prognostic implications in terms of rebleeding, need for surgery, and mortality. As a result, they are integrated in risk assessment scores such as the complete Rockall score, and are further used to determine the need for endoscopic hemostasis. The stigmata of recent bleeding are used to characterize the endoscopic appearance at the base of the bleeding ulcer, and are commonly categorized according to the Forrest classification into high-risk stigmata (HRS) and low-risk stigmata (LRS) (Table 1). HRS comprise active spurting bleeding

Table 1
Forrest classification of stigmata of recent bleeding

Stigmata of Recent Hemorrhage		Forrest Classification
Active spurting bleeding	High-risk stigmata	IA
Active oozing bleeding		IB
Nonbleeding visible vessel		IIA
Adherent clot		IIB
Flat pigmented spot	Low-risk stigmata	IIC
Clean base		III

(Forrest IA), active oozing bleeding (Forrest IB), nonbleeding visible vessel (Forrest IIA), and adherent clot (Forrest IIB). Low-risk lesions that include flat pigmented spots (Forrest IIC) and clean base ulcers (Forrest III) are more prevalent, reaching a prevalence of more than 50%.[3,32,33] Older data predating the routine use of endoscopic hemostasis reveal a natural history with rebleeding rates of 55% (17%–100%) (Forrest IA and IB), 43% (0%–81%) (Forrest IIA), 22% (14%–36%) (Forrest IIB), 10% (0%–13%) (Forrest IIC), and 5% (0%–10%) (Forrest III).[34] Significant interobserver variability has been reported in the identification of endoscopic stigmata.[35] Nonetheless, when ulcer bleeding stigmata are surveyed with sequential endoscopic evaluations, an evolution of stigmata is noted, suggesting various phases of healing whereby a bleeding vessel progressively evolves after endoscopic therapy into a clean base ulcer.[32] Furthermore, most rebleeding episodes were noted within the first 72 hours, consistent with the natural history of ulcer healing.[32]

In patients with LRS ulcers, endoscopic hemostasis has not been shown to alter outcomes.[36,37] The treatment of patients with pigmented spots or clean base ulcers therefore consists of oral acid suppressive pharmacotherapy alone. In contradistinction, endoscopic therapy in ulcer bleeding has been well established to decrease continued or recurrent bleeding, surgery, and mortality, particularly in patients with active bleeding and nonbleeding visible vessel.[36,37] For such patients, the magnitude of improvement in outcome measures from an earlier meta-analysis of 30 RCTs is as follows: further bleeding (OR 0.38; 95% CI 0.32–0.45), surgery (OR 0.36; 95% CI 0.28–0.45), and mortality (OR 0.55; 95% CI 0.40–0.6).[37] The benefits of endoscopic therapy for patients with HRS were confirmed in a more recent meta-analysis demonstrating the superiority of any endoscopic method over pharmacotherapy (which included one trial using high-dose intravenous PPI) for rebleeding (OR 0.35; 95% CI 0.27–0.46), surgery (OR 0.57; 95% CI 0.41–0.81), and mortality (OR 0.57; 95% CI 0.37–0.89).[38] Similarly, Laine and McQuaid[39] found decreased rebleeding and surgery with endoscopic therapy in comparison with no endoscopic therapy for active bleeding and nonbleeding visible vessel. However, they did not detect statistically significant benefits with regard to mortality, or in any outcomes among patients with adherent clots. Endoscopic hemostasis is therefore indicated in all patients with HRS, whereas ulcers with LRS can be managed with pharmacotherapy only, and do not warrant therapy. The more detailed management of lesions with adherent clots is somewhat controversial (see later discussion).

ENDOSCOPIC THERAPY

Endoscopic therapy is indicated in patients presenting with NVUGIB and HRS on endoscopy (see **Table 1**). Meta-analyses have found that endoscopic therapy for ulcers with these features significantly decreased rebleeding, surgery, and mortality.[36,37] In contradistinction, low-risk lesions such as ulcers with flat, pigmented spot (Forrest IIC) or clean based (Forrest III) are associated with lower incidences of rebleeding, and endoscopic therapy has not been shown to be beneficial.[32,34] In terms of endoscopic modalities, there are several techniques that have been developed including injection, thermal, and mechanical therapies and, more recently, hemostatic powders. In addition, several ancillary methods to improve endoscopic risk stratification of bleeding lesions and hemostasis such as Doppler ultrasonography, magnification endoscopy, and chromoendoscopy,[40] have also emerged. The following is an overview of the different endoscopic therapies, with a specific focus on the techniques involved in their successful deployment.

Injection Therapy

Different injectates have been developed, including epinephrine, hypertonic saline, sclerosants (polidocanol, ethanolamine, absolute alcohol, sodium tetradecyl sulfate), and tissue adhesives (cyanoacrylate, thrombin, fibrin). Injection therapy has been widely performed most likely because of its ease of use, availability, and extensive experience with its application by most endoscopists. Injections are delivered through a 25-gauge retractable catheter (**Fig. 1**A). Epinephrine (1:10,000 or 1:20,000 dilution) is the most common injectate used in the control of NVUGIB, and should be performed in increments of 0.5 to 1.5 mL in all 4 quadrants around the ulcer base with or without injections into the center of the ulcerated lesion itself (see **Fig. 1**B).[41] It is important that the main mechanism responsible for successful hemostasis is likely due to the tamponade effect from the volume of the injection rather than the vasoconstrictive mechanism of the epinephrine or resulting platelet aggregation.[34,42] In fact, randomized controlled data suggest that higher total volumes (13–45 mL) per bleeding lesion may decrease rebleeding rates, presumably because of the greater tamponade effect.[43–45] The application of epinephrine is simple and requires little skill, such that its application can be easily performed with both tangential and en-face positioning, and may be the initial agent of choice in massive gastrointestinal (GI) hemorrhage where rapid control of the bleeding field with other modalities can be difficult to achieve because of the obscured view. However injection therapies have been shown to be inferior to monotherapies with both thermal or mechanical modalities and combination therapies.[4,39,46] Pooled data for injection therapy (including trials on epinephrine monotherapy, alcohol monotherapy, and a combination of other injectates) reveals a reduction in rebleeding (OR 0.43; 95% CI 0.24–0.78) compared with pharmacotherapy[38] in patients with HRS. Despite evidence of comparable initial hemostasis success,[39] epinephrine injection is inferior to other monotherapies (thermal, fibrin glue, and clip), as already discussed, with a higher incidence of rebleeding (OR 1.72; 95% CI 1.08–2.78) and surgery (OR 2.27; 95% CI 1.02–5.00) when used alone.[39] In a meta-analysis of 16 RCTs, Calvet and colleagues[46] demonstrated that epinephrine injection, followed by a second modality, provides additional benefits with regard to reducing

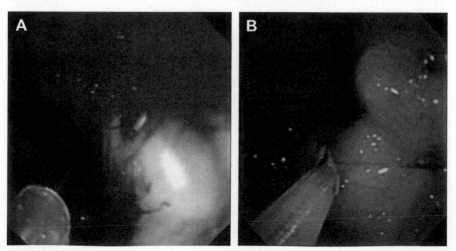

Fig. 1. (A) Injection needle near ulcer with active oozing. (B) Injection of epinephrine in ulcer resulting in mucosal blanching.

rebleeding (OR 0.53; 95% CI 0.40–0.69), surgery (OR 0.64; 95% CI 0.46–0.90), and mortality (OR 0.51; 95% CI 0.31–0.84) when compared with epinephrine monotherapy. Mortality benefits were not reproduced in more recent analyses.[38,39,47] In summary, there is strong evidence suggesting that epinephrine injection should not be used alone for the treatment of ulcer bleeding with HRS.

The role of other injectates, such as sclerosants and tissue adhesives, in the management of NVUGIB are less well defined. Sclerosants including polidocanol, ethanolamine, absolute alcohol, and sodium tetradecyl sulfate are associated with a risk of tissue necrosis, perforation, and vessel thrombosis.[48–53] Sclerosant therapy has nonetheless been associated with significant benefits in reducing rebleeding, surgery, and mortality in comparison with no therapy,[39] and can be considered in the management algorithm of NVUGIB.[4] Tissue adhesives such as cyanoacrylate, thrombin, and fibrin, on the other hand, have not been evaluated as extensively, and are often limited by their high acquisition costs and lack of availability.[54] In comparison with epinephrine, these agents are rarely used in the routine treatment of patients with NVUGIB.

Thermal Therapy

Thermal therapy applies heat or electric current to bleeding lesions, which can lead to coagulation of vessels and successful hemostasis. Thermal treatment can be divided into contact (electrocoagulation or heater probe) and noncontact techniques.

Contact electrocoagulation

Endoscopic contact electrocoagulation is available as monopolar, bipolar (BEC), or multipolar (MEC) electrocautery. Unlike the monopolar modality, the electric circuit with BEC or MEC terminates locally at the tip of the probe and decreases in intensity as the target tissue desiccates with electrocautery, thereby limiting the depth of penetration and decreasing the risk for perforation.[55] Optimal BEC/MEC is best performed using a large-diameter (10F, 3.2 mm) probe with firm, constant pressure on the high-risk lesion and application of low energy (15 W) electrocoagulation for 10 to 12 seconds until flattening of vessels or adequate coagulation of the stigmata (**Fig. 2**).[56] In other words, the goal is to achieve coaptive coagulation, with hemostasis occurring from physical occlusion and tamponade of the vessels in the bed of the bleeding lesion,

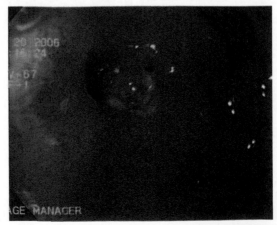

Fig. 2. Appearance of ulcer after thermal therapy, resulting in a footprint with achievement of hemostasis.

followed by thermal coagulation. Data from porcine models suggest that longer duration of electrocoagulation (tamponade station) increases the energy and coagulation, whereas increasing the watt setting does not improve the transfer of coagulation owing to the rapid increase in impedance.[56] Therefore, long-duration (10–12 seconds) and low-energy (15 W) electrocoagulation are preferred for optimal coaptive coagulation.[57,58] In terms of delivery, contact electrocoagulation is easy to use, allows for simultaneous, foot pedal–controlled water irrigation, and is effective in both bleeding and nonbleeding HRS. However, MEC/BEC may be difficult to use in the tangential position given that electric current occurs at the tip of the catheter.

Contact heater probe

The heater probe dissipates heat at the tip and sides of the probe, leading to coagulation of high-risk lesions in both the en-face and tangential position. Similarly to contact electrocoagulation, the application is best performed using a large-diameter probe (10F, 3.2 mm) and requires firm constant pressure with the target lesion; however, unlike BEC or MEC, coagulation is provided in the form of heat energy (25–30 J) and is delivered in a pulsatile fashion (4–5 pulses).[58–60] The main advantage of the heater or gold probe over contact electrocoagulation is its ability to provide coagulation through the tip and sides of the probe, therefore allowing for ease of application in both the tangential and en-face position. The heater probe also allows for foot pedal–controlled water irrigation, and is effective in both bleeding and nonbleeding HRS.[38]

The use of contact thermal therapy, namely heater probe and electrocoagulation, is beneficial in achieving hemostasis in patients with high-risk lesions, as evidenced by reduced rebleeding (OR 0.44; 95% CI 0.36–0.54), surgery (OR 0.39; 95% CI 0.27–0.55), and mortality rates (OR 0.58; 95% CI 0.34–0.98) when compared with no endoscopic treatment,[39] although the impact on mortality was not reproduced in a separate meta-analysis (OR 0.64; 95% CI 0.25–1.65).[38] Aside from the previously discussed benefits over epinephrine monotherapy, comparison of contact thermal therapy with other modalities, alone or in combination, have not yielded consistent results to favor the use of one approach over another.[38,61] It is worth mentioning that although pooled meta-analytical data comparing the combination of injection and thermal therapy with thermal monotherapy did not show any significant differences in rebleeding, subgroup analysis favored combination therapy after the removal of 2 less generalizable trials, resulting in decreased risks of rebleeding (OR 0.37; 95% CI 0.14–0.97).[38] Overall, as data to confidently support the use of one modality over another are lacking, technical considerations may better dictate the use of thermal therapy. In addition, thermocoagulation can be used either alone or in combination with injection therapy.[4]

Noncontact thermal therapy

Argon plasma coagulation (APC) is unique in its ability to deliver electrocautery in a noncontact fashion through the delivery of monopolar, alternating current through ionized argon gas. Electrical current is delivered to the target tissue via electrically charged argon gas that is propelled from the catheter tip. Coagulation is mostly superficial (up to 2.4 mm according to in vitro studies[62]), given that the argon plasma beam shifts away from coagulated tissue, which loses its conduction ability because of increases in electrical resistance with desiccation, therefore preventing further tissue damage and perforation.[57,63,64] In terms of application, the optimal distance between probe and target tissue is estimated to be 2 to 8 mm. Direct contact between the probe and the target lesion should be avoided to prevent submucosal dissection and submucosal argon gas insufflation, which causes significant pain, pneumatosis, and risk of perforation.[65] APC seems to be ideal for shallow and broadly defined bleeding lesions such as angiodysplasia, radiation telangiectasia, and gastric antral vascular ectasia, also known as watermelon stomach.[62,66–69]

The use of APC in ulcer bleeding has been evaluated in several trials that compared this approach with a variety of other modalities including heater probe,[70] sclerotherapy,[71,72] epinephrine in combination with heater probe,[73] endoclips,[74] or polidocanol, with no differences in patient outcomes.[39] However, decreased rebleeding was seen when compared with distilled water injection.[72] A single small randomized trial using epinephrine plus APC versus heater probe in patients with high-risk ulcer bleeding showed improved initial hemostasis in the APC arm.[75]

Endoclips
A wide variety of hemostatic mechanical therapies have been developed over the years; however, the endoscopic deployment of endoclips remains the most extensively studied and widely available technique in the management of NVUGIB. It achieves hemostasis through direct compression or tamponade of vessels and tissue approximation of bleeding stigmata (**Fig. 3**). Moreover, unlike most other endoscopic devices, the use of endoclips is usually associated with minimal to no tissue damage, therefore leading potentially to faster ulcer healing.[76] However, its deployment requires precision, en-face positioning, and may be inadequate in fibrotic ulcer beds given its weak tensile strength.[76] It is also noteworthy that endoclips come in many different sizes, lengths, and shapes, grasping and rotational abilities, and deployment mechanisms. Therefore, familiarity with locally available endoclips should be acquired before their use in emergency situations.

The use of endoclips is effective for ulcer bleeding and can be used alone or in combination with epinephrine, or as an alternative to thermal coagulation.[4] Although endoclips have not been compared with pharmacotherapy alone, several RCTs have assessed the benefit of endoclips with or without epinephrine injection, and in comparison with injection and thermal therapy. Again, benefits in rebleeding (OR 0.22; 95% CI 0.09–0.55) and need for surgery (OR 0.22; 95% CI 0.06–0.83) are significant only when endoclips are compared with epinephrine alone.[39] A meta-analysis evaluating 15 studies including 1156 patients highlighted the important heterogeneity across trials that have compared endoclips with thermocoagulation, with or without injection.[77] Individual trials have reported disparate results regarding the superiority or inferiority of endoclips in comparison with thermal therapy.[39] Furthermore, one meta-analysis demonstrated a benefit of endoclips over thermal therapy for rebleeding (OR 0.24;

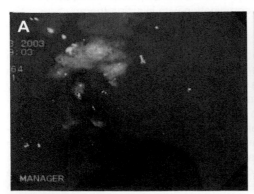
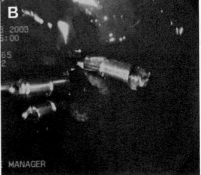

Fig. 3. (*A*) Ulcer with nonbleeding visible vessel. (*B*) Appearance of ulcer after the application of endoclips.

95% CI 0.06–0.95),[38] though statistically less robust. Additional considerations such as ulcer location can help direct the decision to use endoclips rather than another hemostatic modality, as higher endoclip failure is seen for ulcers situated in the posterior wall of the duodenum and gastric body, and along the lesser gastric curvature.[77]

In addition to the general recommendation to avoid epinephrine monotherapy,[4] some organizations have recently suggested that thermal or combination therapy may be favored over endoclips or sclerosants when managing actively bleeding lesions,[78] and that thermal therapy should be used with epinephrine[10] based on lower-quality evidence.

Endoscopic hemostatic powders

Recently, novel endoscopic topical hemostatic powders such as the Ankaferd Blood Stopper (ABS), EndoClot, and TC-325 have been adapted to digestive endoscopy and the management of gastrointestinal bleeding (GIB). ABS (Ankaferd Health Products Ltd, Istanbul, Turkey) is a herbal extract derived from 5 different plants that achieves hemostasis by promoting the formation of a protein network behaving as an anchor for erythrocyte aggregation.[79] This agent, however, is not available in North America.

The EndoClot Polysaccharide Hemostatic System (EndoClot-PHS; EndoClot Plus, Inc, Santa Clara, CA, USA) is another emerging hemostatic powder composed of a biocompatible, nonpyogenic, starch-derived compound. It achieves hemostasis by effecting mechanical tamponade and rapid absorption of water from serum, leading to concentration of platelets and clotting factors and thereby accelerating the clotting cascade.[80] At present, the literature on EndoClot is limited to 1 abstract reporting its successful use as an adjuvant therapy in UGIB in 6 patients.[81] Therefore more data are needed with regard to GIB, and the EndoClot is currently not approved for use in North America. TC-325 (Hemospray; Cook Medical, Winston-Salem, NC, USA) is composed of a proprietary inorganic biologically inert powder that, when put in contact with moisture in the GI tract, becomes coherent, thus serving as a mechanical barrier for hemostasis.[82] In addition, it may provide a scaffold, enhancing platelet aggregation and possibly activating clotting factors.[83] However, the powder only adheres to actively bleeding lesions, so its use in high-risk lesions without active spurting or oozing is likely ineffective in providing appropriate hemostasis. The endoscopic powder is propelled from a canister under CO_2 pressure and is delivered through a catheter onto the bleeding lesion (**Fig. 4**A, B). The TC-325 catheter should be maintained 1 to 2 cm from the high-risk lesion, and application should be performed in a noncontact fashion (see **Fig. 4**C). The endoscopic powder will aggregate immediately when it comes into contact with moisture; therefore, efforts should be made to keep the tip of the catheter dry and to avoid suctioning while it is in use or while the powder is settling. Flushing the accessory channel of the endoscope with a 60-mL syringe of air before TC-325 application is also recommended to ensure that the tip of the catheter does not come into contact with moisture during insertion. With the current second-generation Hemospray delivery system, application of the powder occurs by engaging the trigger button, which results in an initial burst of CO_2 gas followed by the release of the hemostatic powder. The accumulation of CO_2 gas may become uncomfortable for the patient. Advantages associated with TC-325 use include ease of application with a lack of need for precise targeting (although the powder needs to reach the actively bleeding site), noncontact and nontraumatic hemostasis, and ability to cover large surfaces of bleeding. As such it may be the ideal modality for massive NVUGIB where rapid control of the bleeding field is critical, and in hemorrhage arising from GI malignancies where bleeding often stems from friable, irregular, and diffusely bleeding surfaces.

Sung and colleagues[1] first described the use of TC-325 in GIB in a prospective pilot study involving 20 patients with NVUGIB treated with Hemospray, resulting in an

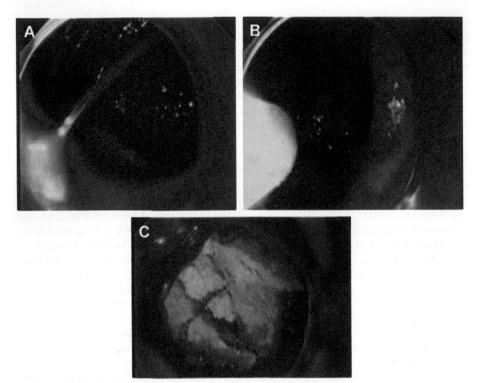

Fig. 4. (*A*) Ulcer with spurting vessel. (*B*) Hemospray catheter advanced near target lesion. (*C*) Appearance of ulcer following the application of Hemospray, resulting in hemostasis.

immediate hemostasis of 95%. Subsequently a multicenter, retrospective study including 63 patients with NVUGIB demonstrated a rate of immediate hemostasis and of 7-day rebleeding with TC-325 therapy for 85% (95% CI 76%–94%) and 15% (95% CI 5%–25%), respectively.[84] More specifically, this study included 25 patients with peptic ulcer bleeding who received TC-325 monotherapy, which resulted in an immediate hemostasis of 76% (95% CI 59%–93%) and a 7-day rebleeding rate of 16% (95% CI 0%–32%). Retrospective data at a single institution recently demonstrated the versatility and effectiveness of TC-325 in both the upper and lower GI tracts in 67 cases of TC-325 therapy in patients with a variety of bleeding disorders including 21 cases of NVUGIB of nonmalignant etiology.[85] The rate of immediate hemostasis and early rebleeding (within 72 hours of TC-325 application) for NVUGIB were 95.2% and 29.4%, respectively. In addition, the powder residency time on the bleeding lesions was demonstrated to be less than 24 hours. Therefore, the current thinking is that TC-325 should not be used as the sole modality in lesions at high risk of rebleeding following the first 24 hours, such as peptic ulcer bleeding with HRS; indeed other modalities, namely thermal or mechanical therapies, should be added to ensure sustained hemostasis. In terms of safety, no major complications, including intestinal obstruction or vascular embolization, have been observed in more than 150 patients treated with TC-325 for GIB.[84–87]

ADHERENT CLOTS

The approach to ulcers with an overlying clot is to irrigate the lesion in an attempt to dislodge the blood clot and reveal the underlying stigma. Vigorous washing for up to

5 minutes is effective in removing the clot in about 40% of lesions.[88] Ulcers with clots resistant to such manipulation are defined as adherent clots (Forrest IIB). These lesions can be further managed by mechanical clot removal without disrupting the pedicle to expose the ulcer base (after preliminary dilute epinephrine injection around the ulcer), followed by endoscopic therapy according to the stigmata of recent bleeding.[4]

The optimal management algorithm for adherent clots remains controversial, as RCTs comparing medical with endoscopic therapy have yielded diverging results. Indeed, some trials have shown that endoscopic therapy decreases rebleeding in adherent clots,[89,90] whereas others,[91,92] including one trial using contemporary high-dose intravenous PPI,[93] have demonstrated low rebleeding rates with acid suppression alone. A previous meta-analysis combining 6 studies with 240 patients suggested a significant reduction in rebleeding with endoscopic hemostasis.[94] However, this work was criticized because of statistical shortcomings and marked heterogeneity of the combined trials, namely differing PPI regimens used in the control arms of the included studies.[95] A more recent meta-analysis failed to detect significant benefits of endoscopic therapy over no endoscopic therapy for adherent clots in terms of rebleeding, need for surgery, or mortality.[39] Consensus guidelines state that endoscopic therapy can be considered while acknowledging that intensive PPI therapy alone may be adequate.[4]

PROTON-PUMP INHIBITORS POSTENDOSCOPIC THERAPY

PPI use in ulcer bleeding improves outcomes. A Cochrane analysis of 31 trials with 5792 patients revealed that PPI use decreases rebleeding (OR 0.45; 95% CI 0.36–0.57), the need for surgery (OR 0.56; 95% CI 0.45–0.70), or repeat endoscopy (OR 0.40; 95% CI 0.30–0.53) regardless of endoscopic hemostasis. A reduction in mortality was achieved only in trials conducted in Asian patients, and more importantly, in patients with active bleeding or nonbleeding visible vessel who had first undergone successful endoscopic hemostasis and who received high-dose intravenous PPIs (80 mg bolus and 8 mg/h infusion for 72 hours).

Another meta-analysis assessing high-dose intravenous PPI as an adjunct to endoscopic hemostasis further supports the observed decrease in rebleeding (OR 0.40; 95% CI 0.28–0.59), surgery (OR 0.43; 95% CI 0.24–0.76), and mortality (OR 0.41; 95% CI 0.20–0.84).[39] Alternative dosing and oral routes have not yielded consistent results to allow for confident routine recommendations of such regimens.[96] All patients with HRS should be treated with high-dose intravenous PPI after endoscopic hemostasis for 72 hours, a period during which most rebleeding occurs.[32] This practice also appears to be cost-effective.[97–99]

SECOND-LOOK ENDOSCOPY

A second-look endoscopy refers to the performance of a preplanned repeat endoscopy 16 to 24 hours following the initial endoscopy, aimed at assessing the need for further endoscopic therapy directed toward any remaining HRS, if present. This practice has previously shown rebleeding benefits,[100,101] although many of the trials did not include concomitant PPI use and used epinephrine monotherapy, a technique now shown to be suboptimal. In fact, in the setting of high-dose intravenous PPI, second-look endoscopy did not provide added benefits.[102] A recent meta-analysis acknowledges the decreased rebleeding conferred by second-look endoscopy in certain high-risk patients with active bleeding, in the absence of high-dose PPI, but discourages against its routine practice in all patients.[103] Consequently, consensus guidelines have concluded that contemporary data do not favor such practice.[4] While further studies are needed to delineate high-risk groups that may benefit from routine second-look endoscopy,[78] the added cost it would entail also needs to be considered.[97] A rebleeding rate exceeding 31% may be needed to offset the cost of a second endoscopy.[104]

In settings where the primary hemostasis is uncertain, and where the initial evaluation was incomplete because of blood clots, repeat endoscopy may be warranted.[105]

PREDICTORS OF FAILURE OF ENDOSCOPIC THERAPY

Rebleeding after endoscopy occurs in 10% to 15% patients presenting with NVU-GIB,[106] although reported values vary in the literature. Data specific to ulcer bleeding vary between 6.3% and 25.2%.[107] Several independent predictors of endoscopic failure have been identified based on both pre-endoscopic and endoscopic features. These predictors include hemodynamic instability (OR 3.30; 95% CI 2.57–4.24), transfusion requirement, and hemoglobin less than 10 g/dL (OR 1.73; 95% CI 1.14–2.62).[107] Active bleeding at endoscopy (OR 1.70; 95% CI 1.31–2.22), the location of bleeding ulcer in either the posterior duodenal wall (OR 3.83; 95% CI 1.38–10.66) or gastric high lesser curvature (OR 2.86; 95% CI 1.69–4.86), in addition to greater ulcer size, particularly larger than 2 cm, also contribute to higher rebleeding rates.[107]

In patients with clinical evidence of rebleeding, a second endoscopy should be attempted to achieve hemostasis. Indeed, comparing endoscopic retreatment with surgery, rates of successful hemostasis in the endoscopy arm reached 73% (35 of 48 patients), with overall lower complication rates, but comparable mortality and length of stay.[108] Failure of repeat endoscopy should be treated with transcatheter arterial embolization or surgery.[109] Details pertaining to such therapies are discussed in articles elsewhere in this issue.

HELICOBACTER PYLORI TESTING

Helicobacter pylori eradication has been demonstrated in a meta-analysis to be significantly more effective than PPI therapy alone in preventing rebleeding from peptic ulcer disease.[110] As such, consensus guidelines have recommended that all patients with peptic ulcer bleeding undergo H pylori evaluation, with subsequent eradication if tested positive.[4,111,112] It is important that if the evaluation for H pylori is negative in the acute setting, repeat testing is indicated. Indeed, a systematic review of 23 studies showed that diagnostic tests for H pylori infection (including serology, histology, urea breath test, rapid urease test, stool antigen, and culture) are associated with high positive predictive values (0.85–0.99) but low negative predictive values (0.45–0.75) in the setting of acute GIB, with 25% to 55% of H pylori–infected patients yielding false-negative results.[113,114] This high false-negative rate in acute bleeding may be related, at least in part, to an alkaline milieu imparted by the presence of blood in the gastric lumen, resulting in proximal migration of the bacterium.[115]

MANAGEMENT OF NONSTEROIDAL ANTI-INFLAMMATORY DRUGS IN PATIENTS WITH PEPTIC ULCER BLEEDING

In patients with previous ulcer bleeding, nonsteroidal anti-inflammatory drugs (NSAIDs) should be discontinued. If absolutely needed, a combination of cyclooxygenase-2 (COX-2) inhibitor with a PPI is recommended.[116,117] Adding a PPI to a traditional NSAID or using a COX-2 inhibitor alone reduces the risk of upper gastrointestinal complications; however, the combination of COX-2 inhibitor with

PPI has been shown to be associated with the greatest reductions in risk.[115,116] RCTs have demonstrated that administration of a COX-2 inhibitor plus a PPI when compared with COX-2 inhibitor alone further decreases the risk of rebleeding following an episode of acute peptic ulcer hemorrhage.[118–120] However, there may be an increased risk of cardiovascular events with the use of COX-2 inhibitors, as demonstrated by 2 meta-analyses.[121,122] As such, when reinstituting NSAID therapy following NVUGIB, the risk of cardiovascular events must be balanced with the risk of GI complications on an individual basis. Following an episode of NVUGIB an alternative to NSAID therapy should first be sought and, if necessary, use of a COX-2 inhibitor with a PPI should be favored.[116]

ACUTE MANAGEMENT OF ANTIPLATELET AND ANTICOAGULATION THERAPY IN PATIENTS WITH PEPTIC ULCER BLEEDING

In the event of acute NVUGIB, ongoing aspirin (acetylsalicylic acid; ASA) intake should be held; however, prolonged discontinuation should be avoided. In a meta-analysis, ASA nonadherence or withdrawal was associated with a 3-fold increase in major cardiac events.[123] Moreover, a recent retrospective cohort study from Sweden demonstrated that prolonged discontinuation of ASA, in the context of secondary cardiovascular prophylaxis following acute GIB, led to a 7-fold increase in cardiovascular events or death.[124] The observed thrombosis time is usually between 7 and 30 days, which is in keeping with the ASA-inhibited platelet circulation time of about 10 days.[125,126] In addition, data from one randomized controlled trial suggest that the cardiovascular protection associated with early reinstitution of ASA outweighs the gastrointestinal bleeding risks.[127] Based on these results, consensus recommendations suggest that ASA therapy should be held in acute peptic ulcer bleeding, and restarted as soon as the risk for cardiovascular complication is thought to outweigh the risk for GIB.[4] Practically the authors recommend that ASA be reintroduced within 3 to 5 days of the index bleed after appropriate endoscopic and pharmacologic therapy, with appropriate discussions among the multidisciplinary treatment team that can include general practitioners, internists, cardiologists, neurologists, gastroenterologists, and intensivists. Data on the optimal management of clopidogrel and dual antiplatelet therapy (DAPT) in the acute context of bleeding are lacking.

Vitamin K antagonists such as warfarin should also be held during the setting of an acute GI bleed, and efforts should be made to correct the coagulopathy. In the Canadian Registry on Non-Variceal Upper Gastrointestinal Bleeding and Endoscopy (RUGBE) cohort of 1869 patients, a presenting international normalized ratio (INR) of greater than 1.5 was associated with an almost 2-fold increased risk of mortality (OR 1.95; 95% CI 1.13–3.41), without any increased risk of rebleeding.[128] Data using a historical cohort comparison showed that correcting an INR to less than 1.8, as part of intensive resuscitation, led to lower mortality and fewer myocardial infarctions.[129] Therefore, current guidelines on NVUGIB support the correction of a coagulopathy; however, this should not delay endoscopy.[4] This recent consensus recommendation is based on the recognition of the benefits of early endoscopic intervention coupled with the decreased tissue damage associated with newer ligation hemostatic techniques such as endoscopic clips or hemostatic powders. Moreover, limited observational data also suggest that endoscopic hemostasis can be safely performed in patients with an elevated INR less than 2.5.[130] Although fresh frozen plasma (FFP) may be administered for the reversal of warfarin-induced coagulopathy in patients presenting with life-threatening hemorrhage, prothrombin complex concentrate (PCC) may be a better adapted blood product in this setting. Contrary to FFP, PCC does not need to be frozen during storage, and therefore can be administered more rapidly without the need for thawing. Furthermore, PCC is associated with more effective warfarin reversal, faster infusion rates, lower volumes of administration, and fewer adverse events including thrombotic complications.[131,132] In addition, the use of PCC may be more cost-effective than FFP in the setting of urgent warfarin reversal.[133]

Lastly, the emergence of direct thrombin and factor Xa inhibitors may present a new challenge in acute GIB, given that neither FFP nor PCC have been found to be effective in reversing these agents[134]; however, PCC may still be considered in severe hemorrhage, based on its variable success in animal and in vitro studies as well as in healthy nonbleeding human volunteers.[135,136] Developments of specific reversal agents for these novel oral anticoagulants (nOAC) are currently under way.

MANAGEMENT OF LONG-TERM ANTIPLATELET THERAPY FOLLOWING PEPTIC ULCER HEMORRHAGE

Peptic ulcer disease (PUD) with or without bleeding is a common complication of long-term ASA administration for cardiothrombotic prophylaxis.[137,138] Both H2 receptor antagonists (H2RA) and PPIs have been used in peptic ulcer prophylaxis. The efficacy of H2RA was demonstrated in an RCT showing that famotidine, 20 mg twice daily, can reduce the incidence of peptic ulcer and erosive esophagitis while on ASA in comparison with placebo-based endoscopic assessment at 12 weeks.[139] Clinical outcomes, however, were not assessed in this study, which only assessed patients at low risk of a GI complication. More recently, an RCT by Ng and colleagues,[140] comparing famotidine 40 mg twice daily with pantoprazole 20 mg daily, demonstrated the superiority of the PPI over H2RA in terms of reducing dyspepsia and upper GIB in patients on long-term ASA and a history of PUD with or without bleeding (these patients are at highest risk of bleeding recurrence). Therefore, current consensus guidelines recommend PPI prophylaxis in patients on ASA and high-risk features for gastrointestinal complications such as a history of PUD with or without bleeding.[4]

In addition to PPI prophylaxis, patients who require long-term ASA following acute peptic ulcer bleeding should undergo testing and eradication of *H pylori*.[4] Data from an RCT demonstrated similar effectiveness in bleeding prophylaxis between *H pylori* eradication and PPI administration following ulcer bleeding in patients requiring chronic ASA over a 6-month period.[141] However, discrepant results, from Lai and colleagues,[142] demonstrated a high rebleeding rate with ASA following an attempt at *H pylori* eradication. This result may be due, at least in part, to the fact that many of the subjects in this group failed eradication therapy. Therefore, *H pylori* testing with eradication coupled with the use of long-term PPI in patients requiring chronic ASA use following an ulcer bleed is recommended.[4] The long-term benefits of sole *H pylori* eradication in patients having bled while on ASA has been shown, in a retrospective cohort study, to be associated with very low rebleeding rates even after a period of 10 years.[143]

Clopidogrel administration following peptic ulcer bleeding is also associated with high rebleeding rates of 9% to 14%,[144,145] and PPI prophylaxis should be considered. RCT data reported by Hsu and colleagues[146] comparing PPI with placebo in patients on clopidogrel and a history of PUD showed a decreased incidence of recurrent PUD when endoscopy was performed at 6-month follow-up. In terms of DAPT, data on PPI gastroprotection, in a patient population at no particularly high risk for bleeding based on history, has been well described in the COGENT trial,[147] showing a significant reduction in GIB (hazard ratio 0.34; 95% CI 0.18–0.63). Therefore, the authors suggest PPI gastroprotection for patients on clopidogrel monotherapy and a history of PUD, whereas societies have suggested that all patients on DAPT should receive PPI routinely, irrespective of previous history of PUD with or without bleeding.[137,138,148]

Pharmacokinetic and platelet ex vivo assay studies have suggested that PPIs may reduce the antiplatelet effects of clopidogrel,[149-151] as have several clinical observational data. However, these findings are confounded by methodological limitations, covariate imbalances in patient characteristics, and the absence of correction for statistical heterogeneity. In fact, following multivariate adjustment, any attenuating effect of PPI on the beneficial clinical effect of clopidogrel seems to be very limited or nonexistent.[152,153] In addition, the COGENT trial comparing DAPT (ASA + clopidogrel) and PPI with DAPT and placebo showed no significant differences in the incidence of major cardiovascular events.[147] However, this trial was terminated prematurely, with a median follow-up time of 133 days, and before the planned full enrollment number was achieved. Lastly, 3 systematic reviews using the best-quality observational studies did not show any significant increase in cardiovascular events with the use of PPI with clopidogrel.[153-155] In summary, high-quality evidence supporting a clinically significant interaction between PPI and clopidogrel is presently lacking. Consequently, most consensus guidelines, including those from the American College of Cardiology, American Heart Association, American College of Gastroenterology (ACG), Canadian Association of Gastroenterology, and the most recent ACG guidelines in the management of gastroesophageal reflux disease,[156] all recommend that patients currently receiving these agents should continue without changing their treatment regimen unless advised by their health care providers.

MANAGEMENT OF LONG-TERM ANTICOAGULATION FOLLOWING PEPTIC ULCER BLEEDING

Warfarin therapy, a vitamin K antagonist, is associated with a significant risk of bleeding, which is accentuated by its narrow therapeutic window. In fact, systematic reviews show that in community practice the therapeutic target (INR 2.0–3.0) is only achieved in 63.6% of patients, with a rate of major hemorrhage (from any source) ranging from 1% to 7.4% per year.[157-159] Controlled data on the benefit of PPI therapy in preventing GIB in patients on warfarin is currently lacking. A population-based, nested case-control study evaluating PPI in patients using antiplatelet therapies and/or oral anticoagulants showed an overall decrease in GIB; however, although there was a trend toward less bleeding in the subgroup analysis of patients on warfarin, it did not reach statistical significance (OR 0.48; 95% CI 0.22–1.04).[160] Nevertheless, the authors recommend that patients on warfarin therapy receive PPI prophylaxis in the presence of previous PUD with or without bleeding.

Triple therapy (ie, DAPT and an oral anticoagulant) is indicated in patients who are at high risk for cardiothrombotic and cardioembolic events. Warfarin combined with DAPT increases the risk of GIB substantially, with one study showing a hazard ratio of 5.0 (95% CI 1.4–17.8) compared with DAPT alone.[161] A randomized controlled trial by Ng and colleagues,[162] comparing PPI with H2RA as gastroprotective agents in patients who presented with acute coronary syndrome and treated with DAPT and enoxaparin or thrombolytics, demonstrated significant reduction in GIB with the use of esomeprazole versus famotidine. More recently, Dewilde and colleagues[163] compared the risk of hemorrhage (from all sources) in an RCT with triple therapy (ASA, clopidogrel, and warfarin/heparin) versus double therapy (anticoagulation and clopidogrel) in patients with high cardioembolic risk factors who underwent percutaneous coronary intervention (PCI). Double therapy was shown to be associated with lower all-cause bleeding except for intracranial hemorrhage. More specifically, in terms of GIB, double therapy was also accompanied by lower bleeding risks when compared with triple therapy, with bleeding rates of 2.9% versus 8.8%, respectively. In addition, withholding ASA was not associated with higher thrombotic events, which is consistent with previous RCTs suggesting similar antithrombotic effectiveness between ASA and warfarin.[164,165] However, the study was underpowered to detect a significant difference in thrombotic complications. In addition, PPI use was unregimented in this study and could have been a major confounder. Overall, the authors recommend that all patients on triple therapy receive PPI prophylaxis regardless of a history of peptic ulcer or GIB. Given a lack of high-level evidence, in patients with previous history of peptic ulcer bleeding a decision to withhold ASA must include consideration of the patient's cardiovascular risks, and appropriate discussions with other appropriate professionals (such as the treating cardiologist) and the patient.

MANAGEMENT OF LONG-TERM NOVEL ANTICOAGULANTS FOLLOWING PEPTIC ULCER BLEEDING

Unlike warfarin, novel anticoagulants, including direct thrombin and factor Xa inhibitors, are not limited by a narrow therapeutic window and do not require routine monitoring of the therapeutic target. Agents such as dabigatran, rivaroxaban, apixaban, and edoxaban are currently used or are undergoing large-scale evaluation in patients with atrial fibrillation, deep vein thrombosis (DVT)/pulmonary embolism, and DVT prophylaxis. However, data from RCTs have shown concerning association with increased risk for GI hemorrhage.[166,167] A recent systematic review of 43 trials showed a modest but significant increase risk for GIB (OR 1.45; 95% CI 1.07–1.97) with the use of nOAC when compared with standard of care (warfarin and/or unfractionated

Table 2			
Antiplatelets and oral anticoagulants (OAC) bleeding risks and recommended gastroprotection			
	Risk of GIB: OR (95% CI)	Routine PPI	PPI Post PUD ± Bleeding
Low-dose ASA	2.07 (1.61–2.66) vs placebo[169]		+[4,78,148]
Clopidogrel	1.67 (1.27–2.20) vs no treatment[170]		+[148]
DAPT	3.90 (2.78–5.47) vs no treatment[170]	+[a,147]	
Warfarin	1.94 (1.61–2.34) vs no treatment[170]		+[148]
Triple therapy: ASA/ clopidogrel/OAC	5.0 (1.4–17.8) vs DAPT[161]	+[a,162]	
Novel OAC	1.45 (1.07–1.97) vs warfarin and/or UFH/LMWH[168]		+[b]

Recommendations based on expert consensus guidelines.

All patients should undergo H pylori testing/eradication post PUD complicated or not, regardless of antiplatelet/OAC use.[4,78,111,112,137,147]

Abbreviations: ASA, aspirin; CI, confidence interval; DAPT, dual antiplatelet therapy; GIB, gastrointestinal bleeding; LMWH, low molecular weight heparin; OAC, oral anticoagulant; OR, odds ratio; PPI, proton-pump inhibitor; PUD, peptic ulcer disease; UFH, unfractionated heparin.

[a] No guideline; refers to the highest-level evidence available.

[b] Recommendations by the authors based on existing evidence discussed in the text.

Data from Refs.[4,78,111,112,137,147]

heparin/low molecular weight heparin).[168] Furthermore, the pooled OR for dabigatran was 1.58 (95% CI 1.29–193) with a number needed to harm of 83, whereas the pooled OR for rivaroxaban was 1.48 (95% CI 1.21–1.82). Neither apixaban nor edoxaban were associated with increased GIB. Of note, no head-to-head evaluations have been completed between these nOACs; therefore, it is premature to conclude which nOAC is associated with the lowest risk for GIB.

With the ongoing large-scale implementation of nOAC, GIB associated with these agents will gain importance in the practice of gastroenterologists. Of note, the nOAC trials to date do not include patients at high risk of GI complications, such as those with a history of GIB or PUD. Moreover, the severity of GIB with nOAC when compared with warfarin is largely unknown, which is especially pertinent considering the lack of effective reversal agents. In terms of GI prophylaxis, the concomitant use of PPI with nOAC has not been evaluated. However, given the benefits of PPI use with ASA, clopidogrel, DAPT, and triple therapy–related GIB, the authors recommend its use in patients on nOAC with a history of PUD, complicated or not, until further data are available (**Table 2**).

SUMMARY

Endoscopic evaluation with hemostasis, if indicated, represents the mainstay in the management of peptic ulcer bleeding. It should be performed within 24 hours of patient presentation, following hemodynamic resuscitation. Endoscopic risk stratification into HRS and LRS further dictates management with the use of either monotherapy or combination endoscopic therapy to achieve hemostasis in patients with high-risk lesions. The choice between injection, thermal, and mechanical modalities, and the use of hemostatic powders, depends on individual preferences, availability, and ulcer characteristics. Epinephrine injection monotherapy should, however, be avoided. All patients with HRS should receive 72 hours of high-dose intravenous PPI after endoscopic hemostasis to further significantly decrease rebleeding, need for surgery, and mortality in high-risk patients. Secondary prophylaxis with regard to *H pylori* testing and eradication, appropriate continued acid suppression, and the optimal management of NSAIDs, ASA, antiplatelets, and anticoagulant agents according to current guidelines is needed to decrease bleeding recurrence.

REFERENCES

1. Laine L, Yang H, Chang SC, et al. Trends for incidence of hospitalization and death due to GI complications in the United States from 2001 to 2009. Am J Gastroenterol 2012;107(8):1190–5. http://dx.doi.org/10.1038/ajg.2012.168 [quiz: 6]. pii:ajg2012168.
2. Hearnshaw SA, Logan RF, Lowe D, et al. Acute upper gastrointestinal bleeding in the UK: patient characteristics, diagnoses and outcomes in the 2007 UK audit. Gut 2011;60(10):1327–35. http://dx.doi.org/10.1136/gut.2010.228437. pii:gut.2010.228437.
3. Enestvedt BK, Gralnek IM, Mattek N, et al. An evaluation of endoscopic indications and findings related to nonvariceal upper-GI hemorrhage in a large multicenter consortium. Gastrointest Endosc 2008;67(3):422–9. http://dx.doi.org/10.1016/j.gie.2007.09.024. pii:S0016-5107(07)02688-0.
4. Barkun AN, Bardou M, Kuipers EJ, et al. International consensus recommendations on the management of patients with nonvariceal upper gastrointestinal bleeding. Ann Intern Med 2010;152(2):101–13. http://dx.doi.org/10.1059/0003-4819-152-2-201001190-00009. pii:152/2/101.

5. Barkun AN, Bardou M, Martel M, et al. Prokinetics in acute upper GI bleeding: a meta-analysis [Systematic reviews and meta-analyses]. Gastrointest Endosc 2010;72(6):1138–45. http://dx.doi.org/10.1016/j.gie.2010.08.011. pii:S0016-5107(10)01967-X.

6. Szary NM, Gupta R, Choudhary A, et al. Erythromycin prior to endoscopy in acute upper gastrointestinal bleeding: a meta-analysis [Systematic reviews and meta-analyses]. Scand J Gastroenterol 2011;46(7–8):920–4. http://dx.doi.org/10.3109/00365521.2011.568520.

7. Bai Y, Guo JF, Li ZS. Meta-analysis: erythromycin before endoscopy for acute upper gastrointestinal bleeding [Systematic reviews and meta-analyses]. Aliment Pharmacol Ther 2011;34(2):166–71. http://dx.doi.org/10.1111/j.1365-2036.2011.04708.x.

8. Altraif I, Handoo FA, Aljumah A, et al. Effect of erythromycin before endoscopy in patients presenting with variceal bleeding: a prospective, randomized, double-blind, placebo-controlled trial. Gastrointest Endosc 2011;73(2):245–50. http://dx.doi.org/10.1016/j.gie.2010.09.043. pii:S0016-5107(10)02181-4.

9. Theivanayagam S, Lim RG, Cobell WJ, et al. Administration of erythromycin before endoscopy in upper gastrointestinal bleeding: a meta-analysis of randomized controlled trials [Systematic reviews and meta-analyses]. Saudi J Gastroenterol 2013;19(5):205–10. http://dx.doi.org/10.4103/1319-3767.118120.

10. NICE. Acute upper gastrointestinal bleeding: management: NHS National Institute for Health and Clinical Excellence. 2012 [cited February 25, 2013]. Available at: http://www.nice.org.uk/nicemedia/live/13762/59549/59549.pdf. Accessed September 9, 2014.

11. Spiegel BM, Vakil NB, Ofman JJ. Endoscopy for acute nonvariceal upper gastrointestinal tract hemorrhage: is sooner better? A systematic review [Systematic reviews and meta-analyses]. Arch Intern Med 2001;161(11):1393–404. pii:ira00052.

12. Cipolletta L, Bianco MA, Rotondano G, et al. Outpatient management for low-risk nonvariceal upper GI bleeding: a randomized controlled trial. Gastrointest Endosc 2002;55(1):1–5. http://dx.doi.org/10.1067/mge.2002.119219.

13. Tsoi KK, Ma TK, Sung JJ. Endoscopy for upper gastrointestinal bleeding: how urgent is it? Nat Rev Gastroenterol Hepatol 2009;6(8):463–9. http://dx.doi.org/10.1038/nrgastro.2009.108. pii:nrgastro.2009.108.

14. Schacher GM, Lesbros-Pantoflickova D, Ortner MA, et al. Is early endoscopy in the emergency room beneficial in patients with bleeding peptic ulcer? A "fortuitously controlled" study. Endoscopy 2005;37(4):324–8. http://dx.doi.org/10.1055/s-2004-826237.

15. Bjorkman DJ, Zaman A, Fennerty MB, et al. Urgent vs. elective endoscopy for acute non-variceal upper-GI bleeding: an effectiveness study. Gastrointest Endosc 2004;60(1):1–8.

16. Targownik LE, Murthy S, Keyvani L, et al. The role of rapid endoscopy for high-risk patients with acute nonvariceal upper gastrointestinal bleeding. Can J Gastroenterol 2007;21(7):425–9.

17. Tai CM, Huang SP, Wang HP, et al. High-risk ED patients with nonvariceal upper gastrointestinal hemorrhage undergoing emergency or urgent endoscopy: a retrospective analysis. Am J Emerg Med 2007;25(3):273–8. http://dx.doi.org/10.1016/j.ajem.2006.07.014.

18. Cooper GS, Chak A, Way LE, et al. Early endoscopy in upper gastrointestinal hemorrhage: associations with recurrent bleeding, surgery, and length of hospital stay. Gastrointest Endosc 1999;49(2):145–52.

19. Cooper GS, Chak A, Connors AF Jr, et al. The effectiveness of early endoscopy for upper gastrointestinal hemorrhage: a community-based analysis. Med Care 1998;36(4):462–74.

20. Lin HJ, Wang K, Perng CL, et al. Early or delayed endoscopy for patients with peptic ulcer bleeding. A prospective randomized study. J Clin Gastroenterol 1996;22(4):267–71.

21. Lim LG, Ho KY, Chan YH, et al. Urgent endoscopy is associated with lower mortality in high-risk but not low-risk nonvariceal upper gastrointestinal bleeding. Endoscopy 2011;43(4):300–6. http://dx.doi.org/10.1055/s-0030-1256110.

22. Academy of Medical Royal Colleges. Upper gastrointestinal bleeding toolkit. 2011 [cited December 15, 2013]. Available at: http://www.aomrc.org.uk/projects/item/upper-gastrointestinal-bleeding-toolkit.html. Accessed September 9, 2014.

23. Barkun AN, Bardou M, Kuipers EJ, et al. How early should endoscopy be performed in suspected upper gastrointestinal bleeding? Am J Gastroenterol 2012;107(2):328–9. http://dx.doi.org/10.1038/ajg.2011.363.

24. Garcia-Tsao G, Sanyal AJ, Grace ND, et al. Prevention and management of gastroesophageal varices and variceal hemorrhage in cirrhosis. Hepatology 2007;46(3):922–38. http://dx.doi.org/10.1002/hep.21907.

25. Hearnshaw SA, Logan RF, Lowe D, et al. Use of endoscopy for management of acute upper gastrointestinal bleeding in the UK: results of a nationwide audit. Gut 2010;59(8):1022–9. http://dx.doi.org/10.1136/gut.2008.174599. pii: gut.2008.174599.

26. Rosenstock SJ, Moller MH, Larsson H, et al. Improving quality of care in peptic ulcer bleeding: nationwide cohort study of 13,498 consecutive patients in the Danish Clinical Register of Emergency Surgery. Am J Gastroenterol 2013; 108(9):1449–57. http://dx.doi.org/10.1038/ajg.2013.162.

27. Jairath V, Kahan BC, Logan RF, et al. Mortality from acute upper gastrointestinal bleeding in the United Kingdom: does it display a "weekend effect"? Am J Gastroenterol 2011;106(9):1621–8. http://dx.doi.org/10.1038/ajg.2011.172.

28. Ananthakrishnan AN, McGinley EL, Saeian K. Outcomes of weekend admissions for upper gastrointestinal hemorrhage: a nationwide analysis. Clin Gastroenterol Hepatol 2009;7(3):296–302.e1. http://dx.doi.org/10.1016/j.cgh.2008.08.013.

29. Shaheen AA, Kaplan GG, Myers RP. Weekend versus weekday admission and mortality from gastrointestinal hemorrhage caused by peptic ulcer disease. Clin Gastroenterol Hepatol 2009;7(3):303–10. http://dx.doi.org/10.1016/j.cgh.2008.08.033.

30. Tsoi KK, Chiu PW, Chan FK, et al. The risk of peptic ulcer bleeding mortality in relation to hospital admission on holidays: a cohort study on 8,222 cases of peptic ulcer bleeding. Am J Gastroenterol 2012;107(3):405–10. http://dx.doi.org/10.1038/ajg.2011.409.

31. Kanwal F, Barkun A, Gralnek IM, et al. Measuring quality of care in patients with nonvariceal upper gastrointestinal hemorrhage: development of an explicit quality indicator set. Am J Gastroenterol 2010;105(8):1710–8. http://dx.doi.org/10.1038/ajg.2010.180.

32. Lau JY, Chung SC, Leung JW, et al. The evolution of stigmata of hemorrhage in bleeding peptic ulcers: a sequential endoscopic study. Endoscopy 1998;30(6):513–8. http://dx.doi.org/10.1055/s-2007-1001336.

33. Marmo R, Koch M, Cipolletta L, et al. Predictive factors of mortality from nonvariceal upper gastrointestinal hemorrhage: a multicenter study. Am J Gastroenterol

2008;103(7):1639–47. http://dx.doi.org/10.1111/j.1572-0241.2008.01865.x [quiz: 48]. pii:AJG1865.

34. Laine L, Peterson WL. Bleeding peptic ulcer. N Engl J Med 1994;331(11): 717–27. http://dx.doi.org/10.1056/NEJM199409153311107.

35. Laine L, Freeman M, Cohen H. Lack of uniformity in evaluation of endoscopic prognostic features of bleeding ulcers. Gastrointest Endosc 1994;40(4):411–7 pii:S0016510794000374.

36. Sacks HS, Chalmers TC, Blum AL, et al. Endoscopic hemostasis. An effective therapy for bleeding peptic ulcers. JAMA 1990;264(4):494–9.

37. Cook DJ, Guyatt GH, Salena BJ, et al. Endoscopic therapy for acute nonvariceal upper gastrointestinal hemorrhage: a meta-analysis [Systematic reviews and meta-analyses]. Gastroenterology 1992;102(1):139–48. pii:S001650859 200009X.

38. Barkun AN, Martel M, Toubouti Y, et al. Endoscopic hemostasis in peptic ulcer bleeding for patients with high-risk lesions: a series of meta-analyses. Gastrointest Endosc 2009;69(4):786–99. http://dx.doi.org/10.1016/j.gie.2008.05.031. pii: S0016-5107(08)01854-3.

39. Laine L, McQuaid KR. Endoscopic therapy for bleeding ulcers: an evidence-based approach based on meta-analyses of randomized controlled trials. Clin Gastroenterol Hepatol 2009;7(1):33–47. http://dx.doi.org/10.1016/j.cgh.2008. 08.016 [quiz: 1–2]. pii:S1542-3565(08)00842-2.

40. Cipolletta L, Bianco MA, Salerno R, et al. Improved characterization of visible vessels in bleeding ulcers by using magnification endoscopy: results of a pilot study. Gastrointest Endosc 2010;72:413–8.

41. Chung SC, Leung JW, Steele RJ, et al. Endoscopic injection of adrenaline for actively bleeding ulcers: a randomised trial. Br Med J (Clin Res Ed) 1988; 296(6637):1631–3.

42. O'Brien JR. Some effects of adrenaline and anti-adrenaline compounds on platelets in vitro and in vivo. Nature 1963;200:763–4.

43. Lin HJ, Hsieh YH, Tseng GY, et al. A prospective, randomized trial of large-versus small-volume endoscopic injection of epinephrine for peptic ulcer bleeding. Gastrointest Endosc 2002;55(6):615–9. pii:S0016510702086480.

44. Liou TC, Lin SC, Wang HY, et al. Optimal injection volume of epinephrine for endoscopic treatment of peptic ulcer bleeding. World J Gastroenterol 2006; 12(19):3108–13.

45. Park CH, Lee SJ, Park JH, et al. Optimal injection volume of epinephrine for endoscopic prevention of recurrent peptic ulcer bleeding. Gastrointest Endosc 2004;60(6):875–80.

46. Calvet X, Vergara M, Brullet E, et al. Addition of a second endoscopic treatment following epinephrine injection improves outcome in high-risk bleeding ulcers. Gastroenterology 2004;126(2):441–50. pii:S0016508503017876.

47. Vergara M, Calvet X, Gisbert JP. Epinephrine injection versus epinephrine injection and a second endoscopic method in high risk bleeding ulcers. Cochrane Database Syst Rev 2007;(2):CD005584. http://dx.doi.org/10.1002/14651858. CD005584.pub2.

48. Benedetti G, Sablich R, Lacchin T. Endoscopic injection sclerotherapy in non-variceal upper gastrointestinal bleeding. A comparative study of polidocanol and thrombin. Surg Endosc 1991;5(1):28–30.

49. Chester JF, Hurley PR. Gastric necrosis: a complication of endoscopic sclerosis for bleeding peptic ulcer. Endoscopy 1990;22(6):287. http://dx.doi.org/10.1055/ s-2007-1012873.

50. Levy J, Khakoo S, Barton R, et al. Fatal injection sclerotherapy of a bleeding peptic ulcer. Lancet 1991;337(8739):504.
51. Loperfido S, Patelli G, La Torre L. Extensive necrosis of gastric mucosa following injection therapy of bleeding peptic ulcer. Endoscopy 1990;22(6):285–6. http://dx.doi.org/10.1055/s-2007-1010728.
52. Randall GM, Jensen DM, Hirabayashi K, et al. Controlled study of different sclerosing agents for coagulation of canine gut arteries. Gastroenterology 1989;96(5 Pt 1):1274–81.
53. Rutgeerts P, Geboes K, Vantrappen G. Experimental studies of injection therapy for severe nonvariceal bleeding in dogs. Gastroenterology 1989;97(3):610–21.
54. Bhat YM, Banerjee S, Barth BA, et al. Tissue adhesives: cyanoacrylate glue and fibrin sealant. Gastrointest Endosc 2013;78(2):209–15. http://dx.doi.org/10.1016/j.gie.2013.04.166.
55. Laine L. Therapeutic endoscopy and bleeding ulcers. Bipolar/multipolar electrocoagulation. Gastrointest Endosc 1990;36(5 Suppl):S38–41.
56. Laine L, Long GL, Bakos GJ, et al. Optimizing bipolar electrocoagulation for endoscopic hemostasis: assessment of factors influencing energy delivery and coagulation. Gastrointest Endosc 2008;67(3):502–8. http://dx.doi.org/10.1016/j.gie.2007.09.025. pii:S0016-5107(07)02689-2.
57. Conway JD, Adler DG, Diehl DL, et al. Endoscopic hemostatic devices. Gastrointest Endosc 2009;69(6):987–96. http://dx.doi.org/10.1016/j.gie.2008.12.251.
58. Kovacs TO, Jensen DM. Endoscopic therapy for severe ulcer bleeding. Gastrointest Endosc Clin N Am 2011;21(4):681–96. http://dx.doi.org/10.1016/j.giec.2011.07.012.
59. Fullarton GM, Birnie GG, Macdonald A, et al. Controlled trial of heater probe treatment in bleeding peptic ulcers. Br J Surg 1989;76(6):541–4.
60. Machicado GA, Jensen DM. Thermal probes alone or with epinephrine for the endoscopic haemostasis of ulcer haemorrhage. Baillieres Best Pract Res Clin Gastroenterol 2000;14(3):443–58. http://dx.doi.org/10.1053/bega.2000.0089.
61. Marmo R, Rotondano G, Piscopo R, et al. Dual therapy versus monotherapy in the endoscopic treatment of high-risk bleeding ulcers: a meta-analysis of controlled trials [Systematic reviews and meta-analyses]. Am J Gastroenterol 2007;102(2):279–89. http://dx.doi.org/10.1111/j.1572-0241.2006.01023.x [quiz: 469]. pii:AJG1023.
62. Johanns W, Luis W, Janssen J, et al. Argon plasma coagulation (APC) in gastroenterology: experimental and clinical experiences. Eur J Gastroenterol Hepatol 1997;9(6):581–7.
63. Farin G, Grund KE. Technology of argon plasma coagulation with particular regard to endoscopic applications. Endosc Surg Allied Technol 1994;2(1):71–7.
64. Watson JP, Bennett MK, Griffin SM, et al. The tissue effect of argon plasma coagulation on esophageal and gastric mucosa. Gastrointest Endosc 2000;52(3):342–5. http://dx.doi.org/10.1067/mge.2000.108412.
65. Ginsberg GG, Barkun AN, Bosco JJ, et al. The argon plasma coagulator: February 2002. Gastrointest Endosc 2002;55(7):807–10.
66. Kwan V, Bourke MJ, Williams SJ, et al. Argon plasma coagulation in the management of symptomatic gastrointestinal vascular lesions: experience in 100 consecutive patients with long-term follow-up. Am J Gastroenterol 2006;101(1):58–63. http://dx.doi.org/10.1111/j.1572-0241.2006.00370.x.
67. Rolachon A, Papillon E, Fournet J. Is argon plasma coagulation an efficient treatment for digestive system vascular malformation and radiation proctitis? Gastroenterol Clin Biol 2000;24(12):1205–10 [in English, French].

68. Kwak HW, Lee WJ, Woo SM, et al. Efficacy of argon plasma coagulation in the treatment of radiation-induced hemorrhagic gastroduodenal vascular ectasia. Scand J Gastroenterol 2013. http://dx.doi.org/10.3109/00365521.2013.865783.

69. Chiu YC, Lu LS, Wu KL, et al. Comparison of argon plasma coagulation in management of upper gastrointestinal angiodysplasia and gastric antral vascular ectasia hemorrhage. BMC Gastroenterol 2012;12:67. http://dx.doi.org/10.1186/1471-230X-12-67.

70. Cipolletta L, Bianco MA, Rotondano G, et al. Prospective comparison of argon plasma coagulator and heater probe in the endoscopic treatment of major peptic ulcer bleeding. Gastrointest Endosc 1998;48(2):191–5.

71. Skok P, Krizman I, Skok M. Argon plasma coagulation versus injection sclerotherapy in peptic ulcer hemorrhage–a prospective, controlled study. Hepatogastroenterology 2004;51(55):165–70.

72. Wang HM, Hsu PI, Lo GH, et al. Comparison of hemostatic efficacy for argon plasma coagulation and distilled water injection in treating high-risk bleeding ulcers. J Clin Gastroenterol 2009;43(10):941–5. http://dx.doi.org/10.1097/MCG.0b013e31819c3885.

73. Chau CH, Siu WT, Law BK, et al. Randomized controlled trial comparing epinephrine injection plus heat probe coagulation versus epinephrine injection plus argon plasma coagulation for bleeding peptic ulcers. Gastrointest Endosc 2003;57(4):455–61. http://dx.doi.org/10.1067/mge.2003.125.

74. Taghavi SA, Soleimani SM, Hosseini-Asl SM, et al. Adrenaline injection plus argon plasma coagulation versus adrenaline injection plus hemoclips for treating high-risk bleeding peptic ulcers: a prospective, randomized trial. Can J Gastroenterol 2009;23(10):699–704.

75. Karaman A, Baskol M, Gursoy S, et al. Epinephrine plus argon plasma or heater probe coagulation in ulcer bleeding. World J Gastroenterol 2011;17(36):4109–12. http://dx.doi.org/10.3748/wjg.v17.i36.4109.

76. Chuttani R, Barkun A, Carpenter S, et al. Endoscopic clip application devices. Gastrointest Endosc 2006;63(6):746–50. http://dx.doi.org/10.1016/j.gie.2006.02.042.

77. Sung JJ, Tsoi KK, Lai LH, et al. Endoscopic clipping versus injection and thermocoagulation in the treatment of non-variceal upper gastrointestinal bleeding: a meta-analysis [Systematic reviews and meta-analyses]. Gut 2007;56(10):1364–73. http://dx.doi.org/10.1136/gut.2007.123976. pii:gut.2007.123976.

78. Laine L, Jensen DM. Management of patients with ulcer bleeding. Am J Gastroenterol 2012;107(3):345–60. http://dx.doi.org/10.1038/ajg.2011.480 [quiz: 61]. pii:ajg2011480.

79. Goker H, Haznedaroglu IC, Ercetin S, et al. Haemostatic actions of the folkloric medicinal plant extract Ankaferd Blood Stopper. J Int Med Res 2008;36(1):163–70.

80. Moosavi S, Chen YI, Barkun AN. TC-325 application leading to transient obstruction of a post-sphincterotomy biliary orifice. Endoscopy 2013;45(Suppl 2 UCTN):E130. http://dx.doi.org/10.1055/s-0032-1326370.

81. Halkerston K, Evans J, Ismail D, et al. PWE-046 Early clinical experience of EndoclotTM in the treatment of acute gastro-intestinal bleeding. Gut 2013;52:A149.

82. Barkun AN, Moosavi S, Martel M. Topical hemostatic agents: a systematic review with particular emphasis on endoscopic application in gastrointestinal bleeding [Systematic reviews and meta-analyses]. Gastrointest Endosc 2013;77(5):692–700.

83. Holster IL, De Maat MP, Ducharme R, et al. In vitro examination of the effects of the hemostatic powder (Hemospray) on coagulation and thrombus formation in humans. Gastrointest Endosc 2012;75:AB240.

84. Smith LA, Stanley AJ, Bergman JJ, et al. Hemospray application in nonvariceal upper gastrointestinal bleeding: results of the survey to evaluate the application of Hemospray in the luminal tract. J Clin Gastroenterol 2013. http://dx.doi.org/10.1097/MCG.0000000000000054.

85. Chen YI, Barkun A, Nolan S. TC-325 in the management of upper and lower GI bleeding: a two-year experience at a single institution. Endoscopy, in press.

86. Chen YI, Barkun AN, Soulellis C, et al. Use of the endoscopically applied hemostatic powder TC-325 in cancer-related upper GI hemorrhage: preliminary experience (with video). Gastrointest Endosc 2012;75(6):1278–81. http://dx.doi.org/10.1016/j.gie.2012.02.009.

87. Soulellis CA, Carpentier S, Chen YI, et al. Lower GI hemorrhage controlled with endoscopically applied TC-325 (with videos). Gastrointest Endosc 2013;77(3):504–7. http://dx.doi.org/10.1016/j.gie.2012.10.014.

88. Laine L, Stein C, Sharma V. A prospective outcome study of patients with clot in an ulcer and the effect of irrigation. Gastrointest Endosc 1996;43(2 Pt 1):107–10. pii:S0016510796000478.

89. Jensen DM, Kovacs TO, Jutabha R, et al. Randomized trial of medical or endoscopic therapy to prevent recurrent ulcer hemorrhage in patients with adherent clots. Gastroenterology 2002;123(2):407–13 pii:S001650850200118X.

90. Bleau BL, Gostout CJ, Sherman KE, et al. Recurrent bleeding from peptic ulcer associated with adherent clot: a randomized study comparing endoscopic treatment with medical therapy. Gastrointest Endosc 2002;56(1):1–6. pii:S0016510702000007.

91. Khuroo MS, Yattoo GN, Javid G, et al. A comparison of omeprazole and placebo for bleeding peptic ulcer. N Engl J Med 1997;336(15):1054–8. http://dx.doi.org/10.1056/NEJM199704103361503.

92. Javid G, Masoodi I, Zargar SA, et al. Omeprazole as adjuvant therapy to endoscopic combination injection sclerotherapy for treating bleeding peptic ulcer. Am J Med 2001;111(4):280–4 pii:S0002-9343(01)00812-9.

93. Sung JJ, Chan FK, Lau JY, et al. The effect of endoscopic therapy in patients receiving omeprazole for bleeding ulcers with nonbleeding visible vessels or adherent clots: a randomized comparison. Ann Intern Med 2003;139(4):237–43. pii:139/4/237.

94. Kahi CJ, Jensen DM, Sung JJ, et al. Endoscopic therapy versus medical therapy for bleeding peptic ulcer with adherent clot: a meta-analysis [Systematic reviews and meta-analyses]. Gastroenterology 2005;129(3):855–62. http://dx.doi.org/10.1053/j.gastro.2005.06.070. pii:S0016-5085(05)01358-2.

95. Laine L. Systematic review of endoscopic therapy for ulcers with clots: can a meta-analysis be misleading? [Systematic reviews and meta-analyses]. Gastroenterology 2005;129(6):2127. http://dx.doi.org/10.1053/j.gastro.2005.10.039 [author reply: 2127–8]. pii:S0016-5085(05)02199-2.

96. Neumann I, Letelier LM, Rada G, et al. Comparison of different regimens of proton pump inhibitors for acute peptic ulcer bleeding. Cochrane Database Syst Rev 2013;(6):CD007999. http://dx.doi.org/10.1002/14651858.CD007999.pub2.

97. Spiegel BM, Ofman JJ, Woods K, et al. Minimizing recurrent peptic ulcer hemorrhage after endoscopic hemostasis: the cost-effectiveness of competing strategies. Am J Gastroenterol 2003;98(1):86–97. http://dx.doi.org/10.1111/j.1572-0241.2003.07163.x. pii:S0002927002058318.

98. Tsoi KK, Lau JY, Sung JJ. Cost-effectiveness analysis of high-dose omeprazole infusion before endoscopy for patients with upper-GI bleeding. Gastrointest Endosc 2008;67(7):1056–63. http://dx.doi.org/10.1016/j.gie.2007.11.056. pii: S0016-5107(07)03199-9.

99. Barkun AN, Herba K, Adam V, et al. High-dose intravenous proton pump inhibition following endoscopic therapy in the acute management of patients with bleeding peptic ulcers in the USA and Canada: a cost-effectiveness analysis. Aliment Pharmacol Ther 2004;19(5):591–600.

100. Marmo R, Rotondano G, Bianco MA, et al. Outcome of endoscopic treatment for peptic ulcer bleeding: is a second look necessary? A meta-analysis [Systematic reviews and meta-analyses]. Gastrointest Endosc 2003;57(1):62–7. http://dx. doi.org/10.1067/mge.2003.48. pii:S0016510703500141.

101. Tsoi KK, Chan HC, Chiu PW, et al. Second-look endoscopy with thermal coagulation or injections for peptic ulcer bleeding: a meta-analysis [Systematic reviews and meta-analyses]. J Gastroenterol Hepatol 2010;25(1):8–13. http://dx. doi.org/10.1111/j.1440-1746.2009.06129.x.

102. Chiu P, Joeng H, Choi C, et al. The effect of scheduled second endoscopy against intravenous high dose omeprazole infusion as an adjunct to therapeutic endoscopy in prevention of peptic ulcer rebleeding-a prospective randomized study. Gastroenterology 2006;130:A121.

103. El Ouali S, Barkun AN, Wyse J, et al. Is routine second-look endoscopy effective after endoscopic hemostasis in acute peptic ulcer bleeding? A meta-analysis [Systematic reviews and meta-analyses]. Gastrointest Endosc 2012;76(2): 283–92. http://dx.doi.org/10.1016/j.gie.2012.04.441. pii:S0016-5107(12)02156-6.

104. Imperiale TF, Kong N. Second-look endoscopy for bleeding peptic ulcer disease: a decision-effectiveness and cost-effectiveness analysis. J Clin Gastroenterol 2012;46(9):e71–5. http://dx.doi.org/10.1097/MCG.0b013e3182410351.

105. Chiu PW, Sung JJ. High risk ulcer bleeding: when is second-look endoscopy recommended? Clin Gastroenterol Hepatol 2010;8(8):651–4. http://dx.doi.org/ 10.1016/j.cgh.2010.01.008 [quiz: e87].

106. Jairath V, Barkun AN. Improving outcomes from acute upper gastrointestinal bleeding. Gut 2012;61(9):1246–9. http://dx.doi.org/10.1136/gutjnl-2011-300019.

107. Garcia-Iglesias P, Villoria A, Suarez D, et al. Meta-analysis: predictors of rebleeding after endoscopic treatment for bleeding peptic ulcer [Systematic reviews and meta-analyses]. Aliment Pharmacol Ther 2011;34(8):888–900. http://dx.doi.org/10.1111/j.1365-2036.2011.04830.x.

108. Lau JY, Sung JJ, Lam YH, et al. Endoscopic retreatment compared with surgery in patients with recurrent bleeding after initial endoscopic control of bleeding ulcers. N Engl J Med 1999;340(10):751–6. http://dx.doi.org/10.1056/ NEJM199903113401002.

109. Lu Y, Loffroy R, Lau JY, et al. Multidisciplinary management strategies for acute non-variceal upper gastrointestinal bleeding. Br J Surg 2014;101(1):e34–50. http://dx.doi.org/10.1002/bjs.9351.

110. Gisbert JP, Khorrami S, Carballo F, et al. *H. pylori* eradication therapy vs. antisecretory non-eradication therapy (with or without long-term maintenance antisecretory therapy) for the prevention of recurrent bleeding from peptic ulcer. Cochrane Database Syst Rev 2004;(2):CD004062. http://dx.doi.org/10.1002/ 14651858.CD004062.pub2.

111. Malfertheiner P, Megraud F, O'Morain CA, et al. Management of *Helicobacter pylori* infection–the Maastricht IV/Florence Consensus Report. Gut 2012;61(5): 646–64. http://dx.doi.org/10.1136/gutjnl-2012-302084.

112. Sung JJ, Chan FK, Chen M, et al. Asia-Pacific Working Group consensus on non-variceal upper gastrointestinal bleeding. Gut 2011;60(9):1170–7. http://dx. doi.org/10.1136/gut.2010.230292.

113. Calvet X, Barkun A, Kuipers EJ, et al. Is *H. pylori* testing clinically useful in the acute setting of upper gastrointestinal bleeding? A systematic review [abstract]. [Systematic reviews and meta-analyses]. Gastroenterology 2009; 136(5):A-605.

114. Gisbert JP, Abraira V. Accuracy of *Helicobacter pylori* diagnostic tests in patients with bleeding peptic ulcer: a systematic review and meta-analysis [Systematic reviews and meta-analyses]. Am J Gastroenterol 2006;101(4):848–63. http://dx.doi.org/10.1111/j.1572-0241.2006.00528.x.

115. McColl KE. Clinical practice. *Helicobacter pylori* infection. N Engl J Med 2010; 362(17):1597–604. http://dx.doi.org/10.1056/NEJMcp1001110.

116. Rostom A, Moayyedi P, Hunt R, Canadian Association of Gastroenterology Consensus Group. Canadian consensus guidelines on long-term nonsteroidal anti-inflammatory drug therapy and the need for gastroprotection: benefits versus risks. Aliment Pharmacol Ther 2009;29(5):481–96. http://dx.doi.org/10. 1111/j.1365-2036.2008.03905.x.

117. Abraham NS, Hlatky MA, Antman EM, et al. ACCF/ACG/AHA 2010 expert consensus document on the concomitant use of proton pump inhibitors and thienopyridines: a focused update of the ACCF/ACG/AHA 2008 expert consensus document on reducing the gastrointestinal risks of antiplatelet therapy and NSAID use. Am J Gastroenterol 2010;105(12):2533–49. http://dx.doi. org/10.1038/ajg.2010.445.

118. Chan FK, Wong VW, Suen BY, et al. Combination of a cyclo-oxygenase-2 inhibitor and a proton-pump inhibitor for prevention of recurrent ulcer bleeding in patients at very high risk: a double-blind, randomised trial. Lancet 2007;369(9573): 1621–6. http://dx.doi.org/10.1016/S0140-6736(07)60749-1.

119. Laine L, Curtis SP, Cryer B, et al. Assessment of upper gastrointestinal safety of etoricoxib and diclofenac in patients with osteoarthritis and rheumatoid arthritis in the Multinational Etoricoxib and Diclofenac Arthritis Long-term (MEDAL) programme: a randomised comparison. Lancet 2007;369(9560):465–73. http://dx. doi.org/10.1016/S0140-6736(07)60234-7.

120. Scheiman JM, Yeomans ND, Talley NJ, et al. Prevention of ulcers by esomeprazole in at-risk patients using non-selective NSAIDs and COX-2 inhibitors. Am J Gastroenterol 2006;101(4):701–10. http://dx.doi.org/10.1111/j.1572-0241.2006. 00499.x.

121. Kearney PM, Baigent C, Godwin J, et al. Do selective cyclo-oxygenase-2 inhibitors and traditional non-steroidal anti-inflammatory drugs increase the risk of atherothrombosis? Meta-analysis of randomised trials [Systematic reviews and meta-analyses]. BMJ 2006;332(7553):1302–8. http://dx.doi.org/10.1136/bmj. 332.7553.1302.

122. Rostom A, Dube C, Lewin G, et al. Nonsteroidal anti-inflammatory drugs and cyclooxygenase-2 inhibitors for primary prevention of colorectal cancer: a systematic review prepared for the U.S. Preventive Services Task Force [Systematic reviews and meta-analyses]. Ann Intern Med 2007;146(5):376–89.

123. Biondi-Zoccai GG, Lotrionte M, Agostoni P, et al. A systematic review and meta-analysis on the hazards of discontinuing or not adhering to aspirin among 50,279 patients at risk for coronary artery disease [Systematic reviews and meta-analyses]. Eur Heart J 2006;27(22):2667–74. http://dx.doi.org/10.1093/ eurheartj/ehl334. pii:ehl334.

124. Derogar M, Sandblom G, Lundell L, et al. Discontinuation of low-dose aspirin therapy after peptic ulcer bleeding increases risk of death and acute cardiovascular events. Clin Gastroenterol Hepatol 2013;11(1):38–42. http://dx.doi.org/10.1016/j.cgh.2012.08.034.

125. Aguejouf O, Eizayaga F, Desplat V, et al. Prothrombotic and hemorrhagic effects of aspirin. Clin Appl Thromb Hemost 2009;15(5):523–8. http://dx.doi.org/10.1177/1076029608319945.

126. Sibon I, Orgogozo JM. Antiplatelet drug discontinuation is a risk factor for ischemic stroke. Neurology 2004;62(7):1187–9.

127. Sung JJ, Lau JY, Ching JY, et al. Continuation of low-dose aspirin therapy in peptic ulcer bleeding: a randomized trial. Ann Intern Med 2010;152(1):1–9. http://dx.doi.org/10.7326/0003-4819-152-1-201001050-00179.   pii:0003-4819-152-1-201001050-00179.

128. Shingina A, Barkun AN, Razzaghi A, et al. Systematic review: the presenting international normalised ratio (INR) as a predictor of outcome in patients with upper nonvariceal gastrointestinal bleeding [Systematic reviews and meta-analyses]. Aliment Pharmacol Ther 2011;33(9):1010–8. http://dx.doi.org/10.1111/j.1365-2036.2011.04618.x.

129. Baradarian R, Ramdhaney S, Chapalamadugu R, et al. Early intensive resuscitation of patients with upper gastrointestinal bleeding decreases mortality. Am J Gastroenterol 2004;99(4):619–22. http://dx.doi.org/10.1111/j.1572-0241.2004.04073.x.

130. Choudari CP, Rajgopal C, Palmer KR. Acute gastrointestinal haemorrhage in anticoagulated patients: diagnoses and response to endoscopic treatment. Gut 1994;35(4):464–6.

131. Ogawa S, Szlam F, Ohnishi T, et al. A comparative study of prothrombin complex concentrates and fresh-frozen plasma for warfarin reversal under static and flow conditions. Thromb Haemost 2011;106(6):1215–23. http://dx.doi.org/10.1160/TH11-04-0240.

132. Hickey M, Gatien M, Taljaard M, et al. Outcomes of urgent warfarin reversal with frozen plasma versus prothrombin complex concentrate in the emergency department. Circulation 2013;128(4):360–4. http://dx.doi.org/10.1161/CIRCULATIONAHA.113.001875.

133. Guest JF, Watson HG, Limaye S. Modeling the cost-effectiveness of prothrombin complex concentrate compared with fresh frozen plasma in emergency warfarin reversal in the United Kingdom. Clin Ther 2010;32(14):2478–93. http://dx.doi.org/10.1016/j.clinthera.2011.01.011.

134. Baron TH, Kamath PS, McBane RD. Management of antithrombotic therapy in patients undergoing invasive procedures. N Engl J Med 2013;368(22):2113–24. http://dx.doi.org/10.1056/NEJMra1206531.

135. Siegal DM, Cuker A. Reversal of novel oral anticoagulants in patients with major bleeding. J Thromb Thrombolysis 2013. http://dx.doi.org/10.1007/s11239-013-0885-0.

136. Alikhan R, Rayment R, Keeling D, et al. The acute management of haemorrhage, surgery and overdose in patients receiving dabigatran. Emerg Med J 2013. http://dx.doi.org/10.1136/emermed-2012-201976.

137. Chan FK. Anti-platelet therapy and managing ulcer risk. J Gastroenterol Hepatol 2012;27(2):195–9. http://dx.doi.org/10.1111/j.1440-1746.2011.07029.x.

138. Almadi MA, Barkun A, Brophy J. Antiplatelet and anticoagulant therapy in patients with gastrointestinal bleeding: an 86-year-old woman with peptic ulcer disease. JAMA 2011;306(21):2367–74. http://dx.doi.org/10.1001/jama.2011.1653.

139. Taha AS, McCloskey C, Prasad R, et al. Famotidine for the prevention of peptic ulcers and oesophagitis in patients taking low-dose aspirin (FAMOUS): a phase III, randomised, double-blind, placebo-controlled trial. Lancet 2009;374(9684): 119–25. http://dx.doi.org/10.1016/S0140-6736(09)61246-0.

140. Ng FH, Wong SY, Lam KF, et al. Famotidine is inferior to pantoprazole in preventing recurrence of aspirin-related peptic ulcers or erosions. Gastroenterology 2010;138(1):82–8. http://dx.doi.org/10.1053/j.gastro.2009.09.063.

141. Chan FK, Chung SC, Suen BY, et al. Preventing recurrent upper gastrointestinal bleeding in patients with *Helicobacter pylori* infection who are taking low-dose aspirin or naproxen. N Engl J Med 2001;344(13):967–73. http://dx.doi.org/10. 1056/NEJM200103293441304.

142. Lai KC, Lam SK, Chu KM, et al. Lansoprazole for the prevention of recurrences of ulcer complications from long-term low-dose aspirin use. N Engl J Med 2002; 346(26):2033–8. http://dx.doi.org/10.1056/NEJMoa012877.

143. Chan FK, Ching JY, Suen BY, et al. Effects of *Helicobacter pylori* infection on long-term risk of peptic ulcer bleeding in low-dose aspirin users. Gastroenterology 2013;144(3):528–35. http://dx.doi.org/10.1053/j.gastro.2012.12.038 pii: S0016-5085(13)00072-3.

144. Chan FK, Ching JY, Hung LC, et al. Clopidogrel versus aspirin and esomeprazole to prevent recurrent ulcer bleeding. N Engl J Med 2005;352(3):238–44. http://dx.doi.org/10.1056/NEJMoa042087.

145. Lai KC, Chu KM, Hui WM, et al. Esomeprazole with aspirin versus clopidogrel for prevention of recurrent gastrointestinal ulcer complications. Clin Gastroenterol Hepatol 2006;4(7):860–5. http://dx.doi.org/10.1016/j.cgh.2006.04.019.

146. Hsu PI, Lai KH, Liu CP. Esomeprazole with clopidogrel reduces peptic ulcer recurrence, compared with clopidogrel alone, in patients with atherosclerosis. Gastroenterology 2011;140(3):791–8. http://dx.doi.org/10.1053/j.gastro.2010.11.056.

147. Bhatt DL, Cryer BL, Contant CF, et al. Clopidogrel with or without omeprazole in coronary artery disease. N Engl J Med 2010;363(20):1909–17. http://dx.doi.org/ 10.1056/NEJMoa1007964.

148. Bhatt DL, Scheiman J, Abraham NS, et al. ACCF/ACG/AHA 2008 expert consensus document on reducing the gastrointestinal risks of antiplatelet therapy and NSAID use: a report of the American College of Cardiology Foundation Task Force on Clinical Expert Consensus Documents. J Am Coll Cardiol 2008; 52(18):1502–17. http://dx.doi.org/10.1016/j.jacc.2008.08.002.

149. Small DS, Farid NA, Payne CD, et al. Effects of the proton pump inhibitor lansoprazole on the pharmacokinetics and pharmacodynamics of prasugrel and clopidogrel. J Clin Pharmacol 2008;48(4):475–84. http://dx.doi.org/10.1177/ 0091270008315310.

150. Gilard M, Arnaud B, Cornily JC, et al. Influence of omeprazole on the antiplatelet action of clopidogrel associated with aspirin: the randomized, double-blind OCLA (Omeprazole CLopidogrel Aspirin) study. J Am Coll Cardiol 2008;51(3): 256–60. http://dx.doi.org/10.1016/j.jacc.2007.06.064.

151. O'Donoghue ML, Braunwald E, Antman EM, et al. Pharmacodynamic effect and clinical efficacy of clopidogrel and prasugrel with or without a proton-pump inhibitor: an analysis of two randomised trials. Lancet 2009;374(9694):989–97. http://dx.doi.org/10.1016/S0140-6736(09)61525-7.

152. Kwok CS, Loke YK. Meta-analysis: the effects of proton pump inhibitors on cardiovascular events and mortality in patients receiving clopidogrel [Systematic reviews and meta-analyses]. Aliment Pharmacol Ther 2010;31(8):810–23. http://dx.doi.org/10.1111/j.1365-2036.2010.04247.x.

153. Siller-Matula JM, Jilma B, Schror K, et al. Effect of proton pump inhibitors on clinical outcome in patients treated with clopidogrel: a systematic review and meta-analysis [Systematic reviews and meta-analyses]. J Thromb Haemost 2010;8(12):2624–41. http://dx.doi.org/10.1111/j.1538-7836.2010. 04049.x.

154. Lima JP, Brophy JM. The potential interaction between clopidogrel and proton pump inhibitors: a systematic review [Systematic reviews and meta-analyses]. BMC Med 2010;8:81. http://dx.doi.org/10.1186/1741-7015-8-81.

155. Kwok CS, Jeevanantham V, Dawn B, et al. No consistent evidence of differential cardiovascular risk amongst proton-pump inhibitors when used with clopidogrel: meta-analysis [Systematic reviews and meta-analyses]. Int J Cardiol 2012. http://dx.doi.org/10.1016/j.ijcard.2012.03.085.

156. Katz PO, Gerson LB, Vela MF. Guidelines for the diagnosis and management of gastroesophageal reflux disease. Am J Gastroenterol 2013;108(3):308–28. http://dx.doi.org/10.1038/ajg.2012.444 [quiz: 29].

157. van Walraven C, Jennings A, Oake N, et al. Effect of study setting on anticoagulation control: a systematic review and metaregression [Systematic reviews and meta-analyses]. Chest 2006;129(5):1155–66. http://dx.doi.org/10.1378/chest. 129.5.1155.

158. Wiedermann CJ, Stockner I. Warfarin-induced bleeding complications - clinical presentation and therapeutic options. Thromb Res 2008;122(Suppl 2):S13–8. http://dx.doi.org/10.1016/S0049-3848(08)70004-5.

159. Levine MN, Raskob G, Beyth RJ, et al. Hemorrhagic complications of anticoagulant treatment: the Seventh ACCP Conference on Antithrombotic and Thrombolytic Therapy. Chest 2004;126(3 Suppl):287S–310S. http://dx.doi.org/10.1378/ chest.126.3_suppl.287S.

160. Lin KJ, Hernandez-Diaz S, Garcia Rodriguez LA. Acid suppressants reduce risk of gastrointestinal bleeding in patients on antithrombotic or anti-inflammatory therapy. Gastroenterology 2011;141(1):71–9. http://dx.doi.org/10.1053/j.gastro. 2011.03.049.

161. DeEugenio D, Kolman L, DeCaro M, et al. Risk of major bleeding with concomitant dual antiplatelet therapy after percutaneous coronary intervention in patients receiving long-term warfarin therapy. Pharmacotherapy 2007;27(5): 691–6. http://dx.doi.org/10.1592/phco.27.5.691.

162. Ng FH, Tunggal P, Chu WM, et al. Esomeprazole compared with famotidine in the prevention of upper gastrointestinal bleeding in patients with acute coronary syndrome or myocardial infarction. Am J Gastroenterol 2012;107(3):389–96. http://dx.doi.org/10.1038/ajg.2011.385.

163. Dewilde WJ, Oirbans T, Verheugt FW, et al. Use of clopidogrel with or without aspirin in patients taking oral anticoagulant therapy and undergoing percutaneous coronary intervention: an open-label, randomised, controlled trial. Lancet 2013;381(9872):1107–15. http://dx.doi.org/10.1016/S0140-6736(12)62177-1.

164. van Es RF, Jonker JJ, Verheugt FW, et al, Antithrombotics in the Secondary Prevention of Events in Coronary Thrombosis-2 Research Group. Aspirin and coumadin after acute coronary syndromes (the ASPECT-2 study): a randomised controlled trial. Lancet 2002;360(9327):109–13. http://dx.doi.org/10.1016/ S0140-6736(02)09409-6.

165. Hurlen M, Abdelnoor M, Smith P, et al. Warfarin, aspirin, or both after myocardial infarction. N Engl J Med 2002;347(13):969–74. http://dx.doi.org/10.1056/ NEJMoa020496.

166. Patel MR, Mahaffey KW, Garg J, et al. Rivaroxaban versus warfarin in nonvalvular atrial fibrillation. N Engl J Med 2011;365(10):883–91. http://dx.doi.org/10.1056/NEJMoa1009638.
167. Connolly SJ, Ezekowitz MD, Yusuf S, et al. Dabigatran versus warfarin in patients with atrial fibrillation. N Engl J Med 2009;361(12):1139–51. http://dx.doi.org/10.1056/NEJMoa0905561.
168. Holster IL, Valkhoff VE, Kuipers EJ, et al. New oral anticoagulants increase risk for gastrointestinal bleeding: a systematic review and meta-analysis [Systematic reviews and meta-analyses]. Gastroenterology 2013;145(1):105–12.e15. http://dx.doi.org/10.1053/j.gastro.2013.02.041 pii:S0016-5085(13)00290-4.
169. Laine L. Review article: gastrointestinal bleeding with low-dose aspirin - what's the risk? Aliment Pharmacol Ther 2006;24(6):897–908. http://dx.doi.org/10.1111/j.1365-2036.2006.03077.x.
170. Delaney JA, Opatrny L, Brophy JM, et al. Drug drug interactions between antithrombotic medications and the risk of gastrointestinal bleeding. Can Med Assoc J 2007;177(4):347–51. http://dx.doi.org/10.1503/cmaj.070186.

Role of Medical Therapy for Nonvariceal Upper Gastrointestinal Bleeding

Kyle J. Fortinsky, MD[a], Marc Bardou, MD, PhD[b],*,
Alan N. Barkun, MD, MSc[c]

KEYWORDS

- Nonvariceal upper gastrointestinal bleeding • Red blood cell transfusions
- Proton pump inhibitors • Erythromycin • Tranexamic acid • Nasogastric lavage
- Iron replacement therapy

KEY POINTS

- Optimal resuscitation should be initiated before any diagnostic or therapeutic procedure.
- Red blood cell transfusion should be offered to patients with a hemoglobin level less than 70 g/L, unless they have preexisting cardiac disease or evidence of an acute coronary syndrome, in which case more liberal transfusion may be appropriate.
- The use of intravenous erythromycin approximately 30 minutes before endoscopy may be useful to improve visualization.
- Preendoscopic high-dose intravenous proton pump inhibitor (PPI) therapy should be offered to all patients, but should not precede adequate resuscitation with crystalloid and/or blood products as necessary.
- Postendoscopic intravenous PPI therapy for 72 hours followed by double-dose oral PPI treatment of 14 days of the next 1 to 2 months prevents recurrence of bleeding in high-risk patients.

INTRODUCTION

The annual incidence of upper gastrointestinal bleeding (UGIB) is 48 to 160 events per 100,000 adults in the United States, where it is the cause of approximately 300,000 hospital admissions per year.[1,2] In Europe, the annual incidence of UGIB in the general

This article originally appeared in Gastrointestinal Endoscopy Clinics, Volume 25, Issue 3, July 2015.

Conflicts of interest: A.N. Barkun declares associations with the following companies: AstraZeneca, Takeda Canada. The other authors declare no competing interests.

[a] Department of Medicine, Toronto General Hospital, University of Toronto, 200 Elizabeth Street, Toronto, Ontario M5G 2C4, Canada; [b] Gastroenterology Department & Centre d'Investigations Clinique CIC1432, CHU de Dijon, 14 rue Gaffarel BP77908, Dijon, Cedex 21079, France; [c] Gastroenterology Department, McGill University Health Centre, Montreal General Hospital Site, Room D7-346, 1650 Cedar Avenue, Montréal, Québec H3G 1A4, Canada
* Corresponding author.
E-mail address: marc.bardou@u-bourgogne.fr

population ranges from $19.4^{3,4}$ to $57.0^{3,5}$ events per 100,000 individuals. There is no formal explanation for the breadth of the range between countries, although differences in health care systems and case recording capacities may be substantial.[4,5] Additional contributing factors may include alcohol intake and *Helicobacter pylori* prevalence. In both North America and Europe, around 80% to 90% of acute UGIB episodes have a nonvariceal cause, with peptic ulcers and gastroduodenal erosions accounting for most such lesions.[6,7]

UGIB-related mortalities have slightly decreased in the past 2 decades, but still range from 2% to 15%.[8–10] Two studies conducted in the United Kingdom highlighted that, despite a notable decrease in mortality in patients with UGIB from 1993 to 2007, mortality from peptic ulcer bleeding is still 10% to 13%.[7,9] A multidisciplinary group of 34 experts from 15 countries published international guidelines in 2010, which were modified and expanded from initial guidelines published in 2003, to help inform clinicians on the optimal management of patients with nonvariceal UGIB.[2]

This article discusses the various management principles of medical therapy in nonvariceal UGIB put forth by guidelines from the multidisciplinary international consensus group in 2010, and the American College of Gastroenterology in 2012.[2,11] When applicable, more recent evidence is included. This article presents the most current evidence and provides recommendations for practice. Overall, this article focuses on providing an evidence-based approach to initial resuscitation, the role of blood transfusion, and both preendoscopic and postendoscopic pharmacologic and nonpharmacologic therapies in patients presenting with nonvariceal UGIB.

REVIEW CRITERIA

We conducted a literature search using the OVID, MEDLINE, EMBASE, PubMed, and ISI Web of Knowledge 4.0 databases to identify articles published in the English or French languages up until December 2014. A highly sensitive search strategy was used to identify randomized controlled trials, cohort studies, and case-control studies conducted in adults, using combinations of search terms, including "UGIB"; "epidemiology," "motility agents," "prokinetics," "erythromycin," "nasogastric," "tranexamic acid," "transfusion," "iron replacement," "*Helicobacter pylori*," "endoscopy," and "proton pump inhibitors" (PPIs). In addition, recursive searches and cross-referencing were performed and manual searches of the reference lists of articles identified in the initial search were completed.

PREENDOSCOPIC MEDICAL MANAGEMENT
Initial Resuscitation

The immediate priority in management is to secure the patient's airway, and tend to breathing and circulation (**Fig. 1**). The patient should be placed in a monitored setting, at which point large-bore venous access should be established. All pertinent blood work (eg, complete blood count, renal function, liver function tests, coagulation testing) should be obtained, in addition to typing and cross-matching.[11] Resuscitation should be initiated for patients with UGIB before any other procedure, and should include stabilization of the blood pressure with appropriate infusion of sufficient fluid volumes.[12,13] In intensive care units, saline or Ringer acetate must be preferred to hydroxyethyl starch (HES), because HES has been shown to increase the need for renal-replacement therapy in intensive care unit patients, and may even increase the risk for severe bleeding.[14] The primary objectives of resuscitation are to restore blood volume and to maintain adequate tissue perfusion, in the hope of preventing hypovolemic shock and ultimately death. No data suggest that any particular type

Initial resuscitation

- Maintain airway, breathing, and circulation
- Ensure large-bore intravenous access and consider monitored setting
- Resuscitate initially with crystalloid solution
- Send blood work including CBC, coagulation studies, and type and cross-matching

Transfusion requirements

- Transfuse red blood cells only if hemoglobin <70g/L, unless symptoms of anemia or significant cardiac disease
- Transfuse platelets only if platelet count <50 x 10^9/L or <100 x 10^9/L with suspected platelet dysfunction

Pre-endoscopic therapy

- Provide erythromycin intravenously 30 minutes prior to endoscopy
- High-dose intravenous proton pump inhibitors should be initiated
- The routine use of nasogastric lavage and/or tranexamic acid is not recommended

Fig. 1. Preendoscopic medical management of nonvariceal UGIB. CBC, complete blood count.

of colloid solution is safer or more effective than any other in patients needing volume replacement.[15] Certain patients require resuscitation with blood products, including red blood cells, platelets, and rarely clotting factors (eg, fresh frozen plasma).

Red Blood Cell Transfusion

The decision whether to transfuse red blood cells is based largely on the presenting hemoglobin level, coupled with symptoms of anemia, patient comorbidities such as cardiac disease, and the initial hemodynamic status. A large Cochrane Review questioned the benefits of red blood cell transfusions in UGIB, showing no overall survival benefit.[16] A recent randomized controlled trial of 921 patients with acute UGIB found a restrictive transfusion strategy (transfusion threshold <70 g/L with target hemoglobin 70–90 g/L) significantly decreased 6-week mortality, length of stay, and transfusion-related adverse events compared with a liberal transfusion strategy (transfusion threshold <90 g/L with target hemoglobin 90 to 110 g/L).[17] The overall mortality benefit conferred by the restrictive transfusion strategy seems to have been driven by results obtained in patients with Child-Pugh class A and B cirrhosis. The subgroup of patients with nonvariceal UGIB did not show a significant decrease in their overall mortality with a restrictive transfusion policy, although there was no suggestion of harm. Moreover, this study excluded all patients presenting with severe hemorrhagic shock, in keeping with consensus guidelines suggesting higher hemoglobin targets for these patients. In addition, patients with acute coronary syndrome, symptomatic peripheral vasculopathy, stroke, transient ischemic attack, or blood transfusion within 30 days were excluded from the study.

The current guidelines suggest that patients with hemoglobin levels less than or equal to 70 g/L should receive blood transfusions to reach a target hemoglobin level of 70 to 90 g/L, provided that the individual has no coronary artery disease, evidence of tissue hypoperfusion, or acute hemorrhage.[2] In patients with acute coronary syndrome, UGIB is associated with a markedly increased mortality, and a higher hemoglobin target level (>100 g/L) may be required to prevent decompensation.[2,18] In contrast, avoidance of unnecessary transfusions reduces the small but real risks attributable to administration of blood components, such as infectious or immune diseases. As part of a recent UK audit, despite 73% of patients with UGIB presenting with a hemoglobin level greater than 80 g/L, approximately 43% nonetheless received red blood cell transfusions.[7,19] A recently published meta-analysis, not restricted to nonvariceal UGIB, suggests that a restrictive transfusion approach reduces health care–associated infections.[20] Additional randomized trials are needed to address the issue of hemoglobin transfusion thresholds in patients with nonvariceal UGIB, and those with preexisting cardiac disease. One large multicentre randomized trial is currently being completed in the United Kingdom, which may help to answer these uncertainties.[21]

Platelet Transfusion

A recent systematic review of 18 studies of platelet transfusion thresholds in patients with UGIB found insufficient evidence supporting an optimal platelet count.[22] However, based primarily on expert opinion, the investigators proposed a platelet transfusion threshold of 50×10^9/L (or 100×10^9/L if altered platelet function is suspected). Additional high-quality data are needed to confirm these recommendations.

Nasogastric Lavage

The routine placement of a nasogastric tube (NGT) in patients with UGIB remains controversial and is not recommended by current guidelines.[2,11] Overall, studies have failed to show any improvement in clinical outcomes attributable to the insertion of an NGT.[23–26] However, there are certain patients in whom the source of gastrointestinal bleeding is unclear and who may benefit from placement of an NGT in order to confirm an upper gastrointestinal source.[27] A recent study investigated the utility of NGT aspirate at predicting UGIB in 64 patients presenting with hematemesis.[28] By using fecal occult blood testing on the aspirate, they were able to accurately identify all cases of UGIB later confirmed on endoscopy, while maintaining a specificity of 94%.[28] Although this study does lend support to the practice of obtaining an NGT aspirate to identify the source of bleeding in certain cases, it is unclear whether the same results would hold true in patients presenting with either coffee-ground emesis or melena. One recent retrospective study of 166 patients was able to predict active bleeding at endoscopy by combining NGT aspirate results with blood pressure and heart rate parameters.[29] Overall, opinions vary because high-quality evidence is lacking to decide whether certain patients benefit from NGT aspiration and lavage to help aid in diagnosing UGIB as well as improving visualization during endoscopy.[30–33]

Prokinetic Agents

The use of prokinetic agents (such as erythromycin) before gastrointestinal endoscopy has been shown to significantly shorten the duration of endoscopy, reduce the need for repeat endoscopy, and decrease the need for blood transfusions.[34–38] In a large, multicentre, randomized controlled trial involving 253 patients presenting with either melena or hematemesis, erythromycin alone was equally efficacious at improving endoscopic visualization as NGT aspirate alone or in combination with erythromycin.[26]

A separate randomized, placebo-controlled trial that involved patients with bleeding esophageal varices found that an erythromycin infusion significantly increased the proportion of empty stomachs at gastroscopy compared with placebo (48.9% with erythromycin vs 23.3% with placebo), reduced the mean endoscopy duration (19 minutes vs 26 minutes), and shortened durations of hospital stay (3.4 days vs 5.1 days).[39]

More recently, another small, low-quality, randomized trial compared NGT aspirate alone versus NGT aspirate with erythromycin, and the combination provided superior visualization, reduced hospital admissions, and decreased blood transfusions.[34] No data suggest that the administration of prokinetic agents can decrease mortality, the risk of rebleeding, or the need for surgery.[35–37,40] Nonetheless, given improved visibility at endoscopy and other potential benefits discussed earlier, especially in light of the favorable benefit-harm profile of erythromycin, current guidelines suggest that, after ruling out contraindications to these agents (such as hypokalemia or a prolonged QT interval), a 250-mg bolus of erythromycin should be administered approximately 30 to 45 minutes before endoscopy in patients with clinical evidence of active hemorrhage (hematemesis or melena) or acute anemia requiring resuscitation, or in those who have recently eaten.[2,26]

Proton Pump Inhibitor Therapy

Despite theoretic pharmacologic differences between the different PPIs, no data support the use of a particular intravenous PPI rather than another when treating patients with UGIB. In this article, "PPI" is therefore used as a generic term for all such agents.

Starting PPI treatment before endoscopy for UGIB remains a controversial practice. A meta-analysis that included 2223 participants from 6 randomized clinical trials found that preendoscopic PPI treatment reduces the proportion of patients identified as having high-risk lesions (active bleeding, nonbleeding visible vessel, and adherent clot) at early endoscopy and the resultant need for endoscopic therapy (ie, there is downstaging of high-risk endoscopic lesions).[41] Despite these advantages, there is no evidence that preendoscopic PPI treatment affects mortality, the risk of rebleeding, or the need for surgery. For this reason, current guidelines recommend initiating PPI therapy on presentation to hospital, although it should never delay optimal resuscitation.[2] PPI therapy is cost-effective in scenarios in which there is an anticipated delay in endoscopy or a high likelihood of a nonvariceal source of bleeding. Current guidelines advise against the use of histamine2 receptor antagonists in acute ulcer bleeding.[2]

No recommendations can be made regarding the optimal dose of PPIs administered preendoscopy. A reasonable strategy may be to adopt a regimen of a high-dose intravenous bolus (eg, Pantoprazole 80 mg) followed by a continuous infusion (eg, Pantoprazole 8 mg/h).[42] This infusion can be continued until endoscopy, at which point reassessment is required, depending on the appearance of the bleeding lesion and the need for therapeutic intervention (discussed later).

Although there is insufficient high-quality evidence to recommend intravenous PPI versus oral PPI, current guidelines suggest high-dose intravenous PPI preendoscopically because this administration has been well studied in multiple randomized controlled trials.[42–44]

A meta-analysis of randomized trials in patients not receiving endoscopic therapy discovered that PPI therapy reduced rebleeding rates and the need for surgery, and may decrease mortality in certain high-risk patients.[45] This approach could be cost-effective if endoscopy is delayed to greater than 16 hours after admission, or if patients have a high likelihood of nonvariceal bleeding, especially in those with high-risk symptoms, such as hematemesis.[46,47] These findings suggest a definite benefit of PPI therapy when endoscopy may be unavailable or delayed.

Somatostatin and Octreotide

Although usually reserved for patients with variceal UGIB, both somatostatin and octreotide may be used in patients presenting with nonvariceal UGIB. One meta-analysis consisting of 1829 patients from 14 randomized controlled trials found that both somatostatin and octreotide reduced the risk of continued nonvariceal UGIB (relative risk [RR], 0.53, 0.43–0.63; number needed to treat [NNT], 5).[48] These trials only compared somatostatin and octreotide with H2-blockers and placebo and none of these patients were on PPI therapy. Current guidelines recommend the use of octreotide or somatostatin in nonvariceal UGIB only as the last resort in patients who are bleeding uncontrollably while waiting for more definitive therapy.[2] Its use in the treatment of gastrointestinal bleeding of unknown origin is controversial.[49]

Tranexamic Acid

The efficacy of tranexamic acid, an antifibrinolytic, has been explored in several randomized trials and a recent meta-analysis.[50] Although the meta-analysis found a significant overall reduction in mortality, there was no reduction in rebleeding rates, the need for surgery, or blood transfusion. Importantly, the mortality benefit of tranexamic acid was absent when current therapy with PPIs and endoscopy were instituted. Although there are currently 2 randomized trials underway (one vs placebo [NCT01713101] and one vs esomeprazole [NCT02071316]) that are investigating the benefit of tranexamic acid in combination with current therapy in UGIB, current guidelines do not support its routine use in UGIB.[51]

POSTENDOSCOPIC MEDICAL MANAGEMENT
Intravenous Proton Pump Inhibitor Therapy

Opinions differ about the optimal time to begin intravenous PPI infusion after endoscopic hemostasis (**Fig. 2**).[13,42,52] The goal of PPI therapy is to increase the gastric pH sufficiently to promote clot stability and to reduce the effect of pepsin and gastric acid.[53] In a study designed to identify the lowest effective dose of PPI, rather than using a high (or low) dose, continuous infusion was the key to maintaining an intragastric pH greater than 6.[54] Two meta-analyses have confirmed that an intravenous PPI bolus followed by continuous PPI infusion over 72 hours reduces the rates of mortality (RR, 0.40, 0.28–0.59; NNT, 12), rebleeding (RR, 0.40, 0.28–0.59; NNT, 12), and surgery (RR, 0.43, 0.24–0.76; NNT, 28). Mortality was only reduced in patients who had previously undergone successful endoscopic hemostasis.[45,55]

A placebo-controlled, randomized trial showed that, in patients with Forrest class Ia to IIb bleeding lesions,[56] intravenous esomeprazole administered as an 80-mg intravenous bolus over 30 minutes followed by continuous infusion of 8 mg/h for 71.5 hours, which was started after successful endoscopic hemostasis and followed by a 40-mg esomeprazole oral regimen for 27 days, significantly reduced rates of rebleeding at 72 hours (5.9% in esomeprazole group compared with 10.3% in the placebo group; RR, 0.57; 95% confidence interval [CI], 0.35–0.94; NNT, 23). The difference in rebleeding rates remained significant at 7 days and 30 days after initial presentation.[57] However, the 30-day mortality was not significantly reduced by the use of a PPI. Because mortality was lower than expected in the placebo group (2.1%), this finding might reflect the exclusion of patients with life-threatening systemic disease (American Society of Anesthesiologists class >3). Cost-effectiveness analyses have shown the economic dominance of high-dose intravenous PPI compared with no treatment strategies.[58]

More recently, a systematic review and meta-analysis compared intermittent versus continuous PPI therapy for the treatment of high-risk bleeding ulcers after endoscopic

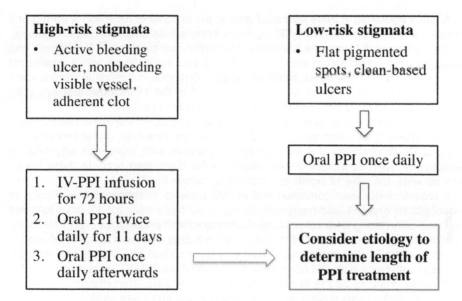

High-risk stigmata	Low-risk stigmata
• Active bleeding ulcer, nonbleeding visible vessel, adherent clot	• Flat pigmented spots, clean-based ulcers

Oral PPI once daily

1. IV-PPI infusion for 72 hours
2. Oral PPI twice daily for 11 days
3. Oral PPI once daily afterwards

⟹ **Consider etiology to determine length of PPI treatment**

H pylori-associated ulcer:
• No need for continuing PPI therapy after eradication of _H pylori_

NSAID-induced ulcer:
• No need for continuing PPI therapy after discontinuation of NSAID
• If NSAID required, consider COX-2 inhibitor with PPI therapy
• Use PPI with low-dose ASA if needed for secondary prevention

Idiopathic ulcers:
• PPI therapy should be prescribed indefinitely

Fig. 2. Postendoscopic medical management of peptic ulcer disease. ASA, acetylsalicylic acid; COX-2, cyclooxygenase-2; IV, intravenous.

therapy.[59] This study revealed that intermittent PPI therapy may be as effective as continuous-infusion high-dose therapy in these high-risk patients, which may have benefits in terms of cost-savings, and the investigators firmly concluded that guidelines should be revised to recommend intermittent PPI therapy. However, overall, current guidelines remain ambivalent toward optimal postendoscopy PPI dosing because of an overall low quality of evidence secondary to a high risk of bias and imprecision in the aforementioned systematic review.[11]

Oral Proton Pump Inhibitor Therapy

High-dose oral PPI treatment after endoscopy was efficacious in early trials conducted in India and Iran, but differences in the physiologic and pharmacokinetic characteristics of the patients, as well as local high _H pylori_ carriage rate and limited comorbidities, make the results of these studies difficult to apply to other populations. The endoscopic treatment administered was also not the current recommended standard.[60]

A study published in 2009 assessed gastric pH in patients receiving a 90-mg oral dose of lansoprazole followed by 30 mg every 3 hours (total dose, 300 mg in 24 hours), following successful endoscopic treatment of peptic ulcer bleeding.[61] The primary end point was the proportion of the 24-hour period that the patients had a gastric pH greater than 6 (median, 55%). However, large differences in this value were evident between individuals (range, 6%–99%), and only 1 of the 14 included patients (7%) reached a pH of more than 6 in at least 80% of this time period.[61]

Accordingly, the evidence is currently insufficient to support the use of oral PPI therapy immediately after endoscopy in high-risk patients. However, current recommendations do recommend oral PPI therapy in patients with lower-risk stigmata on endoscopy, such as a clean-based ulcer or a flat pigmented spot. In these lower-risk patients, the rates of significant rebleeding remain low.[62]

A recent randomized controlled trial of 293 patients investigated the efficacy of double-dose oral PPI (esomeprazole 40 mg orally twice daily for 11 days followed by once-daily dosing for another 14 days) compared with single-dose oral PPI (esomeprazole 40 mg orally once daily for 25 days) after 3 days of intravenous PPI infusion.[63] Patients with a Rockall score greater than or equal to 6 had significantly less rebleeding rates with twice-daily PPI compared with single-dose PPI (10.8% rebleeding in the twice-daily group vs 28.7% in once-daily group; $P = .002$). Surprisingly, rebleeding rates in an earlier study were much lower, whereby patients were randomized to intravenous esomeprazole or placebo for the first 72 hours, followed by oral esomeprazole 40 mg once a day, and reported rebleeding rates were only 1.9% and 5.1%, respectively.[57]

We recommend routinely prescribing double-dose PPI for at least 14 days following intravenous PPI infusion in these high-risk patients and single-dose PPI thereafter. The decision to continue oral PPIs past 28 days must be judged on an individualized basis because there is insufficient evidence to guide practice, and it is determined by the nature of the bleeding lesion. For example, longer courses of PPI therapy may be warranted for patients with bleeding erosive esophagitis compared with patients with duodenal ulcers.

The optimal duration of treatment with oral PPI is unknown and also depends on patient ongoing risk factors, and sometimes the severity of the presentation. For example, a patient treated for peptic ulcer disease related to either H pylori or nonsteroidal antiinflammatory drug (NSAID) use may only require a short course of PPI so long as the H pylori is eradicated or the NSAID discontinued.[2,11] The benefits and risks of ongoing PPI therapy should be discussed with individual patients.

Long-term Safety of Proton Pump Inhibitors

Many patients remain on PPI therapy long after the initial episode of UGIB. The 2 main concerns that have been raised about the long-term safety profile of PPI therapy include infections, such as Clostridium difficile–associated diarrhea (CDAD) and pneumonia, as well as metabolic bone disease.[64]

Gastric acid inhibition predisposes patients to an increased risk of enteric infections because normally the gastric acidity protects against these pathogens. It has been proposed that there is an increased risk of CDAD in patients on PPI therapy, even without exposure to antibiotics.[65] However, a systematic review and meta-analysis recently found only a weak relationship between exposure to PPI therapy and CDAD.[66]

Some evidence suggests that PPI therapy increases the risk of pneumonia, presumably through increased bacteria in the upper gastrointestinal tract that can migrate into the pulmonary system.[67] More recently, a meta-analysis found no increased risk of

CDAD with the use of PPIs.[68] A separate meta-analysis comparing PPI with H2-receptor antagonists for stress ulcer prophylaxis found no difference in rates of nosocomial pneumonia or mortality.[69]

PPI therapy in postmenopáusal women has been associated with an increased risk of hip fracture (RR, 1.30, 1.19–1.43), spine fracture (RR, 1.56, 1.31–1.85), and any-site fracture (RR, 1.16, 1.02–1.32) in the Nurses' Health Study.[70] In the same study, current and former smokers on PPI therapy had a 51% increased risk of hip fracture (hazard ratio, 1.52, 1.20–1.91). Similarly, another meta-analysis found that PPIs increased fracture risk, whereas histamine2 receptor antagonists did not.[71] PPI therapy may directly alter bone metabolism via the vacuolar H^+-ATPase in osteoclasts.[72] Although a recent meta-analysis suggests that PPIs may be linked to a slightly increased risk of fracture (RR, 1.30; 95% CI, 1.13–1.49), this association may be caused by confounding factors such as frailty.[73,74]

Other potential consequences of PPI therapy include hypomagnesaemia, vitamin B_{12} malabsorption, and acute interstitial nephritis.[75–77] The most current US Food and Drug Administration warnings suggest routine screening of magnesium levels before initiating PPI therapy, and occasional monitoring of serum magnesium, especially in those patients at higher risk who are taking digoxin or diuretics. Moreover, interactions with medications, most notably clopidogrel, are a concern, although the most recent high-quality data suggest no clinically significant clopidogrel-PPI interaction.[78–80] Although there are risks involved with long-term PPI therapy, the absolute risks are small. Monitoring magnesium levels periodically, as well as encouraging patients- to stop smoking, may mitigate some of the risk. Overall, physicians should aim to minimize the dose and duration of PPI therapy whenever possible.

Secondary Prophylaxis to Prevent Recurrent Bleeding

In patients with H pylori–associated bleeding ulcers, continuing PPI therapy after H pylori eradication is not required unless there are other ongoing risk factors, including NSAID use or antithrombotic therapy. Similarly, patients with NSAID-induced ulcers do not require long-term PPI therapy unless the ongoing NSAID therapy is warranted. Should NSAID treatment be necessary, the authors recommend considering a cyclooxygenase-2–selective NSAID at the lowest possible dose along with daily PPI therapy. Similarly, in patients with low-dose aspirin–related ulcers, long-term PPI therapy is required if acetylsalicylic acid (ASA) must be continued (eg, secondary prevention of cardiovascular disease).[11,81,82]

Pooled results of 2 randomized trials have shown that ASA with PPI has significantly less risk of rebleeding than clopidogrel alone (OR, 0.06; 95% CI, 0.01–0.32).[2,83,84] Recent guidelines suggest long-term PPI therapy in patients who have idiopathic ulcers (non–H pylori, non-NSAID), in whom the incidence of recurrent ulcer bleeding has been reported at 42%.[11,85]

Helicobacter pylori Eradication

All patients should be tested for infection with H pylori, which is one of the principal causes of bleeding ulcers. Several testing methods are available.[86,87] The low prevalence reported for H pylori infection in patients with UGIB might be related to delay in testing, which is often not performed until 4 weeks after the bleeding episode.[88] Urea breath tests (UBTs) are widely used, but serology is preferable in acute settings because it has the best diagnostic accuracy in this specific condition.[89,90] A second test should be performed if a negative index result is obtained at the time of acute UGIB because false-negative rates in the acute setting reach 55% and are increased for all diagnostic modalities.[2] Real-time polymerase chain reaction (PCR) might improve *H pylori* detection in patients with peptic ulcer bleeding. Real-time PCR testing for a combination of *H pylori* 16S ribosomal RNA and urease A had a sensitivity of 64% and a specificity of 80% in tissue samples that had previously been considered negative by histologic testing alone.[91]

After the completion of antibiotic and PPI treatment, a UBT might be the most convenient approach to assess the effectiveness of *H pylori* eradication treatment, unless repeat endoscopy is indicated, at which time gastric biopsies can be performed. Regardless of the method being used, checking for eradication is mandatory because *H pylori* infection is a major cause of gastric cancer, specifically noncardia gastric cancer.[92,93]

Iron Replacement Therapy

Patients who present with UGIB should have iron studies performed after the acute bleeding episode. Anemic patients and even nonanemic patients with evidence of iron deficiency should be offered iron replacement therapy on discharge from hospital because it may improve their quality of life and cognitive function.[94,95] In one study, only 16% of anemic patients after UGIB were prescribed oral supplementation on discharge from hospital.[96] Correcting anemia rapidly after discharge may be crucial in minimizing both mortality risk and possible need for a transfusion during a rebleeding episode. In a large prospective study, patients discharged after UGIB with hemoglobin values less than 100 g/L had twice the mortality of patients with hemoglobin levels greater than 100 g/L.[97]

However, current international consensus and American College of Gastroenterology guidelines do not discuss the role of iron replacement after UGIB.[2,11] A recent randomized controlled trial of 97 patients highlighted the importance of iron replacement by comparing intravenous iron, oral iron, and placebo in patients with anemia secondary to nonvariceal UGIB.[98] Patients receiving iron therapy had significantly lower rates of anemia (hemoglobin level <120 g/L for women and hemoglobin level <130 g/L for men) compared with patients receiving placebo at 3 months after UGIB (17% on iron therapy vs 70% on placebo; $P<.01$). Importantly, there was no difference in efficacy between 1 dose of intravenous iron and 3 months of oral iron replacement, although compliance in patients taking oral iron was only 56%.

The primary limitation to oral iron supplementation seems to be gastrointestinal tolerability, which is likely attributable to nonabsorbed iron.[99] All iron salts (ferrous sulfate, ferrous fumarate, and ferrous gluconate) showed similar efficacy and side effect profiles in a randomized trial.[100] A certain controlled-release iron preparation (extended-release ferrous sulfate with mucoproteose) has fewer gastrointestinal side effects than the iron salts according to a large meta-analysis.[101] There are currently no studies evaluating the tolerability of the newer polysaccharide-iron complexes, although previous studies evaluating similar formulations (eg, ferric-dextrin complex) have not shown any clear benefit.[102]

SUMMARY

The acute management of patients with nonvariceal UGIB has evolved considerably over the past 10 years, mostly because of earlier endoscopy, improved endoscopic techniques, and enhanced multidisciplinary management of these patients including gastroenterologists, intensivists, radiologists and surgeons. Application of the existing recommendations should lead to improved outcomes. Clinicians are encouraged to monitor ongoing controversies, such as optimal PPI dosing before and after endoscopic therapy, as well as the appropriate use of blood products. All patients should be screened and treated for Helicobacter Pylori and anemic patients should be offered iron therapy upon discharge from hospital.

REFERENCES

1. Button LA, Roberts SE, Evans PA, et al. Hospitalized incidence and case fatality for upper gastrointestinal bleeding from 1999 to 2007: a record linkage study. Aliment Pharmacol Ther 2011;33:64–76.
2. Barkun AN, Bardou M, Kuipers EJ, et al. International consensus recommendations on the management of patients with nonvariceal upper gastrointestinal bleeding. Ann Intern Med 2010;152:101–13.
3. Lau JY, Sung J, Hill C, et al. Systematic review of the epidemiology of complicated peptic ulcer disease: incidence, recurrence, risk factors and mortality. Digestion 2011;84:102–13.
4. Bardhan KD, Williamson M, Royston C, et al. Admission rates for peptic ulcer in the Trent region, UK, 1972–2000. Changing pattern, a changing disease? Dig Liver Dis 2004;36:577–88.
5. Soplepmann J, Peetsalu A, Peetsalu M, et al. Peptic ulcer haemorrhage in Tartu County, Estonia: epidemiology and mortality risk factors. Scand J Gastroenterol 1997;32:1195–200.
6. Barkun A, Sabbah S, Enns R, et al. The Canadian Registry on Nonvariceal Upper Gastrointestinal Bleeding and Endoscopy (RUGBE): endoscopic hemostasis and proton pump inhibition are associated with improved outcomes in a real-life setting. Am J Gastroenterol 2004;99:1238–46.
7. Hearnshaw SA, Logan RF, Lowe D, et al. Acute upper gastrointestinal bleeding in the UK: patient characteristics, diagnoses and outcomes in the 2007 UK audit. Gut 2011;60:1327–35.
8. Liu NJ, Lee CS, Tang JH, et al. Outcomes of bleeding peptic ulcers: a prospective study. J Gastroenterol Hepatol 2007;23(8 Pt 2):e340–7.
9. Crooks C, Card T, West J. Reductions in 28-day mortality following hospital admission for upper gastrointestinal hemorrhage. Gastroenterology 2011;141:62–70.
10. Lanas A, Carrera-Lasfuentes P, Garcia-Rodriguez LA, et al. Outcomes of peptic ulcer bleeding following treatment with proton pump inhibitors in routine clinical practice: 935 patients with high- or low-risk stigmata. Scand J Gastroenterol 2014;49:1181–90.
11. Laine L, Jensen DM. Management of patients with ulcer bleeding. Am J Gastroenterol 2012;107:345–60 [quiz: 61].
12. Greenspoon J, Barkun A. A summary of recent recommendations on the management of patients with nonvariceal upper gastrointestinal bleeding. Pol Arch Med Wewn 2010;120:341–6.
13. Wee E. Management of nonvariceal upper gastrointestinal bleeding. J Postgrad Med 2011;57:161–7.
14. Myburgh JA, Finfer S, Bellomo R, et al. Hydroxyethyl starch or saline for fluid resuscitation in intensive care. N Engl J Med 2012;367:1901–11.
15. Bunn F, Trivedi D, Ashraf S. Colloid solutions for fluid resuscitation. Cochrane Database Syst Rev 2011;(3):CD001319.
16. Jairath V, Hearnshaw S, Brunskill SJ, et al. Red cell transfusion for the management of upper gastrointestinal haemorrhage. Cochrane Database Syst Rev 2010;(9):CD006613.
17. Villanueva C, Colomo A, Bosch A. Transfusion for acute upper gastrointestinal bleeding. N Engl J Med 2013;368:1362–3.

18. Shalev A, Zahger D, Novack V, et al. Incidence, predictors and outcome of upper gastrointestinal bleeding in patients with acute coronary syndromes. Int J Cardiol 2012;157:386–90.

19. Jairath V, Kahan BC, Logan RF, et al. Red blood cell transfusion practice in patients presenting with acute upper gastrointestinal bleeding: a survey of 815 UK clinicians. Transfusion 2011;51:1940–8.

20. Rohde JM, Dimcheff DE, Blumberg N, et al. Health care-associated infection after red blood cell transfusion: a systematic review and meta-analysis. JAMA 2014;311:1317–26.

21. Kahan BC, Jairath V, Murphy MF, et al. Update on the transfusion in gastrointestinal bleeding (TRIGGER) trial: statistical analysis plan for a cluster-randomised feasibility trial. Trials 2013;14:206.

22. Razzaghi A, Barkun AN. Platelet transfusion threshold in patients with upper gastrointestinal bleeding: a systematic review. J Clin Gastroenterol 2012;46:482–6.

23. Pallin DJ, Saltzman JR. Is nasogastric tube lavage in patients with acute upper GI bleeding indicated or antiquated? Gastrointest Endosc 2011;74:981–4.

24. Witting MD. You wanna do what?! Modern indications for nasogastric intubation. J Emerg Med 2007;33:61–4.

25. Palamidessi N, Sinert R, Falzon L, et al. Nasogastric aspiration and lavage in emergency department patients with hematochezia or melena without hematemesis. Acad Emerg Med 2010;17:126–32.

26. Pateron D, Vicaut E, Debuc E, et al. Erythromycin infusion or gastric lavage for upper gastrointestinal bleeding: a multicenter randomized controlled trial. Ann Emerg Med 2011;57:582–9.

27. Barkun A, Bardou M, Marshall JK. Consensus recommendations for managing patients with nonvariceal upper gastrointestinal bleeding. Ann Intern Med 2003; 139:843–57.

28. Colak S, Erdogan MO, Sekban H, et al. Emergency diagnosis of upper gastrointestinal bleeding by detection of haemoglobin in nasogastric aspirate. J Int Med Res 2013;41:1825–9.

29. Iwasaki H, Shimura T, Yamada T, et al. Novel nasogastric tube-related criteria for urgent endoscopy in nonvariceal upper gastrointestinal bleeding. Dig Dis Sci 2013;58(9):2564–71.

30. Aljebreen AM, Fallone CA, Barkun AN. Nasogastric aspirate predicts high-risk endoscopic lesions in patients with acute upper-GI bleeding. Gastrointest Endosc 2004;59:172–8.

31. Gralnek IM, Barkun AN, Bardou M. Management of acute bleeding from a peptic ulcer. N Engl J Med 2008;359:928–37.

32. Pitera A, Sarko J. Just say no: gastric aspiration and lavage rarely provide benefit. Ann Emerg Med 2010;55:365–6.

33. Anderson RS, Witting MD. Nasogastric aspiration: a useful tool in some patients with gastrointestinal bleeding. Ann Emerg Med 2010;55:364–5.

34. Javad Ehsani Ardakani M, Zare E, Basiri M, et al. Erythromycin decreases the time and improves the quality of EGD in patients with acute upper GI bleeding. Gastroenterol Hepatol Bed Bench 2013;6:195–201.

35. Frossard JL, Spahr L, Queneau PE, et al. Erythromycin intravenous bolus infusion in acute upper gastrointestinal bleeding: a randomized, controlled, double-blind trial. Gastroenterology 2002;123:17–23.

36. Barkun AN, Bardou M, Martel M, et al. Prokinetics in acute upper GI bleeding: a meta-analysis. Gastrointest Endosc 2010;72:1138–45.

37. Bai Y, Guo JF, Li ZS. Meta-analysis: erythromycin before endoscopy for acute upper gastrointestinal bleeding. Aliment Pharmacol Ther 2011;34:166–71.
38. Szary NM, Gupta R, Choudhary A, et al. Erythromycin prior to endoscopy in acute upper gastrointestinal bleeding: a meta-analysis. Scand J Gastroenterol 2011;46:920–4.
39. Altraif I, Handoo FA, Aljumah A, et al. Effect of erythromycin before endoscopy in patients presenting with variceal bleeding: a prospective, randomized, double-blind, placebo-controlled trial. Gastrointest Endosc 2011;73:245–50.
40. Coffin B, Pocard M, Panis Y, et al. Erythromycin improves the quality of EGD in patients with acute upper GI bleeding: a randomized controlled study. Gastrointest Endosc 2002;56:174–9.
41. Sreedharan A, Martin J, Leontiadis GI, et al. Proton pump inhibitor treatment initiated prior to endoscopic diagnosis in upper gastrointestinal bleeding. Cochrane Database Syst Rev 2010;(7):CD005415.
42. Lau JY, Leung WK, Wu JC, et al. Omeprazole before endoscopy in patients with gastrointestinal bleeding. N Engl J Med 2007;356:1631–40.
43. Laine L, Shah A, Bemanian S. Intragastric pH with oral vs intravenous bolus plus infusion proton-pump inhibitor therapy in patients with bleeding ulcers. Gastroenterology 2008;134:1836–41.
44. Lin HJ, Lo WC, Cheng YC, et al. Role of intravenous omeprazole in patients with high-risk peptic ulcer bleeding after successful endoscopic epinephrine injection: a prospective randomized comparative trial. Am J Gastroenterol 2006;101:500–5.
45. Leontiadis GI, Sharma VK, Howden CW. Proton pump inhibitor therapy for peptic ulcer bleeding: Cochrane collaboration meta-analysis of randomized controlled trials. Mayo Clin Proc 2007;82:286–96.
46. Al-Sabah S, Barkun AN, Herba K, et al. Cost-effectiveness of proton-pump inhibition before endoscopy in upper gastrointestinal bleeding. Clin Gastroenterol Hepatol 2008;6:418–25.
47. Barkun AN, Bardou M, Kuipers EJ, et al. How early should endoscopy be performed in suspected upper gastrointestinal bleeding? Am J Gastroenterol 2012;107:328–9.
48. Imperiale TF, Birgisson S. Somatostatin or octreotide compared with H2 antagonists and placebo in the management of acute nonvariceal upper gastrointestinal hemorrhage: a meta-analysis. Ann Intern Med 1997;127:1062–71.
49. Arabi Y, Al Knawy B, Barkun AN, et al. Pro/con debate: octreotide has an important role in the treatment of gastrointestinal bleeding of unknown origin? Crit Care 2006;10:218.
50. Bennett C, Klingenberg SL, Langholz E, et al. Tranexamic acid for upper gastrointestinal bleeding. Cochrane Database Syst Rev 2014;(11):CD006640.
51. Manno D, Ker K, Roberts I. How effective is tranexamic acid for acute gastrointestinal bleeding? BMJ 2014;348:g1421.
52. Bardou M, Martin J, Barkun A. Intravenous proton pump inhibitors: an evidence-based review of their use in gastrointestinal disorders. Drugs 2009;69:435–48.
53. Ghassemi KA, Kovacs TO, Jensen DM. Gastric acid inhibition in the treatment of peptic ulcer hemorrhage. Curr Gastroenterol Rep 2009;11:462–9.
54. Vorder Bruegge WF, Peura DA. Stress-related mucosal damage: review of drug therapy. J Clin Gastroenterol 1990;12(Suppl 2):S35–40.
55. Laine L, McQuaid KR. Endoscopic therapy for bleeding ulcers: an evidence-based approach based on meta-analyses of randomized controlled trials. Clin Gastroenterol Hepatol 2009;7:33–47 [quiz: 1–2].

56. Forrest JA, Finlayson ND, Shearman DJ. Endoscopy in gastrointestinal bleeding. Lancet 1974;2:394–7.

57. Sung JJ, Barkun A, Kuipers EJ, et al. Intravenous esomeprazole for prevention of recurrent peptic ulcer bleeding: a randomized trial. Ann Intern Med 2009;150: 455–64.

58. Barkun AN, Adam V, Sun-g JJ, et al. Cost effectiveness of high-dose intravenous esomeprazole for peptic ulcer bleeding. Pharmacoeconomics 2010;28:217–30.

59. Sachar H, Vaidya K, Laine L. Intermittent vs continuous proton pump inhibitor therapy for high-risk bleeding ulcers: a systematic review and meta-analysis. JAMA Intern Med 2014;174:1755–62.

60. Leontiadis GI, Sharma VK, Howden CW. Systematic review and meta-analysis: enhanced efficacy of proton-pump inhibitor therapy for peptic ulcer bleeding in Asia–a post hoc analysis from the Cochrane Collaboration. Aliment Pharmacol Ther 2005;21:1055–61.

61. Hoie O, Stallemo A, Matre J, et al. Effect of oral lansoprazole on intragastric pH after endoscopic treatment for bleeding peptic ulcer. Scand J Gastroenterol 2009;44:284–8.

62. Laine L, Peterson WL. Bleeding peptic ulcer. N Engl J Med 1994;331:717–27.

63. Cheng HC, Wu CT, Chang WL, et al. Double oral esomeprazole after a 3-day intravenous esomeprazole infusion reduces recurrent peptic ulcer bleeding in high-risk patients: a randomised controlled study. Gut 2014;63:1864–72.

64. Yang YX, Metz DC. Safety of proton pump inhibitor exposure. Gastroenterology 2010;139:1115–27.

65. Dial S, Delaney JA, Barkun AN, et al. Use of gastric acid-suppressive agents and the risk of community-acquired *Clostridium difficile*-associated disease. JAMA 2005;294:2989–95.

66. Tleyjeh IM, Bin Abdulhak AA, Riaz M, et al. Association between proton pump inhibitor therapy and *Clostridium difficile* infection: a contemporary systematic review and meta-analysis. PLoS One 2012;7:e50836.

67. Eom CS, Jeon CY, Lim JW, et al. Use of acid-suppressive drugs and risk of pneumonia: a systematic review and meta-analysis. CMAJ 2011;183:310–9.

68. Filion KB, Chateau D, Targownik LE, et al. Proton pump inhibitors and the risk of hospitalisation for community-acquired pneumonia: replicated cohort studies with meta-analysis. Gut 2014;63:552–8.

69. Barkun AN, Bardou M, Pham CQ, et al. Proton pump inhibitors vs. histamine 2 receptor antagonists for stress-related mucosal bleeding prophylaxis in critically ill patients: a meta-analysis. Am J Gastroenterol 2012;107:507–20 [quiz: 21].

70. Khalili H, Huang ES, Jacobson BC, et al. Use of proton pump inhibitors and risk of hip fracture in relation to dietary and lifestyle factors: a prospective cohort study. BMJ 2012;344:e372.

71. Yu EW, Bauer SR, Bain PA, et al. Proton pump inhibitors and risk of fractures: a meta-analysis of 11 international studies. Am J Med 2011;124:519–26.

72. Jo Y, Park E, Ahn SB, et al. A proton pump inhibitor's effect on bone metabolism mediated by osteoclast action in old age: a prospective randomized study. Gut Liver 2014. [Epub ahead of print].

73. Moayyedi P, Yuan Y, Leontiadis G, et al. Canadian Association of Gastroenterology position statement: hip fracture and proton pump inhibitor therapy–a 2013 update. Can J Gastroenterol 2013;27:593–5.

74. Leontiadis GI, Moayyedi P. Proton pump inhibitors and risk of bone fractures. Curr Treat Options Gastroenterol 2014;12:414–23.

75. Hess MW, Hoenderop JG, Bindels RJ, et al. Systematic review: hypomagnesaemia induced by proton pump inhibition. Aliment Pharmacol Ther 2012;36:405–13.
76. Lam JR, Schneider JL, Zhao W, et al. Proton pump inhibitor and histamine 2 receptor antagonist use and vitamin B12 deficiency. JAMA 2013;310:2435–42.
77. Muriithi AK, Leung N, Valeri AM, et al. Biopsy-proven acute interstitial nephritis, 1993–2011: a case series. Am J Kidney Dis 2014;64:558–66.
78. Ghebremariam YT, LePendu P, Lee JC, et al. Unexpected effect of proton pump inhibitors: elevation of the cardiovascular risk factor asymmetric dimethylarginine. Circulation 2013;128:845–53.
79. Lima JP, Brophy JM. The potential interaction between clopidogrel and proton pump inhibitors: a systematic review. BMC Med 2010;8:81.
80. Schneider-Lindner V, Filion KB, Brophy JM. Adverse outcomes associated with use of proton pump inhibitors and clopidogrel. JAMA 2009;302:29–30 [author reply: 1].
81. Lai KC, Lam SK, Chu KM, et al. Lansoprazole for the prevention of recurrences of ulcer complications from long-term low-dose aspirin use. N Engl J Med 2002; 346:2033–8.
82. Sung JJ, Lau JY, Ching JY, et al. Continuation of low-dose aspirin therapy in peptic ulcer bleeding: a randomized trial. Ann Intern Med 2010;152:1–9.
83. Lai KC, Chu KM, Hui WM, et al. Esomeprazole with aspirin versus clopidogrel for prevention of recurrent gastrointestinal ulcer complications. Clin Gastroenterol Hepatol 2006;4:860–5.
84. Chan FK, Ching JY, Hung LC, et al. Clopidogrel versus aspirin and esomeprazole to prevent recurrent ulcer bleeding. N Engl J Med 2005;352:238–44.
85. Wong GL, Wong VW, Chan Y, et al. High incidence of mortality and recurrent bleeding in patients with *Helicobacter pylori*-negative idiopathic bleeding ulcers. Gastroenterology 2009;137:525–31.
86. Talley NJ, Li Z. *Helicobacter pylori*: testing and treatment. Expert Rev Gastroenterol Hepatol 2007;1:71–9.
87. Sfarti C, Stanciu C, Cojocariu C, et al. 13C-urea breath test for the diagnosis of *Helicobacter pylori* infection in bleeding duodenal ulcer. Rev Med Chir Soc Med Nat Iasi 2009;113:704–9.
88. Sanchez-Delgado J, Gene E, Suarez D, et al. Has *H. pylori* prevalence in bleeding peptic ulcer been underestimated? A meta-regression. Am J Gastroenterol 2011;106:398–405.
89. Gisbert JP, Abraira V. Accuracy of *Helicobacter pylori* diagnostic tests in patients with bleeding peptic ulcer: a systematic review and meta-analysis. Am J Gastroenterol 2006;101:848–63.
90. Stenstrom B, Mendis A, Marshall B. *Helicobacter pylori*-the latest in diagnosis and treatment. Aust Fam Physician 2008;37:608–12.
91. Ramirez-Lazaro MJ, Lario S, Casalots A, et al. Real-time PCR improves *Helicobacter pylori* detection in patients with peptic ulcer bleeding. PLoS One 2011;6: e20009.
92. Fock KM. Review article: the epidemiology and prevention of gastric cancer. Aliment Pharmacol Ther 2014;40:250–60.
93. Plummer M, Franceschi S, Vignat J, et al. Global burden of gastric cancer attributable to *Helicobacter pylori*. Int J Cancer 2015;136:487–90.
94. Verdon F, Burnand B, Stubi CL, et al. Iron supplementation for unexplained fatigue in non-anaemic women: double blind randomised placebo controlled trial. BMJ 2003;326:1124.

95. Bruner AB, Joffe A, Duggan AK, et al. Randomised study of cognitive effects of iron supplementation in non-anaemic iron-deficient adolescent girls. Lancet 1996;348:992–6.
96. Bager P, Dahlerup JF. Lack of follow-up of anaemia after discharge from an upper gastrointestinal bleeding centre. Dan Med J 2013;60:A4583.
97. Rockall TA, Logan RF, Devlin HB, et al. Risk assessment after acute upper gastrointestinal haemorrhage. Gut 1996;38:316–21.
98. Bager P, Dahlerup JF. Randomised clinical trial: oral vs. intravenous iron after upper gastrointestinal haemorrhage–a placebo-controlled study. Aliment Pharmacol Ther 2014;39:176–87.
99. Bayraktar UD, Bayraktar S. Treatment of iron deficiency anemia associated with gastrointestinal tract diseases. World J Gastroenterol 2010;16:2720–5.
100. Hallberg L, Ryttinger L, Solvell L. Side-effects of oral iron therapy. A double-blind study of different iron compounds in tablet form. Acta Med Scand Suppl 1966;459:3–10.
101. Cancelo-Hidalgo MJ, Castelo-Branco C, Palacios S, et al. Tolerability of different oral iron supplements: a systematic review. Curr Med Res Opin 2013;29: 291–303.
102. Sas G, Nemesanszky E, Brauer H, et al. On the therapeutic effects of trivalent and divalent iron in iron deficiency anaemia. Arzneimittelforschung 1984;34: 1575–9.

Dyspepsia

Maryann Katherine Overland, MD

KEYWORDS

- Functional dyspepsia • *Helicobacter pylori* test and treat • Peptic ulcer disease
- Gastroesophageal reflux disease

KEY POINTS

- Dyspepsia is a complex disease with multiple potential pathophysiologic mechanisms including abnormal gut motility, visceral hypersensitivity, genetic, infectious/postinfectious, and psychosocial factors.
- Although serious pathology is rare in patients presenting with dyspepsia, physicians should be aware of alarm features and refer those patients promptly for endoscopy or subspecialty care.
- A trial of antisecretory therapy, such as a proton pump inhibitor or histamine-2 receptor antagonist, should be provided to patients without alarm features, especially if their primary symptom is epigastric burning.
- A test-and-treat strategy for *Helicobacter pylori* infection is a cost-effective intervention and provides symptomatic relief for some patients with dyspepsia.
- Patients with depression, anxiety, or a history of abuse should be offered antidepressant therapy and psychotherapy.

INTRODUCTION

Dyspepsia is not a single disease, but rather a complex of symptoms that often overlap with other disease entities.[1] The investigation of undifferentiated dyspepsia poses a diagnostic dilemma for primary care physicians. Because evidence to guide best practices is sparse, it is challenging for the primary care physician to decide the optimal diagnostic and therapeutic plan. Although life-threatening conditions are rare in this setting, a missed diagnosis of esophageal cancer or other serious upper gastrointestinal pathology could be devastating. For this reason, invasive diagnostic tests, including endoscopies, are common in the evaluation of uninvestigated dyspepsia. Given the high prevalence of dyspepsia around the world, developing a prudent and evidence-based method of investigation and treatment of dyspepsia is of the utmost importance to prevent potential harm and unnecessary medical expense.

This article originally appeared in Medical Clinics, Volume 98, Issue 3, May 2014.
Division of General Internal Medicine, Primary Care Clinic, VA Puget Sound Health Care System, University of Washington, 1660 South Columbian Way, Seattle, WA 98108, USA
E-mail address: Maryann.Overland@va.gov

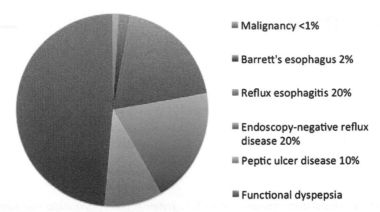

Fig. 1. Causes of dyspepsia. (*Data from* Zagari RM, Fuccio L, Bazzoli F. Investigating dyspepsia. BMJ 2008;337:1–5.)

Dyspepsia affects 25% to 40% of the population over a lifetime and accounts for 3% to 5% of all primary care clinic visits,[2] estimated at 4 million primary care visits a year in the United States alone.[3] One study found that 50% of European and North American patients with dyspepsia are on medication for it, and more than 30% report ever missing work or school because of burdensome symptoms.[4] Another study reported 12.4% of patients with dyspepsia missed work because of their symptoms over a 1-year period.[5] Among active workers with dyspepsia, more than 32% reported their symptoms caused them to be absent from work, and 78% reported reduced productivity because of dyspepsia (presenteeism). That study did not find a difference in lost productivity between those with organic versus those with functional dyspepsia (FD).[6] Nearly 62% of the patients in one study had consulted a physician for their dyspeptic symptoms, and 74% of those went more than once. More than two-thirds of those patients who had consulted

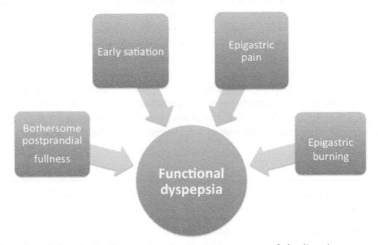

Fig. 2. Functional dyspepsia diagnostic criteria. One or more of the listed symptoms, in the absence of structural disease. Criteria must be fulfilled for the last 3 months with symptom onset at least 6 months before diagnosis.

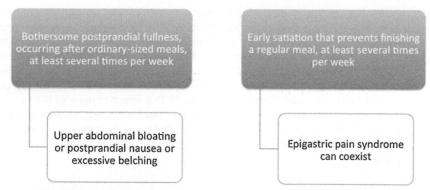

Fig. 3. Postprandial distress syndrome.

a physician were taking medications for their dyspepsia, and 36% underwent endoscopy.[5]

Of patients presenting with dyspepsia symptoms, 50% to 60% have no biochemical or structural lesion to explain their symptoms (**Fig. 1**). FD, previously referred to as "nonulcer dyspepsia," describes these symptoms in the absence of an identifiable organic, systemic, or metabolic etiology (**Fig. 2**).[2,7–9] FD is divided into two categories by the Rome III criteria, although there is considerable overlap between the two. The first is postprandial distress syndrome (**Fig. 3**), characterized by bothersome postprandial fullness and early satiation; the second is epigastric pain syndrome (**Fig. 4**), characterized by epigastric pain and burning, with onset of at

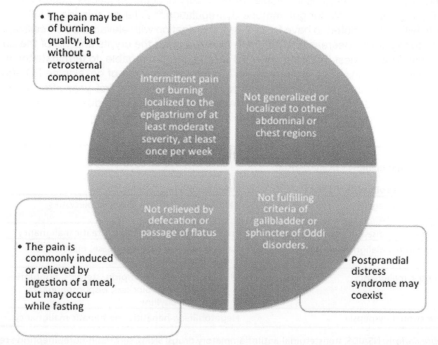

Fig. 4. Epigastric pain syndrome.

least 6 months ago, and present during the last 3 months.[9] The symptoms are usually aggravated by meals. Some older definitions of FD include symptoms of gastroesophageal reflux, such as heartburn and belching, whereas the newer Rome III definition does not include these symptoms. However, there is a great degree of overlap between FD and coexisting reflux disease. One study revealed 37% of patients complaining of symptoms that could be characterized as FD actually had esophageal acid reflux proved by pH monitoring.[10] The exact causes of FD remain unknown[9] but symptoms are more common in women,[5] smokers, aspirin users,[11] and those with a history of acute gastroenteritis.[12] Coffee and alcohol are not definitively associated with FD, and the role of *Helicobacter pylori* infection in FD is still up for debate.

PATHOPHYSIOLOGY

The pathophysiology of FD is not completely understood, with abnormal gut motility, visceral hypersensitivity, genetic, infectious/postinfectious, and psychosocial factors playing a role.

Delayed gastric emptying occurs in 20% to 50% of patients with FD.[13] Up to two-thirds may have abnormalities of either antral or duodenal motility.[14] Those patients with delayed gastric emptying predominantly have symptoms of postprandial fullness, nausea, and vomiting.[15] Up to 40% of patients with symptoms of early satiety and weight loss have impaired gastric accommodation, which suggests those patients' dyspeptic symptoms could be caused by increased intragastric pressure after ingestion of a meal.[16–18] Studies using capsaicin have shown increased sensitivity to visceral stimulation in patients with FD.[19,20] Several genetic polymorphisms are associated with visceral hypersensitivity and other upper abdominal symptoms in FD.[21]

FD occurs at higher rates in people with a history of acute infectious gastroenteritis (IGE), suggesting a role for gut immune dysregulation.[22] After an episode of IGE, patients with FD are noted to have focal T-cell aggregation with elevated CD8+ cells and macrophages and decreased CD4+ cells in and around the crypts and villi of the duodenum. This suggest that patients with FD are slower, or unable, to terminate the inflammatory response.[23] A meta-analysis investigating the risk of developing FD after an episode of acute IGE found an odds ratio of 4.76 in the first year after a self-reported episode of IGE and 1.97 thereafter, with an overall odds ratio of nearly 2.2.[12] Several studies have also linked eradication of *H pylori* to improvement in FD.

Table 1
Differential diagnosis of dyspepsia

Upper Gastrointestinal Tract	Other Sources
Gastroesophageal reflux with or without esophagitis	Gallbladder: cholelithiasis or cholecystitis
Peptic ulcer disease: gastric or duodenal	Pancreas: pancreatitis or pancreatic malignancy
Esophageal malignancy	Vascular: ischemic heart disease, mesenteric ischemia
Gastric malignancy	Medications: NSAIDS, aspirin, steroids, antibiotics, calcium channel blockers, bisphosphonates, SNRIs, theophylline
Functional dyspepsia	Hepatobiliary: hepatitis and hepatic malignancy

Abbreviations: NSAIDS, nonsteroidal antiinflammatory drugs; SNRIs, serotonin-norepinephrine reuptake inhibitors.

FD is more common in patients with concomitant depression or anxiety, and those with a history of abuse. A recent prospective cohort study of nearly 1200 patients demonstrated that high baseline levels of anxiety were an independent predictor of developing FD in the future.[24] Patients with anxiety and depression are more likely to seek treatment of their dyspepsia,[25] and are also more likely to experience their symptoms as more severe than those without a comorbid psychiatric condition.[26] As with any functional gastrointestinal disorder, somatization is a potential cause (**Table 1**).[27]

GASTROESOPHAGEAL REFLUX DISEASE

Gastroesophageal reflux disease (GERD) is one of the most common upper gastrointestinal disorders in the developed world. It is caused by prolonged gastric acid exposure in the esophagus due to poor esophageal motility, decreased lower esophageal sphincter tone, and impairments in gastroesophageal junctions. Obesity, smoking, alcohol, pregnancy, certain foods, and a recumbent position shortly after eating can all cause GERD or make it worse.[28] There is a great deal of overlap between GERD and FD. A study of prevalence of pathologic esophageal acid reflux in patients with FD found that nearly 32% of patients with FD had pathologic esophageal acid reflux. The prevalence is approximately 50% in patients who complained predominantly of epigastric burning.[10]

The hallmark of GERD is heartburn and regurgitation, particularly after meals. Patients may also have extraesophageal symptoms, such as cough or laryngitis. Endoscopy is 90% to 100% specific for diagnosing esophagitis in reflux disease. However, 50% to 70% of patients with the classic heartburn and regurgitation symptoms of GERD have no esophagitis on endoscopy,[29] making it a rather insensitive screening tool. When typical heartburn and regurgitation occur together, a diagnosis of GERD can be made without further testing with greater than 90% accuracy.[30] A study comparing a 2-week course of high-dose omeprazole versus 24-hour esophageal pH monitoring found the two interventions to be equally sensitive in diagnosing GERD in patients with erosive esophagitis.[31,32] Thus, for those patients presenting with heartburn and regurgitation, an empiric therapeutic trial of a standard-dose proton pump inhibitor (PPI) for 2 weeks or a double-dose of PPI therapy for 1 week is appropriate. If patients respond to an appropriate trial of antisecretory therapy, a diagnosis can be made and no further testing is warranted. However, if patients do not respond to empiric therapy, have chronic symptoms, or have alarm symptoms, endoscopy should be considered to evaluate for Barrett esophagus, stricture, ulcers, or malignancy.[30]

Dietary and lifestyle modifications are often recommended as first-line treatment of GERD. Suggested dietary changes include avoiding foods and drinks that decrease lower esophageal sphincter pressure, delay gastric emptying, or provoke reflux symptoms. These foods include chocolate, mint, alcohol, tomato, citrus juice, carbonated beverages, garlic, onions, and fatty meals. Additionally, instituting behavioral modifications might also decrease reflux symptoms. These modifications include elevating the head of the bed while sleeping, avoiding a recumbent position for 3 hours after meals, sleeping in the left lateral position, smoking cessation, and avoidance of alcohol.[28] Although these recommendations are almost universally accepted, the evidence to support their effectiveness is not strong.

After the diagnosis of GERD is made, patients and providers can engage in shared decision making to determine if a step-up or a step-down approach to therapy is appropriate. A step-up approach starts with over-the-counter therapy with an H_2-receptor antagonist (H_2RA) and steps up therapy to medications with a

Table 2 Standard-dose and high-dose PPIs		
Drug	Standard Dose	High Dose
Dexlansoprazole	30 mg daily	30 mg twice daily
Esomeprazole	20 mg daily	40 mg daily
Lansoprazole	15–30 mg daily	30 mg twice daily
Omeprazole	20–40 mg daily	20–40 mg twice daily
Pantoprazole	20–40 mg daily	40 mg twice daily
Rabeprazole	20 mg daily	20 mg twice daily

Data from Wolfe MM, Sachs G. Acid suppression: optimizing therapy for gastroduodenal ulcer healing, gastroesophageal reflux disease, and stress-related erosive syndrome. Gastroenterology 2000;118:S9–31.

higher degree of efficacy (standard-dose PPI, then high-dose PPI) if symptoms persist (**Table 2**). A step-down approach to therapy starts with daily or twice-daily PPI therapy and steps down to therapies with lower degree of efficacy as symptoms allow. With each model, the therapy is maintained at the lowest level that completely controls symptoms.[28] Clinicians should choose the most cost-effective medication at the lowest effective dose for the shortest amount of time possible.

HELICOBACTER PYLORI AND PEPTIC ULCER DISEASE

Helicobacter pylori infection is associated with 90% to 95% of duodenal ulcers and 60% to 80% of gastric ulcers. The prevalence of *H pylori* ranges from 20% in North America and western Europe to more than 80% in eastern Europe, Asia, and most of the developing world.[33] *H pylori* can progress rapidly in high-prevalence areas or slowly in low-prevalence areas toward atrophic gastritis. A fast rate of progression toward gastritis is associated with a higher incidence of gastric cancer, whereas a slower rate of progression is more closely associated with peptic (duodenal) ulcer disease.[34] *H pylori* are a known carcinogen. The International Agency for Research on Cancer estimates 43% of the global burden of gastric cancer to be related to *H pylori*,[35] and this is likely an underestimation.

There is, however, some uncertainty as to whether chronic *H pylori* infection plays a role in dyspepsia in the absence of peptic ulcer disease or gastric cancer. Indeed, multiple systematic reviews and meta-analyses have looked into this question with conflicting results. One trial of *H pylori* eradication found that patients with complete or satisfactory response to a proton pump–based eradication therapy had decreased gastritis and improvement of dyspepsia symptoms at 1 year.[36] Some randomized controlled trials have shown a test-and-treat strategy is equally as effective as prompt endoscopy in reducing the severity of dyspepsia symptoms but with much lower medical costs. Recently, the HEROES trial identified *H pylori*–positive adults with FD by Rome III criteria, and randomized them to *H pylori* triple therapy or omeprazole plus placebo. The main outcome was at least 50% symptomatic improvement at 12 months. Forty-nine percent of the patients in the antibiotics group reached the primary outcome, as opposed to 36.5% in the PPI plus placebo group.[37] Overall, 78% in the antibiotics group and 67.5% in the control group reported some symptomatic improvement. Based on a large Cochrane review, the number needed to treat to achieve a complete symptomatic response in one patient is 14.[38] Some studies suggest a trend toward higher symptom response by *H pylori* eradication treatment in high-prevalence populations.[39] However, a recent meta-analysis of randomized

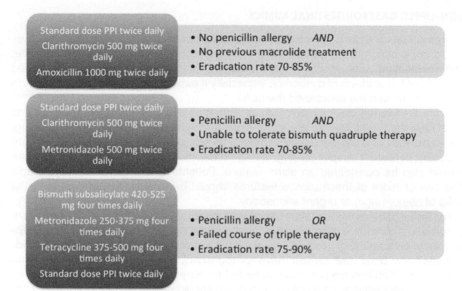

Standard dose PPI twice daily Clarithromycin 500 mg twice daily Amoxicillin 1000 mg twice daily	• No penicillin allergy AND • No previous macrolide treatment • Eradication rate 70-85%
Standard dose PPI twice daily Clarithromycin 500 mg twice daily Metronidazole 500 mg twice daily	• Penicillin allergy AND • Unable to tolerate bismuth quadruple therapy • Eradication rate 70-85%
Bismuth subsalicylate 420-525 mg four times daily Metronidazole 250-375 mg four times daily Tetracycline 375-500 mg four times daily Standard dose PPI twice daily	• Penicillin allergy OR • Failed course of triple therapy • Eradication rate 75-90%

Fig. 5. *Helicobacter pylori* treatment regimens. (*Data from* Chey WD, Wong BC. American College of Gastroenterology Guideline on the Management of *Helicobacter pylori* Infection. Am J Gastroenterol 2007;102:1808–25.)

controlled trials of *H pylori* eradication therapy on symptoms of FD demonstrated improvement in symptoms and a similar rate of response across Asian, European, and American populations.[40] Test-and-treat will cure most cases of underlying peptic ulcer disease, and will prevent most cases of gastric cancer. Although it does not resolve most cases of FD, at least a significant minority of patients will have significant improvements in their dyspepsia symptoms with this intervention. A test-and-treat strategy for *H pylori*, especially in populations with a high prevalence of the disease, is a reasonable approach (**Fig. 5**).

The ^{13}C-urea breath test is 95% sensitive and specific for *H pylori*; however, it is not universally available. The *H pylori* stool antigen test has similar sensitivity (91%) and specificity (93%), but patients have to remain off their PPI therapy for 2 weeks, and antibiotics for 4 weeks, before performing either of these tests. *H pylori* serology is widely available but is considerably less sensitive and specific (85% and 79%, respectively) than the other testing (**Table 3**).[2] However, patients do not need to be off therapies to obtain serology, and the ease with which it is administered (a simple blood draw) makes for improved adherence. In populations with a high prevalence of *H pylori* and challenges with follow through, *H pylori* serology is a reasonable compromise.

Table 3
Sensitivity and specificity of *Helicobacter pylori* tests

Test	Sensitivity (%)	Specificity (%)
^{13}C-urea breath test	95	95
Stool antigen test	91	93
Serology	85	79

From Zagari RM, Fuccio L, Bazzoli F. Investigating dyspepsia. BMJ 2008;337:1–5.

NON–UPPER GASTROINTESTINAL MIMICS

Diseases that can mimic symptoms of dyspepsia include cholelithiasis and cholecystitis, chronic pancreatitis, cardiac and mesenteric ischemia, irritable bowel syndrome, and medication side effects. These alternate diagnoses should be considered throughout the work-up of dyspepsia, especially if patients are not reporting symptom improvement with the prescribed therapies.

There are five key decision points in investigating dyspepsia (**Fig. 6**). The first, and most important, is to identify any alarm signs and symptoms. They include bleeding, iron-deficiency anemia, persistent vomiting, an epigastric mass, unexplained weight loss, and persistent dysphagia (**Fig. 7**). Age older than 55 years at the time of onset should also be considered an alarm feature. Patients who present with dysphagia and one or more of these clinical features should be referred for emergent (in the case of hemorrhage) or urgent endoscopy.

For those patients without alarm signs and symptoms, the other key questions are as follows: (1) Are there other possible mimics of the dyspepsia, such as cardiac, hepatobiliary, pancreatic, or vascular? (2) Is the patient on any potentially offending medications? (3) Does the patient have predominant symptoms of heartburn and regurgitation? (4) Has the patient been tested for *H pylori*? Those who are determined to have an alternative source of their dyspepsia should be treated accordingly. If a patient is found to be taking a potentially offending medication, all efforts should be made to find alternative therapies. If this is not possible, then antisecretory therapy, such as a PPI, should be added to the patient's therapy.

Those who have symptoms of heartburn or regurgitation, even if they also have symptoms of epigastric pain and postprandial fullness, deserve a 4- to 6-week trial of a PPI. All others should be tested, and treated if positive, for *H pylori* with the

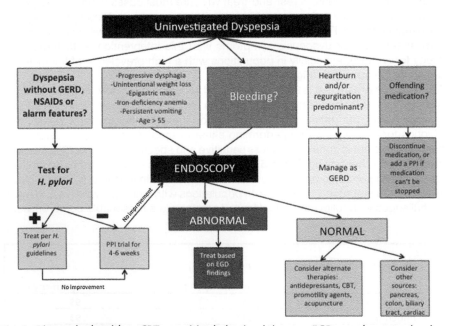

Fig. 6. Diagnosis algorithm. CBT, cognitive behavioral therapy; EGD, esophagastroduodenoscopy; GERD, gastroesophageal reflux disease; *H. pylori*, *Helicobacter pylori*; NSAIDs, nonsteroidal antiinflammatory drugs; PPI, proton pump inhibitor.

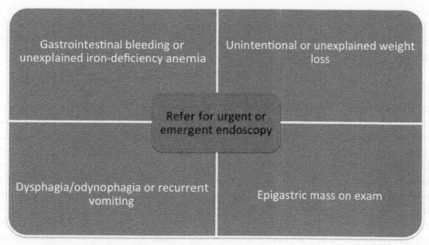

Fig. 7. Dyspepsia alarm signs and symptoms. (*Data from* Zagari RM, Fuccio L, Bazzoli F. Investigating dyspepsia. BMJ 2008;337:1–5.)

most sensitive and specific test available. Those who are negative for *H pylori* should be given a 4- to 6-week trial of antisecretory therapy. If patients fail to respond to these measures, endoscopy is an appropriate next step, and if the endoscopy is negative, gastric emptying studies can be considered. A gastric emptying study can help guide therapy if it demonstrates rapid or delayed emptying. After that, alternate therapies can be explored, including antidepressants, psychotherapy, cognitive behavioral therapy, hypnosis, and acupuncture.

TREATMENT OF FD

Fewer than 60% of patients with FD improve with medication alone.[41]

Acid-suppression Therapy

Various forms of acid-suppression therapy are available, including over-the-counter antacids, H_2RAs, and PPIs. Antacids are commonly used but have the least compelling evidence for effectiveness, and PPIs have the strongest evidence of effectiveness.

The evidence to support the use of H_2RAs for FD is conflicting. Some trials have demonstrated superiority of H_2RAs over placebo, whereas others have not. In a small crossover study, nizatidine was shown to improve postprandial fullness and early satiation over placebo (70% response vs 10% response). The treatment also improved gastroesophageal reflux symptoms over placebo (53% vs 0%). This study evaluated gastric motility and ghrelin levels, and found that the H_2RA improved gastric emptying but had no impact on ghrelin levels.[42] A Cochrane review from 2006 showed H_2RAs improved dyspepsia symptoms in 54% of patients, compared with 40% for placebo. However, some of the studies included in this meta-analysis were of poor quality.[43]

PPIs have been shown to be effective in the treatment of FD in several placebo-controlled, randomized controlled trials. Symptom improvement ranges from 32% in one study[44] to 68% in another.[45] Notably, the response to PPIs tends to be higher in patients with reflux-like dyspepsia, epigastric pain, or burning.[46] The subset of patients with postprandial distress symptoms did not tend to respond to PPI therapy.[47]

Interestingly, the response rate to placebo across several studies ranged from 19% to 49%, which overlaps considerably with the range of responders to PPI therapy.[43–48] A Cochrane review demonstrated overall symptom relief rates of 34% in patients receiving PPI therapy, compared with 25% in patients receiving placebo.[43]

Prokinetics

A brief randomized controlled trial comparing efficacy of PPIs versus prokinetic therapy in relieving the symptoms of patients with FD did not demonstrate a difference between the two, with 50.6% of the PPI group and 47.85% of the prokinetic group achieving meaningful symptom relief. The therapeutic response did not differ in subgroup analyses of patients fulfilling criteria of either epigastric pain syndrome or postprandial distress syndrome.[49] A meta-analysis of 27 randomized, controlled trials of prokinetic agents for treatment of FD symptoms found the prokinetics were significantly more likely to improve symptoms over placebo. However, most of the trials included in this analysis studied cisapride, which is off the market, and domperidone, which is not available in the United States. Only one of the studies included metoclopramide.[50] Thus, although prokinetic agents are likely equally efficacious to PPIs for the treatment of FD, given the risk of tardive dyskinesia with use of metoclopramide, this medication is not generally recommended for prolonged use.

Acotiamide, an acetylcholinesterase inhibitor that works by accelerating gastric motility,[51] has been shown in several placebo-controlled trials to improve FD symptoms and gastric emptying. The number need to treat to improve symptoms was six, and the number needed to treat to eliminate symptoms was 16.[52–54] This medication is still undergoing investigation and has not yet been approved by the Food and Drug Administration.

Anxiolytics and Antidepressants

Several studies have shown possible efficacy of anxiolytics and antidepressants for treatment of FD. A systematic review of studies comparing antidepressants and anxiolytics with placebo in the treatment of FD found benefit with the study drugs. Although there were limitations to the studies included in the review, the therapies (which included tricyclic antidepressant agents, levosulpiride [a dopamine-2 receptor agonist], and anticholinergic and anxiolytic medications) were approximately equivalent to studies of antisecretory agents and prokinetic agents (overall relative risk reduction of 0.45).[55] A more recent review again showed that antidepressants and anxiolytics are associated with significant pain reduction in patients with FD, and are as effective as classic antisecretory and prokinetic agents.[56] Several randomized controlled trials have demonstrated modest efficacy of tricyclic antidepressants in treating FD.[57,58]

Theoretically, serotonin-norepinephrine reuptake inhibitors and tricyclic antidepressants should decrease neuropathic pain and address underlying psychiatric issues, which would address at least two of the potential pathophysiologic mechanisms of FD. Furthermore, selective serotonin reuptake inhibitors may enhance gut transit and alter gastric accommodation.[59] However, study data to support the use of newer antidepressants for FD have been mixed. A randomized clinical trial of venlafaxine, a serotonin-norepinephrine reuptake inhibitor, failed to demonstrate improvement over placebo.[60] The Functional Dyspepsia Treatment Trial, an international multicenter, parallel group, randomized, double-blind, placebo-controlled trial, is ongoing to evaluate whether 12 weeks of treatment with escitalopram or amitriptyline improves FD symptoms compared with treatment with placebo.[61]

Buspirone, an anxiolytic medication with fundus-relaxing properties, was compared with placebo in a small double-blind, randomized, controlled crossover trial. Patients were given the study drug 15 minutes before meals. Buspirone significantly reduced the overall severity of dyspepsia symptoms, including postprandial fullness, early satiation, and upper abdominal bloating. Buspirone increased gastric accommodation but did not alter the rate of gastric emptying.[62]

Other Medications

An industry-sponsored study out of France of 276 general practice patients with dyspepsia compared a combination pill (simethicone, activated charcoal, and magnesium oxide) with placebo. Those receiving the study drug had decreased postprandial fullness, epigastric pain, epigastric burning, and abdominal bloating compared with placebo. The number needed to treat to achieve a 70% decrease in overall dyspeptic symptoms was seven.[63] Although this combination pill is not commercially available in the United States, an interested patient or practitioner could conceivably prescribe the components separately.

Psychotherapy

A recent study out of Japan randomized patients with FD to medical therapy alone or medical therapy with brief psychodynamic therapy. The results demonstrated brief psychodynamic therapy improved all gastrointestinal symptoms, including heartburn, nausea, postprandial fullness, bloating, and upper and lower abdominal pain, over medical therapy alone.[64] Another randomized, controlled trial compared cognitive psychotherapy with usual care and found the intervention group had fewer days of epigastric pain, and less nausea, heartburn, and diarrhea.[65] A randomized controlled trial of psychodynamic-interpersonal therapy versus supportive therapy demonstrated significant improvement with psychodynamic-interpersonal therapy over supportive therapy. However, the differences had disappeared at 1-year poststudy, unless the group with severe heartburn was excluded, in which case the psychodynamic-interpersonal group still did better.[66] However, a systematic review of psychological therapies for FD found insufficient evidence on the efficacy of psychological therapies for FD, noting that the sample sizes were small and the study designs variable. All of the included studies in that review had to adjust for baseline differences to achieve statistical significance.[67]

Acupuncture

Some research has suggested that acupuncture might improve gastric emptying and accommodation.[68] A Cochrane review is underway to survey the available evidence on the effectiveness and safety of this intervention for FD.

SUMMARY

Dyspepsia is a complex disorder with several distinct pathophysiologic mechanisms that are still poorly understood (**Fig. 8**). Patients who experience dyspepsia have a high burden of disease, with significant personal and economic costs. Although serious pathology presenting as dyspepsia is rare, clinicians need to be aware of alarm features that should trigger prompt referral for subspecialty care. Those without alarm features can be managed in a rational way with either empiric antisecretory therapy, test-and-treat for *H pylori* eradication, antidepressants, and psychotherapy, or a combination of these. Given the heterogeneity of symptoms and large variability in

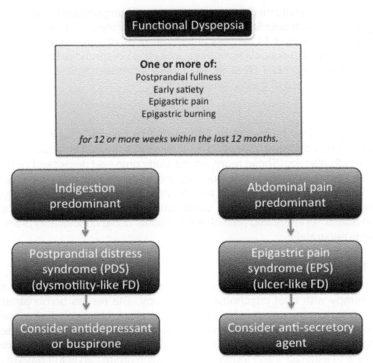

Fig. 8. Functional dyspepsia.

response to different treatments, more research into specific pathophysiologic mechanisms will likely help guide diagnosis and treatment choices in the future.

REFERENCES

1. Van Zanten S, Flook N, Chiba N. An evidence-based approach to the management of uninvestigated dyspepsia in the era of *Helicobacter pylori*. CMAJ 2000; 162(Suppl 12):S3–23.
2. Zagari R, Fuccio L, Bazzoli F. Investigating dyspepsia. BMJ 2008;337:11400.
3. Peery AF, Dellon ES, Lund J, et al. Burden of gastrointestinal disease in the United States: 2012 update. Gastroenterology 2012;143:1179–87.
4. Haycox A, Einarson T, Eggleston A. The health economic impact of upper gastrointestinal symptoms in the general population: results from the Domestic/International Gastroenterology Surveillance Study (DIGEST). Scand J Gastroenterol Suppl 1999;231(Suppl):38–47.
5. Piessevaux H, De Winter B, Louis E, et al. Dyspeptic symptoms in the general population: a factor and cluster analysis of symptom groupings. Neurogastroenterol Motil 2009;21:378–88.
6. Sander GB, Mazzoleni LE, Francesconi CF, et al. Influence of organic and functional dyspepsia on work productivity: the HEROES-DIP study. Value Health 2011;14:S126–9.
7. Talley NJ, American Gastroenterological Association. American Gastroenterological Association medical position statement: evaluation of dyspepsia. Gastroenterology 2005;129(5):1753–5.

8. National Institute for Health and Clinical Excellence (NICE). Dyspepsia: managing dyspepsia in adults in primary care. London: National Institute for Health and Clinical Excellence (NICE); 2004.

9. Tack J, Talley NJ, Camilleri M, et al. Functional gastroduodenal disorders. Gastroenterology 2006;130(5):1466–79.

10. Xiao YL, Peng S, Tao J, et al. Prevalence and symptom pattern of pathologic esophageal acid reflux in patients with functional dyspepsia based on the Rome III criteria. Am J Gastroenterol 2010;105:2626–31.

11. Nandurkar S, Talley NJ, Xia H, et al. Dyspepsia in the community is linked to smoking and aspirin use but not to *Helicobacter pylori* infection. Arch Intern Med 1998;158:1427–33.

12. Pike B, Porter C, Sorrell T, et al. Acute gastroenteritis and the risk of functional dyspepsia: a systemic review and meta-analysis. Am J Gastroenterol 2013; 108(10):1558–63.

13. Talley NJ, Locke GR III, Lahr BD, et al. Functional dyspepsia, delayed gastric emptying and impaired quality of life. Gut 2006;55:933–9.

14. Sha W, Pasricha PJ, Chen JD. Correlations among electrogastrogram, gastric dysmotility, and duodenal dysmotility in patients with functional dyspepsia. J Clin Gastroenterol 2009;43:716–22.

15. Perri F, Clemente R, Festa V, et al. Patterns of symptoms in functional dyspepsia: role of *Helicobacter pylori* infection and delayed gastric emptying. Am J Gastroenterol 1998;93:2082–8.

16. Kindt S, Tack J. Impaired gastric accommodation and its role in dyspepsia. Gut 2006;55(12):1685–91.

17. Quartero AO, de Wit NJ, Lodder AC, et al. Disturbed solid phase gastric emptying in functional dydpepsia: a meta-analysis. Dig Dis Sci 1998;43:2028–32.

18. Stanghellini V, Tossetti C, Paternico A, et al. Risk indicators of delayed gastric emptying of solids in patients with functional dyspepsia. Gastroenterology 1996;110:1036–42.

19. Führer M, Vogelsang H, Hammer J. A placebo-controlled trial of an oral capsaicin load in patients with functional dyspepsia. Neurogastroenterol Motil 2011; 23(10):918–28.

20. Li X, Cao Y, Wong RK, et al. Visceral and somatic sensory function in functional dyspepsia. Neurogastroenterol Motil 2013;25(3):246–53.

21. Holtmann G, Siffert W, Haag S, et al. G-protein beta 3 subunit 825 CC genotype is associated with unexplained (functional) dyspepsia. Gastroenterology 2004; 126:971–9.

22. Mearin F, Perez-Oliveras M, Perello A, et al. Dyspepsia and irritable bowel syndrome after a *Salmonella* gastroenteritis outbreak: one-year follow up cohort study. Gastroenterology 2005;129:98–104.

23. Kindt S, Tertychnyy A, de Hertogh G, et al. Intestinal immune activation in presumed post-infectious functional dyspepsia. Neurogastroenterol Motil 2009;21: 832–8.

24. Koloski NA, Jones M, Kalantar J, et al. The brain-gut pathway in functional gastrointestinal disorders is bidirectional: a 12-year prospective population-based study. Gut 2012;61:1284–90.

25. Talley NJ, Zinmeister AR, Schleck CD, et al. Dyspepsia and dyspepsia subgroups: a population-based study. Gastroenterology 1992;102:1259–68.

26. Konekes K, Jackson JL, Chamberlin J. Depressive and anxiety disorders in patients presenting with physical complaints: clinical predictors and outcomes. Am J Med 1997;103:339–47.

27. Clauwaert N, Jones MP, Holvoet L, et al. Associations between gastric sensori-motor function, depression, somatization, and symptom-based subgroups in functional gastroduodenal disorders: are all symptoms equal? Neurogastroenterol Motil 2012;24:1088–95.

28. Wilson J. Gastroesophageal reflux disease. Ann Intern Med 2008;149(3):ITC(2) 1–15.

29. Tefera L, Fein M, Ritter MP, et al. Can the combination of symptoms and endoscopy confirm the presence of gastroesophageal reflux disease? Am Surg 1997; 63:933–6.

30. DeVault KR, Castell DO. Updated guidelines for the diagnosis and treatment of gastroesophageal reflux disease. Am J Gastroenterol 2005;100:190–200.

31. Fass R, Ofman IJ, Samplinter RE, et al. The omeprazole test is as sensitive as 24-h oesophageal pH monitoring in diagnosing gastrooesophageal reflux disease in symptomatic patients with erosive esophagitis. Aliment Pharmacol Ther 2000;14:389–96.

32. Schenk BE, Kuipers EJ, Klinkenberg-Knol EC, et al. Omeprazole as a diagnostic tool in gastroesophageal reflux disease. Am J Gastroenterol 1997;92: 1997–2000.

33. Breuer T, Halaty HM, Graham DY. The epidemiology of H. pylori-associated gastroduodenal disease. In: Ernst P, Michetti P, Smith PD, editors. The immunobiology of H. pylori from pathogenesis to prevention. Philadelphia: Lippincott-Raven; 1997. p. 1–14.

34. Forman D, Graham DY. Review article: impact of Helicobacter pylori on society: role for a strategy of 'search and eradicate. Aliment Pharmacol Ther 2004; 19(Suppl 1):17–21.

35. Parkin DM, Pisani P, Munoz N. The global burden of cancer. Cancer Surv 1999; 33:5–33.

36. Kim S, Park Y, Kim N, et al. Effect of Helicobacter pylori eradication on functional dyspepsia. J Neurogastroenterol Motil 2013;19:233–43.

37. Mazzoleni L, Sander G, Francesconi C, et al. Helicobacter pylori eradication in functional dyspepsia. Arch Intern Med 2011;171:1929–35.

38. Moayyedi P, Soo S, Deeks J, et al. Eradication of Helicobacter pylori for non-ulcer dyspepsia. Cochrane Database Syst Rev 2006;(2):CD002096.

39. Den Hollander W, Sostres C, Kuipers E, et al. Helicobacter pylori and nonmalignant disease. Helicobacter 2013;18(Suppl 1):24–7.

40. Zhao B, Zhao J, Cheng WF, et al. Efficacy of Helicobacter pylori eradication therapy on functional dyspepsia: a meta-analysis of randomized controlled studies with 12-month follow up. J Clin Gastroenterol 2014;48(3):241–7.

41. Mönkemüller K, Malfertheiner P. Drug treatment of functional dyspepsia. World J Gastroenterol 2006;12(17):2694–700.

42. Futagami S, Shimpuku M, Song JM, et al. Nizatidine improves clinical symptoms and gastric emptying in patients with functional dyspepsia accompanied by impaired gastric emptying. Digestion 2012;86(2):114–21.

43. Moayyedi P, Shelly S, Deeks JJ, et al. WITHDRAWN: pharmacological interventions for non-ulcer dyspepsia. Cochrane Database Syst Rev 2011;(2): CD001960.

44. Van Zanten SV, Armstrong D, Chiba N, et al. Esomeprazole 40 mg once a day in patients with functional dyspepsia: the randomized, placebo-controlled "ENTER" trial. Am J Gastroenterol 2006;101:2096–106.

45. Meineche-Schmidt V, Christensen E, Bytzer P. Randomised clinical trial: identification of responders to short-term treatment with esomeprazole for dyspepsia

in primary care: a randomized, placebo-controlled study. Aliment Pharmacol Ther 2011;33:41–9.

46. Talley NJ, Meineche-Schmidt V, Pare P, et al. Efficacy of omeprazole in functional dyspepsia: double-blind, randomized, placebo-controlled trials (the Bond and Opera studies). Aliment Pharmacol Ther 1998;12:1055–65.

47. Bolling-Sternevald E, Lauritsen K, Talley NJ, et al. Is it possible to predict treatment response to a proton pump inhibitor in functional dyspepsia? Aliment Pharmacol Ther 2003;18:117–24.

48. Peura DA, Kovacs TO, Metz DC, et al. Lansoprazole in the treatment of functional dyspepsia: two double-blind, randomized, placebo-controlled trials. Am J Med 2004;116:740–8.

49. Hsu YC, Liou JM, Yang TH, et al. Proton pump inhibitor therapy versus prokinetic therapy in patients with functional dyspepsia: is therapeutic response predicted by Rome III subgroups? J Gastroenterol 2011;46(2):183–90.

50. Hiyama T, Yoshihara M, Matsuo K, et al. Meta-analysis of the effects of prokinetic agents in patients with functional dyspepsia. J Gastroenterol Hepatol 2007;22: 304–10.

51. Yoshii K, Hirayami M, Nakamura T, et al. Mechanism for distribution of acotiamide, a novel gastroprokinetic agent for the treatment of functional dyspepsia, in rat stomach. J Pharm Sci 2011;100:4965–73.

52. Matsueda K, Hongo M, Tack J, et al. A placebo-controlled trial of acotiamide for meal-related symptoms of functional dyspepsia. Gut 2012;61(6):821–8.

53. Kusunoki H, Haruma K, Manabe N, et al. Therapeutic efficacy of acotiamide in patients with functional dyspepsia based on enhanced postprandial gastric accommodation and emptying: randomized controlled study evaluation by real-time ultrasonography. Neurogastroenterol Motil 2012;24(6):540–5.

54. Altan E, Masaoka T, Farré R, et al. Acotiamide, a novel gastroprokinetic for the treatment of patients with functional dyspepsia: postprandial distress syndrome. Expert Rev Gastroenterol Hepatol 2012;6(5):533–44.

55. Hojo M, Miwa H, Yokoyama T, et al. Treatment of functional dyspepsia with anti-anxiety or antidepressive agents: systematic review. J Gastroenterol 2005; 40(11):1036–42.

56. Passos MC, Duro D, Fregni F. CNS or classic drugs for the treatment of pain in functional dyspepsia? A systematic review and meta-analysis of the literature. Pain Physician 2008;11:597–609.

57. Grover M, Drossman DA. Psychotropic agents in functional gastrointestinal disorders. Curr Opin Pharmacol 2008;8:715–23.

58. Braak B, Klooker TK, Wouters MM, et al. Randomized clinical trial: the effects of amitriptyline on drinking capacity and symptoms in patients with functional dyspepsia, a double-blind placebo-controlled study. Aliment Pharmacol Ther 2011;34:638–48.

59. Moshiree B, Barboza J, Talley NJ. An update on current pharmacotherapy options for dyspepsia. Expert Opin Pharmacother 2013;14:1737–53.

60. Van Kerkhoven LA, Laheij RJ, Aparicio N, et al. Effect of the antidepressant venlafaxine in functional dyspepsia: a randomized, double-blind, placebo-controlled trial. Clin Gastroenterol Hepatol 2008;6:746–52.

61. Talley NJ, Locke GR III, Herrick LM, et al. Functional Dyspepsia Treatment Trial (FDTT): a double-blind, randomized, placebo-controlled trial of antidepressants in functional dyspepsia, evaluating symptoms, psychopathology, pathophysiology and pharmacogenetics. Contemp Clin Trials 2012;33(3): 523–33.

62. Tack J, Janssen P, Masaoka T. Efficacy of buspirone, a fundus-relaxing drug, in patients with functional dyspepsia. Clin Gastroenterol Hepatol 2012;10(11):1239–45.

63. Coffin B, Bortolloti C, Bourgeois O, et al. Efficacy of a smiethicone, activated charcoal and magnesium oxide combination (Carbosymag) in functional dyspepsia: results of a general practice-based randomized trial. Clin Res Hepatol Gastroenterol 2011;35(6–7):494–9.

64. Faramarzi M, Azadfallah P, Book HE, et al. A randomized controlled trial of brief psychoanalytic psychotherapy in patients with functional dyspepsia. Asian J Psychiatr 2013;6(3):228–34.

65. Haug T, Wilhelmsen I, Svebak S, et al. Psychotherapy in functional dyspepsia. J Psychosom Res 1994;38:735–44.

66. Hamilton J, Guthrie E, Creed F, et al. A randomized controlled trial of psychotherapy in patients with chronic functional dyspepsia. Gastroenterology 2000; 119:662–9.

67. Soo S, Forman D, Delaney B, et al. A systematic review of psychological therapies for nonulcer dyspepsia. Am J Gastroenterol 2004;99:1817–22.

68. Xu S, Zha H, Hou X, et al. Electroacupuncture accelerates solid gastric emptying in patients with functional dyspepsia. Gastroenterology 2004;126: A-437.

Eosinophilic Esophagitis
Overview of Clinical Management

Alain M. Schoepfer, MD[a], Ikuo Hirano, MD[b],*, David A. Katzka, MD[c]

KEYWORDS

- Eosinophilic esophagitis • Gastroesophageal reflux disease • Dysphagia
- Treatment end points • Patient-reported outcomes

KEY POINTS

- Recommended therapeutic end points in eosinophilic esophagitis (EoE) include symptoms (eg, dysphagia, chest pain), histologic activity, and endoscopic activity (especially strictures). Symptom assessment should examine meal modification and food-avoidance behaviors.
- Evidence is accumulating that maintenance therapy for EoE, by means of either swallowed topical corticosteroids or elimination diets, leads to a reduction of symptoms and esophageal remodeling processes that are associated with food bolus impactions.
- Esophageal dilation can offer long-lasting symptom improvement for EoE patients with esophageal remodeling not responsive to medical or diet therapy.

INTRODUCTION

This article covers several clinically relevant topics in the clinical management of eosinophilic esophagitis (EoE). First, which end points should be assessed in daily practice and in clinical trials are discussed. Second, the existing evidence to support maintenance treatment is highlighted, and the different therapeutic options discussed. Third, treatment options for patients refractory to standard therapies and for asymptomatic patients with esophageal eosinophilia are addressed. Finally, a therapeutic algorithm is presented.

This article originally appeared in Gastroenterology Clinics, Volume 43, Issue 2, June 2014.
Disclosures: A.M. Schoepfer received consulting fees and/or speaker fees and/or research grants from AstraZeneca, AG, Switzerland, Aptalis Pharma, Inc, Dr Falk Pharma, GmbH, Germany, Glaxo Smith Kline, AG, Nestlé S. A., Switzerland, and Novartis, AG, Switzerland. D.A. Katzka has no relevant financial, professional, or personal relationships to disclose. I. Hirano received consulting fees and/or speaker fees and/or research grants from Meritage Pharma, Inc, Aptalis Pharma, Inc, and Receptos, Inc.
^a Division of Gastroenterology and Hepatology, Centre Hospitalier Universitaire Vaudois/CHUV, Rue de Bugnon 44, 07/2409, 1011 Lausanne, Switzerland; ^b Division of Gastroenterology, Esophageal Center, Northwestern University Feinberg School of Medicine, 676 North Saint Clair, Suite 1400, Chicago, IL 60611, USA; ^c Division of Gastroenterology and Hepatology, Mayo Clinic, 200 First Avenue, Southwest, Rochester, MN 55905, USA
* Corresponding author.
E-mail address: i-hirano@northwestern.edu

Clinics Collections 7 (2015) 235–250
http://dx.doi.org/10.1016/j.ccol.2015.06.016

END POINTS TO ASSESS TREATMENT EFFICACY
General Considerations

EoE has been defined as a clinicopathologic entity with symptoms of esophageal dysfunction and eosinophil-predominant esophageal inflammation.[1]

EoE activity can be assessed by patient-reported outcomes (PRO) in addition to biological markers, including endoscopic and histologic alterations as well as serologic biomarkers. One should discriminate between the use of outcomes in daily clinical practice and in clinical trials. For daily clinical practice the relevant outcomes are EoE-related symptoms, esophageal eosinophilia, and endoscopic features, especially the presence of esophageal strictures. In addition to these outcomes, quality of life and different biomarkers can become relevant in clinical trials.

Fig. 1 provides an overview of the different dimensions in which EoE activity can be measured. There is an ongoing debate as to whether EoE activity should be assessed based on PRO, biological components, or both dimensions. Which measures most accurately reflect disease activity depends on the impact of the disease's natural history on either PRO or biological markers. This concept is further illustrated by **Fig. 2**. In diseases such as migraine (PRO = headache; biological marker = abnormalities in functional magnetic resonance imaging [MRI]) or low back pain (PRO = pain; biological marker = MRI findings), activity assessment is mainly based on PRO measurement. At the other end of the spectrum there exist diseases in which patients may remain without any symptom for a long time but whereby appropriate biomarkers exist for activity assessment that are associated with distinct clinical outcomes, such as myocardial infarction in arterial hypertension (PRO = eg, quality of life; biological marker = blood pressure). In between these two poles there are diseases such as inflammatory bowel diseases (PRO = eg, bowel frequency, abdominal pain; biological marker = severity of endoscopically assessed inflammation) in which activity is determined by both PRO and biological markers.

Straumann and colleagues,[2] the first to publish on the natural history of 30 adult EoE patients, demonstrated that symptoms and eosinophil-predominant esophageal inflammation persisted over time. Several recent publications have demonstrated

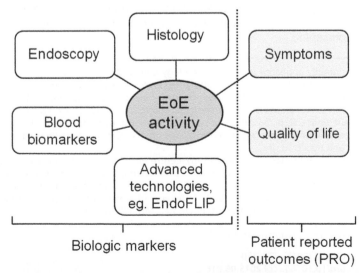

Fig. 1. Dimensions in which eosinophilic esophagitis (EoE) activity can be assessed.

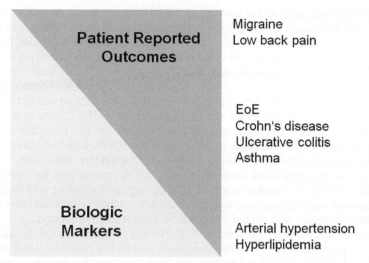

Migraine
Low back pain

EoE
Crohn's disease
Ulcerative colitis
Asthma

Arterial hypertension
Hyperlipidemia

Fig. 2. Patient-reported outcomes and biological markers in activity assessment of various diseases.

that long-standing eosinophil-predominant esophageal inflammation leads to deposition of subepithelial fibrous tissue, and that this remodeling process is associated with stricturing complications.[3–6] Current understanding suggests that symptom generation in EoE depends on active, eosinophil-predominant esophageal inflammation and associated esophageal remodeling processes. These observations support the recommendation that EoE activity assessment in daily practice and clinical trials should be performed using a combination of PRO and biological markers.[7]

There is currently no validated activity index to measure EoE activity in the different dimensions. Such an index is urgently needed to define end points for clinical trials, observational studies, and daily clinical practice. Several therapeutic trials have reported either a correlation or a dissociation between EoE-related symptoms and esophageal eosinophil counts, which might be related to the use of different, mostly nonvalidated instruments for symptom assessment.[8–11] The lack of a standardized, validated PRO instrument to assess EoE-associated symptom severity has several important implications. First, the results of different clinical trials are difficult to compare. Second, several therapeutic trials have documented heterogeneous associations between changes in PRO and biological markers. As such, the current situation poses a challenge for regulatory authorities to approve therapies for EoE management.[12–14] The US Food and Drug Administration (FDA) has identified the deficiency of clinically meaningful end points in EoE, calling for effective collaboration involving different interest groups (patients, physicians, researchers, pharmaceutical industry, and regulatory authorities).[13,14]

Current Status Regarding the Development of PRO Instruments

The development and validation of a PRO instrument to assess symptom severity in pediatric and adult EoE patients represents a challenge for several reasons. First, the leading EoE symptoms typically change in the pediatric population with ongoing age.[1,15] Second, again for pediatric patients, a cutoff age has to be chosen from which children are able to report on symptoms themselves; moreover, up to which age symptom reporting should be performed by parents must be decided. Third, the severity and frequency of dysphagia, which represents the leading symptom in adolescent and adult EoE patients, strongly depends on the ingested food consistencies; therefore, symptoms should be assessed according to defined food categories. Fourth, symptom severity may depend on food avoidance, food modification, or the time to ingest a standardized meal. These behavioral modifications should also be taken into account when developing a PRO instrument. Fifth, a distinct symptom-recall period has to be chosen for symptom assessment. The choice of the optimal symptom-recall period depends, among other factors, on the intended use of the PRO, the patient's ability to recall the required information, and the extent to which the patient is burdened by his or her EoE when completing the instrument.[16] All these factors should be considered when developing a PRO instrument for pediatric and adult EoE patients. The performance of an esophageal stress test with ingestion of a standardized meal to measure symptom severity bears the potential risk of acute food bolus impaction, and should therefore be exercised with caution.

Several PROs are being evaluated for EoE. The Dysphagia Symptom Questionnaire (DSQ) is a 3-item electronic PRO that was developed for the purpose of a pharmaceutical trial for EoE.[17] The DSQ is administered daily to assess the frequency and intensity of dysphagia caused by eating solid food.[17] The Eosinophilic Esophagitis Activity Index (EEsAI) study group is currently developing and validating a PRO instrument to assess EoE symptom severity. The EEsAI PRO instrument evaluates dysphagia severity according to 8 distinct food consistencies, and also takes into account behavioral adaptations such as food avoidance, food modification, and time to eat a regular meal (clinicaltrials.gov, NCT00939263). In 2011 Taft and colleagues[18] published a quality-of-life questionnaire for adult EoE patients. The Adult EoE Quality of Life (EoO-QOL-A) Questionnaire demonstrated good internal consistency and test-retest reliability.[18] Franciosi and colleagues[19] reported in 2011 on the qualitative methods of the Pediatric Eosinophilic Esophagitis Symptom Score (PEESS, version 2.0). The same group recently published a quality-of-life instrument for pediatric EoE patients.[20]

Overview of the Current Status Regarding the Development of Biological Measures

A classification and grading system for endoscopic assessment of esophageal features in EoE was recently published.[21] The EoE Endoscopic REFerence Score (EREFS) assesses 5 characteristic features of exudates, rings, edema (loss of vascular markings), furrows (longitudinal markings), and stricture. Definitions for endoscopic remission and mild, moderate, or severe endoscopic activity still need to be established.

The assessment of histologic activity is mainly based on the peak eosinophil count per high-power field (hpf) or the eosinophil load.[8–11] Additional histologic findings such as papillary elongation, basal layer hyperplasia, eosinophil degranulation, or subepithelial fibrosis have also been reported as parameters of histologic outcome. Dellon and colleagues[22] have shown that the number of reported peak eosinophil counts may not be necessarily comparable, as different microscope types with specific hpf sizes are being used. One way to overcome this issue would be the reporting of peak eosinophil counts standardized to mm^2. In analogy to the reporting of endoscopic severity, definitions regarding histologic remission and different semiquantitative degrees of histologic activity still need to be established.[7]

Furuta and colleagues[23] have recently evaluated the esophageal string test as a minimally invasive tool to assess the correlation between esophageal eosinophil counts and eosinophil granule proteins attached to the string. Excellent correlations were found between the level of eosinophil granule proteins extracted from the string and esophageal tissue eosinophilia.[23] Long-standing eosinophil-predominant inflammation leads to esophageal remodeling, resulting in stricture formation.[5,6] The EndoFLIP, an impedance planimetry catheter–based device, measures esophageal compliance and distensibility and is thereby able to provide quantitative information on remodeling consequences in EoE.[24]

MAINTENANCE THERAPY

Only recently have studies begun to address the need and management options for long-term maintenance therapy in EoE. In examining the topic of maintenance therapy, limitations to existing assumptions should be acknowledged. (1) Although EoE is considered a chronic and lifelong disease, only 10 to 20 years of data exist, and spontaneous remission could occur. (2) The concept that untreated disease leads to a progressive fibrosis and stricture formation is largely based on retrospective data. (3) The current focus on control of esophageal eosinophilia as the end point of therapy ignores other potentially significant inflammatory pathways (eg, eosinophil degranulation proteins) and cells (eg, mast cells, basophils, lymphocytes).

Why is Maintenance Needed?

As in any chronic disease, the decision to use maintenance therapy balances the benefits of symptom control and prevention of disease progression with costs, side effects, and complications of long-term therapy. In the case of EoE, those in favor of observation and periodic treatment of symptom exacerbations might point out that many patients with EoE adapt to their disease, weight loss is uncommon, the disease remains isolated to the esophagus, and there are no neoplastic consequences.

On the other hand, EoE may be associated with morbidity. For example, food impaction is common, occurring in up to 35% of patients.[25–28] Patients with food impaction are indubitably at risk for perforation and aspiration. Furthermore, spontaneous perforation during food impaction (Boerhaave syndrome) has been reported.[26,29] Perforation may also occur with endoscopic bolus disimpaction and esophageal dilation. Although uncommonly requiring surgical repair, esophageal perforation results in chest pain, and careful inpatient observation is necessary.[30,31] The impact of EoE on the quality of life is now being examined.[32] Patients are commonly anxious or embarrassed by their slow eating and/or diet restrictions. As a result, important events such as business meals or social gatherings may be avoided. This scenario is particularly problematic among teenagers and young adults, a common demographic of the disease, of an age at which social stigmatisms are easily perceived.

The reason such complications ensue is the high rate of stricture formation. Indeed, once patients with EoE become or are diagnosed as young adults, the rate of esophageal stenosis reaches up to 40%.[33] In untreated patients, the natural history of persistent esophageal eosinophilia and increased collagen deposition supports the risk of progression.[2] In patients with initial successful treatment, disease regression is uncommon.[20,34] In a recent study from the Swiss EoE database, the duration of untreated disease (as measured through years of untreated symptoms) corresponded to the chance of stricture formation.[5] Specifically, after 30 years of untreated symptoms of EoE, 80% of patients had esophageal stricture formation.[5] Of note, these strictures were diagnosed with endoscopy. If one uses more sensitive tests to diagnose esophageal fibrosis, such as barium esophagography, endoscopic ultrasonography, or the EndoFLIP, the prevalence of strictures is even higher, including patients with a normal-appearing esophagus or alterations limited only to rings.[35–37] Studies with the EndoFLIP, a measurement of esophageal distensibility whereby patients may demonstrate a marked decrease in esophageal compliance presumably long before endoscopic strictures are evident, are particularly enlightening.[37]

There is also a good foundation of basic research that accounts for esophageal stricture formation in EoE. Specifically, careful analysis of tissue and inflammatory mediators in EoE has demonstrated the profibrotic process that results from the eosinophil-mediated inflammation in EoE.[38–41] For example, subepithelial collagen deposition is a common finding in these patients.[41] Moreover, many of the inflammatory mediators released from eosinophils are profibrotic. As a result, one of the main justifications for the use of maintenance therapy is to control esophageal inflammation and thereby prevent stricture formation.

Disease chronicity is a strong argument in favor of maintenance therapy. Prospective data demonstrate disease relapse in most, if not all patients, following cessation on initial therapy.[2,42] However, there are only limited data demonstrating that maintenance therapy prevents or reverses existing esophageal strictures.

What is the Goal of Maintenance Therapy?

The goal of maintenance therapy may focus on symptoms, control of histologic inflammation, or both. For symptom relief, periodic esophageal dilation may be as effective as swallowed fluticasone in reducing dysphagia.[43,44] Esophageal inflammation, however, is not lessened with dilation alone.[31] Thus, from a pathophysiologic point of view, the goal of maintenance medical therapy is to reduce esophageal eosinophilia and adverse consequences of esophageal remodeling. Unfortunately, as yet there are no data that can guide to what degree esophageal eosinophilia must be reduced, or even whether the eosinophil is the primary determinant of fibrotic change. More specifically, it is not known whether complete elimination of esophageal eosinophils is necessary or if fewer than 5, fewer than 10, or fewer than 15 eosinophils per hpf is sufficient. Indeed, in other chronic inflammatory diseases that lead to fibrosis, such as inflammatory bowel disease, investigators have long debated the appropriate end point of medical therapy, with more recent data suggesting that endoscopic demonstration of mucosal healing predicts sustained control of disease.[45] EoE is now approached in a similar manner, with the desired goal of sustained and complete elimination of eosinophilic inflammation.

Which Patients with EoE Should Be Considered for Maintenance Therapy?

Should all patients with EoE be treated with maintenance therapy? To some degree this depends on the safety and tolerability of the therapy. A patient whose esophageal inflammation remains under control with avoidance of a limited number of foods might continue with diet therapy indefinitely. On the other hand, for patients who use topical steroids, in whom the risk of long-term side effects is unclear, a more selective strategy may be appropriate. As a result, it may be important to identify subsets of EoE patients who are at greater risk of developing esophageal strictures or in whom clinically significant strictures already exist. Such patients might include those with repeated food impactions, those who relapse quickly with symptoms and/or esophageal eosinophilia off therapy, patients who cannot maintain their weight owing to severe diet restrictions, or those with narrow or small-caliber esophagus. It must be borne in mind that given the lack of data in this area, it is not known whether all or any of these specific subsets of EoE patients will respond to therapy. Patients with narrow-caliber esophagus or multiple severe atoplc comorbidities may be less responsive to conventional therapies.[46]

What Potential Maintenance Treatments Exist and Are They Effective?

The potential treatments to maintain remission in EoE include steroids and elimination diet therapy. There are several reasons for which the use of steroids for maintenance therapy is an attractive option. First, there are clear data demonstrating excellent control of inflammatory change and reduction of tissue eosinophilia.[7] Second, studies in EoE have shown downregulation of genes associated with tissue remodeling following steroid therapy.[4,40,47,48] Furthermore, there are some clinical data suggesting an increase in stricture diameter with steroids based on endoscopic and/or radiologic assessment.[35,49] There are additional data demonstrating that steroids are effective in suppressing some of the key pathways and genes that mediate esophageal injury in EoE[50] and the abnormal transcriptome of EoE,[51,52] thus holding a mechanistic potential to reverse fibrosis.[4] In favor of diet therapy is the lack of concern for side effects as long as daily nutritional requirements are met. On the other hand, diet therapy poses greater challenges with identification of triggering food antigens and in lifelong avoidance of these antigens, particularly when multiple and/or common table foods are implicated.[33,53] This latter point is particularly relevant given the commonality of milk and wheat allergy identified in these patients. Elemental diets, though also effective,[54] are limited by tolerability and expense.

Another emerging issue in maintenance therapy is whether control of extraesophageal allergies positively affects esophageal disease. This contention is suggested in animal models by induction of esophageal eosinophilia through an initial priming mechanism of allergy in the lung or skin.[55] It is supported in humans by the finding of years of preceding airway allergies in most patients[56] as well as the inconsistent finding of flares of EoE during respiratory allergy seasons.[57] On identification of risk factors for EoE in patients with asthma, patients most typically have an allergic phenotype such as presence of allergic asthma and peripheral eosinophilia.[58] However, no controlled trials have been performed that demonstrate a beneficial effect of therapy directed toward extraesophageal allergic disease on EoE.

Data on Maintenance Therapy

Despite the theoretical benefits of maintenance steroid therapy, there is a distinct paucity of data available. In a randomized controlled trial conducted by Straumann and colleagues,[11] 28 patients were randomized to 0.25 mg of budesonide twice daily or placebo for 50 weeks. The favorable results from this trial demonstrated that budesonide reduced markers of inflammation, epithelial cell apoptosis, and remodeling events, without adverse side effects. Unfortunately, eosinophil count and symptoms significantly increased on both placebo and budesonide. A higher maintenance dosing of budesonide may have improved the therapeutic gain. These findings provide valuable data for defining an adequate maintenance dose, but further work needs to be performed to refine this approach.

Another looming issue on maintenance therapy is the potential long-term side effects of oral steroid therapies. In the Straumann trial, measurement of the effects of long-term budesonide on adrenal function are not discussed.[11] In a 3-month trial examining the use of swallowed topical steroids in children with EoE, there was no clear evidence of adrenal suppression.[59] Similarly, in another pediatric randomized study comparing prednisone with fluticasone, systemic effects such as Cushingoid features were only identified with systemic steroid administration.[60] When inhaled steroids are used for maintenance therapy in patients with asthma, both fluticasone and budesonide have been shown to slightly increase the risk for adrenal suppression.[61] One has to be careful in extrapolating the effects of steroid therapy in asthma to

EoE, as the distal esophagus venous network drains through the portal vein, exposing the drugs to hepatic first-pass metabolism. One also needs to consider that although it is assumed that little small-bowel or esophageal absorption occurs with the oral route of a topical steroid preparation, this is also not well studied.

Diet therapy has more robust and longer-term data on maintenance, albeit uncontrolled. In a series of 562 children studied for up to 14 years and treated mostly with diet, only 11 children remained in remission as defined by absence of esophageal eosinophilia.[57] On the other hand, improvement in symptoms and histology occurred in 98% of 381 patients studied long term and maintained on diet therapy, including 16% maintained on an elemental diet.[42] Lucendo and colleagues[33] reported that adult EoE patients on an empiric 6-food elimination diet had prolonged clinical and histopathologic remission for up to 3 years of follow-up.

Conclusions on Maintenance Therapy

Current data support the conceptual and clinical benefits of long-term maintenance therapy in EoE. At present, however, the appropriate patients to use maintenance therapy, the proper end point of therapy that will prevent and perhaps reverse complications of EoE, and the type of therapy that will provide the greatest benefit-to-risk ratio are unanswered questions. Nevertheless, it is reasonable to discuss the potential benefits of maintenance therapy in all patients with EoE, particularly those who have already evidenced disease complications. For those patients who have responded and are able to adhere to elimination diet therapy, maintenance is relatively straightforward. For those patients who have responded to short-term topical steroids, options include reduced-dose maintenance steroids, intermittent steroids, and clinical observation without therapy. Esophageal dilation, discussed next, may offer a long-term symptom improvement in selected patients.

ESOPHAGEAL DILATION

Esophageal dilation was one of the first therapies used to treat stricturing EoE.[62,63] Recent publications on the natural history of EoE have demonstrated that persisting eosinophil-predominant inflammation leads to the formation of esophageal strictures.[5,6] More than one-third of EoE patients suffer from one or several food bolus impactions necessitating endoscopic removal as an emergency procedure.[25,64] Esophageal dilation can be performed using either through-the-scope inflatable balloons or wire-guided Savary bougies. Strictures are readily recognized if a standard, diagnostic endoscope does not traverse the esophagus. It is not yet clear as to how accurate gastroenterologists are in detecting and reporting lower grades of esophageal strictures. It can be hypothesized that mild strictures or generalized esophageal narrowing will be underappreciated by the endoscopist.

A study by Schoepfer and colleagues[31] of 474 dilations in 207 EoE patients treated by esophageal dilation found that 67% of patients reported an improvement or absence of dysphagia following esophageal dilation. Patient acceptance for dilation was high.[31] Similarly, Dellon and colleagues[65] reported on a series of 36 EoE patients who were treated by a total of 70 dilations with a symptom response of 83%. A recently reported meta-analysis on 860 EoE patients, of whom 525 underwent at least 1 esophageal dilation and a total of 992 dilations, showed a clinical improvement in 75% of patients.[66]

Esophageal dilation may also be associated with several limitations, the first of which is the occurrence of postprocedural thoracic pain.[31] Postdilational pain may last for some days and responds favorably to analgesics.[31] Hospitalizations resulting from postprocedural pain are rare (about 1%).[66] A second limitation is that dilation does not influence the severity of eosinophil-predominant esophageal inflammation.[31] As a third limitation, dilation may be associated with esophageal perforation. Whereas earlier case series have reported a high complication rate,[67] subsequent studies consistently showed a lower perforation rate, approximating estimates of perforation risk for dilation for other benign esophageal disorders. Jung and colleagues[30] evaluated 293 dilations in 167 patients, and found a perforation rate of 1% (3 cases). In a series of 207 dilated patients (mean 2 dilations per patient), no case of esophageal perforation was documented.[31] A 2010 meta-analysis that included 468 patients having undergone 671 dilations found only 1 perforation (0.1%).[68] This result is comparable to that of the meta-analysis by Moawad and colleagues[66] reporting on 3 perforations during 992 dilations (0.3% perforation rate).

It is unknown as to which defined esophageal diameter should be targeted by dilation, but most patients show considerable symptomatic improvement when a diameter of 16 to 18 mm has been reached.[31] It has been recommended that the progression of dilation per session should be limited to 3 mm or less.[30] Mucosal tears or lacerations following dilation should not be regarded as a complication but rather as evidence of effective therapy.[68] Dilation-related esophageal bleedings that necessitate an endoscopic intervention do occur on rare occasion.[66]

PATIENTS REFRACTORY TO STANDARD THERAPIES

Patients with EoE with a limited or lack of response to initial diet or medical therapy include those with persistent symptoms, persistent esophageal inflammation, or both symptoms and inflammation. In addition, patients may demonstrate both symptoms and histologic response but have persistent esophageal luminal stenosis. As discussed earlier, the definition of symptom and histologic response has yet to be determined in either daily practice or clinical trials. With this caveat in mind, when both symptoms and inflammation persist, the initial therapy needs to be examined.

Patients not responding to topical steroids should be questioned as to adherence, dosing, and appropriate method of administration. Adherence to medications can be challenging for adolescent and adult patients, most of whom are unaccustomed to the use of medications on a long-term basis. Dose escalation of topical steroids is a consideration, as higher response rates have been reported in studies using fluticasone 880 μg twice daily compared with those using 440 μg twice daily.[8] Prospective studies comparing various dosing regimens are lacking, however. Anecdotal reports have noted patients failing to respond to swallowed fluticasone by inhaler administration who responded to liquid budesonide. This observation may be the result of inadvertent inhalation instead of swallowing of the aerosolized steroid. A randomized controlled trial compared swallowed budesonide administered via a nebulizer with a liquid suspension.[69] Although superiority was apparent with the liquid suspension, steroid formulations studied in clinical trials and used in clinical practice are delivered by metered dose inhalation, not nebulizers. Systemic steroids are often considered superior to topical steroids. A randomized trial, however, found similar efficacy in terms of the primary end point of a histopathology score for topical fluticasone compared with oral prednisone in a pediatric cohort.[60] The study did find that a secondary end point of histologic normalization was significantly greater with systemic steroids, supporting a potential role for systemic steroids in patients unresponsive to topical steroids.

Dietary therapy is an option for patients unresponsive to topical steroids, although there are only anecdotal reports regarding the effectiveness of this crossover strategy.

Several uncontrolled, retrospective studies indicate a greater response to elemental formula diets compared with empiric or allergy testing–directed elimination diet therapy. However, the tolerability and acceptability of elemental diets limits their widespread use. Other medical therapies including montelukast, cromolyn sodium, or antihistamines have shown limited benefits in a few small uncontrolled studies, and are considered second-line agents.[1] The effectiveness of therapies combining steroids, diet, montelukast, and antihistamines has not been reported.

Patients with resolution of eosinophilia but continued dysphagia with evidence of esophageal stenosis are candidates for esophageal dilation. The reversibility of esophageal remodeling in EoE with medical or diet therapies is discussed in an article elsewhere in this issue.[47–49] It should be noted that the reversal of esophageal submucosal fibrosis and remodeling in EoE may require prolonged therapy, whereas the epithelial inflammatory response may respond rapidly (within 2 weeks) with topical corticosteroid administration. Available studies have demonstrated modest improvement in esophageal lamina propria fibrosis and stricture in adults with EoE with short-term and intermediate-term (1 year) therapy with topical steroids.[11]

Novel biologic therapies have emerged for the treatment of EoE. Anti–immunoglobulin E, anti–interleukin (IL)-5, anti-IL-13, anti–tumor necrosis factor, and CRTH2-antagonist therapies have been reported in small studies.[70–72] Several of these studies included patients who were refractory or dependent on corticosteroid therapy. Significant histologic response was seen in pediatric studies of anti–IL-5 therapy, but symptom response was more difficult to demonstrate. Analogous to their use in inflammatory bowel disease, biologics therapy offers the potential of disease-modifying and steroid-sparing agents. More data on their use as monotherapy or in combination with existing therapies is needed.

TREATMENT OF ASYMPTOMATIC PATIENTS

Based on current consensus recommendations and clinical guidelines, patients with significant esophageal eosinophilia on biopsy but without symptoms would not meet the definition of EoE.[1] However, patients may have substantial esophageal luminal stenoses but do not report dysphagia, because of careful mastication, prolonged meal times, and/or food avoidance. The same situation may be encountered in patients initially diagnosed with EoE but achieving symptom but not histologic remission following medical or dietary therapy. At present, there is limited evidence to support additional treatment of such individuals. A more proactive approach might be considered in asymptomatic patients with esophageal eosinophilia and higher degrees of esophageal stenosis, and in treated patients without symptoms but with esophageal eosinophilia who have a history of disease complications such as food impaction or esophageal stricture. Given the uncertainties regarding the natural history of EoE, clinical follow-up for patients with esophageal eosinophilia even in the absence of symptoms is reasonable. Growing evidence supports the concept that untreated disease leads to higher degrees of esophageal stricture over time.[5]

THERAPEUTIC ALGORITHM

Given the many unknowns in EoE therapy and outcome assessment, it may seem venturesome to provide a therapy algorithm for clinical practice. Nevertheless, the authors provide here their approach in EoE patient management that is in line with recent clinical consensus recommendations and guidelines (**Fig. 3**).[1,7] Relevant end points

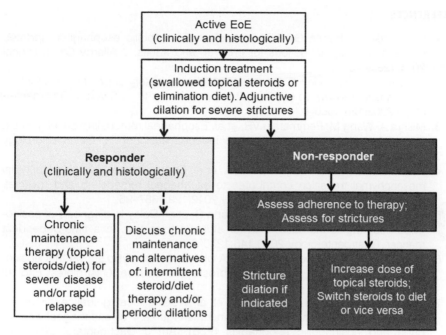

Fig. 3. Eosinophilic esophagitis (EoE) therapy algorithm.

for daily practice include EoE-related symptoms and esophageal eosinophilic inflammation. Patient history in adult EoE patients should not only include dysphagia and thoracic pain but also behavioral modifications such as food avoidance, food modification, and time taken to eat a regular meal. Dysphagia should be assessed according to distinct food consistencies, especially meat, rice, and bread. Endoscopic features, especially the presence of strictures, should be taken into account when establishing a therapy plan. Symptomatic EoE patients with esophageal eosinophilic inflammation should be treated either with swallowed topical corticosteroids or elimination diets. A reasonable clinical goal is to achieve an important reduction in EoE-related symptoms as well as esophageal eosinophilic inflammation. How much of residual esophageal eosinophilic inflammation can be tolerated is currently unknown. Evidence is increasing to support a maintenance therapy. In EoE patients in symptomatic remission, the authors recommend a yearly disease monitoring with symptom, endoscopic, and histologic assessments of sustained treatment response. In cases of persistent symptomatic esophageal strictures, esophageal dilation is an effective and safe approach.

SUMMARY

For clinical practice, therapeutic goals in EoE include relief of esophageal symptoms and improvement in eosinophilic inflammation and endoscopic features, particularly strictures. EoE activity indices that incorporate PROs are currently being validated and evaluated in the context of randomized, controlled clinical trials. Maintenance therapies are an important consideration for both pediatric and adult patients with EoE, especially in light of recent data reporting a substantial risk for esophageal stricture development in the setting of prolonged untreated disease.

REFERENCES

1. Liacouras CA, Furuta GT, Hirano I, et al. Eosinophilic esophagitis: updated consensus recommendations for children and adults. J Allergy Clin Immunol 2011;128:3–20.
2. Straumann A, Spichtin HP, Grize L, et al. Natural history of primary eosinophilic esophagitis: a follow-up of 30 adult patients for up to 11.5 years. Gastroenterology 2003;125:1660–9.
3. Mishra A, Wang M, Pemmaraju VR, et al. Esophageal remodeling develops as a consequence of tissue specific IL-5 induced eosinophilia. Gastroenterology 2008;134:204–14.
4. Kagalwalla AF, Akhtar N, Woodruff SA, et al. Eosinophilic esophagitis: epithelial mesenchymal transition contributes to esophageal remodeling and reverses with treatment. J Allergy Clin Immunol 2012;129:1387–96.
5. Schoepfer AM, Safroneeva E, Bussmann C, et al. Delay in diagnosis of eosinophilic esophagitis increases risk for stricture formation, in a time-dependent manner. Gastroenterology 2013;145:1230–6.
6. Dellon ES, Kim HP, Sperry SL, et al. A phenotypic analysis shows that eosinophilic esophagitis is a progressive fibrostenotic disease. Gastrointest Endosc 2013. [Epub ahead of print].
7. Dellon ES, Gonsalves N, Hirano I, et al. ACG clinical guideline: evidence based approach to the diagnosis and management of esophageal eosinophilia and eosinophilic esophagitis (EoE). Am J Gastroenterol 2013;108:679–92.
8. Alexander JA, Jung KW, Arora AS, et al. Swallowed fluticasone improves histologic but not symptomatic response of adults with eosinophilic esophagitis. Clin Gastroenterol Hepatol 2012;10:742–9.
9. Pentiuk S, Putnam PE, Collins MH, et al. Dissociation between symptoms and histological severity in pediatric eosinophilic esophagitis. J Pediatr Gastroenterol Nutr 2009;48:152–60.
10. Straumann A, Conus S, Degen L, et al. Budesonide is effective in adolescent and adult patients with active eosinophilic esophagitis. Gastroenterology 2010;139:1526–37.
11. Straumann A, Conus S, Degen L, et al. Long-term budesonide maintenance treatment is partially effective for patients with eosinophilic esophagitis. Clin Gastroenterol Hepatol 2011;9:400–9.
12. US Food and Drug Administration. Patient-reported outcome measures: use in medical product development to support labeling claims. Available at: www.fda.gov/downloads/Drugs/Guidances/UCM193282.pdf. Accessed December 3, 2013.
13. Fiorentino R, Liu G, Pariser AR, et al. Cross-sector sponsorship of research in eosinophilic esophagitis: a collaborative model for rational drug development in rare diseases. J Allergy Clin Immunol 2012;130:613–6.
14. Rothenberg ME, Aceves S, Bonis PA, et al. Working with the US Food and Drug Administration: progress and timelines in understanding and treating patients with eosinophilic esophagitis. J Allergy Clin Immunol 2012;130:617–9.
15. Noel RJ, Putnam PE, Rothenberg ME. Eosinophilic esophagitis. N Engl J Med 2004;351:940–1.
16. Norquist JM, Girman C, Fehnel S, et al. Choice of recall period for patient-reported outcome (PRO) measures: criteria for consideration. Qual Life Res 2012;21:1013–20.

17. Dellon ES, Irani AM, Hill MR, et al. Development and field testing of a novel patient-reported outcome measure of dysphagia in patients with eosinophilic esophagitis. Aliment Pharmacol Ther 2013;38:634–42.

18. Taft TH, Kern E, Kwiatek MA, et al. The adult eosinophilic esophagitis quality of life questionnaire: a new measure of health-related quality of life. Aliment Pharmacol Ther 2011;34:790–8.

19. Franciosi JP, Hommel KA, DeBrosse CW, et al. Development of a validated patient-reported symptom metric for pediatric eosinophilic esophagitis: qualitative methods. BMC Gastroenterol 2011;11:126.

20. Franciosi JP, Hommel KA, Bendo CB, et al. PedsQL eosinophilic esophagitis module: feasibility, reliability, and validity. J Pediatr Gastroenterol Nutr 2013;57:57–66.

21. Hirano I, Moy N, Heckman MG, et al. Endoscopic assessment of the oesophageal features of eosinophilic oesophagitis: validation of a novel classification and grading system. Gut 2013;62:489–95.

22. Dellon ES, Aderoju A, Woosley JT, et al. Variability in diagnostic criteria for eosinophilic esophagitis: a systematic review. Am J Gastroenterol 2007;102:2300–13.

23. Furuta GT, Kagalwalla AF, Lee JJ, et al. The oesophageal string test: a novel, minimally invasive method measures mucosal inflammation in eosinophilic oesophagitis. Gut 2013;62:1395–405.

24. Kwiatek MA, Hirano I, Kahrilas PJ, et al. Mechanical properties of the esophagus in eosinophilic esophagitis. Gastroenterology 2011;140:82–90.

25. Straumann A, Bussmann C, Zuber M, et al. Eosinophilic esophagitis: analysis of food impaction and perforation in 251 adolescent and adult patients. Clin Gastroenterol Hepatol 2008;6:598–600.

26. Desai TK, Goldstein NS, Stecevic V, et al. Esophageal eosinophilia is common among adults with esophageal food impaction. Gastroenterology 2002;122:343.

27. Kerlin P, Jones D, Remedios M, et al. Prevalence of eosinophilic esophagitis in adults with food bolus obstruction of the esophagus. J Clin Gastroenterol 2007;41:356–61.

28. Prasad GA, Talley NJ, Romero Y, et al. Prevalence and predictive factors of eosinophilic esophagitis in patients presenting with dysphagia: a prospective study. Am J Gastroenterol 2007;102:2627–32.

29. Cohen MS, Kaufman A, Dimarino AJ, et al. Eosinophilic esophagitis presenting as spontaneous esophageal rupture (Boerhaave's syndrome). Clin Gastroenterol Hepatol 2007;5:A24.

30. Jung KW, Gundersen N, Kopacova J, et al. Occurrence and risk factors for complications after endoscopic dilation in eosinophilic esophagitis. Gastrointest Endosc 2011;73:15–21.

31. Schoepfer AM, Gonsalves N, Bussmann C, et al. Esophageal dilation in eosinophilic esophagitis: effectiveness, safety, and impact on the underlying inflammation. Am J Gastroenterol 2010;105:1062–70.

32. DeBrosse CW, Franciosi JP, King EC, et al. Long-term outcomes in pediatric-onset esophageal eosinophilia. J Allergy Clin Immunol 2011;128:132–8.

33. Lucendo AJ, Arias A, Gonzalez-Cervera J, et al. Empiric 6-food elimination diet induced and maintained prolonged remission in patients with adult eosinophilic esophagitis: a prospective study on the food cause of the disease. J Allergy Clin Immunol 2013;131:797–804.

34. Helou EF, Simonson J, Arora AS. Three-year follow-up of topical corticosteroid treatment for eosinophilic esophagitis in adults. Am J Gastroenterol 2008;103:2194–9.

35. Lee J, Huprich J, Kujath C, et al. Esophageal diameter is decreased in some patients with eosinophilic esophagitis and might increase with topical corticosteroid therapy. Clin Gastroenterol Hepatol 2012;10:481–6.

36. Fox VL, Nurko S, Teitelbaum JE, et al. High-resolution EUS in children with eosinophilic "allergic" esophagitis. Gastrointest Endosc 2003;57:30–6.

37. Roman S, Hirano I, Kwiatek MA, et al. Manometric features of eosinophilic esophagitis in esophageal pressure topography. Neurogastroenterol Motil 2011;23:208–14.

38. Aceves SS, Newbury RO, Dohil R, et al. Esophageal remodeling in pediatric eosinophilic esophagitis. J Allergy Clin Immunol 2007;119:206–12.

39. Aceves SS. Tissue remodeling in patients with eosinophilic esophagitis: what lies beneath the surface? J Allergy Clin Immunol 2011;128:1047–9.

40. Lucendo AJ, Arias A, De Rezende LC, et al. Subepithelial collagen deposition, profibrogenic cytokine gene expression, and changes after prolonged fluticasone propionate treatment in adult eosinophilic esophagitis: a prospective study. J Allergy Clin Immunol 2011;128:1037–46.

41. Lee S, de Boer WB, Naran A, et al. More than just counting eosinophils: proximal oesophageal involvement and subepithelial sclerosis are major diagnostic criteria for eosinophilic oesophagitis. J Clin Pathol 2010;63:644–7.

42. Liacouras CA, Spergel JM, Ruchelli E, et al. Eosinophilic esophagitis: a 10-year experience in 381 children. Clin Gastroenterol Hepatol 2005;3: 1198–206.

43. Bohm M, Richter JE, Kelsen S, et al. Esophageal dilation: simple and effective treatment for adults with eosinophilic esophagitis and esophageal rings and narrowing. Dis Esophagus 2010;23:377–85.

44. Bohm ME, Richter JE. Review article: oesophageal dilation in adults with eosinophilic oesophagitis. Aliment Pharmacol Ther 2011;33:748–57.

45. Schnitzler F, Fidder H, Ferrante M, et al. Mucosal healing predicts long-term outcome of maintenance therapy with infliximab in Crohn's disease. Inflamm Bowel Dis 2009;15:1295–301.

46. Noel RJ, Putnam PE, Collins MH, et al. Clinical and immunopathologic effects of swallowed fluticasone for eosinophilic esophagitis. Clin Gastroenterol Hepatol 2004;2:568–75.

47. Aceves SS, Newbury RO, Chen D, et al. Resolution of remodeling in eosinophilic esophagitis correlates with epithelial response to topical corticosteroids. Allergy 2010;65:109–16.

48. Caldwell JM, Blanchard C, Collins MH, et al. Glucocorticoid-regulated genes in eosinophilic esophagitis: a role for FKBP51. J Allergy Clin Immunol 2010;125: 879–88.

49. Lucendo AJ, Pascual-Turrion JM, Navarro M, et al. Endoscopic, bioptic, and manometric findings in eosinophilic esophagitis before and after steroid therapy: a case series. Endoscopy 2007;39:765–71.

50. Hsu Blatman KS, Gonsalves N, Hirano I, et al. Expression of mast cell-associated genes is upregulated in adult eosinophilic esophagitis and responds to steroid or dietary therapy. J Allergy Clin Immunol 2011;127:1307–8.

51. Lu TX, Lim EJ, Wen T, et al. MiR-375 is downregulated in epithelial cells after IL-13 stimulation and regulates an IL-13-induced epithelial transcriptome. Mucosal Immunol 2012;5:388–96.

52. Sherrill JD, Rothenberg ME. Genetic dissection of eosinophilic esophagitis provides insight into disease pathogenesis and treatment strategies. J Allergy Clin Immunol 2011;128:23–32 [quiz: 33–4].

53. Gonsalves N, Yang GY, Doerfler B, et al. Elimination diet effectively treats eosinophilic esophagitis in adults; food reintroduction identifies causative factors. Gastroenterology 2012;142:1451–9.e1 [quiz: e14–5].
54. Peterson K, Clayton F, Vinson LA, et al. Utility of an elemental diet in adult eosinophilic esophagitis. Gastroenterology 2011;140(Suppl 1):S180.
55. Rothenberg ME, Mishra A, Collins MH, et al. Pathogenesis and clinical features of eosinophilic esophagitis. J Allergy Clin Immunol 2001;108:891–4.
56. Simon D, Marti H, Heer P, et al. Eosinophilic esophagitis is frequently associated with IgE-mediated allergic airway diseases. J Allergy Clin Immunol 2005;115: 1090–2.
57. Spergel JM, Brown-Whitehorn TF, Beausoleil JL, et al. 14 years of eosinophilic esophagitis: clinical features and prognosis. J Pediatr Gastroenterol Nutr 2009;48:30–6.
58. Harer KN, Enders FT, Lim KG, et al. An allergic phenotype and the use of steroid inhalers predict eosinophilic oesophagitis in patients with asthma. Aliment Pharmacol Ther 2013;37:107–13.
59. Dohil R, Newbury R, Fox L, et al. Oral viscous budesonide is effective in children with eosinophilic esophagitis in a randomized, placebo-controlled trial. Gastroenterology 2010;139:418–29.
60. Schaefer ET, Fitzgerald JF, Molleston JP, et al. Comparison of oral prednisone and topical fluticasone in the treatment of eosinophilic esophagitis: a randomized trial in children. Clin Gastroenterol Hepatol 2008;6:165–73.
61. Clark DJ, Grove A, Cargill RI, et al. Comparative adrenal suppression with inhaled budesonide and fluticasone propionate in adult asthmatic patients. Thorax 1996;51:262–6.
62. Attwood SE, Smyrk TC, Demeester TR, et al. Esophageal eosinophilia with dysphagia, a distinct clinicopathologic syndrome. Dig Dis Sci 1993;38: 109–16.
63. Straumann A, Spichtin HP, Bernoulli R, et al. Idiopathic eosinophilic esophagitis: a frequently overlooked disease with typical clinical aspects and discrete endoscopic findings. Schweiz Med Wochenschr 1994;124:1419–29 [in German with English abstract].
64. Lucendo AJ, Friginal-Ruiz AB, Rodriguez B. Boerhaave's syndrome as the primary manifestation of adult eosinophilic esophagitis. Two case reports and a review of the literature. Dis Esophagus 2011;24:E11–5.
65. Dellon ES, Gibbs WS, Rubinas TC, et al. Esophageal dilation in eosinophilic esophagitis: safety and predictors of clinical response and complications. Gastrointest Endosc 2010;71:706–12.
66. Moawad FJ, Cheatham JG, DeZee KJ. Meta-Analysis: the safety and efficacy of dilation in eosinophilic esophagitis. Aliment Pharmacol Ther 2013;38:713–20.
67. Hirano I. Dilation in eosinophilic esophagitis: to do or not to do? Gastrointest Endosc 2010;71:713–4.
68. Jacobs JW Jr, Spechler SJ. A systematic review of the risk of perforation during esophageal dilation for patients with eosinophilic esophagitis. Dig Dis Sci 2010; 55:1512–5.
69. Dellon ES, Sheikh A, Speck O, et al. Viscous topical is more effective than nebulized steroid therapy for patients with eosinophilic esophagitis. Gastroenterology 2012;143:321–4.
70. Straumann A, Conus S, Grzonka P, et al. Anti-interleukin-5 antibody treatment (mepolizumab) in active eosinophilic esophagitis: a randomised, placebo-controlled, double-blind trial. Gut 2010;59:21–30.

71. Straumann A, Bussmann C, Conus S, et al. Anti-TNF-alpha (infliximab) therapy for severe adult eosinophilic esophagitis. J Allergy Clin Immunol 2008;122: 425–7.
72. Straumann A, Hoesli S, Bussmann C, et al. Anti-eosinophil activity and clinical efficacy of the CRTH2 antagonist OC000459 in eosinophilic esophagitis. Allergy 2013;68:375–85.

Eosinophilic Esophagitis
Clinical Presentation in Children

Chris A. Liacouras, MD[a],*, Jonathan Spergel, MD[b], Laura M. Gober, MD[c]

KEYWORDS

- Eosinophil • Esophagitis • EoE • Children • Pediatric

KEY POINTS

- Symptoms of eosinophilic esophagitis (EoE) vary by age. They range from failure to thrive in toddlers, to abdominal pain in school age children, to dysphagia in adolescents.
- Symptom overlap exists between EoE and other disorders, including gastroesophageal reflux disease, asthma, and primary eating disorders.
- Diagnosis is made by clinical history combined with results of upper endoscopy with biopsy.

INTRODUCTION

Our understanding of eosinophilic esophagitis (EoE) has evolved over the past 30 years from isolated case reports of patients with prominent esophageal eosinophilia (often misclassified as gastroesophageal reflux [GERD]) to a well-defined clinical disorder. In the past, EoE was described differently, including allergic esophagitis, primary EoE, or idiopathic EoE. We now know that EoE is a distinct disease. It is defined as a clinicopathologic diagnosis characterized by a localized eosinophilic inflammation of the esophagus (with no other gastrointestinal involvement), symptoms of esophageal dysfunction, the presence of 15 or more eosinophils in the most severely involved high-powered field (HPF) isolated to the esophagus, and failure to respond to adequate proton-pump inhibitor (PPI) therapy. Other recognized causes of esophageal eosinophilia should be excluded before making the diagnosis (**Box 1**).

This article originally appeared in Gastroenterology Clinics, Volume 43, Issue 2, June 2014.
[a] Division of Gastroenterology, Hepatology and Nutrition, The Children's Hospital of Philadelphia, Perelman School of Medicine, University of Pennsylvania, 3401 Civic Center Boulevard, Philadelphia, PA 19104, USA; [b] Division of Allergy, Immunology, and Infectious Diseases, The Children's Hospital of Philadelphia, Perelman School of Medicine, University of Pennsylvania, 3401 Civic Center Boulevard, Philadelphia, PA 19104, USA; [c] Division of Allergy, Immunology, and Infectious Diseases, Center for Pediatric Eosinophilic Disorders, The Children's Hospital of Philadelphia, 3401 Civic Center Boulevard, Philadelphia, PA 19104, USA
* Corresponding author.
E-mail address: liacouras@email.chop.edu

Box 1
Causes of esophageal eosinophilia

- EoE
- GERD
- PPI-responsive esophageal eosinophilia
- Celiac disease
- Eosinophilic gastroenteritis
- Crohn disease
- Hypereosinophilic syndrome
- Achalasia
- Vasculitis
- Pemphigus
- Connective tissue disease
- Infection
- Graft-versus-host disease

DEMOGRAPHICS

EoE is characterized by eosinophilia of the esophagus, an organ typically devoid of eosinophils, without infiltration in other parts of the gastrointestinal tract.[1,2] First described in 1993, EoE has been increasing in incidence and prevalence in Western nations with an estimated annual incidence equal to Crohn disease.[3–8] The increase in EoE mirrors the increased prevalence of allergic diseases (asthma, allergic rhinitis, atopic dermatitis, and food allergy) over the last few decades. Data from the CDC National Health Information Survey (NHIS) confirm the increase in all atopic diseases.[9,10] The reported prevalence of asthma increased from 3% in 1990% to 7.7% in 2007.[11] An estimated 25% to 30% of the population in industrialized countries has atopic dermatitis, food allergy, or allergic rhinitis.[12] EoE has now been reported in every continent.[12–15] Five to 10% of pediatric patients and 6% of adult patients with poorly controlled GERD are thought to have EoE.[16–18] In our cohort at The Children's Hospital of Philadelphia, the authors have seen a 70-fold increase, from 1994 to 2011.[19] In Olten Country, Switzerland, this increase has also been observed in the adult population with increased prevalence from 2 per 100,000 in 1989 to 23 per 100,000 in 2004.[5] Patients who have EoE typically are male (by a 3:1 ratio)[8,19] and 75% have a personal history of atopy.[19–22] Like other atopic diseases, such as asthma and eczema, EoE is a chronic disease. Most patients will continue to have the disease into adulthood. In a 12-year study of adults, no patients had remission.[23] In a 14-year study of pediatric patients, only 2% had remission of disease.[19]

CLINICAL PRESENTATION: GENERAL CONSIDERATIONS

EoE should be suspected in patients describing symptoms consistent with GERD but not responding to adequate reflux medications. Presentation in children varies depending on the age of the child. Characteristic symptoms in infants and young children are feeding difficulties, failure to thrive, and classic GERD symptoms. In contrast, school-aged children are more likely to present with vomiting, abdominal pain, and regurgitation. Dysphagia and food impaction are more prevalent in adolescents and adults.[1,19,20,22,24–26] One study looked at age of presenting symptoms over a 14-year span and found feeding difficulties or failure to thrive in young children (median age 2.8 years), vomiting and GERD symptoms in older children (median age 5.1 years), abdominal pain in young adolescents (median age 9.0 years), and dysphagia and food impaction (median age 11.1 years) in older adolescents.[19] Food impaction can be a presenting symptom especially if dysphagia is intermittent and mild in nature. In adults, the percent of patients who present with dysphagia and who are diagnosed with EoE has risen by 15% from 1999 to 2009.[27] In addition, adult reports have also suggested that the probability of developing fibrostenosis increases over time (especially when not properly treated).[28] It is easy to postulate that chronic untreated inflammation in children may lead to the esophageal dysfunction and dysphagia seen in older adolescents and adults. In addition, a select cohort of patients with abdominal pain on initial presentation who refused therapy all returned 6 years later with symptoms changed to dysphagia.[19] Mechanical obstruction can be the cause for dysphagia.[29] It is unclear whether variable presentations represent different disease phenotypes or the natural history of the untreated disease.

VOMITING AND PAIN

Vomiting is a common symptom in younger children. It can be mistaken for GERD but, unlike GERD, vomiting associated with EoE usually is not diagnosed before 6 months of life. It can be sporadic in occurrence and not associated with meals. If occurring after ingestion of particular foods, vomiting can be mistaken for food protein-induced enterocolitis or IgE-mediated food allergy especially in children with other food allergies. Although vomiting can present early on in infancy, especially in a highly atopic child, it is more likely after the introduction of solid food into the diet. Some children may induce vomiting if they have dysphagia and feel something is stuck in their throat.

Children may complain of abdominal pain, in particular localizing to the epigastrium despite only having esophageal disease. Adolescents and adults are more likely to localize pain to the chest or complain of heartburn. The pain, which is spasmodic, can be severe enough to lead patients to seek emergency evaluation and lead to cardiac evaluation.

DYSPHAGIA AND FOOD IMPACTION

Dysphagia associated with EoE is intermittent and some patients may experience it for more than 2 years before presentation.[29,30] How patients report dysphagia varies, as can be expected, especially in different age groups. Patients may describe difficultly initiating swallowing, food going down the esophagus too slowly, or food being stuck in the throat. Food impaction can lead to patient anxiety. Patients gradually learn techniques for compensating for dysphagia, including taking small bites, eating slowly with excessive chewing, and drinking fluids after each bite. Some may even jump up and down to help food pass. Patients may also avoid certain food textures or types (eg, meat) due to difficulty swallowing these in the past. In younger children and infants, it is unclear if symptoms such as gagging, choking, feeding difficulties, and food aversions are secondary to current dysphagia and the associated pain or due to previous negative feeding experiences and the related anxiety toward eating. In adolescents, patients with EoE have been misdiagnosed with eating disorders because of symptoms of food-related anxiety, vomiting, and food aversion. Barium radiographic studies are extremely useful in patients who complain of dysphagia. These studies can demonstrate fixed strictures, small caliber esophagus, transient or fixed rings, or a normal esophagus (suggesting that dysphagia is due to secondary esophageal dysmotility). These findings are especially important for the gastroenterologist before an endoscopy is performed.

EoE patients with dysphagia may have a mechanical obstruction. Strictures can be seen, even in infants.[1] Strictures are, however, less common in children who usually do not have radiographic evidence of obvious mechanical obstruction.[29] One study found that 8 out of 18 children found to have Schatzki rings via radiographic images had EoE. Those having EoE did not have rings on endoscopy but, most likely, had a focal spasm at time of imaging. In contrast, strictures, rings, narrowing of the esophagus, and Schatzki rings have all been described in adults with EoE and dysphagia.[31] A biopsy should be performed on patients with mechanical obstruction, including foreign bodies (eg, food, coins), to rule out EoE.

One active area of research in EoE, as well as other atopic conditions, is tissue remodeling. In atopic dermatitis, skin can become lichenified and thick over time.[32] In poorly controlled asthmatics, a permanent decline in lung function may occur.[33] Patients with EoE can have narrowing of the esophagus or stricture formation secondary to untreated EoE.[25,26,33] However, narrowing occurs in only a very small percentage of adult patients because strictures are only seen in 5% to 15% of adult series and these are usually only in patients with longstanding untreated disease.[23,34] This progression of complications is attributed to fibrous remodeling associated with the natural history of untreated EoE.[35] Delayed diagnosis of EoE is associated with an increased risk of stricture formation in a time-dependent manner.[36] Children with untreated EoE have basement membrane thickening and increased vascular activation, similar to changes seen in airway remodeling with increased SMAD2/3 and transforming growth factor (TGF)-β.[37,38]

CORRELATION OF SYMPTOMS WITH ENDOSCOPY AND HISTOLOGY

The appearance of mucosal rings, furrowing, strictures, and white plaques are often seen on visual inspection.[20,23–26,39] However, up to one-third of patients with active EoE may have a normal appearing esophagus.[25] There is poor correlation between biopsies and symptoms. Patients can have normal biopsies and still have symptoms and the converse. For example, in the largest clinical trial for EoE with 240 subjects, there was no correlation between symptoms and eosinophils found on esophageal biopsies. Subjects on placebo had symptom resolution without improvement in esophageal eosinophilia.[22] Currently, serial endoscopies of the esophagus are unavoidable for EoE because there are no other available testing options. One study followed 330 subjects with at least 1 year of clinical follow-up (average 3.2 years). These subjects had 2526 total biopsies with an average of 4.5 esophagogastroduodenoscopies (EGDs) per subject. At time of presentation, 144 subjects also required lower endoscopies.[19] Disease burden, including financial, would be eased if there was a reliable, easily obtainable (eg, blood, stool) biomarker for EoE that would lessen the frequency of EGDs.

OTHER CLINICAL PRESENTATIONS

In children with asthma, chest pain and cough may be mistaken for an asthma exacerbation; however when these patients do not respond to aggressive asthma treatment, after asking a careful history, EoE should be considered. The diagnosis of EoE has also been made in children with airway anomalies such as subglottic stenosis and laryngeal cleft.[40]

Eosinophilic gastroenteritis is eosinophilic inflammation at extraesophageal gastrointestinal sites. This entity usually does not respond to dietary therapies and it is treated with corticosteroids. EoE has also been described in conjunction with other gastrointestinal disorders such as Crohn disease and celiac disease. The prevalence of EoE in children with confirmed celiac disease is 1% to 4%.[41,42] In general, EoE is not typically in remission with removal of gluten-containing foods alone.

Connective tissue disorders (CTDs) have been recently associated with a greater risk for EoE. A recent retrospective study noted an eightfold increase in EoE (1.3% prevalence) in patients with CTDs at their institution.[43] This included patients with Marfan syndrome, Ehlers-Danlos syndrome, joint hypermobility syndrome, and Loeys-Dietz syndrome. Patients had dysmorphic scaphocephalic facial features, hypermobility of hands and large joints, and high rate of atopic diseases. Esophageal biopsies from EoE patients with CTDs were indistinguishable from those without CTDs but this cohort was more likely to have significant eosinophilic gastrointestinal inflammatory disease affecting other sites such as stomach, duodenum, and colon. On a molecular level, the EoE transcriptome for EoE-CTD was not unique. However, two genes (CD200R1 and SAMSN1) had higher expression and two genes (PTGFRN and COL8A2) had lower expression in this group. This association may further support that TGF-β signaling plays a role in EoE pathogenesis and help target future pharmacotherapies.

EoE has been described in neurologic disorders such as seizure disorders, cerebral palsy, migraines, and Chiari malformation. Certain antiepileptic drugs have been linked to the development of EoE in the setting of a hypersensitivity reaction involving other organ systems.[44] There is no evidence for a causal relationship between EoE and neurodevelopmental disorders such as pervasive developmental delays or sensory integration disorders.

PSYCHOSOCIAL DYSFUNCTION

A recent retrospective study at a tertiary care EoE program evaluated patients and families for psychosocial dysfunction.[45] Most children (69%) evaluated suffered from difficulties in at least one area assessed (sleep, social, school, anxiety, and depression). Children who had pain or eating difficulties were more likely to have difficulties across multiple assessed areas. Anxiety (41%) and depression (28%) increased with age. Children with gastrostomy tubes had more social (64%), school (26%), and psychological adjustment (44%) disorders. Adjustment problems were more likely in older children, whereas sleep problems (33%) were seen almost exclusively in younger children. In addition, 48% of families and children had concerns about feeding refusal or poor appetite, predominantly in younger children. Another study found that caregivers (98% were mothers) of children with eosinophilic gastrointestinal disorders reported stress and psychological distress from caring for their child.[46] These studies support the need for psychosocial evaluation and support for children with EoE as well as their families.

GROWTH AND NUTRITIONAL CONCERNS

Long-term elimination diets pose significant challenges to patients and families, so nonadherence must be ruled out. In particular, milk and wheat generally are the most difficult allergens to remove because they make up a large part of children's diets. Their removal also results in the greatest nutritional impact and has a significant affect on quality of life of children and their families. In children, a nutritionist needs to be closely involved with family when multiple foods are removed to assess risk of malnutrition and calcium, iron, vitamin D, vitamin E, and zinc deficiencies.[47] Children with milk allergy or children with two or more food allergies were shorter, based on height-for-age percentiles than those with only one food allergy (not cow's milk). In addition, children with cow's milk allergy or multiple food allergies consumed less dietary calcium than did children without cow's milk allergy and/or one food allergy.[48]

A frequent barrier in children with EoE is acceptance of amino acid formulas whenever a strict amino acid based diet is warranted. The use of amino acids as the main protein source renders the formulas significantly less palatable than their intact protein counterparts are. Flavors of these formulas have improved in recent years, although this remains, as expected, largely a matter of the child's opinion. If elemental formulas are essential, enteral tube feeds may be inevitable and should be managed in conjunction with an experienced dietician. Micronutrient supplementation may be required, depending up the volume of formula consumed. Fiber supplementation may be required because elemental formulas do not contain dietary fiber; these are especially useful for children with constipation, or those dependent on elemental formula with little solid food in diet for a prolonged period.

Not all patients require elemental formulas for treatment of their EoE. Dietary restriction may be based on individual testing or empiric removal of foods. A history is obtained from the family and then testing to foods in the child's diet is recommended. One approach involves using skin prick testing (identifying IgE-mediated reactions) and patch testing (identifying non–IgE-mediated reactions) in guiding food removal; upwards of 75% improve symptomatically and histologically with this approach.[49] Another approach is empiric removal of foods. Empiric removal of the six most common food allergens (milk, soy, egg, peanut, tree nuts, wheat, and seafood) has also been used with reported success of 74% in one study.[50] However, removal of the most common food allergens did not reduce eosinophils to a normal range (13.6 eosinophils per HPF).[50] When effective, elimination diets (based on a combination of skin prick testing and patch testing) reduced counts to 1.1 eosinophils per HPF.[49,51] Elemental diets reduced eosinophil counts to 0 eosinophils per HPF.[25] Even with elemental diets there is a small percentage (<10%) of patients who do not have resolution of esophageal eosinophilia. In these patients, it is important to review adherence to diet and compliance with reflux medications, and to rule out other causes of eosinophilia in the gastrointestinal tract, including aeroallergens.

ATOPIC COMORBIDITIES

Children with EoE have a higher rate of atopy compared with normal children. Approximately 30% to 50% of children with EoE have asthma compared with 10% in the normal population. Similarly, 50% to 75% have allergic rhinitis compared with 30% in normal children. In addition, 10% to 20% of children with EoE have IgE-mediated food allergy (urticaria and anaphylaxis) compared with 1% to 5% in normal children. These data suggest EoE has a superatopic phenotype. However, it does not appear to be IgE-mediated because skin testing or specific IgE do not identify foods, and murine models of EoE do not require IgE to produce symptoms or esophageal eosinophilia.[19] These rates of atopy (asthma, allergic rhinitis, and atopic dermatitis) are approximately three times higher than what is expected in the general population. Other studies of pediatric and adult patients with EoE have confirmed the higher prevalence of environmental and/or food allergies, approximately 50% higher than the general population.[20,21,52] Similar to asthma and atopic dermatitis,[53–56] 14% of patients with EoE have a single nucleotide polymorphism (SNP) inferring a possible genetic component.[16] Furthermore, there is a strong familial association with EoE.[57–59]

ROLE OF ALLERGENS IN PEDIATRIC EoE

In almost all cases of pediatric EoE, an underlying food allergy has been found to be the culprit. Convincing work from Kelly and colleagues[14] revealed the use of an elemental diet and a few basic foods in 10 patients with refractory EoE, six of whom had Nissen fundoplications. All children improved and eight of the original children had complete resolution on biopsy. Other studies have corroborated this data showing success rates of 98% with elemental diets.[25,60]

A few studies have suggested that aeroallergens may play a causative role in the development of EoE in humans. A seasonal variation in cases of newly diagnosed EoE has been described, with fewer cases diagnosed in the winter when the air contains less pollen.[61] During pollen season there are increased numbers of eosinophils in subjects with allergic rhinitis compared with normal controls, although the number of eosinophils observed was lower than values typically seen in patients who have EoE.[62] In a case report, full disease control was achieved only during seasons without pollen and symptoms and esophageal eosinophilia worsened during seasons with pollen.[19] There are various case reports of immunotherapy for birch pollen and dust mite aeroallergens leading to symptomatic improvement of EoE.[63,64] Food allergies were still the primary cause of disease in these patients. However, in a few patients, during pollen season in the spring or fall, biopsy-confirmed exacerbation of disease without change in diet have been documented. In these patients, disease control was improved during seasons without pollen and on proper dietary therapy.[19] Assuming that environmental allergens cause EoE, the mechanism of action could be either that direct deposition of pollens onto the esophageal mucosa cause esophageal eosinophilia or that aeroallergens stimulate eotaxin secretion leading to eosinophil migration into the esophagus. Eotaxin overexpression was noted in subjects with EoE.[16] Intranasal steroid therapy has decreased nasal secretion of eotaxin in subjects who have allergic rhinitis,[65] thus aggressive treatment of allergic rhinitis with intranasal steroids is highly recommended in patients with EoE.[66]

More recently, sublingual immunotherapy to aeroallergens has been shown to induce EoE.[67] Oral immunotherapy (OIT) has shown to be effective for treatment of IgE-mediated food allergies but one of the reported side effects is the development of EoE in patients having undergone OIT to milk and egg. This confirms that IgE-mediated food allergy and EoE have different disease mechanisms.[68–70] In these cases, EoE resolved once the food was removed again from the diet.

SUMMARY

The prevalence of EoE is increasing in children. Characteristic symptoms in infants and young children are feeding difficulties, failure to thrive, and classic GERD symptoms in contrast to school-aged children who are more likely to present with vomiting, abdominal pain, and regurgitation. Dysphagia and food impaction are more prevalent in adolescents and adults. Atopic comorbidities, growth or nutritional deficiencies, psychosocial impact, and recently recognized associations with CTDs are concerns in pediatric patients with EoE. Although food elimination diets can effectively treat most children with this disease, there is a lack of allergy testing with high specificity to identify foods that trigger the disease. Food reintroduction can be difficult because endoscopies are required to identify trigger foods. Earlier research studies failed to correlate noninvasive biomarkers with biopsy findings. Currently, in asymptomatic children with abnormal biopsies, the standard of care is to treat because of the risk of tissue remodeling and fibrosis resulting in stricture formation with potential need for dilatation.

REFERENCES

1. Furuta GT, Liacouras CA, Collins MH, et al. Eosinophilic esophagitis in children and adults: a systematic review and consensus recommendations for diagnosis and treatment. Gastroenterology 2007;133(4):1342–63.

2. Liacouras CA, Furuta GT, Hirano I, et al. Eosinophilic esophagitis: updated consensus recommendations for children and adults. J Allergy Clin Immunol 2011;128(1):3–20.
3. Prasad GA, Alexander JA, Schleck CD, et al. Epidemiology of eosinophilic esophagitis over three decades in Olmsted County, Minnesota. Clin Gastroenterol Hepatol 2009;7(10):1055–61.
4. Noel RJ, Putnam PE, Rothenberg ME. Eosinophilic esophagitis. N Engl J Med 2004;351(9):940–1.
5. Straumann A, Simon HU. Eosinophilic esophagitis: escalating epidemiology? J Allergy Clin Immunol 2005;115(2):418–9.
6. Hruz P, Straumann A, Bussmann C, et al. Escalating incidence of eosinophilic esophagitis: a 20-year prospective, population-based study in Olten County, Switzerland. J Allergy Clin Immunol 2011;128(6):1349–50.
7. Cherian S, Smith NM, Forbes DA. Rapidly increasing prevalence of eosinophilic oesophagitis in Western Australia. Arch Dis Child 2006;91(12):1000–4.
8. van Rhijn BD, Verheij J, Smout AJ, et al. Rapidly increasing incidence of eosinophilic esophagitis in a large cohort. Neurogastroenterol Motil 2013;25(1): 47–52.
9. Branum AM, Lukacs SL. Food allergy among U.S. children: trends in prevalence and hospitalizations. NCHS Data Brief 2008;10:1–8.
10. Mannino DM, Homa DM, Pertowski CA, et al. Surveillance for asthma—United States, 1960–1995. MMWR CDC Surveill Summ 1998;47(1):1–27.
11. Brim SN, Rudd RA, Funk RH, et al. Asthma prevalence among US children in underrepresented minority populations: American Indian/Alaska Native, Chinese, Filipino, and Asian Indian. Pediatrics 2008;122(1):217–22.
12. Kiyohara C, Tanaka K, Miyake Y. Genetic susceptibility to atopic dermatitis. Allergol Int 2008;57(1):39–56.
13. Riou PJ, Nicholson AG, Pastorino U. Esophageal rupture in a patient with idiopathic eosinophilic esophagitis. Ann Thorac Surg 1996;62(6):1854–6.
14. Kelly KJ, Lazenby AJ, Rowe PC, et al. Eosinophilic esophagitis attributed to gastroesophageal reflux: improvement with an amino acid-based formula. Gastroenterology 1995;109(5):1503–12.
15. Straumann A, Spichtin HP, Bernoulli R, et al. Idiopathic eosinophilic esophagitis: a frequently overlooked disease with typical clinical aspects and discrete endoscopic findings. Schweiz Med Wochenschr 1994;124(33):1419–29.
16. Blanchard C, Wang N, Stringer KF, et al. Eotaxin-3 and a uniquely conserved gene-expression profile in eosinophilic esophagitis. J Clin Invest 2006;116(2): 536–47.
17. Markowitz JE, Liacouras CA. Ten years of eosinophilic oesophagitis: small steps or giant leaps? Dig Liver Dis 2006;38(4):251–3.
18. Fox VL, Nurko S, Furuta GT. Eosinophilic esophagitis: it's not just kid's stuff. Gastrointest Endosc 2002;56(2):260–70.
19. Spergel JM, Brown-Whitehorn TF, Beausoleil JL, et al. 14 years of eosinophilic esophagitis: clinical features and prognosis. J Pediatr Gastroenterol Nutr 2009;48(1):30–6.
20. Assa'ad AH, Putnam PE, Collins MH, et al. Pediatric patients with eosinophilic esophagitis: an 8-year follow-up. J Allergy Clin Immunol 2007;119(3): 731–8.
21. Simon D, Marti H, Heer P, et al. Eosinophilic esophagitis is frequently associated with IgE-mediated allergic airway diseases. J Allergy Clin Immunol 2005;115(5): 1090–2.

22. Spergel JM, Brown-Whitehorn TF, Cianferoni A, et al. Identification of causative foods in children with eosinophilic esophagitis treated with an elimination diet. J Allergy Clin Immunol 2012;130(2):461–7.

23. Straumann A, Spichtin HP, Grize L, et al. Natural history of primary eosinophilic esophagitis: a follow-up of 30 adult patients for up to 11.5 years. Gastroenterology 2003;125(6):1660–9.

24. Orenstein SR, Shalaby TM, Di Lorenzo C, et al. The spectrum of pediatric eosinophilic esophagitis beyond infancy: a clinical series of 30 children. Am J Gastroenterol 2000;95(6):1422–30.

25. Liacouras CA, Spergel JM, Ruchelli E, et al. Eosinophilic esophagitis: a 10-year experience in 381 children. Clin Gastroenterol Hepatol 2005;3(12):1198–206.

26. Baxi S, Gupta SK, Swigonski N, et al. Clinical presentation of patients with eosinophilic inflammation of the esophagus. Gastrointest Endosc 2006;64(4):473–8.

27. Kidambi T, Toto E, Ho N, et al. Temporal trends in the relative prevalence of dysphagia etiologies from 1999–2009. World J Gastroenterol 2012;18(32):4335–41.

28. Dellon ES, Kim HP, Sperry SL, et al. A phenotypic analysis shows that eosinophilic esophagitis is a progressive fibrostenotic disease. Gastrointest Endosc 2013;79(4):57–85.

29. Khan S, Orenstein SR, Di Lorenzo C, et al. Eosinophilic esophagitis: strictures, impactions, and dysphagia. Dig Dis Sci 2003;48(1):22–9.

30. Nurko S, Teitelbaum JE, Husain K, et al. Association of Schatzki ring with eosinophilic esophagitis in children. J Pediatr Gastroenterol Nutr 2004;38(4):436–41.

31. Vasilopoulos S, Murphy P, Auerbach A, et al. The small-caliber esophagus: an unappreciated cause of dysphagia for solids in patients with eosinophilic esophagitis. Gastrointest Endosc 2002;55(1):99–106.

32. Bieber T. Atopic dermatitis. N Engl J Med 2008;358(14):1483–94.

33. Hoshino M, Nakamura Y, Sim J, et al. Bronchial subepithelial fibrosis and expression of matrix metalloproteinase-9 in asthmatic airway inflammation. J Allergy Clin Immunol 1998;102(5):783–8.

34. Attwood SE, Smyrk TC, Demeester TR, et al. Esophageal eosinophilia with dysphagia. A distinct clinicopathologic syndrome. Dig Dis Sci 1993;38(1):109–16.

35. Aceves SS, Ackerman SJ. Relationships between eosinophilic inflammation, tissue remodeling, and fibrosis in eosinophilic esophagitis. Immunol Allergy Clin North Am 2009;29:197–211.

36. Schoepfer AM, Safroneeva E, Bussmann C, et al. Delay in diagnosis of eosinophilic esophagitis increases risk for stricture formation in a time-dependent manner. Gastroenterology 2013;145(6):1230–6.

37. Aceves SS, Furuta GT, Spechler SJ. Integrated approach to treatment of children and adults with eosinophilic esophagitis. Gastrointest Endosc Clin N Am 2008;18(1):195–217.

38. Aceves SS, Newbury RO, Dohil R, et al. Esophageal remodeling in pediatric eosinophilic esophagitis. J Allergy Clin Immunol 2007;119(1):206–12.

39. Siafakas CG, Ryan CK, Brown MR, et al. Multiple esophageal rings: an association with eosinophilic esophagitis: case report and review of the literature. Am J Gastroenterol 2000;95(6):1572–5.

40. Goldstein NA, Putnam PE, Dohar JE. Laryngeal cleft and eosinophilic gastroenteritis: report of 2 cases. Arch Otolaryngol Head Neck Surg 2000;126(2):227–30.

41. Leslie C, Mews C, Charles A, et al. Celiac disease and eosinophilic esophagitis: a true association. J Pediatr Gastroenterol Nutr 2010;50(4):397–9.

42. Ooi CY, Day AS, Jackson R, et al. Eosinophilic esophagitis in children with celiac disease. J Gastroenterol Hepatol 2008;23(7):1144–8.
43. Abonia JP, Wen T, Stucke EM, et al. High prevalence of eosinophilic esophagitis in patients with inherited connective tissue disorders. J Allergy Clin Immunol 2013;132:378–86.
44. Balatsinou C, Milano A, Caldarella MP, et al. Eosinophilic esophagitis is a component of the anticonvulsant hypersensitivity syndrome: description of two cases. Dig Liver Dis 2008;40(2):145–8.
45. Harris RF, Menard-Katcher C, Atkins D, et al. Psychosocial dysfunction in children and adolescents with eosinophilic esophagitis. J Pediatr Gastroenterol Nutr 2013;57(4):500–5.
46. Taft TH, Ballou S, Keefer L. Preliminary evaluation of maternal caregiver stress in pediatric eosinophilic gastrointestinal disorders. J Pediatr Psychol 2012;37:523–32.
47. Spergel JM, Shuker M. Nutritional management of eosinophilic esophagitis. Gastrointest Endosc Clin N Am 2008;18(1):179–94.
48. Christie L, Hine RJ, Parker JG, et al. Food allergies in children affect nutrient intake and growth. J Am Diet Assoc 2002;102:1648–51.
49. Spergel JM, Beausoleil JL, Mascarenhas M, et al. The use of skin prick tests and patch tests to identify causative foods in eosinophilic esophagitis. J Allergy Clin Immunol 2002;109(2):363–8.
50. Kagalwalla AF, Sentongo TA, Ritz S, et al. Effect of six-food elimination diet on clinical and histologic outcomes in eosinophilic esophagitis. Clin Gastroenterol Hepatol 2006;4(9):1097–102.
51. Spergel JM, Brown-Whitehorn T. The use of patch testing in the diagnosis of food allergy. Curr Allergy Asthma Rep 2005;5(1):86–90.
52. Roy-Ghanta S, Larosa DF, Katzka DA. Atopic characteristics of adult patients with eosinophilic esophagitis. Clin Gastroenterol Hepatol 2008;6(5):531–5.
53. Weidinger S, O'Sullivan M, Illig T, et al. Filaggrin mutations, atopic eczema, hay fever, and asthma in children. J Allergy Clin Immunol 2008;121(5):1203–9.
54. Weiss ST, Raby BA, Rogers A. Asthma genetics and genomics 2009. Curr Opin Genet Dev 2009;19(3):279–82.
55. Flory JH, Sleiman PM, Christie JD, et al. 17q12-21 variants interact with smoke exposure as a risk factor for pediatric asthma but are equally associated with early-onset versus late-onset asthma in North Americans of European ancestry. J Allergy Clin Immunol 2009;124(3):605–7.
56. Steinke JW, Rich SS, Borish L. 5. Genetics of allergic disease. J Allergy Clin Immunol 2008;121(Suppl 2):S384–7.
57. Meyer GW. Eosinophilic esophagitis in a father and a daughter. Gastrointest Endosc 2005;61(7):932.
58. Patel SM, Falchuk KR. Three brothers with dysphagia caused by eosinophilic esophagitis. Gastrointest Endosc 2005;61(1):165–7.
59. Zink DA, Amin M, Gebara S, et al. Familial dysphagia and eosinophilia. Gastrointest Endosc 2007;65(2):330–4.
60. Markowitz JE, Spergel JM, Ruchelli E, et al. Elemental diet is an effective treatment for eosinophilic esophagitis in children and adolescents. Am J Gastroenterol 2003;98(4):777–82.
61. Wang FY, Gupta SK, Fitzgerald JF. Is there a seasonal variation in the incidence or intensity of allergic eosinophilic esophagitis in newly diagnosed children? J Clin Gastroenterol 2007;41(5):451–3.

62. Onbasi K, Sin AZ, Doganavsargil B, et al. Eosinophil infiltration of the oesophageal mucosa in patients with pollen allergy during the season. Clin Exp Allergy 2005;35(11):1423–31.
63. De Swert L, Veereman G, Bublin M, et al. Eosinophilic gastrointestinal disease suggestive of pathogenesis-related class 10 (PR-10) protein allergy resolved after immunotherapy. J Allergy Clin Immunol 2013;131(2):600–2.
64. Ramirez RM, Jacobs RL. Eosinophilic esophagitis treated with immunotherapy to dust mites. J Allergy Clin Immunol 2013;132(2):503–4.
65. Greiff L, Petersen H, Mattsson E, et al. Mucosal output of eotaxin in allergic rhinitis and its attenuation by topical glucocorticosteroid treatment. Clin Exp Allergy 2001;31(8):1321–7.
66. Fogg MI, Ruchelli E, Spergel JM. Pollen and eosinophilic esophagitis. J Allergy Clin Immunol 2003;112(4):796–7.
67. Miehlke S, Alpan O, Schröder S, et al. Induction of eosinophilic esophagitis by sublingual pollen immunotherapy. Case Rep Gastroenterol 2013;7(3):363–8.
68. Narisety SD, Skripak JM, Steele P, et al. Open-label maintenance after milk oral immunotherapy for IgE-mediated cow's milk allergy. J Allergy Clin Immunol 2009;124(3):610–2.
69. Sanchez-Garcia S, Rodriguez del Rio P, Escudero C, et al. Possible eosinophilic esophagitis induced by milk oral immunotherapy. J Allergy Clin Immunol 2012; 124(4):1155–7.
70. Ridolo E, De Angelis GL, Dall'aglio P. Eosinophilic esophagitis after specific oral tolerance induction for egg protein. Ann Allergy Asthma Immunol 2011;106(1): 73–4.

Clinical Presentation and Pathophysiology of Gastroparesis

Linda Anh Nguyen, MD[a],*, William J. Snape Jr, MD[b],*

KEYWORDS

- Gastroparesis • Pathophysiology • Gastric motor function • Gastric emptying
- Visceral hypersensitivity • Gastric accommodation

KEY POINTS

- Symptoms of gastroparesis go beyond delay in gastric emptying.
- There is significant overlap between idiopathic gastroparesis and functional dyspepsia in terms of symptoms and pathophysiology.
- Abdominal pain is an under-recognized symptom of gastroparesis that is associated with decreased quality of life.

Gastroparesis is a heterogeneous disorder defined as delayed gastric emptying in the absence of a mechanical obstruction. Symptoms of gastroparesis include nausea, vomiting, bloating, early satiety, and/or abdominal pain.[1]

ETIOLOGIES OF GASTROPARESIS

The most common forms of gastroparesis are idiopathic, diabetic, and postsurgical.[2] In earlier studies, idiopathic gastroparesis comprised approximately 35% of all gastroparetic patients. However, a larger multicenter study found that 67% of patients had idiopathic gastroparesis.[3] Additionally, other conditions can lead to gastroparesis (**Table 1**). Independent of etiology, gastroparesis affects women more commonly than men.

CLINICAL MANIFESTATIONS

Symptoms of gastroparesis are variable and include nausea, vomiting, early satiety, bloating, postprandial fullness, abdominal pain/discomfort, and anorexia (**Table 2**).[1–4] However, despite its prevalence in gastroparesis, consensus publications have traditionally not considered pain as a predominant factor.[1] Additionally, there is significant overlap between symptoms of gastroparesis and functional dyspepsia. In a recent

This article originally appeared in Gastroenterology Clinics, Volume 44, Issue 1, March 2015.
Disclosures: None.
[a] Division of Gastroenterology, Department of Medicine, Stanford University, 900 Blake Wilbur Drive, 2nd Floor, Palo Alto, CA 94305, USA; [b] Division of Gastroenterology, Department of Medicine, California Pacific Medical Center, 2340 Clay Street, Suite 210, San Francisco, CA 94115, USA
* Corresponding authors.
E-mail addresses: nguyenLB@stanford.edu; snapew@sutterhealth.org

Clinics Collections 7 (2015) 263–272
http://dx.doi.org/10.1016/j.ccol.2015.06.018

Table 1 Etiologies of gastroparesis			
Etiology	N = 146	%	Female (%)
Idiopathic Postviral	52 (12)	35.6 (8.2)	90.4
Diabetes	42	28.8	76.2
Postsurgical	19	13.0	73.7
Parkinson disease	11	7.5	81.8
Collagen vascular disease Scleroderma Systemic lupus erythematosus Raynaud	7	4.8	85.7
Intestinal pseudo-obstruction	6	4.1	66.7
Miscellaneous Stiffman syndrome Charcot-Marie-Tooth syndrome Wardenburg syndrome Superior mesenteric artery syndrome Median arcuate ligament syndrome Paraneoplastic syndrome Systemic mastocytosis	9	6.2	55.6

Data from Soykan I, Sivri B, Saroseik I, et al. Demography, clinical characteristics, psychological and abuse profiles, treatment, and long-term follow-up of patients with gastroparesis. Dig Dis Sci 1998;43(11):2398–404.

multicenter study, 86% of patients with idiopathic gastroparesis met Rome III criteria for functional dyspepsia.[5] Likewise, delayed gastric emptying has been found to present in 23% to 33% of patients with functional dyspepsia.[6,7] Many of the patients had a previous cholecystectomy prior to the diagnosis of gastroparesis.[8] Cholecystectomy was more common in patients with type 2 diabetes and idiopathic gastroparesis than in patients with type 1 diabetes. Patients who had a cholecystectomy had a higher prevalence of comorbidities including chronic fatigue, fibromyalgia, depression, and anxiety. These symptoms led to a worse quality of life.

Patients with type 1 diabetes mellitus had increased vomiting and retching, whereas the idiopathic gastroparesis group had increased prevalence of early satiety, postprandial fullness, and abdominal pain (**Table 3**).

Table 2 Gastroparesis symptom prevalence	
Symptom	%
Nausea	80–92
Vomiting	66–84
Bloating	55–75
Early satiety	54–60
Abdominal pain	46–68

Data from Soykan I, Sivri B, Saroseik I, et al. Demography, clinical characteristics, psychological and abuse profiles, treatment, and long-term follow-up of patients with gastroparesis. Dig Dis Sci 1998;43(11):2398–404; and Parkman H, Yates K, Hasler WL, et al. Similarities and differences between diabetic and idiopathic gastroparesis. Clin Gastroenterol Hepatol 2011;9(12):1056–64.

Table 3
Symptom pattern—idiopathic versus diabetic gastroparesis

Symptom	Idiopathic (%)	Type 1 DM (%)	Type 2 DM (%)
Nausea	84.3	84.6	94.9[a]
Vomiting	59.8	88.5[a]	91.5[a]
Bloating	57.5	56.4	62.7
Early satiety	57.5	47.4	74.6[a]
Abdominal pain	76.0	60.3[a]	69.5
Weight loss	46.5	52.6	52.5

[a] $P<.05$ when compared with idiopathic gastroparesis.
Data from Parkman H, Yates K, Hasler WL, et al. Similarities and differences between diabetic and idiopathic gastroparesis. Clin Gastroenterol Hepatol 2011;9(12):1056–64.

Not all patients with chronic nausea and vomiting have a delay in gastric emptying.[9] The Gastroparesis Registry enrolled 106 patients (25%) with normal emptying and chronic nausea and vomiting. The symptoms in patients with normal gastric emptying, including nausea, vomiting and abdominal pain, had a similar severity as in patients with delayed gastric emptying. The majority of patients in either the normal or delayed gastric emptying group satisfied Rome III criteria for functional dyspepsia. Both groups remained equally symptomatic at 48-week follow-up.

In addition to nausea and vomiting, abdominal pain is a major symptom in patients with gastroparesis.[10] Abdominal pain often has been an overlooked symptom in patients with gastroparesis. Classical teaching dictates that patients with pain predominance should undergo additional evaluation for other causes. This in part may be due to the overlap between idiopathic gastroparesis and functional dyspepsia and the broad differential diagnoses for abdominal pain. However, in a large multicenter cohort study, the prevalence of moderate-to-severe abdominal pain (approximately 60%) was similar between patients with idiopathic and diabetic gastroparesis.[10] In this study, 20% of patients with gastroparesis reported pain predominance compared with 44% reporting nausea/vomiting predominance. The presence of pain predominance was associated with decreased quality of life and increased depression and anxiety. The delay in gastric emptying was similar in patients with predominant pain and predominant nausea and vomiting. Moderate-to-severe abdominal pain was more prevalent in idiopathic gastroparesis and in those patients who did not have an infectious prodrome. Compared with patients with predominant nausea/vomiting, the patients with pain had greater use of opiates and less use of antiemetics.

MEASURES OF SYMPTOM SEVERITY

The Patient Assessment of Upper Gastrointestinal Disorders Symptoms (PAGI-SYM) was developed to assess symptom severity of upper gastrointestinal (GI) symptoms in patients with gastroesophageal reflux disease (GERD), dyspepsia, and gastroparesis.[11] The PAGI-SYM consists of 20 questions and 6 subscales: heartburn/regurgitation, nausea/vomiting, postprandial fullness/early satiety, bloating, upper abdominal pain, and lower abdominal pain. The subscale scores are calculated by taking the mean of the items in each of the subscales.

The Gastroparesis Cardinal Symptom Index (GCSI) is derived from the PAGI-SYM and validated as a tool to assess patient-derived symptom severity in patients with upper gut symptoms.[12] Based on review of the literature, physician interviews, and patient focus groups, the GCSI was constructed with 9 items that categorized gastroparesis into 3 subscales: nausea/vomiting, postprandial fullness/early satiety, and bloating. The purpose of the GCSI is to provide a patient-reported tool that can be used in clinical trials to assess patient responses to therapy. However, the GCSI does not address the impact of pain on treatment outcomes.

Psychological dysfunction is associated with increased severity of symptoms as measured with the Beck Depression Inventory and the State–Trait Anxiety Inventory.[13] All 3 indexes were greater for GCSI scores greater than 3.1. The measures of psychological dysfunction were not different for diabetic or idiopathic gastroparesis and were not related to the severity of gastric retention. Nausea, vomiting, bloating, and postprandial fullness were increased in patients with higher depression or anxiety inventories.

NORMAL GASTRIC MOTOR FUNCTION

Normal GI function depends on a complex coordination between smooth muscles of the gastric fundus, antrum, pylorus, and duodenum under the control of the enteric (intrinsic) and central (extrinsic) nervous systems. Central nervous system control of digestion is mediated through the autonomic nervous system. Parasympathetic control is mediated through the vagus, while sympathetic control is mediated through the spinal cord at T5 to T10 via the celiac ganglia.[14] Vagal efferents arise from the dorsal motor nucleus and terminate in the myenteric plexus. The vagus effects gastric motility indirectly via the enteric nervous system rather than direct innervation of gastric smooth muscles.

Distention of the antrum by a solid meal triggers the fundus to relax to store food as the rest of the meal enters the stomach.[15] This accommodation response effectively increases the gastric volume without raising the intragastric pressure. Tonic contractions of the proximal stomach transfer food to the gastric antrum, where high amplitude contractions break down the food into particles 1 to 2 mm in size through trituration.[16] These particles are able to pass through the pylorus into the duodenum. Particles greater than 2 mm that cannot pass the pylorus during the postprandial phase are cleared during the interdigestive period by phase 3 of the migrating motor complexes (MMCs), which are cyclical contractions of the antrum and small bowel that propel undigestable solids distally.[17]

Motor dysfunction anywhere in the stomach may delay gastric emptying.

PATHOPHYSIOLOGY OF DELAYED GASTRIC EMPTYING
Impaired Gastric Accommodation

Regulation of proximal gastric tone and accommodation is vagally mediated through activation of nonadrenergic, noncholinergic myenteric neurons that release nitric oxide (NO).[18,19] NO produced by neuronal NO synthase in nitregic neurons diffuses to the smooth muscle cells and inhibits gastric tone via guanosine $3',5'$-cyclic monophospate (cGMP).[15] Inhibition of cholinergic pathways can also increase gastric accommodation. There are presynaptic inhibitory α2-adrenoceptors and 5-HT1A receptors on cholinergic neurons in the stomach.[20] Disruption of these can lead to impaired gastric accommodation. The impaired accommodation may increase sensory afferent input into the chemoreceptor's trigger zone, causing nausea and vomiting.

Antral Hypomotility

The antrum is responsible for the trituration and emptying of solid foods from the stomach.[16] Postprandial antral hypomotility occurs in 70% of patients with unexplained nausea and vomiting[21] and 46% of patients with delayed gastric emptying.[22]

The presence of acute hyperglycemia is associated with antral hypomotility, especially at glucose levels of at least 250 mg/dL, but it can occur at levels as low as 140 mg/dL.[23]

Pylorospasm

In a preliminary study, 58% of DM patients had elevated pyloric tone,[24] which correlates with the number of patients who had improvement in symptoms and gastric emptying at 2 and 6 weeks after injection of botulinum toxin.[24–26] These studies suggest that pyloric pressure, including both tonic and phasic contractions, can be elevated in patients with gastroparesis. However, double-blind trials, which may have been underpowered, did not demonstrate improvement in symptoms in patients with gastroparesis.[27,28]

Duodenal Dysmotility

Coordination of antral and duodenal contractions is important in gastric emptying.[29] In this study of 12 patients with gastroparesis, simultaneous gastric emptying scintigraphy and antropyloroduodenal manometry found that postprandial coordination of antroduodenal contractions was impaired. Cisapride stimulated increased frequency of coordinated antroduodenal contractions that was associated with faster gastric emptying.

Autonomic Dysfunction

Dysfunction of the autonomic nervous system, including the parasympathetic and sympathetic systems, may contribute to gastroparesis. Vagal afferents convey sensory signals from the upper GI tract to the central nervous system (CNS). Vagal efferents mediate smooth muscle contraction and motility. Patients with orthostatic intolerance frequently have chronic GI complaints, most commonly abdominal pain, nausea, and vomiting.[30] However, the nausea often resolves with treatment of the orthostasis. Autonomic dysfunction can cause symptoms by altering either afferent or efferent pathways.

Visceral Hypersensitivity

Gastric sensation is mediated by mechano- and chemoreceptors in the stomach that transmit signals to the CNS.[31] Mechanosensitivity can be studied using the gastric barostat, which can deliver isobaric or isovolumetric distentions of the stomach during fasting or postprandially. Visceral hypersensitivity or a lowered gastric sensory threshold can be measured using the gastric barostat. The presence of visceral hypersensitivity has been described in functional dyspepsia.[19] Similarly, in a small study of patients with diabetic gastroparesis, 55% demonstrated hypersensitivity to pressure distention during fasting, while all patients exhibited hypersensitivity to distention in the postprandial state.[32]

PATHOPHYSIOLOGY OF SYMPTOMS

There is poor correlation between severity of gastroparesis symptoms and the degree of delayed gastric emptying.[33–35] Additionally, changes in gastric emptying correlated poorly with symptom response in treatment trials.[36–38] It is postulated that the presence of visceral hypersensitivity and/or impaired gastric accommodation may explain part of this disparity.

Because of the vague and heterogeneous nature of symptoms, classifying patients based on symptom predominance was proposed, in hopes of providing a framework for treating gastroparesis symptoms and gaining a better understanding of the pathophysiology. A study validating the classification of gastroparesis subgroups (**Table 4**)

Table 4
Definition of symptom subtypes

Symptom Subtype	Definition of Most Bothersome Symptom(s)
Nausea/vomiting predominant	Nausea, vomiting and/or retching
Pain/dyspepsia predominant	Upper abdominal pain/discomfort or fullness
Regurgitation predominant	Effortless regurgitation of food or heartburn

Data from Harrell S, Studts JL, Dryden GW, et al. A novel classification scheme for gastroparesis based on predominant-symptom presentation. J Clin Gastroenterol 2008;42(5):455–9; and Hasler W, Wilson LA, Parkman HP, et al. Factors related to abdominal pain in gastroparesis: contrast to patients with predominant nausea and vomiting. Neurogastroenterol Motil 2013;25(5):427–38.

found that there was concordance between patient and physician classifications. Additionally, when comparing symptom predominance with a validated 20-item symptom severity questionnaire (PAGI-SYM), there was good correlation between vomiting predominance with the nausea/vomiting subscale and regurgitation predominance with the heartburn/regurgitation subscale. However, the dyspepsia predominant group did not correlate well with any of the PAGI-SYM subscales.[39] This study also found that regurgitation predominant patients were heavier than the other 2 groups, while vomiting predominant patients were younger.

Nausea and Vomiting

Nausea and vomiting are the most common symptoms in patients with gastroparesis, with over 40% of patients reporting that these are the most bothersome symptoms.[10] However, the pathogenesis of these symptoms is heterogeneous and often multifactorial.

Centrally, the receptor site for vomiting is located in the area postrema at the base of the fourth ventricle (chemoreceptor trigger zone). Peripheral receptor sites include the vagus and vestibular apparatus. Stimulation of vagal afferents triggers emesis.[40]

Early Satiety/Fullness

Early satiety and fullness are common symptoms among patients with idiopathic and diabetic gastroparesis, especially those with type 2 diabetes.[3] Impaired gastric accommodation has been found in 43% of patients with idiopathic gastroparesis, and it contributes to patients' inability to complete eating a normal meal.[35] In this group of patients, symptoms of early satiety and weight loss were more prevalent. Similarly, impaired gastric accommodation was found in 40% of patients with functional dyspepsia.[41] A smaller study of 10 diabetic gastroparesis patients who were refractory to prokinetic therapy found that 90% of patients had impaired gastric accommodation.[32]

Several medications have been shown to increase gastric accommodation in healthy subjects as well as patients with functional dyspepsia (see **Table 5**). Moreover,

Table 5
Medications that stimulate gastric accommodation

Medication	Mechanism of Action
Sildenafil[43]	Phosphodiesterase inhibitor
Paroxetine[44]	Selective serotonin reuptake inhibitor
Cisapride[45]	5-HT4 agonist, 5-HT3 antagonist
Tegaserod[46]	Partial 5-HT4 agonist
Clonidine[20]	α2-adrenoceptor agonist
Buspirone[47]	5-HT1A agonist

Table 6 Mechanisms of bloating	
Functional Gastrointestinal Disorder	**Pathophysiology**
Functional dyspepsia[51]	Abnormal intragastric distribution of food to the distal half of the stomach
IBS with visible distention[52]	Lower sensory threshold
IBS-C[53]	Delayed colonic and/or orocecal transit

buspirone also resulted in improvement in functional dyspepsia symptoms, notably postprandial fullness, bloating, and early satiety.[42]

Bloating

Bloating is a common symptom among functional GI disorders (**Table 6**) including gastroparesis, irritable bowel syndrome (IBS), and functional dyspepsia.[48] There is no association between rate of gastric emptying and severity of bloating.[49] The presence of bloating is associated with a poor response to medical therapy.[50] A large multicenter study including 335 patients found bloating was present in 76% of patients with gastroparesis, with 41% suffering severe symptoms.[49] This study also found an association between use of norepinephrine reuptake inhibitors (predominantly tricyclic antidepressants) and minimal symptoms of bloating.

Abdominal Pain

Although a common feature of gastroparesis, abdominal pain studies have consistently shown that the severity of pain does not correlate with the severity of the delay in gastric emptying.[10,35] Patient defined pain predominance was found in approximately 20% of patients referred to the NIDDK (National Institute of Diabetes and Digestive and Kidney Diseases) Gastroparesis Clinical Research Consortium.[10]

Visceral hypersensitivity, defined as lowered threshold for eliciting visceral pain, is common among functional GI disorders, including functional dyspepsia and IBS. The presence of visceral hypersensitivity was found in 29% of patients with idiopathic gastroparesis[35] and 55% of patients with diabetic gastroparesis.[32] The presence of hypersensitivity to intragastric balloon distention was associated with a higher prevalence of abdominal pain, early satiety, and weight loss. Among these patients, the presence of hypersensitivity was also associated with greater symptom severity.

SUMMARY

There is significant overlap between idiopathic gastroparesis and functional dyspepsia in terms of symptoms and pathophysiology. This suggests that idiopathic gastroparesis and functional dyspepsia are on a spectrum a single disorder. Once thought to be a minor aspect of gastroparesis, abdominal pain is common and associated with decreased quality of life. Approximately 20% of patients describe pain as their predominant symptom. Patients with a severe delay in gastric emptying have a greater correlation between emptying and symptoms. Patients with less severe delays in emptying may benefit in classification by symptom to direct therapy.

REFERENCES

1. Parkman HP, Hasler WL, Fisher RS. American Gastroenterological Association medical position statement: diagnosis and treatment of gastroparesis. Gastroenterology 2004;127(5):1589–91.

2. Soykan I, Sivri B, Sarosiek I, et al. Demography, clinical characteristics, psychological and abuse profiles, treatment, and long-term follow-up of patients with gastroparesis. Dig Dis Sci 1998;43(11):2398–404.

3. Parkman HP, Yates K, Hasler WL, et al. Similarities and differences between diabetic and idiopathic gastroparesis. Clin Gastroenterol Hepatol 2011;9(12): 1056–64 [quiz: e133–4].

4. Hoogerwerf WA, Pasricha PJ, Kalloo AN, et al. Pain: the overlooked symptom in gastroparesis. Am J Gastroenterol 1999;94(4):1029–33.

5. Parkman HP, Yates K, Hasler WL, et al. Clinical features of idiopathic gastroparesis vary with sex, body mass, symptom onset, delay in gastric emptying, and gastroparesis severity. Gastroenterology 2011;140(1):101–15.

6. Sarnelli G, Caenepeel P, Geypens B, et al. Symptoms associated with impaired gastric emptying of solids and liquids in functional dyspepsia. Am J Gastroenterol 2003;98(4):783–8.

7. Stanghellini V, Tosetti C, Paternico A, et al. Risk indicators of delayed gastric emptying of solids in patients with functional dyspepsia. Gastroenterology 1996;110(4):1036–42.

8. Parkman HP, Yates K, Hasler WL, et al. Cholecystectomy and clinical presentations of gastroparesis. Dig Dis Sci 2013;58(4):1062–73.

9. Pasricha PJ, Colvin R, Yates K, et al. Characteristics of patients with chronic unexplained nausea and vomiting and normal gastric emptying. Clin Gastroenterol Hepatol 2011;9(7):567–76.e1-4.

10. Hasler WL, Wilson LA, Parkman HP, et al. Factors related to abdominal pain in gastroparesis: contrast to patients with predominant nausea and vomiting. Neurogastroenterol Motil 2013;25(5):427–38.

11. Rentz AM, Kahrilas P, Stanghellini V, et al. Development and psychometric evaluation of the patient assessment of upper gastrointestinal symptom severity index (PAGI-SYM) in patients with upper gastrointestinal disorders. Qual Life Res 2004; 13(10):1737–49.

12. Revicki DA, Rentz AM, Dubois D, et al. Development and validation of a patient-assessed gastroparesis symptom severity measure: the gastroparesis cardinal symptom index. Aliment Pharmacol Ther 2003;18(1):141–50.

13. Hasler WL, Parkman HP, Wilson LA, et al. Psychological dysfunction is associated with symptom severity but not disease etiology or degree of gastric retention in patients with gastroparesis. Am J Gastroenterol 2010;105(11):2357–67.

14. Wood JD, Alpers DH, Andrews PL. Fundamentals of neurogastroenterology. Gut 1999;45(Suppl 2):II6–16.

15. Kindt S, Tack J. Impaired gastric accommodation and its role in dyspepsia. Gut 2006;55(12):1685–91.

16. Camilleri M, Malagelada JR, Brown ML, et al. Relation between antral motility and gastric emptying of solids and liquids in humans. Am J Physiol 1985;249(5 Pt 1): G580–5.

17. Takahashi T. Interdigestive migrating motor complex -its mechanism and clinical importance. J Smooth Muscle Res 2013;49:99–111.

18. Azpiroz F. Control of gastric emptying by gastric tone. Dig Dis Sci 1994;39(Suppl 12):18S–9S.

19. Carbone F, Tack J. Gastroduodenal mechanisms underlying functional gastric disorders. Dig Dis 2014;32(3):222–9.

20. Thumshirn M, Camilleri M, Choi MG, et al. Modulation of gastric sensory and motor functions by nitrergic and alpha2-adrenergic agents in humans. Gastroenterology 1999;116(3):573–85.

21. Kerlin P. Postprandial antral hypomotility in patients with idiopathic nausea and vomiting. Gut 1989;30(1):54–9.
22. Camilleri M, Brown ML, Malagelada JR. Relationship between impaired gastric emptying and abnormal gastrointestinal motility. Gastroenterology 1986;91(1): 94–9.
23. Barnett JL, Owyang C. Serum glucose concentration as a modulator of interdigestive gastric motility. Gastroenterology 1988;94(3):739–44.
24. Mearin F, Camilleri M, Malagelada JR. Pyloric dysfunction in diabetics with recurrent nausea and vomiting. Gastroenterology 1986;90(6):1919–25.
25. Ezzeddine D, Jit R, Katz N, et al. Pyloric injection of botulinum toxin for treatment of diabetic gastroparesis. Gastrointest Endosc 2002;55(7):920–3.
26. Miller LS, Szych GA, Kantor SB, et al. Treatment of idiopathic gastroparesis with injection of botulinum toxin into the pyloric sphincter muscle. Am J Gastroenterol 2002;97(7):1653–60.
27. Arts J, Holvoet L, Caenepeel P, et al. Clinical trial: a randomized-controlled crossover study of intrapyloric injection of botulinum toxin in gastroparesis. Aliment Pharmacol Ther 2007;26(9):1251–8.
28. Friedenberg FK, Palit A, Parkman HP, et al. Botulinum toxin A for the treatment of delayed gastric emptying. Am J Gastroenterol 2008;103(2):416–23.
29. Fraser RJ, Horowitz M, Maddox AF, et al. Postprandial antropyloroduodenal motility and gastric emptying in gastroparesis–effects of cisapride. Gut 1994; 35(2):172–8.
30. Sullivan SD, Hanauer J, Rowe PC, et al. Gastrointestinal symptoms associated with orthostatic intolerance. J Pediatr Gastroenterol Nutr 2005;40(4):425–8.
31. Camilleri M, Coulie B, Tack JF. Visceral hypersensitivity: facts, speculations, and challenges. Gut 2001;48(1):125–31.
32. Kumar A, Attaluri A, Hashmi S, et al. Visceral hypersensitivity and impaired accommodation in refractory diabetic gastroparesis. Neurogastroenterol Motil 2008;20(6):635–42.
33. Horowitz M, Su YC, Rayner CK, et al. Gastroparesis: prevalence, clinical significance and treatment. Can J Gastroenterol 2001;15(12):805–13.
34. Talley NJ, Verlinden M, Jones M. Can symptoms discriminate among those with delayed or normal gastric emptying in dysmotility-like dyspepsia? Am J Gastroenterol 2001;96(5):1422–8.
35. Karamanolis G, Caenepeel P, Arts J, et al. Determinants of symptom pattern in idiopathic severely delayed gastric emptying: gastric emptying rate or proximal stomach dysfunction? Gut 2007;56(1):29–36.
36. Talley NJ, Verlinden M, Snape W, et al. Failure of a motilin receptor agonist (ABT-229) to relieve the symptoms of functional dyspepsia in patients with and without delayed gastric emptying: a randomized double-blind placebo-controlled trial. Aliment Pharmacol Ther 2000;14(12):1653–61.
37. Silvers D, Kipnes M, Broadstone V, et al. Domperidone in the management of symptoms of diabetic gastroparesis: efficacy, tolerability, and quality-of-life outcomes in a multicenter controlled trial. DOM-USA-5 Study Group. Clin Ther 1998;20(3):438–53.
38. Arts J, Caenepeel P, Verbeke K, et al. Influence of erythromycin on gastric emptying and meal related symptoms in functional dyspepsia with delayed gastric emptying. Gut 2005;54(4):455–60.
39. Harrell SP, Studts JL, Dryden GW, et al. A novel classification scheme for gastroparesis based on predominant-symptom presentation. J Clin Gastroenterol 2008; 42(5):455–9.

40. Urayama Y, Yamada Y, Nakamura E, et al. Electrical and chemical stimulation of the nucleus raphe magnus inhibits induction of retching by afferent vagal fibers. Auton Neurosci 2010;152(1–2):35–40.
41. Tack J, Piessevaux H, Coulie B, et al. Role of impaired gastric accommodation to a meal in functional dyspepsia. Gastroenterology 1998;115(6):1346–52.
42. Tack J, Janssen P, Masaoka T, et al. Efficacy of buspirone, a fundus-relaxing drug, in patients with functional dyspepsia. Clin Gastroenterol Hepatol 2012; 10(11):1239–45.
43. Sarnelli G, Sifrim D, Janssens J, et al. Influence of sildenafil on gastric sensori-motor function in humans. Am J Physiol Gastrointest Liver Physiol 2004;287(5): G988–92.
44. Tack J, Broekaert D, Coulie B, et al. Influence of the selective serotonin re-uptake inhibitor, paroxetine, on gastric sensorimotor function in humans. Aliment Pharmacol Ther 2003;17(4):603–8.
45. Tack J, Broekaert D, Coulie B, et al. The influence of cisapride on gastric tone and the perception of gastric distension. Aliment Pharmacol Ther 1998;12(8):761–6.
46. Tack J, Janssen P, Bisschops R, et al. Influence of tegaserod on proximal gastric tone and on the perception of gastric distention in functional dyspepsia. Neurogastroenterol Motil 2011;23(2):e32–9.
47. Van Oudenhove L, Kindt S, Vos R, et al. Influence of buspirone on gastric sensorimotor function in man. Aliment Pharmacol Ther 2008;28(11–12):1326–33.
48. Jiang X, Locke GR 3rd, Choung RS, et al. Prevalence and risk factors for abdominal bloating and visible distention: a population-based study. Gut 2008;57(6): 756–63.
49. Hasler WL, Wilson LA, Parkman HP, et al. Bloating in gastroparesis: severity, impact, and associated factors. Am J Gastroenterol 2011;106(8):1492–502.
50. Anaparthy R, Pehlivanov N, Grady J, et al. Gastroparesis and gastroparesis-like syndrome: response to therapy and its predictors. Dig Dis Sci 2009;54(5): 1003–10.
51. Troncon LE, Bennett RJ, Ahluwalia NK, et al. Abnormal intragastric distribution of food during gastric emptying in functional dyspepsia patients. Gut 1994;35(3): 327–32.
52. Agrawal A, Houghton LA, Lea R, et al. Bloating and distention in irritable bowel syndrome: the role of visceral sensation. Gastroenterology 2008;134(7):1882–9.
53. Agrawal A, Houghton LA, Reilly B, et al. Bloating and distension in irritable bowel syndrome: the role of gastrointestinal transit. Am J Gastroenterol 2009;104(8): 1998–2004.

Other Forms of Gastroparesis
Postsurgical, Parkinson, Other Neurologic Diseases, Connective Tissue Disorders

Eamonn M.M. Quigley, MD, FRCP, FRCPI

KEYWORDS

- Gastroparesis • Parkinson disease • Multiple sclerosis • Motor neuron disease
- Neurologic • Post-surgical • Fundoplication • Scleroderma

KEY POINTS

- Fundoplication, bariatric procedures, and pancreatic surgeries are nowadays the surgical approaches most commonly complicated by gastroparesis.
- Virtually any neurologic disorder may be complicated by gastroparesis, and its development may affect nutrition and drug availability.
- Gastroparesis is a common feature of gastrointestinal involvement in scleroderma and other connective tissue disorders.

POSTSURGICAL GASTROPARESIS

Although acute gastroparesis may be a component of the ileus syndrome that can complicate many surgical procedures and of the acute pseudo-obstruction syndrome that may accompany severe sepsis and multiorgan failure, this review focuses on chronic manifestations of gastric dysmotility.[1] In contrast to chronic gastroparesis, whose pathophysiology is often poorly understood, inflammatory processes seem fundamental to the inhibition of motility in the acute form.

Gastroparesis and other disorders of gastric sensorimotor function may complicate specific surgical procedures.[2] In the important Olmstead County study of the community prevalence of gastroparesis, 7.2% of all cases of definite gastroparesis were related to prior gastrectomy or fundoplication.[3] Rates of postsurgical gastroparesis vary widely depending on many factors, including the site and nature of the surgical procedure. For example, in their comprehensive review, Dong and colleagues[4] noted that rates ranged from 0.4% to 5% following gastrectomy, from 20% to 50% after

This article originally appeared in Gastroenterology Clinics, Volume 44, Issue 1, March 2015.
The author has nothing to disclose.
Division of Gastroenterology and Hepatology, Houston Methodist Hospital, Well Cornell Medical College, 6550 Fannin Street, SM 1001, Houston, TX 77030, USA
E-mail address: equigley@tmhs.org

Clinics Collections 7 (2015) 273–285
http://dx.doi.org/10.1016/j.ccol.2015.06.019

pylorus-preserving pancreaticoduodenectomy, and from 50% to 70% after cryoablation therapy for pancreatic cancer.

Vagotomy

Although vagotomy is infrequently performed nowadays in the management of acid-peptic disease, inadvertent vagal injury may complicate other interventions, rendering an understanding of the complex effects of vagotomy on gastric motor function still relevant. Receptive relaxation, a vagally mediated reflex, is impaired. As a consequence, the early phase of liquid emptying is accelerated. This acceleration causes rapid emptying of hyperosmolar solutions into the proximal small intestine and may result in the early dumping syndrome. By contrast, and as a consequence of impaired antropyloric function, the later phases of liquid and solid emptying are prolonged by vagotomy. Other motor effects of vagotomy include an impairment of the motor response to feeding (which contributes to the pathophysiologic mechanisms of postvagotomy diarrhea) and a suppression of the antral component of the migrating motor complex. The latter phenomenon is particularly prevalent among individuals who have symptomatic postvagotomy gastroparesis.

The now standard addition of a drainage procedure, such as a pyloroplasty or gastroenterostomy, has tended to negate the effects of vagotomy alone. In most patients, the net result of the combined procedure is little alteration in the gastric emptying of liquids or solids. Thus, prolonged postoperative gastroparesis (ie, lasting longer than 3–4 weeks) is, in fact, rare (<2.5% of patients after either vagotomy and pyloroplasty or vagotomy and antrectomy).[5] Significant postoperative gastroparesis may occur, however, in patients who have a prior history of prolonged gastric outlet obstruction. In this circumstance, normal gastric emptying may not return for several weeks.

Longitudinal studies suggest that vagotomy-related gastroparesis tends to resolve over time, with one study suggesting gastric emptying rates in those who had undergone either a truncal or a highly selective vagotomy being similar by 12 months after the procedure.[6]

Persisting postsurgical gastric motor dysfunction often presents a formidable management challenge. Therapeutic responses to prokinetic agents have proved particularly disappointing in this group. In these resistant cases, a completion gastrectomy may be the best alternative. It should be noted, however, that in one large series this approach was deemed successful in only 43% of patients.[7]

Gastrectomy

Antral resection by removing the antral mill renders the stomach incontinent to solids and leads to accelerated emptying, and symptomatic "dumping" may occur in up to 50% of patients after Billroth I or II gastrectomy.[8] Late dumping symptoms occur 90 to 120 minutes after a meal and are a consequence of reactive hypoglycemia. The accommodation reflex is impaired among symptomatic patients.[9] By contrast, delayed gastric emptying sometimes occurs after a Billroth II gastrectomy as a result of a large atonic gastric remnant.[8] Meng and colleagues[10] reported a 6.9% frequency of gastroparesis among 563 patients who underwent radical gastrectomy for gastric cancer in their unit in Shanghai, China. Preoperative gastric outlet obstruction and the performance of a Billroth II anastomosis were the principal risk factors for the occurrence of gastroparesis. Of note, they documented a similar rate of gastroparesis (3.7%) among a smaller group of patients who underwent a laparoscopic gastrectomy.[10] Laparoscopy-assisted, pylorus-preserving gastrectomy represents a less radical operative approach to early gastric cancer; gastric stasis is the most common complication of this procedure, occurring in 6.2% of cases.[11] In one series, and in contrast to the aforementioned experience with this procedure following vagotomy, completion gastrectomy resulted in significant symptomatic improvement among subjects with postgastrectomy gastroparesis.[12]

Roux-en-Y Syndrome

The creation of a Roux-en-Y gastroenterostomy may be associated with a specific clinical entity, the Roux syndrome.[13] Severe symptoms of postprandial abdominal pain, bloating, and nausea many develop. Studies have variably described impaired gastric motor function[14] and a functional obstruction within the duodenal Roux limb as a result of motor asynchrony.[13,15] The latter can be revealed by manometry, but the status of these motility patterns in the pathophysiologic processes of this syndrome remains unclear.[16]

Pancreatectomy

Pancreatectomy and pylorus-preserving pancreaticoduodenectomy, in particular, have been associated with a high incidence of postoperative gastric stasis. The principal predictor of gastric emptying delay after these operations is the occurrence of other postoperative complications.[17,18] Operative technique seems, in general, to be of less importance, although there is a suggestion that an antecolic anastomosis may be associated with less emptying delay. Accordingly in what has been, perhaps, the largest series (N = 711) to date, Parmar and colleagues[19] documented an overall rate of delayed gastric emptying following pancreaticoduodenectomy of 20%. The occurrence of gastroparesis did not seem to be influenced by such technical factors as pylorus preservation or whether the gastrojejunostomy was antecolic or retrocolic, but was associated with fistula formation, postoperative sepsis, and reoperation. These results contrast with those of a prior systematic review, which found that antecolic reconstruction was linked to lower rates of gastroparesis.[20] Furthermore, others have suggested that the use of a Billroth II rather than a gastrojejunostomy for reconstruction following this procedure may reduce the risk of gastric emptying delay.[21] Preoperative diabetes has been identified as an additional risk factor.[22] Gastroparesis has also been reported following pancreas transplantation.[23]

Antireflux Operations

The physiology of the lower esophageal sphincter and the proximal stomach are intimately related in health; it should come as no surprise, therefore, that a variety of antireflux procedures can influence gastric sensorimotor function.[24] Fundoplication, as expected, affects sensorimotor function of the proximal stomach.[25–27] Most, but not all,[28] studies have demonstrated impaired relaxation of the proximal stomach, in response to meal ingestion, following this surgical procedure. Although the usual effect of fundoplication is to accelerate, rather than delay, gastric emptying,[26] instances of gastroparesis have been described following antireflux surgery and endoscopic antireflux procedures.[29] Given the high frequency with which the procedure is now performed, it should come as no surprise that Nissen fundoplication was the most common cause of postsurgical gastroparesis in the audit performed by the National Institute of Diabetes and Digestive and Kidney Diseases gastroparesis consortium.[30] The pathophysiologic process leading to these occurrences is unclear. In some, postsurgical gastroparesis may represent the overt appearance of an unrecognized preoperative disorder; in others there is compelling evidence to incriminate vagal injury, which is especially likely in relation to redo procedures and may contribute to persistent gas-bloat symptoms.[31] In rare instances, postfundoplication gastroparesis may be persistent and severe. Although gastric resection does not seem to offer much help for these unfortunate patients,[32] some success has been reported with an approach that combines conversion to a partial fundoplication with a pyloroplasty.[33]

Bariatric Surgery

Ardila-Hani and Soffer[34] comprehensively reviewed the impact of bariatric (or metabolic) surgical procedures on gastrointestinal motor function. Esophageal problems were by far the most common. Gastric emptying did not appear to be affected by laparoscopic adjustable gastric banding and tended to accelerate following Roux-en-Y gastric bypass. However, instances of gastroparesis, at times severe and persistent, have been reported following the latter procedure. Salameh and colleagues,[35] for example, described successful treatment of 6 patients with intractable gastroparesis following Roux-en-Y gastric bypass for morbid obesity using gastric electrical stimulation. In an uncontrolled trial, endoscopic injection of the pylorus with botulinum toxin A produced symptomatic improvement in a small series of patients with postvagotomy gastroparesis, which was thought to result from fundoplication in the vast majority.[36]

Other Procedures

Virtually any procedure that could compromise the vagi or affect upper gastrointestinal motor function could result in gastroparesis. Clinically significant gastroparesis has, therefore, been reported not only in association with a wide range of gastric procedures but also in relation to esophageal resection,[37] botulinum toxin injection for achalasia,[38] lung transplantation, and even hepatic surgery. Sutcliffe and colleagues[37] noted a 12% rate of gastric emptying delay following esophagectomy in their series; in another report, gastroparesis was more common after minimally invasive than open esophagectomy.[39] Gastroparesis in relation to lung transplantation is especially ominous, as its presence preoperatively has been associated with an increased risk for the development of bronchiolitis obliterans syndrome.[40] Though common before surgery,[40] new-onset gastroparesis was documented in 6% of subjects after transplantation in one large series.[41] In the lung transplant patient gastroparesis may trigger or exacerbate gastroesophageal reflux, from which these patients have no protection. For this reason there is a low threshold for the performance of fundoplication in this patient population, and gastric electrical stimulation has been added to address concomitant gastroparesis.[42]

Although cholecystectomy, per se, has not been incriminated as a cause of gastroparesis,[43] a prior cholecystectomy seems to negatively affect the natural history of both diabetic and idiopathic gastroparesis.[44]

PARKINSON DISEASE AND OTHER NEUROLOGIC DISORDERS

As populations age the prevalence of neurologic disease in the community continues to increase, and consultations relating to gastrointestinal motility problems in the patient afflicted with a neurologic disorder become ever more common.

The high prevalence of gastroparesis and other disturbances of gut motor function in neurologic diseases is based on similarities in morphology and function between the neuromuscular apparatus of the gut and that of the somatic nervous system. First, it is now recognized that the enteric and central nervous systems share many similarities, both morphologic and functional. The basic organization of the enteric nervous system (ENS) (neurons, ganglia, glia, and ENS-blood barrier), and the ultrastructure of its components, are similar to those of the central nervous system (CNS), and almost all neurotransmitters identified within the CNS are also found in enteric neurons; the concept of ENS involvement in neurologic disease should not, therefore, come as a great surprise. Second, given the prevalence of dysfunction in the autonomic nervous system (an important modulator of enteric neuromuscular function) in several neurologic syndromes, in addition to the existence of several primary and secondary disorders of autonomic function, disturbed autonomic modulation of gut motor function may be an important contributory factor to symptomatology in some scenarios. Third, it is now evident that the gut has important sensory functions; though usually subconscious, gut sensation may be relayed to and perceived within the CNS. Sensory input is also fundamental to several reflex events in the gut, such as the viscerovisceral reflexes that coordinate function along the gut. However, the role of sensory dysfunction in the mediation of common symptoms, such as abdominal pain and nausea, in the patient with CNS disease with gastrointestinal manifestations has not been extensively investigated.

PATHOGENESIS OF GASTROINTESTINAL DYSFUNCTION IN NEUROLOGIC DISEASE

Although a whole range of disease processes affecting central, peripheral, and autonomic nervous systems may affect gut motor function, the 2 predominant neurologic disorders encountered in gastrointestinal practice are cerebrovascular disease and parkinsonism.

Cerebrovascular Disease

In contrast to swallowing function, gastric, small intestinal, colonic, and anorectal motor or sensory function have been little studied in the context of stroke and, therefore, the pathophysiology of complications involving these parts of the gastrointestinal tract is less clearly understood. Nevertheless, there is some indirect evidence to suggest that gastric emptying may be delayed following an acute stroke[45] and may have implications for feeding and drug administration.

Parkinson Disease

Idiopathic Parkinson disease (PD) causes widespread and sometimes severe derangement of gastrointestinal motility.[46–49] There are 2 basic contributors to gastrointestinal dysfunction in PD. First, striatal muscle dysfunction in the oropharynx, proximal esophagus, and anal canal is based on the same neurologic abnormalities that cause the cardinal manifestations of this disorder. The second component, namely dysfunction in the smooth muscle parts of the gastrointestinal tract, is less well understood but may reflect abnormality in the autonomic and/or enteric nervous systems.[50–53] Indeed, neuropathologic changes reminiscent of CNS Parkinson features, such as dopamine depletion[52] and the presence of Lewy neuritis[53] and α-synuclein,[54,55] has been demonstrated in the myenteric and submucosal plexi.

The pathophysiology of dysphagia and constipation in PD has received some attention, but little is known of the pathogenesis of symptoms arising from the stomach and small intestine, despite their high prevalence.[56] The contribution of autonomic dysfunction is illustrated by the higher prevalence of gastrointestinal symptoms and postural instability among patients with a PD variant, multiple system atrophy, in whom autonomic dysfunction is especially common.[57,58] For some symptoms, such as nausea, the contribution of antiparkinsonian medications and dopaminergics, in particular, must be borne in mind.

Delayed gastric emptying has been well documented in PD[59–65] and delayed emptying of solids has been linked, in some studies, to the severity of motor impairment.[60,62] Here again, the impact of levodopa must be accounted for.[62] The association between gastric emptying delay and the presence of levodopa response fluctuations,[61] coupled with irregular patterns of drug absorption[66] and the documentation of improved symptom control with intrajejunal[67] or transdermal[68] administration of antiparkinsonian drugs, underlines the potential clinical relevance of gastric emptying delay: by retarding drug delivery and absorption, gastroparesis could induce or further exacerbate response fluctuations. Several factors, however, limit the interpretation of reports of delayed gastric emptying and its association with upper gastrointestinal symptoms in PD.[60] These factors include variations in the patient population studied (eg, age, gender, disease severity, study location), the definition of gastroparesis, and the methodology used to assess the gastric emptying rate (meal, test technique, study protocol, and manner of interpretation). Variations between studies in these parameters make it very difficult to attempt real comparisons or draw firm conclusions. Nevertheless, delayed gastric emptying may occur in as many as 70% to 100% of PD patients attending specialist neurology clinics; the prevalence of symptomatic gastroparesis, in PD, however, remains unknown. Indeed, there has been a lack of a consistent correlation between gastric emptying rate and upper gastrointestinal symptoms in PD. While it is reasonable to assume that gastroparesis may contribute to the weight loss that has been so well documented in PD,[69] it is unclear as to whether nutrient delivery is affected by delayed gastric emptying, and a relationship between delayed gastric emptying and weight loss is yet to be demonstrated. Electrogastrography has also been used to study gastric motor activity in PD, but correlations with symptoms have been poor.[70,71] Parenthetically, it is of interest to note the suggestion that *Helicobacter pylori* and *Helicobacter heilmannii* infection are implicated in contributing to, not only gastrointestinal symptoms and weight loss in PD[72], but also systemic proinflammatory cytokine activation,[73] and even the pathogenesis of PD itself.[74]

Multiple Sclerosis

Delayed gastric emptying,[75] isolated cases of gastroparesis,[76–79] and even an instance of gastric perforation[80] have been reported in multiple sclerosis, with their cause attributed to autonomic dysfunction of central origin.[81] In one small series, parallel improvements in neurologic and gastric emptying function were documented in response to corticosteroid therapy.[79]

Autonomic and Peripheral Neuropathies

Given its ever increasing worldwide prevalence, diabetic autonomic neuropathy is by far the most common autonomic neuropathy encountered in clinical practice; diabetic gastroparesis is dealt with in detail by Koch and Calles-Escandón, elsewhere in this issue. Gastrointestinal involvement occurs to a variable extent in the many other types of autonomic peripheral neuropathies.[82] Upper gastrointestinal symptoms (early satiety, nausea and vomiting) are common in autoimmune autonomic neuropathies.[83]

Autonomic dysfunction is commonly detectable in Guillain-Barré syndrome (GBS) but is usually of minor clinical importance.[84] Delayed gastric emptying, gastroparesis, constipation, diarrhea, and fecal incontinence have all been described in GBS.[85] The gastrointestinal tract has a role in the pathogenesis of GBS; 15% to 40% of cases of GBS in the West have followed infection with *Campylobacter jejuni*.[86]

Muscle Disease

Myopathy and muscular dystrophy

Gastrointestinal involvement has been described in several muscular dystrophies,[87–90] but has been most extensively documented in myotonic dystrophy and Duchenne muscular dystrophy. Symptoms suggestive of gastroparesis, such as early satiety, nausea, vomiting, and epigastric pain, are common in myotonic dystrophy.[91,92] Of these, abdominal pain, dysphagia, vomiting, diarrhea, coughing while eating, and fecal incontinence were the most common in one survey[92]; up to 25% of patients consider gastrointestinal involvement as the most disabling feature of their disease.[93] Delayed gastric emptying and gastroparesis have indeed been well documented,[94–96] and instances of gastric volvulus described.[97] In Duchenne dystrophy, gastric motor dysfunction is an early feature,[98] resulting in hypomotility and gastroparesis,[99] which can be profound and result in acute gastroparesis and gastric dilatation.[100,101]

MANAGEMENT OF GASTROPARESIS IN PARKINSON DISEASE AND OTHER NEUROLOGIC DISORDERS

A multidisciplinary team (neurologist/neurosurgeon, gastroenterologist, nutritionist, therapist, specialist nurse), aware of the wishes and needs of the family and their carers, and mindful of the nature and the natural history of the underlying disease process, is best placed to assess and manage gastroparesis and other gastrointestinal problems in the patient with neurologic disease.

For the patient with PD and gastric emptying delay it is critical to avoid metoclopramide, in view of its central antidopaminergic effects; domperidone and mosapride, if available, may provide some potential therapeutic solutions. The main aim of pharmacologic therapy in correcting delayed gastric emptying in PD is primarily to reduce response fluctuations rather than deal with upper gastrointestinal symptoms. If pharmacologic approaches do not work, jejunal or transdermal delivery of L-dopa is an interesting option, although jejunal delivery may be technically challenging. The role of gastric electrical stimulation has not been defined in this population.

CONNECTIVE TISSUE DISORDERS

Gastroparesis and related symptoms may be prominent features of any disorder associated with autonomic neuropathy, and may also be components of both primary and secondary intestinal pseudo-obstruction syndromes. In scleroderma, one of the most common causes of pseudo-obstruction, gastroparesis is common, and gastric involvement tends to parallel that of the esophagus.[102] In the Olmstead County study, 10.8% of all cases of definite gastroparesis were associated with the presence of a connective tissue disorder.[2] In scleroderma, gastric involvement has been documented in anywhere from 10% to 75% of all patients and delayed gastric emptying in 50% to 75% of those with scleroderma who have gastrointestinal symptoms. Gastroparesis has important clinical consequences in scleroderma, including malnutrition and exacerbation of gastroesophageal reflux. The latter is of critical importance, given the predilection of these patients to severe and complicated reflux resulting from severe lower esophageal sphincter hypotension and markedly impaired esophageal peristaltic amplitude. Using the relatively noninvasive ^{13}C-octonoic acid breath test, Marie and colleagues[103] documented delayed gastric emptying in 47% of 57 consecutive scleroderma patients. Furthermore, they described a close correlation between a gastrointestinal symptom score and gastric emptying delay.[103]

Using the same approach, Hammar and colleagues[104] discovered gastroparesis in 29% of their 28 patients with primary Sjögren syndrome.

Most recently, a reported association between Ehlers-Danlos syndrome type III (the joint hypermobility syndrome) and a variety of functional gastrointestinal symptoms, including those that may be based on gastric emptying delay, has begun to emerge.[105–107] In some studies, gastroparesis has been documented.[105]

REFERENCES

1. Aderinto-Adike AO, Quigley EM. Gastrointestinal motility problems in critical care: a clinical perspective. J Dig Dis 2014;15:335–44.
2. Shafi MA, Pasricha PJ. Post-surgical and obstructive gastroparesis. Curr Gastroenterol Rep 2007;9:280–5.
3. Jung HK, Choung RS, Locke GR 3rd, et al. The incidence, prevalence, and outcomes of patients with gastroparesis in Olmsted County, Minnesota, from 1996 to 2006. Gastroenterology 2009;136:1225–33.
4. Dong K, Yu XJ, Li B, et al. Advances in mechanisms of postsurgical gastroparesis syndrome and its diagnosis and treatment. Chin J Dig Dis 2006;7:76–82.
5. Fich A, Neri M, Camilleri M, et al. Stasis syndromes following gastric surgery: clinical and motility features of sixty symptomatic patients. J Clin Gastroenterol 1990;12:505–12.
6. Chang TM, Chen TH, Tsou SS, et al. Differences in gastric emptying between highly selective vagotomy and posterior truncal vagotomy combined with anterior seromyotomy. J Gastrointest Surg 1999;3:533–6.
7. Forstner-Barthell AW, Murr MM, Nitecki S, et al. Near-total completion gastrectomy for severe postvagotomy gastric stasis: analysis of early and long-term results in 62 patients. J Gastrointest Surg 1999;3:15–21.
8. Akkermans LM, Hendrikse CA. Post-gastrectomy problems. Dig Liver Dis 2000; 32(Suppl 3):S263–4.
9. Le Blanc-Louvry I, Savoye G, Maillot C, et al. An impaired accommodation of the proximal stomach to a meal is associated with symptoms after distal gastrectomy. Am J Gastroenterol 2003;98:2642–7.
10. Meng H, Zhou D, Jiang X, et al. Incidence and risk factors for postsurgical gastroparesis syndrome after laparoscopic and open radical gastrectomy. World J Surg Oncol 2013;11:144.
11. Jiang X, Hiki N, Nunobe S, et al. Postoperative pancreatic fistula and the risk factors of laparoscopy-assisted distal gastrectomy for early gastric cancer. Ann Surg Oncol 2012;19:115–21.
12. Speicher JE, Thirlby RC, Burggraaf J, et al. Results of completion gastrectomies in 44 patients with postsurgical gastric atony. J Gastrointest Surg 2009;13: 874–80.
13. Mathias JR, Fernandez A, Sninsky CA, et al. Nausea, vomiting and abdominal pain after Roux-en-Y anastomosis: motility of the jejunal limb. Gastroenterology 1985;88:101–7.
14. Hinder RA, Esser MB, DeMeester TR. Management of gastric emptying disorders following the Roux-en-Y procedure. Surgery 1988;104:765–72.
15. Vantrappen G, Coremans G, Janssens J, et al. Inversion of the slow wave frequency gradient in symptomatic patients with Roux-en-Y anastomosis. Gastroenterology 1991;101:1282–8.
16. Miedema BW, Kelly KA, Camilleri M, et al. Human gastric and jejunal transit and motility after Roux gastrojejunostomy. Gastroenterology 1992;103:1133–43.

17. Fabre JM, Burgel JS, Navarro F, et al. Delayed gastric emptying after pancreaticoduodenectomy and pancreaticogastrostomy. Eur J Surg 1999;165:560–5.
18. Horstmann O, Becker H, Post S, et al. Is delayed gastric emptying following pancreaticoduodenectomy related to pylorus preservation? Langenbecks Arch Surg 1999;384:354–9.
19. Parmar AD, Sheffield KM, Vargas GM, et al. Factors associated with delayed gastric emptying after pancreaticoduodenectomy. HPB (Oxford) 2013;15: 763–72.
20. Su AP, Cao SS, Zhang Y, et al. Does antecolic reconstruction for duodenojejunostomy improve delayed gastric emptying after pylorus-preserving pancreaticoduodenectomy? a systematic review and meta-analysis. World J Gastroenterol 2012;18:6315–23.
21. Shimoda M, Kubota K, Katoh M, et al. Effect of Billroth II or Roux-en-Y reconstruction for the gastrojejunostomy on delayed gastric emptying after pancreaticoduodenectomy: a randomized controlled study. Ann Surg 2013;257: 938–42.
22. Qu H, Sun GR, Zhou SQ, et al. Clinical risk factors of delayed gastric emptying in patients after pancreaticoduodenectomy: a systematic review and meta-analysis. Eur J Surg Oncol 2013;39:213–23.
23. Ben-Youssef R, Baron PW, Franco E, et al. Intrapyloric injection of botulinum toxin a for the treatment of persistent gastroparesis following successful pancreas transplantation. Am J Transplant 2006;6:214–8.
24. Penagini R, Alloca M, Cantu P, et al. Relationship between motor function of the proximal stomach and transient lower oesophageal sphincter relaxation after morphine. Gut 2004;53:1227–31.
25. Vu MK, Straathof JW, van der Schaar PJ, et al. Motor and sensory function of the proximal stomach in reflux disease and after laparoscopic Nissen fundoplication. Am J Gastroenterol 1999;94:1481–9.
26. Vu MK, Ringers J, Arndt JW, et al. Prospective study of the effect of laparoscopic hemifundoplication on motor and sensory function of the proximal stomach. Br J Surg 2000;87:338–43.
27. Lindeboom MY, Vu MK, Ringers J, et al. Function of the proximal stomach after partial versus complete laparoscopic fundoplication. Am J Gastroenterol 2003; 98:284–90.
28. Scheffer RC, Tatum RP, Shi G, et al. Reduced tLESR elicitation in response to gastric distention in fundoplication patients. Am J Physiol Gastrointest Liver Physiol 2003;284:G815–20.
29. Richards WO, Scholz S, Khaitan L, et al. Initial experience with the Stretta procedure for the treatment of gastroesophageal reflux disease. J Laparoendosc Adv Surg Tech A 2001;11:267–73.
30. Sarosiek I, Yates KP, Abell PL, et al. Interpreting symptoms suggesting gastroparesis in patients after gastric and esophageal surgeries. Gastroenterology 2011;140:S-813.
31. Richter JE. Gastroesophageal reflux disease treatment: side effects and complications of fundoplication. Clin Gastroenterol Hepatol 2013;11:465–71.
32. Clark CJ, Sarr MG, Arora AS, et al. Does gastric resection have a role in the management of severe postfundoplication gastric dysfunction? World J Surg 2011;35:2045–50.
33. Masqusi S, Velanovich V. Pyloroplasty with fundoplication in the treatment of combined gastroesophageal reflux disease and bloating. World J Surg 2007; 31:332–6.

34. Ardila-Hani A, Soffer EE. Review article: the impact of bariatric surgery on gastrointestinal motility. Aliment Pharmacol Ther 2011;34:825–31.
35. Salameh JR, Schmieg RE Jr, Runnels JM, et al. Refractory gastroparesis after Roux-en-Y gastric bypass: surgical treatment with implantable pacemaker. J Gastrointest Surg 2007;11:1669–72.
36. Reddymasu SC, Singh S, Sankula R, et al. Endoscopic pyloric injection of botulinum toxin-A for the treatment of postvagotomy gastroparesis. Am J Med Sci 2009;337:161–4.
37. Sutcliffe RP, Forshaw MJ, Tandon R, et al. Anastomotic strictures and delayed gastric emptying after esophagectomy: incidence, risk factors and management. Dis Esophagus 2008;21:712–7.
38. Radaelli F, Paggi S, Terreni N, et al. Acute reversible gastroparesis and megaduodenum after botulinum toxin injection for achalasia. Gastrointest Endosc 2010;71:1326–7.
39. Nafteux P, Moons J, Coosemans W, et al. Minimally invasive oesophagectomy: a valuable alternative to open oesophagectomy for the treatment of early oesophageal and gastro-oesophageal junction carcinoma. Eur J Cardiothorac Surg 2011;40:1455–63.
40. Raviv Y, D'Ovidio F, Pierre A, et al. Prevalence of gastroparesis before and after lung transplantation and its association with lung allograft outcomes. Clin Transplant 2012;26:133–42.
41. Paul S, Escareno CE, Clancy K, et al. Gastrointestinal complications after lung transplantation. J Heart Lung Transplant 2009;28:475–9.
42. Filichia LA, Baz MA, Cendan JC. Simultaneous fundoplication and gastric stimulation in a lung transplant recipient with gastroparesis and reflux. JSLS 2008; 12:303–5.
43. Vignolo MC, Savassi-Rocha PR, Coelho LG, et al. Gastric emptying before and after cholecystectomy in patients with cholecystolithiasis. Hepatogastroenterology 2008;55:850–4.
44. Parkman HP, Yates K, Hasler WL, et al. Cholecystectomy and clinical presentations of gastroparesis. Dig Dis Sci 2013;58:1062–73.
45. Schaller BJ, Graf R, Jacobs AH. Pathophysiological changes of the gastrointestinal tract in ischemic stroke. Am J Gastroenterol 2006;101:1655–65.
46. Quigley EM. Gastrointestinal dysfunction in Parkinson's disease. Semin Neurol 1996;16:245–50.
47. Jost WH. Gastrointestinal dysfunction in Parkinson's disease. J Neurol Sci 2010; 289:69–73.
48. Gallagher DA, Lees AJ, Schrag A. What are the most important nonmotor symptoms in patients with Parkinson's disease? Mov Disord 2010;25:2493–500.
49. Pfeiffer RF. Gastrointestinal dysfunction in Parkinson's disease. Parkinsonism Relat Disord 2011;17:10–5.
50. Lebouvier T, Chaumette T, Paillusson S, et al. The second brain and Parkinson's disease. Eur J Neurosci 2009;30:735–41.
51. Natale G, Pasquali L, Ruggieri S, et al. Parkinson's disease and the gut: a well known clinical association in need of an effective cure and explanation. Neurogastroenterol Motil 2008;20:741–9.
52. Singaram C, Ashraf W, Gaumnitz EA, et al. Depletion of dopaminergic neurons in the colon in Parkinson's disease. Lancet 1995;346:861–86.
53. Lebouvier T, Neunlist M, Bruley des Varannes S, et al. Colonic biopsies to assess the neuropathology of Parkinson's disease and its relationship with symptoms. PLoS One 2010;5:e12728.

54. Shannon KM, Keshavarzian A, Mutlu E, et al. Alpha-synuclein in colonic submucosa in early untreated Parkinson's disease. Mov Disord 2012;27:709–15.
55. Gold A, Turkalp ZT, Munoz DG. Enteric alpha-synuclein expression is increased in Parkinson's disease but not Alzheimer's disease. Mov Disord 2013;28: 237–40.
56. Edwards L, Pfeiffer RF, Quigley EM, et al. Incidence of gastrointestinal symptoms in Parkinson's disease. Mov Disord 1991;6:151–6.
57. Colosimo C, Morgante L, Antonini A, et al, PRIAMO Study Group. Non-motor symptoms in atypical and secondary parkinsonism: the PRIAMO study. J Neurol 2010;257:5–14.
58. Antonini A, Barone P, Marconi R, et al. The progression of non-motor symptoms in Parkinson's disease and their contribution to motor disability and quality of life. J Neurol 2012;259:2621–31.
59. Marrinan S, Emmanuel AV, Burn DJ. Delayed gastric emptying in Parkinson's disease. Mov Disord 2014;29:23–32.
60. Heetun ZS, Quigley EM. Gastroparesis and Parkinson's disease: a systematic review. Parkinsonism Relat Disord 2012;18:433–40.
61. Djaldetti R, Baron J, Ziv I, et al. Gastric emptying in Parkinson's disease: patients with and without response fluctuations. Neurology 1996;46:1051–4.
62. Hardoff R, Sula M, Tamir A, et al. Gastric emptying time and gastric motility in patients with Parkinson's disease. Mov Disord 2001;16:1041–7.
63. Goetze O, Wieczorek J, Mueller T, et al. Impaired gastric emptying of a solid test meal in patients with Parkinson's disease using ^{13}C-sodium octanoate breath test. Neurosci Lett 2005;375:170–3.
64. Thomaides T, Karapanaayiotides T, Zoukos Y, et al. Gastric emptying after semi-solid food in multiple system atrophy and Parkinson disease. J Neurol 2005;25:1055–9.
65. Goetze O, Nikodem AB, Wieczorek J, et al. Predictors of gastric emptying in Parkinson's disease. Neurogastroenterol Motil 2006;18:369–75.
66. Nyholm D, Lennernas H. Irregular gastrointestinal drug absorption in Parkinson's disease. Expert Opin Drug Metab Toxicol 2008;4:193–203.
67. Eggert K, Schrader C, Hahn M, et al. Continuous jejunal levodopa infusion in patients with advanced Parkinson disease: practical aspects and outcome of motor and non-motor complications. Clin Neuropharmacol 2008;31:151–66.
68. Steiger M. Constant dopaminergic stimulation by transdermal delivery of dopaminergic drugs: a new treatment paradigm in Parkinson's disease. Eur J Neurol 2008;15:6–15.
69. Kashihara K. Weight loss in Parkinson's disease. J Neurol 2006;253(Suppl 7): VII38–41.
70. Naftali T, Gadoth N, Huberman M, et al. Electrogastrography in patients with Parkinson's disease. Can J Neurol Sci 2005;32:82–6.
71. Chen CL, Lin HH, Chen SY, et al. Utility of electrogastrography in differentiating Parkinson's disease with or without gastrointestinal symptoms: a prospective controlled study. Digestion 2005;71:187–91.
72. Dobbs RJ, Dobbs SM, Weller C, et al. Role of chronic infection and inflammation in the gastrointestinal tract in the etiology and pathogenesis of idiopathic parkinsonism. Part 1: eradication of Helicobacter in the cachexia of idiopathic parkinsonism. Helicobacter 2005;10:267–75.
73. Bjarnason IT, Charlett A, Dobbs RJ, et al. Role of chronic infection and inflammation in the gastrointestinal tract in the etiology and pathogenesis of idiopathic parkinsonism. Part 2: response of facets of clinical idiopathic parkinsonism

to *Helicobacter pylori* eradication. A randomized, double-blind, placebo-controlled efficacy study. Helicobacter 2005;10:276–87.

74. Weller C, Charlett A, Oxlade NL, et al. Role of chronic infection and inflammation in the gastrointestinal tract in the etiology and pathogenesis of idiopathic parkinsonism. Part 3: predicted probability and gradients of severity of idiopathic parkinsonism based *H. pylori* antibody profile. Helicobacter 2005;10:288–97.

75. El-Maghraby TA, Shalaby NM, Al-Tawdy MH, et al. Gastric motility dysfunction in patients with multiple sclerosis assessed by gastric emptying scintigraphy. Can J Gastroenterol 2005;19:141–5.

76. Gupta YK. Gastroparesis with multiple sclerosis. JAMA 1984;252:42.

77. Read SJ, Leggett BA, Pender MP. Gastroparesis with multiple sclerosis. Lancet 1995;346:1228.

78. Raghav S, Kipp D, Watson J, et al. Gastroparesis in multiple sclerosis. Mult Scler 2006;12:243–4.

79. Reddymasu SC, Bonino J, McCallum RW. Gastroparesis secondary to a demyelinating disease: a case series. BMC Gastroenterol 2007;7:3.

80. Ben-Zvi JS, Daniel SJ. Painless gastric perforation in a patient with multiple sclerosis. Am J Gastroenterol 1988;83:1008–11.

81. Haensch CA, Jorg J. Autonomic dysfunction in multiple sclerosis. J Neurol 2006; 253(Suppl 1):I3–9.

82. Freeman R. Autonomic peripheral neuropathy. Lancet 2005;365:1259–70.

83. Klein CM, Vernino S, Lennon VA, et al. The spectrum of autoimmune autonomic neuropathies. Ann Neurol 2003;53:752–8.

84. Van Doorn PA, Ruts L, Jacobs BC. Clinical features, pathogenesis, and treatment of Guillain-Barré syndrome. Lancet Neurol 2008;7:939–50.

85. McDougall AJ, McLeod JG. Autonomic neuropathy, I. Clinical features, investigation, pathophysiology, and treatment. J Neurol Sci 1996;137:79–88.

86. Sivadon-Tardy V, Orlokowski D, Rozenberg F, et al. Guillain-Barré syndrome, greater Paris area. Emerg Infect Dis 2006;12:990–3.

87. Simpson AJ, Khilnani MT. Gastrointestinal manifestations of the muscular dystrophies. Am J Roentgenol Radium Ther Nucl Med 1975;125:948–55.

88. Nowak TV, Ionasescu V, Anuras S. Gastrointestinal manifestations of the muscular dystrophies. Gastroenterology 1982;82:800–10.

89. Karasick D, Karasick S, Mapp E. Gastrointestinal radiologic manifestations of proximal spinal muscular atrophy (Kugelberg-Welander syndrome). J Natl Med Assoc 1982;74:475–8.

90. Staiano A, Del Giudice E, Romano A, et al. Upper gastrointestinal tract motility in children with progressive muscular dystrophy. J Pediatr 1992;121:720–4.

91. Bellini M, Biagi S, Stasi S, et al. Gastrointestinal manifestations in myotonic muscular dystrophy. World J Gastroenterol 2006;12:1821–8.

92. Ronnblom A, Forsberg H, Danielsson A. Gastrointestinal symptoms in myotonic dystrophy. Scand J Gastroenterol 1996;31:654–7.

93. Tieleman AA, van Vliet J, Jansen JB, et al. Gastrointestinal involvement is frequent in myotonic dystrophy type 2. Neuromuscul Disord 2008;18:646–9.

94. Bellini M, Alduini P, Costa F, et al. Gastric emptying in myotonic dystrophy patients. Dig Liver Dis 2002;34:484–8.

95. Ronnblom A, Andersson S, Hellstrom PM, et al. Gastric emptying in myotonic dystrophy. Eur J Clin Invest 2002;32:570–4.

96. Horowitz M, Maddox A, Maddern GJ, et al. Gastric and esophageal emptying in dystrophia myotonica. Effect of metoclopramide. Gastroenterology 1987;92:570–7.

97. Kusunoki M, Hatada T, Ikeuchi H, et al. Gastric volvulus complicating myotonic dystrophy. Hepatogastroenterology 1992;39:586–8.
98. Borrelli O, Salvia G, Mancini V, et al. Evolution of gastric electrical features and gastric emptying in children with Duchenne and Becker muscular dystrophy. Am J Gastroenterol 2005;100:695–702.
99. Barohn RJ, Levine EJ, Olson JO, et al. Gastric hypomotility in Duchenne's muscular dystrophy. N Engl J Med 1988;319:15–8.
100. Bensen ES, Jaffe KM, Tarr PI. Acute gastric dilatation in Duchenne muscular dystrophy: a case report and review of the literature. Arch Phys Med Rehabil 1996;77:512–4.
101. Chung BC, Park HJ, Yoon SB, et al. Acute gastroparesis in Duchenne's muscular dystrophy. Yonsei Med J 1998;39:175–9.
102. Marie I, Levesque H, Ducrotté P, et al. Gastric involvement in systemic sclerosis: a prospective study. Am J Gastroenterol 2001;96:77–83.
103. Marie I, Gourcerol G, Leroi AM, et al. Delayed gastric emptying determined using the 13C-octanoic acid breath test in patients with systemic sclerosis. Arthritis Rheum 2012;64:2346–55.
104. Hammar O, Ohlsson B, Wollmer P, et al. Impaired gastric emptying in primary Sjögren's syndrome. J Rheumatol 2010;37:2313–8.
105. Zarate N, Farmer AD, Grahame R, et al. Unexplained gastrointestinal symptoms and joint hypermobility: is connective tissue the missing link? Neurogastroenterol Motil 2010;22:252–252.e78.
106. Fikree A, Grahame R, Aktar R, et al. A prospective evaluation of undiagnosed joint hypermobility syndrome in patients with gastrointestinal symptoms. Clin Gastroenterol Hepatol 2014;12:1680–7.
107. Kovacic K, Chelimsky TC, Sood MR, et al. Joint hypermobility: a common association with complex functional gastrointestinal disorders. J Pediatr 2014; 165:973–8.

Symptomatic Management for Gastroparesis

Antiemetics, Analgesics, and Symptom Modulators

William L. Hasler, MD

KEYWORDS

- Antiemetic medications • Opiates • Tricyclic antidepressants
- Neuropathic pain modulators • Fundus relaxants

KEY POINTS

- A recent series reported reduced nausea and vomiting caused by open-label transdermal granisetron, a 5-hydroxytryptamine-3 (5-HT$_3$) receptor antagonist, in patients with gastroparesis.
- Opiate analgesics are often taken for pain control; however, caution should be exercised because these agents worsen nausea and vomiting and further delay gastric emptying.
- As with antiemetics, support for use of neuromodulatory agents was restricted to individual cases; however, the largely negative findings from a multicenter, randomized, placebo-controlled trial of the tricyclic antidepressant nortriptyline in patients with idiopathic gastroparesis raise doubts about the effectiveness of neuromodulators in this condition.
- Postulated benefits of antiemetic and neuromodulatory therapies must be weighed against adverse outcomes during gastroparesis treatment, which recently have stressed neurologic and cardiac toxicities of these drugs.
- Placebo-controlled trials must be conducted to characterize the usefulness of these drug classes in managing gastroparesis symptoms.

INTRODUCTION

Gastroparesis presents with a range of symptoms referable to the upper gut including nausea, vomiting, early satiety, postprandial fullness, bloating, distention, and upper abdominal pain or discomfort. Although increased gastric retention is mandated for diagnosis, gastroparesis symptom severity correlates poorly with the degree of gastric

This article originally appeared in Gastroenterology Clinics, Volume 44, Issue 1, March 2015.
Disclosure statement: Dr W.L. Hasler receives research funding from the National Institute of Diabetes and Digestive and Kidney Diseases (grant U01DK073983) as part of the Gastroparesis Clinical Research Consortium. He also receives funding from Given Imaging, Inc (grant MA-501) for a clinical trial validating the WMC recording system as a diagnostic test for delayed gastric emptying. In the past 24 months, Dr W.L. Hasler has been a consultant to Janssen Pharmaceuticals, Inc; Novartis Pharmaceuticals; GSK; and Salix Pharmaceuticals, Inc.
Division of Gastroenterology, University of Michigan Health System, 3912 Taubman Center, SPC 5362, Ann Arbor, MI 48109, USA
E-mail address: whasler@umich.edu

emptying delay. In a large gastroparesis cohort comprising both diabetic and idiopathic patients from the multicenter National Institute of Diabetes and Digestive and Kidney Diseases Gastroparesis Consortium, gastric retention measured at 2 and 4 hours showed no relation to overall or individual symptom intensities among 319 patients with delayed emptying and 106 with normal emptying.[1] Likewise in functional dyspepsia, emptying parameters show no correlation or are only weakly associated with fullness but not nausea, pain, or bloating. One investigation calculated that only 10% of the variance in dyspeptic symptoms relates to gastric emptying rates.[2] Other physiologic defects are proposed to contribute to symptom development. In studies in which combined gastric emptying and barostat testing was performed in dyspeptic patients, delayed gastric emptying correlated with nausea, vomiting, and postprandial fullness, whereas impaired gastric fundic accommodation associated with epigastric pain, early satiety, and weight loss.[3] In a different report, the prevalence of hypersensitivity to gastric distention was greatest (44%) among patients who rated abdominal pain as their predominant symptom.[4]

Because of the importance of delayed emptying in diagnosing gastroparesis, the main focus of treating this condition has been on prokinetic agents that promote gastric evacuation. However, in gastroparesis and functional dyspepsia, metoclopramide and domperidone reduce symptoms over the long term even when there is diminution of initial prokinetic effects with time.[5] Many benefits of these agents may therefore stem from antiemetic effects in the central nervous system. Furthermore, agents with only prokinetic treatments without central antiemetic effects (erythromycin, pyloric botulinum toxin) may be less effective than therapies with combined prokinetic and antiemetic action. One systematic review calculated benefits in only 43% of patients with gastroparesis receiving erythromycin.[6]

These investigations raise the possibility that pharmaceuticals with actions unrelated to gastrokinesis may be beneficial for some gastroparesis manifestations. Medications with only antiemetic mechanisms of action would theoretically be effective with prominent vomiting (and nausea). In contrast, central analgesics or drugs targeting other sensorimotor defects, such as enhanced sensitivity or impaired accommodation, might be useful for discomfort or pain.

MANAGEMENT GOALS

Given the disconnect between symptoms and gastric emptying, it is reasonable to propose that the primary goal of treating gastroparesis should focus on symptom reductions rather than stimulation of gastric emptying. Pharmacologic agents in diverse drug classes are available that decrease nausea, vomiting, and abdominal pain by acting as antiemetics, analgesics, or modulators of enteric neuronal function. These medications represent the sole forms of treatment of some individuals or may complement gastric prokinetic drugs in others. Little controlled investigation has been performed to define benefits of these agents in gastroparesis. Thus, use of these medications is based on pathophysiologic plausibility and expert opinion.

PHARMACOLOGIC STRATEGIES

The benefits of antiemetic, analgesic, and neuromodulatory medications in gastroparesis are unproved and may be modest in scope. Because of these limitations, decisions on any gastroparesis therapies rely on defining and assessing the severity of symptoms that represent the target of treatment. Introduction of validated surveys to measure numerical symptom intensity represents an advance in quantifying gastroparesis severity. The Gastroparesis Cardinal Symptom Index (GCSI) comprises

9 questions in 3 domains (nausea/vomiting, fullness/early satiety, bloating/distention) rated from 0 (no symptoms) to 5 (very severe) and shows good test-retest reliability and treatment response.[7] The GCSI–Daily Diary adds a pain/discomfort domain to this survey and is administered daily.[8] In comprehensive evaluations of a large patient cohort from the Gastroparesis Consortium followed for 48 weeks, overall GCSI scores decreased only by an average of 0.3 points while subjects were under the care of clinicians with expertise in managing this condition.[9] Subjects with predominant nausea and/or vomiting more often improved than those with predominant upper abdominal pain. Future controlled investigations of novel therapies will determine whether medications targeting nausea and vomiting are more effective than those that are designed to reduce other gastroparesis symptoms.

Antiemetic Agents

Nausea is the most prevalent gastroparesis symptom, being experienced by 90% to 95% of patients, whereas 55% to 80% report vomiting.[10] Nausea and/or vomiting represent the predominant symptoms, prompting specialist referral of 44% of patients (**Table 1**).[11] In a single-center study, nausea scores averaged 3.4 (on a scale from 0 to 5) over 8 hours daily in patients with both diabetic and idiopathic gastroparesis.[10] Mean daily vomiting frequencies ranged from 3.5 with idiopathic disease to 7.3 for diabetics with gastroparesis. Vomiting with gastroparesis often occurs 30 to 120 minutes after eating. The vomitus may contain partially digested food residue from meals ingested days before.

Because of the prevalence and severity of nausea and vomiting in gastroparesis, antiemetic agents commonly are prescribed. In data on 416 patients from the Gastroparesis Consortium, antiemetics were used similarly with idiopathic disease (61%) and gastroparesis from type 1 (70%) and type 2 (66%) diabetes.[12] However, symptom improvements are not different between gastroparetics who take versus do not take antiemetic drugs over 48 weeks of care.[9] Although not specifically investigated, this suggests that antiemetics provide no more than modest benefits to gastroparetics referred to centers specializing in motility disorders.

Antiemetic drugs acting on several receptor subtypes have been developed for clinical conditions with nausea and vomiting (**Table 2**). Histamine H_1 antagonists (eg, promethazine, meclizine, dimenhydrinate) are useful for vomiting in conditions with activation of the vestibular system (motion sickness, labyrinthitis), uremia, and postoperative settings. Side effects of antihistamines include sedation and mouth dryness. Nonsedating newer antihistamines (astemizole, cetirizine, fexofenadine) are less effective antiemetics. Muscarinic M_1 antagonists given orally or as transdermal patches (scopolamine) also are best characterized in labyrinthine conditions, including motion sickness, and can elicit side effects including sedation, dryness of the eyes and mouth, constipation, urinary retention, and headaches. Dopamine D_2 antagonists in the phenothiazine (eg, prochlorperazine) and butyrophenone (eg, droperidol, haloperidol) classes exert beneficial effects with vomiting from acute gastroenteritis, medication and cancer chemotherapy, radiation therapy, and surgery. Therapy with dopamine antagonists may cause sleep disturbances, mood changes, anxiety, and movement disorders, and gynecomastia, galactorrhea, or menstrual irregularities from drug-induced hyperprolactinemia. Some agents with antidopaminergic activity also evoke antihistaminic and antimuscarinic side effects. Serotonin 5-hydroxytryptamine-3 (5-HT_3) antagonists (eg, ondansetron, granisetron, dolasetron, palonosetron) can be swallowed, dissolved within the mouth, administered intravenously, or applied transdermally. 5-HT_3 antagonists are effective for prophylaxis of emesis and postoperative vomiting induced by chemotherapy and radiotherapy but also have been used

Table 1
Gastroparesis patient-reported symptom predominance

Predominant Symptom Subscale	Predominant Symptom	Individual Symptom (N)	Individual Symptom (%)	Symptom Subscale (N)	Symptom Subscale (%)
Abdominal pain/discomfort	Upper abdominal pain	27	7	81	21
	Abdominal pain location not specified	42	11		
	Lower abdominal pain	6	2		
	Upper abdominal discomfort	2	0.5		
	Abdominal discomfort location not specified	2	0.5		
	Lower abdominal discomfort	2	0.5		
Nausea/vomiting	Nausea	135	34	172	44
	Vomiting	36	9		
	Retching	1	0.3		
Postprandial fullness/early satiety	Stomach fullness	26	7	47	12
	Not able to finish normal-sized meal	8	2		
	Feeling excessively full after meals	8	2		
	Loss of appetite	5	1		
Bloating/distention	Bloating	26	7	27	7
	Stomach or belly visibly larger	1	0.3		
Esophageal symptoms	Heartburn during the day	1	0.3	32	8
	Heartburn, did not specify day vs when lying down	5	1		
	Feeling of discomfort inside chest during day	1	0.3		
	Feeling of discomfort inside chest, did not specify day vs lying down	4	1		
	Regurgitation or reflux during day	4	1		
	Regurgitation or reflux lying down	3	1		
	Regurgitation or reflux, did not specify day vs lying down	12	3		
	Bitter, acid, or sour taste in mouth	2	0.5		
Bowel habit abnormalities	Constipation	18	5	33	8
	Diarrhea	15	4		
Miscellaneous	No symptom specified	1	0.3	1	0.3

From Hasler WL, Wilson LA, Parkman HP, et al. Factors related to abdominal pain in gastroparesis: contrast to patients with predominant nausea and vomiting. Neurogastroenterol Motil 2013;25:433; with permission.

Table 2
Antiemetic medications and gastroparesis

Medication Class	Examples	Published Data in Gastroparesis
Histamine H_1 antagonist	Dimenhydrinate Meclizine Promethazine	None
Muscarinic (cholinergic) M_1 antagonist	Scopolamine	None
Dopamine D_2 antagonist	Prochlorperazine Trimethobenzamide	1 case report (thiethylperazine)
Serotonin 5-HT_3 antagonist	Ondansetron Granisetron Dolasetron	1 case report (intraperitoneal ondansetron) 1 case series (36 patients, granisetron)
Neurokinin NK_1 antagonist	Aprepitant	2 case reports
Cannabinoid CB_1 agonist	Dronabinol	None

Abbreviation: 5-HT, 5-hydroxytryptamine.

for bulimia nervosa, emesis caused by hepatic or renal disease, and nausea with human immunodeficiency virus infection.[13] In contrast, 5-HT_3 antagonists offer only limited benefits to prevent nausea instead of vomiting. 5-HT_3 antagonist use is complicated by constipation, headaches, increased liver chemistries, and cardiac rhythm disturbances secondary to QTc interval prolongation. Neurokinin -1 receptor subtype (NK_1) antagonists show potent antiemetic effects for chemotherapy-induced nausea and vomiting, postoperative nausea and vomiting, and motion sickness given orally (aprepitant) or intravenously (fosaprepitant).[13] Unlike 5-HT_3 antagonists, NK_1 antagonists are effective at reducing nausea as well as vomiting. Side effects of these agents include bowel habit changes, anorexia, and singultus. Cannabinoid-1 receptor subtype (CB1) agonists (eg, dronabinol) are approved for preventing chemotherapy-induced vomiting but side effects include sedation, euphoria, impaired cognition, and rarely syncope and hallucinations in the elderly. A cannabinoid hyperemesis syndrome mimicking cyclic vomiting syndrome occurs with long-standing use of large amounts of cannabis, but this condition has not been reported with prescription agents like dronabinol.[14]

Case reports and series have suggested the utility of selected antiemetic agents for treating gastroparesis. The dopamine D_2 antagonist thiethylperazine produced symptom benefits in 1 diabetic with gastroparesis.[15] In a 32-year-old type 1 diabetic gastroparetic on continuous cycling peritoneal dialysis, long-term intraperitoneal administration of the 5-HT_3 antagonist ondansetron in the dialysate greatly reduced nausea and vomiting without adverse effects.[16] A recent open-label study of a transdermal patch that delivers 3.1 mg per 24 hours of the 5-HT_3 antagonist granisetron for 7 days was performed in 36 patients with gastroparesis and nausea and vomiting unresponsive to standard antiemetics (**Fig. 1**).[17] On therapy, 18 patients reported symptoms that were somewhat better or moderately better, whereas 15 remained the same, 2 worsened, and 1 discontinued therapy because of poor adhesive adherence to the skin. Side effects included constipation (4 cases), rash (3 patients), and headache (2 individuals). Two cases describing antiemetic benefits of the NK_1 antagonist aprepitant in gastroparesis have been published. In the first, a 31-year-old type 1 diabetic with vomiting refractory to cyclizine, haloperidol, metoclopramide, erythromycin, and pyloric botulinum toxin injection experienced 4 months free of nausea

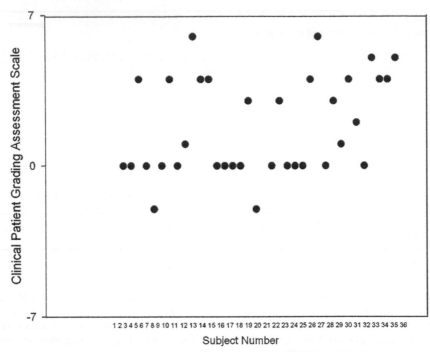

Fig. 1. Responses to a granisetron transdermal patch are shown for individuals with gastroparesis as measured by the Clinical Patient Grading Assessment Scale, ranging from −7 (completely worse) to 0 (no change) to +7 (completely better). Approximately half the patients reported being somewhat to moderately better on therapy. (*From* Simmons K, Parkman HP. Granisetron transdermal system improves refractory nausea and vomiting in gastroparesis. Dig Dis Sci 2014;59:1233; with permission.)

and vomiting on daily aprepitant.[18] In the second case, a 41-year-old woman with idiopathic gastroparesis with vomiting unresponsive to metoclopramide, ondansetron, and promethazine reported significant reductions in symptoms over 2 months on aprepitant before the therapy was withdrawn because of cost.[19] A 4-week placebo-controlled phase 3 trial assessing aprepitant efficacy in patients with chronic nausea and vomiting of presumed gastric origin is being conducted by the Gastroparesis Consortium.

Other prescription pharmaceuticals show antiemetic activity. Corticosteroids and benzodiazepines are frequently included as components of antiemetic programs to prevent delayed chemotherapy-induced emesis or postoperative vomiting. Mechanisms of their antivomiting effects are poorly characterized.

Analgesic and Neuromodulatory Medications

Gastroparesis often presents with symptoms other than nausea and vomiting. Single-center studies report abdominal pain prevalences in gastroparesis ranging from 42% to 89%.[11,20,21] In a report from the Gastroparesis Consortium, upper abdominal pain and discomfort were predominant in 21% of patients (see **Table 1**). Case series have described pain location (epigastric in 36%–43%), timing (postprandial in 24%–80%; nocturnal in 80%), frequency (daily in 43%; weekly in 38%; intermittent in 24%–62%), and characteristics (burning, vague, crampy, sharp, pressure).[20,21] Investigators observe more severe vomiting in diabetics with gastroparesis, whereas pain may be more prominent in idiopathic patients.[10,11] Two-thirds of gastroparetics note

GCSI pain scores of 3 to 5, indicating moderate to very severe intensity, which is associated with impaired quality of life and increased depression and anxiety.[11] The pathophysiology of gastroparesis pain is poorly understood. Most studies, including from the Gastroparesis Consortium, show no relation of pain to gastric emptying.[11,20,21] In diabetics, pain severity does not correlate with neuropathic complications or glycemic control. Twelve percent of gastroparetics report predominant postprandial fullness, early satiety, or anorexia, whereas 7% note bloating or visible distention as their main symptom (see **Table 1**).[11] Extragastric symptoms dominate, with 16% reporting predominance of esophageal symptoms (including heartburn, chest discomfort, regurgitation, or a sour taste in the throat) or bowel habit disturbances.

Because of the prominence of symptoms other than nausea and vomiting, it is reasonable to consider other medication classes that might be beneficial in gastroparesis. Analgesic drugs would be most useful for pain or discomfort. Neuromodulatory agents that act by blunting visceral perception or altering proximal gastric function might also be effective for epigastric pain, but could show utility for fullness, nausea, and vomiting. In data from the Gastroparesis Consortium, 43% of idiopathic patients were taking opiate medications on initial evaluation, compared with 46% of type 1 and 48% of type 2 diabetics with gastroparesis.[12] Higher percentages of patients who reported predominant pain or discomfort expressed opiate use versus those with predominant nausea or vomiting (60% vs 40%).[11] Sixteen percent of idiopathic gastroparetics were on neuropathic pain modulators (duloxetine, gabapentin, pregabalin) versus 27% and 29% of type 1 and 2 diabetics. Use of antidepressants in other classes was reported by 33% to 38%; however, this categorization was not subdivided among agents with versus without analgesic effects.

Prokinetics produce inconsistent reductions in gastroparesis pain, thus agents with analgesic actions often are empirically prescribed.[22] Nonsteroidal antiinflammatory drugs show some beneficial effects on gastric myoelectric function in older studies, but can induce mucosal ulceration or impair renal function. Although often given, opioid agonists retard gastric, small intestinal, and colonic transit and elicit nausea and vomiting.[12,23] In data from the Gastroparesis Consortium, antiemetic agent use was more prevalent among patients with higher abdominal pain scores, perhaps from induction of nausea by the pain or from the opiates prescribed for the pain.[11] Some experts advocate use of weaker opiates like tramadol and tapentadol or longer-acting medications, such as methadone or transdermal fentanyl, to minimize these effects.[23]

Neuromodulatory medications in several classes reduce perception of gastric stimulation or enhance fundic accommodation to meal ingestion (**Table 3**). Many actions relate to modification of serotonergic nerve function in the gut. Tricyclic antidepressants are norepinephrine and serotonin reuptake inhibitors with variable inhibition of dopamine reuptake. In experimental models, tricyclic agents reduce gut sensitivity to mechanical and electrical stimulation.[24] Likewise, prolonged dosing of selective serotonin reuptake inhibitors reduces perception of gut distention, possibly from receptor desensitization to continued serotonin exposure.[25] Other serotonin receptor subtypes represent potential neuromodulatory targets. The 5-HT$_{1A}$ partial agonist buspirone decreases fundic tone, whereas the 5-HT$_{1B/1D/1P}$ agonist sumatriptan augments gastric accommodation and blunts perception of distention in functional dyspepsia.[26]

Because of actions on gastric sensorimotor function, tricyclic medications were thought to have promise in gastroparesis. These drugs showed efficacy in initial uncontrolled reports in related conditions. In a small study in functional dyspepsia, amitriptyline reduced symptoms without altering perception of gastric distention.[27]

Table 3
Neuromodulatory medications and gastroparesis

Medications	Mechanisms of Action	Published Data in Gastroparesis
Tricyclic antidepressants (nortriptyline, amitriptyline, desipramine)	Norepinephrine reuptake inhibition with variable serotonin (and dopamine) reuptake inhibition	Case series in diabetics with nausea and vomiting (29% with delayed emptying) Controlled trial in idiopathic gastroparesis
Mirtazapine	Indirect CNS 5-HT_{1A} agonism, 5-HT_2 antagonism, 5-HT_{2C} inverse agonism, 5-HT_3 antagonism, alpha-2 antagonism, H_1 inverse agonism	Several case reports Preliminary controlled trial in functional dyspepsia
Olanzapine	5-HT_2 inverse agonism, 5-HT_3 antagonism, M_1 antagonism, M_3 antagonism, D_2 antagonism, H_1 inverse agonism	None
Buspirone	5-HT_1 partial agonist, presynaptic D_2 antagonist, alpha-1 partial agonist	Controlled trial in functional dyspepsia

Abbreviation: CNS, central nervous system.

Tricyclic antidepressants also reduce functional vomiting in retrospective reports.[28] In a follow-up analysis of 24 diabetics with refractory nausea and vomiting, tricyclics at median doses of 50 mg reduced symptoms in 88% and abolished them in nearly one-third.[29] Twenty-nine percent of patients showed delayed gastric emptying. Taken together, these observations suggested potential utility of tricyclics to reduce nausea, vomiting, and pain in gastroparesis.

In the most comprehensive assessment of the utility of neuromodulatory therapy for gastroparesis published to date, investigators from the 7 centers of the Gastroparesis Consortium tested benefits of the tricyclic agent nortriptyline versus placebo in a cohort of patients with idiopathic gastroparesis.[30] One-hundred and thirty patients with symptoms for longer than or equal to 6 months, overall GCSI scores greater than or equal to 21 (mean $\geq$2.33 for 9 symptoms), and delayed emptying (>10% 4-hour retention and/or >60% 2-hour retention) were randomized to nortriptyline or placebo in a 15-week trial. Nortriptyline dosing escalated from 10 mg for 3 weeks, 25 mg for 3 weeks, 50 mg for 3 weeks, and 75 mg at bedtime for 6 weeks if tolerated. Dosage reductions were permitted for medication side effects. The mean baseline GCSI symptom scores were 3.8 for nausea, 3.9 for early satiety, 3.7 for bloating, and 3.4 for upper abdominal pain/discomfort. Sixty-five percent of patients on nortriptyline tolerated the 75 mg dose, 11% reached 50 mg, 11% achieved 25%, and 14% were only able to take 10 mg nightly. A strict primary outcome was set: greater than or equal to 50% reduction in overall GCSI scores on 2 consecutive assessments compared with baseline values. Using this measure, improvements on nortriptyline (23%; 95% confidence interval [CI], 14%–35%) and placebo (21%; 95% CI, 12%–34%) were not different (relative risk of improvement, 1.06; 95% CI, 0.56–2.00; $P = .86$). On assessing secondary outcomes, GCSI loss of appetite scores improved more on nortriptyline (−1.6; 95% CI, −2.1 to −1.1) versus placebo (−0.9; 95% CI, −1.4 to −0.5; $P = .03$). Other secondary measures favoring nortriptyline therapy included GCSI inability to finish a meal scores, Gastrointestinal Symptom Rating Scale abdominal pain scores, and overall symptom relief scores on the Clinical Global Patient

Impression survey. Trends to greater increases in body mass index were observed with nortriptyline (0.5 kg/m^2; 95% CI, 0.1–0.8) versus placebo (0.0 kg/m^2; 95% CI, −0.3 to 0.3; P = .06). However, other important GCSI symptom subscores, especially nausea and vomiting, showed no differential improvement on nortriptyline (**Fig. 2**). Treatment was stopped more frequently with nortriptyline (29%; 95% CI, 19%–42%) than placebo (9%; 95% CI, 3%–19%; P = .007). Five serious adverse events were reported with nortriptyline compared with 1 with placebo. Despite the few positive findings on secondary data analysis, the overall negative trial findings raise doubts about the utility of this neuromodulator class in treating idiopathic gastroparesis.

Another antidepressant, mirtazapine, has been considered as a potential neuromodulatory therapy for gastroparesis. Mirtazapine exerts a complex interaction with several receptors, including indirect central nervous system 5-HT$_{1A}$ agonism, 5-HT$_2$ antagonism, 5-HT$_{2C}$ inverse agonism, 5-HT$_3$ antagonism, alpha-2 antagonism, and H$_1$ inverse agonism.[31] Several case reports have observed gastroparesis symptom reductions with open-label mirtazapine. In an initial report, mirtazapine 15 mg decreased emesis and allowed discontinuation of metoclopramide and lorazepam for 3 months in a 27-year-old diabetic with gastroparesis.[32] Likewise, 3 months of mirtazapine 15 mg nightly reduced nausea and vomiting and promoted adequate oral

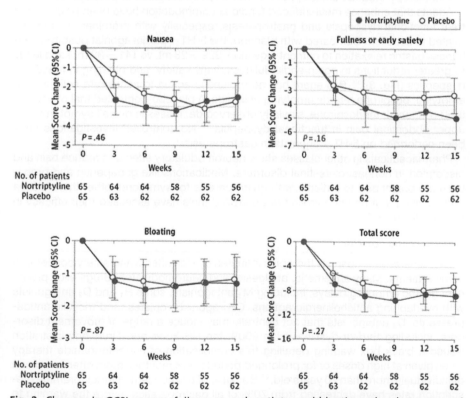

Fig. 2. Changes in GCSI nausea, fullness or early satiety, and bloating subscale scores, and total GCSI scores are shown for nortriptyline versus placebo over 15 weeks. There were no differences in individual or overall symptoms on nortriptyline and placebo (all P = nonsignificant). (*From* Parkman HP, Van Natta ML, Abell TL, et al. Effect of nortriptyline on symptoms of idiopathic gastroparesis: the NORIG randomized clinical trial. JAMA 2013;310:2646; with permission.)

intake in a 52-year-old man with postsurgical gastroparesis.[33] Mirtazapine 30 mg similarly evoked significant antiemetic actions with associated weight gain and improved oral intake in a 34-year-old woman with postinfectious gastroparesis.[34] Mirtazapine has not been investigated in gastroparesis in a controlled fashion, but a preliminary study was reported for functional dyspepsia.[35] Thirty-four functional dyspeptics with greater than or equal to 10% loss of body weight were given mirtazapine 15 mg nightly versus placebo for 8 weeks. Compared with baseline, mirtazapine reduced overall symptoms (on a 24-point scale) from 10.9 ± 0.9 to 7.5 ± 1.1 ($P = .02$), whereas placebo did not produce statistical benefits. Reductions in early satiety and weight increases were better on mirtazapine than placebo. If confirmed, these observations warrant controlled testing in gastroparesis. The mechanisms of mirtazapine on gastric sensorimotor function remain uncertain. Mirtazapine accelerated gastric emptying in healthy dogs and in a canine model of delayed emptying induced by rectal distention.[36] Such prokinetic effects have not been proved in gastroparesis, although mirtazapine reduced gastric residuals during gastrostomy feedings in an 87-year-old diabetic with gastroparesis.[37] Another antidepressant agent with antiemetic effects, olanzapine, acts via $5\text{-}HT_2$ inverse agonism, $5\text{-}HT_3$ antagonism, M_1 antagonism, M_3 antagonism, D_2 antagonism, and H_1 inverse agonism.[38] This agent has efficacy in chemotherapy-induced emesis, but has not been investigated in gastroparesis.

Agents that enhance meal-induced fundic accommodation have been proposed to treat functional dyspepsia and gastroparesis, especially with prominent symptoms related to satiation. Compared with placebo, the $5\text{-}HT_{1A}$ partial agonist buspirone enhances gastric relaxation to nutrient ingestion (229 ± 28 mL vs 141 ± 32 mL) and leads to greater reductions in postprandial fullness, early satiety, and bloating in functional dyspeptics (**Fig. 3**).[39] This agent has no prokinetic action to accelerate solid gastric emptying; buspirone retards emptying of liquids. A placebo-controlled trial of another $5\text{-}HT_{1A}$ agonist, tandospirone, similarly observed decreases in overall symptoms and upper abdominal pain in functional dyspepsia.[40] No controlled investigations have been performed on $5\text{-}HT_{1A}$ agonists in gastroparesis.

Pharmaceuticals in other classes show neuromodulatory effects to reduce pain and discomfort in nongastrointestinal disorders. Medications like gabapentin and pregabalin are prescribed to patients with gastroparesis for symptoms other than nausea and vomiting, but no uncontrolled or controlled trials have assessed their efficacy in this condition.[21,22]

Potential Drug Toxicity

Use of several gastroparesis therapies is limited by side effects and safety concerns in some patients. Many antiemetic, analgesic, and neuromodulatory drugs elicit prominent gastric emptying delays, including M_1 antagonists, some H_1 and D_2 antagonists with overlapping anticholinergic actions, CB_1 agonists, opiates, and tricyclic antidepressants. D_2 antagonists that act centrally may induce a range of movement disorders, including tardive dyskinesia. In 2009, the US Food and Drug Administration issued a black box warning detailing this complication of metoclopramide therapy when given at high doses or for prolonged periods (>18 months), most often in women or individuals more than 70 years old.[41] Because of this concern, metoclopramide prescription rates have decreased from 70% of all gastroparetics before the warning to 24% in 2013.[42] The other prominent safety concern that has been a focus of attention is medication induction of dangerous cardiac rhythm disturbances such as torsades de pointes, most often with electrocardiographic QTc interval prolongation (>450 milliseconds in men, >470 milliseconds in women). This complication has been associated with prokinetics currently in use worldwide (domperidone) or withdrawn except

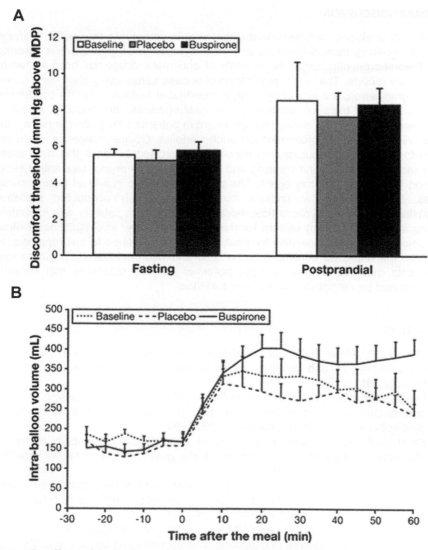

Fig. 3. The effects of the 5-HT$_{1A}$ agonist buspirone are shown on gastric sensitivity to distention (*A*) and gastric accommodation after eating (*B*) in patients with functional dyspepsia. Buspirone had no effect on sensation but enhanced meal-induced gastric relaxation. (*From* Tack J, Janssen P, Masaoka T, et al. Efficacy of buspirone, a fundus-relaxing drug, in patients with functional dyspepsia. Clin Gastroenterol Hepatol 2012;10:1243; with permission.)

in regulated patient-assistance programs (cisapride). QTc prolongation also has been attributed to other antiemetic and neuromodulatory drugs used for gastroparesis, including 5-HT$_3$ receptor antagonists and tricyclic antidepressants.[43] Although increases in sudden cardiac death have been reported, no similar black box warnings have been issued for these medications. Consideration has been advocated for surveillance monitoring of electrolytes and electrocardiographic testing in selected clinical settings during use of some of these drugs.

SUMMARY/DISCUSSION

Antiemetic, analgesic, and neuromodulatory agents commonly are used to manage nausea, vomiting, pain, discomfort, and other symptoms of gastroparesis. Despite their theoretic benefits, evidence for utility of antiemetic drugs has been limited to a few case reports. The recent publication of a case series using short-term transdermal granisetron, a 5-HT$_3$ antagonist, in open-label fashion supports conduct of more controlled trials of antiemetics in gastroparesis. An ongoing placebo-controlled trial of the NK$_1$ antagonist aprepitant in patients with gastroparesis symptoms will provide new information on such benefits. Opiate analgesics are often taken for pain control, but caution should be exercised because this drug class can exacerbate nausea and vomiting and retard gastric emptying. Like antiemetics, support for neuromodulatory agents has been restricted to individual gastroparesis cases. However, negative findings from a meticulously conducted placebo-controlled trial of the tricyclic antidepressant nortriptyline in patients with idiopathic gastroparesis dampen enthusiasm for this type of therapy. Investigations of other neuromodulators are proceeding for treating conditions related to gastroparesis. In addition, the unproved benefits of antiemetic and neuromodulatory gastroparesis treatments must be weighed against potential adverse outcomes that recently have focused on neurologic and cardiac toxicities.

REFERENCES

1. Pasricha PJ, Colvin R, Yates K, et al. Characteristics of patients with chronic unexplained nausea and vomiting and normal gastric emptying. Clin Gastroenterol Hepatol 2011;9:567–76.
2. Delgado-Aros S, Camilleri M, Cremonini F, et al. Contributions of gastric volumes and gastric emptying to meal size and postmeal symptoms in functional dyspepsia. Gastroenterology 2004;127:1685–94.
3. Karamanolis G, Caenepeel P, Arts J, et al. Determinants of symptom pattern in idiopathic severely delayed gastric emptying: gastric emptying rate or proximal stomach dysfunction? Gut 2007;56:29–36.
4. Karamanolis G, Caenepeel P, Arts J, et al. Association of the predominant symptom with clinical characteristics and pathophysiological mechanisms in functional dyspepsia. Gastroenterology 2006;130:296–303.
5. Schade RR, Dugas MC, Lhotsky DM, et al. Effect of metoclopramide on gastric liquid emptying in patients with diabetic gastroparesis. Dig Dis Sci 1985;30:10–5.
6. Maganti K, Onyemere K, Jones MP. Oral erythromycin and symptomatic relief of gastroparesis: a systematic review. Am J Gastroenterol 2003;98:259–63.
7. Revicki DA, Rentz AM, Dubois D, et al. Development and validation of a patient-assessed gastroparesis symptom severity measure: the Gastroparesis Cardinal Symptom Index. Aliment Pharmacol Ther 2003;18:141–50.
8. Revicki DA, Camilleri M, Kuo B, et al. Evaluating symptom outcomes in gastroparesis clinical trials: validity and responsiveness of the Gastroparesis Cardinal Symptom Index—Daily Diary (GCSI-DD). Neurogastroenterol Motil 2012;24: 456–63.
9. Pasricha PJ, Nguyen LA, Snape WJ, et al. Changes in quality of life and symptoms in a large cohort of patients with gastroparesis followed prospectively for 48 weeks [abstract]. Gastroenterology 2010;138:1069.
10. Cherian D, Parkman HP. Nausea and vomiting in diabetic and idiopathic gastroparesis. Neurogastroenterol Motil 2012;24:217–22.

11. Hasler WL, Wilson LA, Parkman HP, et al. Factors related to abdominal pain in gastroparesis: contrast to patients with predominant nausea and vomiting. Neurogastroenterol Motil 2013;25:427–38.
12. Parkman HP, Yates K, Hasler WL, et al. Similarities and differences between diabetic and idiopathic gastroparesis. Clin Gastroenterol Hepatol 2011;9:1056–64.
13. Navavi RM. Management of chemotherapy-induced nausea and vomiting: focus on newer agents and new uses for older agents. Drugs 2013;73:249–62.
14. Galli JA, Sawaya RA, Friedenberg FK. Cannabinoid hyperemesis syndrome. Curr Drug Abuse Rev 2011;4:241–9.
15. Lossos IS, Mevorach D, Oren R. Thiethylperazine treatment of gastroparesis diabeticorum. Ann Pharmacother 1992;26:1016.
16. Amin K, Bastani B. Intraperitoneal ondansetron hydrochloride for intractable nausea and vomiting due to diabetic gastroparesis in a patient on peritoneal dialysis. Perit Dial Int 2002;22:539–40.
17. Simmons K, Parkman HP. Granisetron transdermal system improves refractory nausea and vomiting in gastroparesis. Dig Dis Sci 2014;59:1231–4.
18. Chong K, Dharariya K. A case of severe, refractory diabetic gastroparesis managed by prolonged use of aprepitant. Nat Rev Endocrinol 2009;5:285–8.
19. Fahler J, Wall GC, Leman BI. Gastroparesis-associated refractory nausea treated with aprepitant. Ann Pharmacother 2012;46:e38.
20. Cherian D, Sachdeva P, Fisher RS, et al. Abdominal pain is a frequent symptom of gastroparesis. Clin Gastroenterol Hepatol 2010;8:676–81.
21. Bielefeldt K, Raza N, Zickmund SL. Different faces of gastroparesis. World J Gastroenterol 2009;15:6052–60.
22. Anaparthy R, Pehlivanov N, Grady J, et al. Gastroparesis and gastroparesis-like syndrome: response to therapy and its predictors. Dig Dis Sci 2009;54:1003–10.
23. Maurer AH, Krevsky B, Knight LC, et al. Opioid and opioid-like drug effects on whole-gut transit measured by scintigraphy. J Nucl Med 1996;37:818–22.
24. Peghini PL, Katz PO, Castell DO. Imipramine decreases oesophageal pain perception in human male volunteers. Gut 1998;42:807–13.
25. Coates MD, Johnson AC, Greenwood-Van Meerveld B, et al. Effects of serotonin transporter inhibition on gastrointestinal motility and colonic sensitivity in the mouse. Neurogastroenterol Motil 2006;18:464–71.
26. Tack J, Vanden Berghe P, Coulie B, et al. Sumatriptan is an agonist at 5-HT1P receptors on myenteric neurons in the guinea pig gastric antrum. Neurogastroenterol Motil 2007;19:39–46.
27. Mertz H, Fass R, Kodner A, et al. Effect of amitriptyline on symptoms, sleep, and visceral perception in patients with functional dyspepsia. Am J Gastroenterol 1998;93:160–5.
28. Prakash C, Lustman PJ, Freedland KE, et al. Tricyclic antidepressants for functional nausea and vomiting: clinical outcome in 37 patients. Dig Dis Sci 1998;43:1951–6.
29. Sawhney MS, Prakash C, Lustman PJ, et al. Tricyclic antidepressants for chronic vomiting in diabetic patients. Dig Dis Sci 2007;52:418–24.
30. Parkman HP, Van Natta ML, Abell TL, et al. Effect of nortriptyline on symptoms of idiopathic gastroparesis: the NORIG randomized clinical trial. JAMA 2013;310:2640–9.
31. Fernández J, Alonso JM, Andrés JI, et al. Discovery of new tetracyclic tetrahydrofuran derivatives as potential broad-spectrum psychotropic agents. J Med Chem 2005;48:1709–12.
32. Kim SW, Shin IS, Kim JM, et al. Mirtazapine for severe gastroparesis unresponsive to conventional prokinetic treatment. Psychosomatics 2006;47:440–2.

33. Johnstone M, Buddhdev P, Peter M, et al. Mirtazapine: a solution for postoperative gastroparesis? BMJ Case Rep 2009. http://dx.doi.org/10.1136/bcr.02.2009.1579.

34. Kundu S, Rogal S, Alam A, et al. Rapid improvement in post-infectious gastroparesis symptoms with mirtazapine. World J Gastroenterol 2014;20:6671–4.

35. Ly HG, Carbone F, Holvoet L, et al. Mirtazapine improves early satiation, nutrient intake, weight recovery and quality of life in functional dyspepsia with weight loss: a double-blind, randomized, placebo-controlled pilot study (abstract). Gastroenterology 2013;144:161.

36. Yin J, Song J, Lei Y, et al. Prokinetic effects of mirtazapine on gastrointestinal transit. Am J Physiol Gastrointest Liver Physiol 2014;306:G796–801.

37. Gooden JY, Takahashi PY. Mirtazapine treatment of diabetic gastroparesis as a novel method to reduce tube-feed residual: a case report. J Med Case Rep 2013;7:38.

38. Kaneishi K, Kawabata M, Morita T. Olanzapine for the relief of nausea in patients with advanced cancer and incomplete bowel obstruction. J Pain Symptom Manage 2012;44:604–7.

39. Tack J, Janssen P, Masaoka T, et al. Efficacy of buspirone, a fundus-relaxing drug, in patients with functional dyspepsia. Clin Gastroenterol Hepatol 2012;10:1239–45.

40. Miwa H, Nagahara A, Tominaga K, et al. Efficacy of the 5-HT$_{1A}$ agonist tandospirone citrate in improving symptoms of patients with functional dyspepsia: a randomized controlled trial. Am J Gastroenterol 2009;104:2779–87.

41. Lee A, Kuo B. Metoclopramide in the treatment of diabetic gastroparesis. Expert Rev Endocrinol Metab 2010;5:653–62.

42. Ehrenpreis ED, Deepak P, Sifuentes H, et al. The metoclopramide black box warning for tardive dyskinesia: effect on clinical practice, adverse event reporting, and prescription drug lawsuits. Am J Gastroenterol 2013;108:866–72.

43. Keller GA, Ponte ML, Di Girolamo G. Other drugs acting on nervous system associated with QT-interval prolongation. Curr Drug Saf 2010;5:105–11.

Prokinetics in Gastroparesis

Andres Acosta, MD, PhD, Michael Camilleri, MD*

KEYWORDS

- Domperidone • Erythromycin • Ghrelin • Metoclopramide • Pharmacology
- Pyridostigmine • Receptor • Relamorelin • Serotonin

KEY POINTS

- Prokinetic agents are medications that enhance coordinated gastrointestinal motility and transit of content in the gastrointestinal tract, mainly by amplifying and coordinating the gastrointestinal muscular contractions.
- Prokinetic therapy should be considered as a means to improve gastric emptying and symptoms of gastroparesis.
- Metoclopramide remains the first-line prokinetic therapy, because it is the only approved medication for gastroparesis in the United States.
- Other medications for gastroparesis should be used by balancing benefits and risks of treatment.
- There are newer agents being developed for the management of gastroparesis targeting different pathways: 5-hydroxytryptamine type 4 (receptor agonists), new motilin receptors agonists, and ghrelin agonists.

INTRODUCTION

Gastroparesis is defined as objectively delayed gastric emptying in the absence of mechanical obstruction and in the presence of upper gastrointestinal symptoms including early satiety, postprandial fullness, nausea, vomiting, bloating, and upper abdominal pain.[1,2] The most common causes of gastroparesis are diabetes mellitus, postsurgical, and idiopathic; less common causes are iatrogenic, extrinsic neuronal (such as parkinsonism and paraneoplastic disease), and infiltrative disorders (such as scleroderma).[1,3–7] The management of gastroparesis is based on dietary therapy;

This article originally appeared in Gastroenterology Clinics, Volume 44, Issue 1, March 2015.
Funding: Dr M. Camilleri is supported by grants R01-DK92179 and R01-DK67071 from National Institutes of Health.
Conflicts of interest: None.
Clinical Enteric Neuroscience Translational and Epidemiological Research (C.E.N.T.E.R.), Mayo Clinic, 200 First Street Southwest, Rochester, MN 55905, USA
* Corresponding author. Mayo Clinic, 200 First Street Southwest, Charlton Building, Room 8-110, Rochester, MN 55905.
E-mail address: camilleri.michael@mayo.edu

restoration of fluid and electrolyte balance; nutritional support; treating the underlying cause, such as optimization of glycemic control in diabetics; and stimulation of gastric emptying (**Fig. 1**).[2]

This article discusses in detail the prokinetic agents available or under evaluation for the treatment of gastroparesis.

PROKINETICS: DEFINITIONS AND CLASSIFICATIONS

Prokinetic agents are medications that enhance coordinated gastrointestinal motility and transit of content in the gastrointestinal tract, mainly by amplifying and

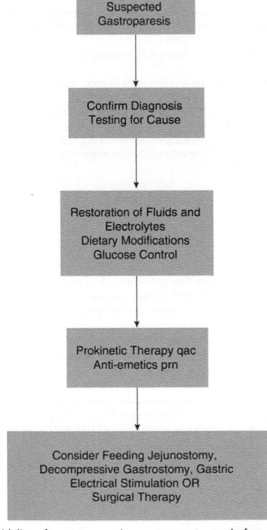

Fig. 1. Clinical guidelines for gastroparesis management. qac, before every meal; prn, as required or needed. (*From* Camilleri M, Parkman HP, Shafi MA, et al. Clinical guideline: management of gastroparesis. Am J Gastroenterol 2013;108(1):18–37; with permission.)

coordinating the gastrointestinal muscular contraction. Prokinetics enhance coordination among the segments of the gut, which is necessary for propulsion of luminal contents. Prokinetics may be either selective to certain areas of the gastrointestinal tract or more generalized, and this reflects the distribution of the receptor targets of the different compounds.

Acetylcholine (Ach), released from primary motor neurons in the myenteric plexus, is the principal excitatory transmitter mediating muscle contractility; other excitatory transmitters are the tachykinins (such as substance P), motilin, and ghrelin. To date, most of the clinically useful prokinetic agents act upstream of Ach, at receptor sites on the motor neuron, or on neurons or nonneuronal cells that synapse with cholinergic neurons. Prokinetic agents are pharmacologically and chemically diverse; they release excitatory neurotransmitters at the nerve-muscle junction without interfering with the normal physiologic patterns and rhythms of motility.

The gastric prokinetics (their main effect is to enhance gastric contractility) include dopamine receptor antagonists, motilin receptor agonists, serotonin (5-hydroxytryptamine [5-HT] type 4 [5-HT$_4$]) receptor agonists, cholinesterase inhibitors, and ghrelin agonists. This article categorizes medications as approved or under evaluation.

PROKINETICS IN MANAGEMENT GUIDELINES FOR GASTROPARESIS

The American College of Gastroenterology (ACG) guidelines, published in 2013, documented the evidence for the pharmacologic management of gastroparesis and used the GRADE (Grades of Recommendation Assessment, Development and Evaluation) system to evaluate the strength of the recommendations (strong, moderate, or weak if the desirable effects on an intervention clearly outweigh the undesirable effects, and as conditional if there is uncertainty) and the overall quality of evidence (high, moderate, low, or very low).[8]

The most recently published guidelines for the pharmacologic management of gastroparesis[2] are shown in **Box 1**.

APPROVED MEDICATIONS (INCLUDING OFF-LABEL USE)
Dopamine Receptor Antagonists

There are 2 dopamine receptor antagonists available for the management of gastroparesis: metoclopramide and domperidone. Metoclopramide should be the first-line treatment and is the only medication approved by the US Food and Drug Administration (FDA) for the indication of gastroparesis, with recommended use for less than 12 weeks. Domperidone can be prescribed through the FDA's Expanded Access to Investigational Drugs program. Both agents are dopamine2 (D2) receptor antagonists. Dopamine inhibits the release of Ach, thus decreasing gastric and proximal small bowel motility.[9] A D2 antagonist reverses the inhibitory effects of endogenous dopamine.

Metoclopramide
Chemistry and pharmacokinetics Metoclopramide, or 4-amino-5-chloro-N-(2-(diethylamino)ethyl)-2-methoxybenzamide, is a substituted benzamide derivative, with a chemical structure similar to procainamide, but without antiarrhythmic effects.[10] Metoclopramide is metabolized mainly by CYP2D6 and to a lesser extent by the CYP3A4 and CYP1A3[11]; up to 30% of the drug is excreted unchanged in the urine.[12]

Mechanism of action Metoclopramide has dual activity as a D2 receptor antagonist and a 5-HT$_4$ agonist, decreasing effects of dopamine and thereby stimulating the

> **Box 1**
> **Recommendations in ACG 2013 guidelines for gastroparesis**
>
> - In addition to dietary therapy, prokinetic therapy should be considered to improve gastric emptying and gastroparesis symptoms, taking into account benefits and risks of treatment (strong recommendation, moderate level of evidence).
>
> - Metoclopramide is the first line of prokinetic therapy and should be administered at the lowest effective dose in a liquid formulation to facilitate absorption. The risk of tardive dyskinesia has been estimated to be less than 1%. Patients should be instructed to discontinue therapy if they develop side effects including involuntary movements (moderate recommendation, moderate level of evidence).
>
> - For patients unable to use metoclopramide, domperidone can be prescribed with investigational new drug clearance from the US Food and Drug Administration and has been shown to be as effective as metoclopramide in reducing symptoms without the propensity for causing central nervous system side effects; given the propensity of domperidone to prolong corrected QT interval on electrocardiogram, a baseline electrocardiogram is recommended and treatment withheld if the corrected QT is greater than 470 milliseconds in men and greater than 450 milliseconds in women. Follow-up electrocardiogram on treatment with domperidone is also advised (moderate recommendation, moderate level of evidence).
>
> - Erythromycin improves gastric emptying and symptoms from delayed gastric emptying. Administration of intravenous erythromycin should be considered when intravenous prokinetic therapy is needed in hospitalized patients. Oral treatment with erythromycin also improves gastric emptying. However, the long-term effectiveness of oral therapy is limited by tachyphylaxis (strong recommendation, moderate level of evidence).
>
> - Treatment with antiemetic agents should be given for improvement of associated nausea and vomiting, but does not result in improved gastric emptying (conditional recommendation, moderate level of evidence).
>
> - Tricyclic antidepressants can be considered for refractory nausea and vomiting in gastroparesis, but do not result in improved gastric emptying and may potentially retard gastric emptying (conditional recommendation, low level of evidence).
>
> *From* Camilleri M, Parkman HP, Shafi MA, et al. Clinical guideline: management of gastroparesis. Am J Gastroenterol 2013;108(1):18–37; with permission.

cholinergic receptors. This effect promotes the release of Ach, which increases lower esophageal sphincter and gastric tone, increases intragastric pressure, improves antroduodenal coordination, and accelerates gastric emptying.[10] The dual effects on gastric contractility and the centrally mediated antiemetic effect are considered responsible for the improved symptoms of gastroparesis (**Fig. 2**). The antiemetic effect is mainly mediated from inhibition of D2 and 5-HT$_3$ receptors within the nausea or vomiting centers in the brainstem, especially the chemoreceptor trigger zone and the area postrema.

Pharmacodynamics and clinical pharmacology The effect of metoclopramide on gastric emptying has been shown in short-term (less than 4 weeks) studies (**Table 1**).[13–18] Metoclopramide significantly increased gastric motor activity in patients with gastroparesis, often triggering an intense burst of motor activity in the stomach.[19] Metoclopramide improved gastric emptying by 56% in patients with gastroparesis compared with 37% in the placebo group.[20] These short-term studies showed generally poor correlation of acceleration of gastric emptying with symptom improvement.

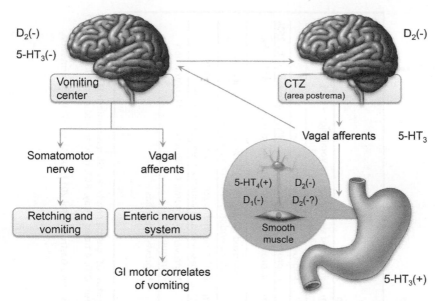

Fig. 2. Dual mechanism of action of metoclopramide. GI, gastrointestinal. (*From* Lee A, Kuo B. Metoclopramide in the treatment of diabetic gastroparesis. Expert Rev Endocrinol Metab 2010;5(5):653–62; with permission.)

Formulations Metoclopramide is available in multiple formulations: oral, orally disinte-grating sublingual, intranasal, subcutaneous injections, and intravenous. The last 3 formulations have the advantage of bypassing the first-pass elimination in the liver and are ideal in patients with limited absorption caused by recurrent vomiting.[10]

Dosing The current guidelines recommend starting with liquid formulation at 5 mg orally, 30 minutes before meals and at bedtime. If needed, the doses can be increased to 10 mg, up to 4 times per day, but it is recommended to avoid doses higher than 40 mg daily to avoid side effects.

Adverse effects Metoclopramide is associated with reversible or irreversible side ef-fects, and the FDA has placed a Black Box warning on the use of metoclopramide (http://www.fda.gov/newsevents/newsroom/pressannouncements/ucm149533.htm). Metoclopramide's central nervous system (CNS) side effects are secondary to easy crossing of the blood-brain barrier and are observed in up to 30% of patients.[2] Thus the most common side effects are related to the dopaminergic effects on the CNS. The reversible side effects, which resolve once the drug is discontinued, are mainly drowsiness, fatigue, lethargy, hyperprolactinemia, and worsening depression.[10]

  The extrapyramidal reactions associated with metoclopramide are acute dystonic reactions, such as facial spasms, torticollis, oculogyric crisis, trismus, abdominal ri-gidity, or spasm of the entire body; these effects usually are reversible.[21] The irrevers-ible and most concerning side effect is tardive dyskinesia, which typically occurs at doses higher than 40 mg daily. The overall frequency of all extrapyramidal side effects associated with metoclopramide is 0.2%.[10,22,23] Treatment recommendations and careful monitoring are described by Rao and Camilleri.[23]

  In addition, metoclopramide may increase the half-life of other drugs metabolized by CYP2D6. Hence, the use of metoclopramide in combination with other neuroleptic

Table 1
Trials of metoclopramide for gastroparesis

Reference #	Design	#, Cause	Dose	Duration	Results
20	DB, PC, XO, RCT	10 DG	10 mg QID	3 wk/arm	Improved symptoms and vomiting; ~60% acceleration in GE liquid 150-kcal meal
13	DB, PC, PG, RCT	28: 5 DM, 4 PSG, 19 IG	10 mg QID	3 wk	Improved symptoms by 29%
15	PC, RCT	18 DG	10 mg QID	3 wk	Improved symptom score by 29%, improved GE by 25%
16	DB, PC, XO, RCT	13 DG with GE accelerated by metoclopramide	10 mg QID	3 wk/arm	Improved symptoms with mean reduction of 52.6%
17	DB, RCT, domperidone controlled	45 DG	10 mg QID	4 wk	Improved symptoms by 39%; similar efficacy with domperidone, which had fewer AEs
18	DB, XO, erythromycin-control RCT	13 DG	10 mg TID	3 wk/arm	Both treatments accelerated GE compared with baseline and improved symptoms score
56	Open	1 DG	15 mg QID	6 mo	Improved symptoms, GE liquids, antral contraction frequency
57	Open	10 GI symptomatic (N,V) type 1 DM; 6 asymptomatic T1DM, 18 controls	10 mg once	acute	Improved GE solids

Abbreviations: AE, adverse events; DB, double-blind; DG, diabetic gastroparesis; DM, diabetes mellitus; GE, gastric emptying; GI, gastrointestinal; IG, idiopathic gastroparesis; N, nausea; PC, placebo-controlled; PG, parallel group; PSG, postsurgical gastroparesis; QID, 4 times a day; RCT, randomized controlled trial; TID, 3 times a day; T1DM, type 1 diabetes mellitus; V, vomitting; XO, crossover.

From Camilleri M, Parkman HP, Shafi MA, et al. Clinical guideline: management of gastroparesis. Am J Gastroenterol 2013;108(1):18–37; with permission.

drugs, such as haloperidol, thioridazine, chlorpromazine, perphenazine, and risperidone, can increase the risk of extrapyramidal symptoms. Polymorphisms in *CYP2D6*, *KCNH2*, and *HTR4* genes were associated with side effects, whereas polymorphisms in *KCNH2* and *ADRA1D* genes were associated with clinical response.[24]

Domperidone

Chemistry and pharmacokinetics Domperidone is a D2 receptor antagonist with similar efficacy to metoclopramide as an antiemetic and prokinetic. However, domperidone has poor penetration of the blood-brain barrier with limited to no CNS side effects. Domperidone structure is based on butyrophenones, and the drug has a low oral bioavailability (15%) that can be further decreased by increasing gastric pH.[25] Domperidone has high affinity for gastrointestinal tissue, and high concentrations of the drug are found in the esophagus, stomach, and small intestine after oral administration.[26] Approximately 90% of domperidone is bound to plasma proteins. It has a half-life of 7.5 hours, is mainly metabolized by the liver, and 32% of the drug is excreted in the urine.[27]

Mechanism of action Domperidone increases the amplitude of esophageal motor function and antroduodenal contractions, coordinates peristalsis across the pylorus, and accelerates gastric emptying.[28,29] The effect of domperidone on gastric emptying has been shown in short-term studies (**Table 2**).

Dosing The current guidelines recommend starting with 10 mg 3 times a day, and increasing to 20 mg 3 times a day and at bedtime. Patients should have a baseline electrocardiogram and another when on medication, because domperidone can prolong the QTc interval. Domperidone should be avoided if the corrected QTc interval is greater than 470 milliseconds in men and greater than 450 milliseconds in women.

Although available for the past 25 years in most countries (and a recent recommendation from European Medicines Agency (EMA) made it also available over the counter in Europe), it is only available in the United States through compassionate clearance for patients with refractory gastroparesis (http://www.fda.gov/cder/news/domperidone.htm).

Adverse effects Side effects with oral administration of domperidone occur in less than 7% of patients and include headaches, dry mouth, diarrhea, anxiety, and hyperprolactinemia. As with metoclopramide, domperidone inhibits the CYP2D6 enzyme, and drug-drug interactions should be considered.[30] There are polymorphisms that predispose to potentially higher drug levels of domperidone and cardiac toxicity; nevertheless, the opinion of the European Medicines Agency's Pharmacovigilance Risk Assessment Committee was that the benefits outweighed risks when given in the short term and in low doses to treat nausea or vomiting, but not for bloating or heartburn. The recommended doses are 10 mg up to 3 times daily by mouth for adults and adolescents weighing 35 kg or more, and 0.25 mg/kg bodyweight up to 3 times daily for children or patients weighing less than 35 kg.[31]

Motilin Receptor Agonists

The most common motilin receptor agonists are the macrolides, a class of antibiotics that stimulates the motilin receptors in the gastrointestinal tract. Erythromycin is the most commonly studied macrolide. These agents improve gastric emptying and symptoms; however, in the medium or long term, they are associated with tachyphylaxis caused by downregulation of the motilin receptor, typically starting within 2 weeks of the onset of therapy.[32]

Table 2
Trials of domperidone in gastroparesis

Reference #	Type of Study	N, Cause	Duration	Symptom Improvement vs Baseline (Open) vs Placebo (RCT)	Δ Gastric Emptying	Adverse Effects
58	Open, 10 mg QID	3 DG	1 wk	Yes, not quantified	Improved, not quantified	NA
59	Open	12 IG; 3 DG, 2 PSG	48 mo	68.3% (P<.05)	34.5% (P<.05)	↑ Prolactin (100%), symptoms (17.6%)
60	Retrospective	57 DM	377 d	70% patients improved	NA	16%
61	Open	6 DG	6 mo	79.2% (P<.01)	26.9% (NS)	NA
62	Open	12 DG	Single oral dose	Chronic oral administration (35–51 d) reduced symptoms	↑ Solid and liquid emptying (P<.005)	NA
63	RCT, PG, withdrawal study	208 DG: 105 DOM, 103 PLA	4 wk	53.8% lower overall score with domperidone (P = .025)	NA	2%–3% ↑ prolactin, similar to placebo
64	RCT, PC, XO	13 DG	8 wk	↓ In symptom frequency and intensity vs placebo (P<.03)	NA	NA
65	RCT, PC, XO	6 DG	Single 10 mg IV	NA	↑ Homogenized solid emptying	NA
66	RCT, PC, XO	8 IG; 3 DG	4 wk	No overall benefit compared with placebo; 2 of 3 DM improved	NA	Gas pains, skin rash
67	RCT, PG vs cisapride, 14 per group	Total 31 pediatric DG; 3 excluded for poor compliance	8 wk	Domperidone improved vs baseline (P<.001); domperidone vs cisapride (P<.01)	Domperidone significantly more effective than placebo in reducing the gastric emptying time measured by ultrasonography	None recorded
17	RCT, PG, vs metoclopramide	95 DG	4 wk	41.19% improved vs baseline (NA); NS vs metoclopramide	NA	CNS effects more severe and common with metoclopramide: somnolence, mental acuity (49% metoclopramide vs 29% DOM)

Abbreviations: CNS, central nervous system; DG, diabetic gastroparesis; DM, diabetes-mellitus; DOM, domperidone; IG, idiopathic gastroparesis; IV, intravenously; NA, not assessed; NS, nonsignificant; PC, placebo-controlled; PG, parallel group; PLA, placebo; PSG, postsurgical gastroparesis; QID, 4 times a day; RCT, randomized controlled trial; XO, crossover.

From Camilleri M, Parkman HP, Shafi MA, et al. Clinical guideline: management of gastroparesis. Am J Gastroenterol 2013;108(1):18–37; with permission.

Erythromycin

Mechanism of action Erythromycin induces phasic contractions in the antrum by cholinergic activity and promotes pyloric relaxation through action on the inhibitory nerves of the pylorus.[33–35] High-dose erythromycin (eg, 2–3 mg/kg intravenously [IV]) stimulates migrating motor complex activities, whereas lower dosing (eg, 1 mg/kg IV) activates phasic stomach and small bowel motility similar to a fed pattern.[2,33,36] The lack of a long-term effect, mainly explained by tachyphylaxis,[32] precludes medium-term efficacy in clinical practice, and there have been no long-term, randomized, placebo-controlled trials.

Dosing

The current recommended doses are 1.5 to 3 mg/kg IV (by infusion over 45 minutes) every 6 hours in patients admitted to hospital with gastroparesis, and 125 mg, twice a day, orally in liquid formulation, for outpatient gastroparesis management. The oral regimen may provide benefit for a few weeks.

Adverse effects Side effects of erythromycin include abdominal pain, nausea, and diarrhea. Erythromycin also may induce drug interactions with agents that alter or are metabolized by CYP3A4, and they should be used carefully in combination with diltiazem or verapamil because of an increased risk for sudden cardiac death.[37]

Other macrolides, such as azithromycin and clarithromycin

Other macrolides, such as azithromycin and clarithromycin, accelerate gastric emptying.[38,39] However, there are no randomized controlled trials comparing these drugs with placebo or other medications, and their use should be balanced with the potential for tachyphylaxis, cardiac risk, and antibiotic resistance.

5-Hydroxytryptamine Type 4 Receptor Agonists

5-HT$_4$ receptors are distributed throughout the gastrointestinal tract and have been extensively studied in gastrointestinal motility disorders.

Cisapride and tegaserod

In the past, 2 5-HT$_4$ receptor agonists, cisapride and tegaserod, were on the market for indications of gastroparesis and chronic constipation, respectively. However, their poor receptor selectivity and cisapride's high affinity for the heart voltage-gated K$^+$ (hERG-K$^+$) channel caused drug-induced ventricular arrhythmias.

Prucalopride, naronapride, velusetrag, and YKP10811

A new generation of 5-HT$_4$ receptor agonists, such as prucalopride, naronapride, velusetrag, and YKP10811, have lower affinity for the hERG-K$^+$ channel and higher selectivity for the 5-HT$_4$ receptor.[40,41]

Prucalopride Prucalopride is approved by the EMA for the treatment of chronic constipation. In addition, prucalopride accelerates gastric emptying and small bowel transit in patients with chronic constipation[42] and could be considered as a potential agent for gastroparesis. However, the use of prucalopride for gastroparesis is not supported by any clinical evidence or trials to date. Prucalopride is currently not approved by the FDA for any indication.

YKP10811 YKP10811 accelerated gastrointestinal and colonic transit and gastric empting, and improved bowel functions, compared with placebo, in an 8-day study in patients with functional constipation.[41]

Cholinesterase Inhibitors

Neostigmine
Neostigmine is a cholinesterase inhibitor that induced an irregular increase in gastro-duodenal motor activity, sometimes characterized by propagated and nonpropagated clustered contractions,[43] and accelerated liquid gastric emptying in critically ill patients with delayed gastric emptying.[44] Neostigmine is only available in parenteral formulation and may be used in the hospital setting.

Pyridostigmine
Pyridostigmine may have similar efficacy to neostigmine; it is used off-label in liquid formulation at a dose of 60 mg, 3 times a day. However, there are no clinical trials to support its use in gastroparesis.

MEDICATIONS CURRENTLY UNDER EVALUATION
New Motilin Receptor Agonist

GSK962040 (Camicinal)
GSK962040 is a nonmotilide motilin receptor agonist with low molecular mass that increases gastrointestinal motility in dogs.[45] It selectively activates the motilin receptor in humans and specifically activates the antrum preferentially relative to the fundus, small intestine, or colon in human tissue in vitro.[46] This medication has been evaluated to determine safety and tolerability in humans.[47] It is currently being investigated in phase 2 clinical trials (ClinicalTrials.gov trial NCT01262898).

Ghrelin Agonists

Ghrelin is a 28-amino residue peptide secreted mainly in the stomach and, through the ghrelin receptor, it promotes gastric motility in mice, rats, dogs, and humans.[48–50] Synthetic ghrelin agonists, predominantly small molecules, are being developed as prokinetic agents that may prove useful in the treatment of gastrointestinal dysmotility disorders such as gastroparesis.[51] Actions and therapeutic pathways of ghrelin for gastrointestinal disorders have been reviewed elsewhere.[52]

Relamorelin
Relamorelin, a pentapeptide synthetic ghrelin agonist, has similar characteristics to native ghrelin but with improved stability, a longer plasma half-life, and greater potency. Results from 2 small, phase 1b, placebo-controlled, single-dose (100 μg), 2-period, crossover studies in patients with type 2 diabetes mellitus and type 1 diabetes mellitus and prior documentation of delayed gastric emptying indicated that relamorelin was generally well tolerated. Relamorelin significantly accelerated gastric emptying of solids at 1 and 2 hours (**Fig. 3**). The most common adverse events included hyperhidrosis, dizziness, fatigue, abdominal pain/cramping, decreased blood pressure, hunger, feeling cold, and muscular weakness.[53]

A subsequent randomized, double-blind, placebo-controlled, adaptive-design, parallel-group, 28-day, phase 2 study was conducted in patients with diabetic gastroparesis. Compared with baseline, relamorelin, 10 μg, twice a day, resulted in significant acceleration of gastric emptying ($P<.03$). There were also significant improvements in vomiting end points on relamorelin treatment compared with placebo; these effects were most evident in the 58.3% of patients who had vomiting during the baseline period.[54]

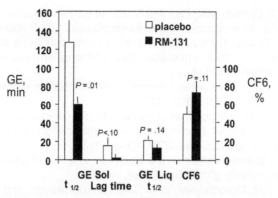

Fig. 3. Effects of Relamorelin (RM-131) in patients with type 2 diabetic gastroparesis with previously documented delayed gastric emptying (GE). CF6, colonic filling 6 hr; Liq, liquid; Sol, solid. (*From* Shin A, Camilleri M, Busciglio I, et al. The ghrelin agonist RM-131 accelerates gastric emptying of solids and reduces symptoms in patients with type 1 diabetes mellitus. Clin Gastroenterol Hepatol 2013;11(11):1453–59; with permission.)

Ulimorelin (TZP-102)

Ulimorelin is a ghrelin receptor agonist that accelerates gastric emptying and improves upper gastrointestinal symptoms in diabetic patients with gastroparesis.[55] In a phase 2a study, ulimorelin improved gastroparesis symptoms without correlation or improvement in gastric emptying. However, in a phase 2b study, ulimorelin efficacy was not shown compared with placebo.

SUMMARY

Prokinetic agents should be the first line of treatment of patients with gastroparesis. Metoclopramide remains the only approved medication in the United States for the indication of gastroparesis. The use of metoclopramide should be limited to less than 12 weeks; this limitation is a challenge for patients and their physicians, because gastroparesis often lasts several years. Other medications, including domperidone, require special FDA approval or off-label use. Promising new agents being developed for the management of gastroparesis include 5-HT$_4$ agonists and the ghrelin agonist, relamorelin.

REFERENCES

1. Camilleri M, Bharucha AE, Farrugia G. Epidemiology, mechanisms, and management of diabetic gastroparesis. Clin Gastroenterol Hepatol 2011;9(1):5–12 [quiz: e7].
2. Camilleri M, Parkman HP, Shafi MA, et al. Clinical guideline: management of gastroparesis. Am J Gastroenterol 2013;108(1):18–37 [quiz: 38].
3. Choung RS, Locke GR 3rd, Schleck CD, et al. Risk of gastroparesis in subjects with type 1 and 2 diabetes in the general population. Am J Gastroenterol 2012; 107(1):82–8.
4. Parkman HP, Yates K, Hasler WL, et al. Clinical features of idiopathic gastroparesis vary with sex, body mass, symptom onset, delay in gastric emptying, and gastroparesis severity. Gastroenterology 2011;140(1):101–15.
5. Camilleri M. Clinical practice. Diabetic gastroparesis. N Engl J Med 2007;356(8): 820–9.

6. Frantzides CT, Carlson MA, Zografakis JG, et al. Postoperative gastrointestinal complaints after laparoscopic Nissen fundoplication. JSLS 2006;10(1):39–42.
7. Bityutskiy LP, Soykan I, McCallum RW. Viral gastroparesis: a subgroup of idiopathic gastroparesis–clinical characteristics and long-term outcomes. Am J Gastroenterol 1997;92(9):1501–4.
8. Atkins D, Best D, Briss PA, et al. Grading quality of evidence and strength of recommendations. BMJ 2004;328(7454):1490.
9. Tonini M, Cipollina L, Poluzzi E, et al. Review article: clinical implications of enteric and central D2 receptor blockade by antidopaminergic gastrointestinal prokinetics. Aliment Pharmacol Ther 2004;19(4):379–90.
10. Lee A, Kuo B. Metoclopramide in the treatment of diabetic gastroparesis. Expert Rev Endocrinol Metab 2010;5(5):653–62.
11. Desta Z, Wu GM, Morocho AM, et al. The gastroprokinetic and antiemetic drug metoclopramide is a substrate and inhibitor of cytochrome P450 2D6. Drug Metab Dispos 2002;30(3):336–43.
12. Bateman DN. Clinical pharmacokinetics of metoclopramide. Clin Pharmacokinet 1983;8(6):523–9.
13. Perkel MS, Moore C, Hersh T, et al. Metoclopramide therapy in patients with delayed gastric emptying: a randomized, double-blind study. Dig Dis Sci 1979; 24(9):662–6.
14. Perkel MS, Hersh T, Moore C, et al. Metoclopramide therapy in fifty-five patients with delayed gastric emptying. Am J Gastroenterol 1980;74(3):231–6.
15. McCallum RW, Ricci DA, Rakatansky H, et al. A multicenter placebo-controlled clinical trial of oral metoclopramide in diabetic gastroparesis. Diabetes Care 1983;6(5):463–7.
16. Ricci DA, Saltzman MB, Meyer C, et al. Effect of metoclopramide in diabetic gastroparesis. J Clin Gastroenterol 1985;7(1):25–32.
17. Patterson D, Abell T, Rothstein R, et al. A double-blind multicenter comparison of domperidone and metoclopramide in the treatment of diabetic patients with symptoms of gastroparesis. Am J Gastroenterol 1999;94(5):1230–4.
18. Erbas T, Varoglu E, Erbas B, et al. Comparison of metoclopramide and erythromycin in the treatment of diabetic gastroparesis. Diabetes Care 1993;16(11):1511–4.
19. Malagelada JR, Rees WD, Mazzotta LJ, et al. Gastric motor abnormalities in diabetic and postvagotomy gastroparesis: effect of metoclopramide and bethanechol. Gastroenterology 1980;78(2):286–93.
20. Snape WJ Jr, Battle WM, Schwartz SS, et al. Metoclopramide to treat gastroparesis due to diabetes mellitus: a double-blind, controlled trial. Ann Intern Med 1982; 96(4):444–6.
21. Ganzini L, Casey DE, Hoffman WF, et al. The prevalence of metoclopramide-induced tardive dyskinesia and acute extrapyramidal movement disorders. Arch Intern Med 1993;153(12):1469–75.
22. Bateman DN, Rawlins MD, Simpson JM. Extrapyramidal reactions with metoclopramide. Br Med J (Clin Res Ed) 1985;291(6500):930–2.
23. Rao AS, Camilleri M. Review article: metoclopramide and tardive dyskinesia. Aliment Pharmacol Ther 2010;31(1):11–9.
24. Parkman HP, Mishra A, Jacobs M, et al. Clinical response and side effects of metoclopramide: associations with clinical, demographic, and pharmacogenetic parameters. J Clin Gastroenterol 2012;46(6):494–503.
25. Reddymasu SC, Soykan I, McCallum RW. Domperidone: review of pharmacology and clinical applications in gastroenterology. Am J Gastroenterol 2007;102(9): 2036–45.

26. Van Nueten JM, Ennis C, Helsen L, et al. Inhibition of dopamine receptors in the stomach: an explanation of the gastrokinetic properties of domperidone. Life Sci 1978;23(5):453–7.
27. Champion MC, Hartnett M, Yen M. Domperidone, a new dopamine antagonist. CMAJ 1986;135(5):457–61.
28. Weihrauch TR, Forster CF, Krieglstein J. Evaluation of the effect of domperidone on human oesophageal and gastroduodenal motility by intraluminal manometry. Postgrad Med J 1979;55(Suppl 1):7–10.
29. Valenzuela JE. Dopamine as a possible neurotransmitter in gastric relaxation. Gastroenterology 1976;71(6):1019–22.
30. Parkman HP, Jacobs MR, Mishra A, et al. Domperidone treatment for gastroparesis: demographic and pharmacogenetic characterization of clinical efficacy and side-effects. Dig Dis Sci 2011;56(1):115–24.
31. EMA-webpage. 2014. Available at: http://www.ema.europa.eu/docs/en_GB/document_library/Referrals_document/Domperidone_31/Recommendation_provided_by_Pharmacovigilance_Risk_Assessment_Committee/WC500162559.pdf. Accessed September 4, 2014.
32. Richards RD, Davenport K, McCallum RW. The treatment of idiopathic and diabetic gastroparesis with acute intravenous and chronic oral erythromycin. Am J Gastroenterol 1993;88(2):203–7.
33. Janssens J, Peeters TL, Vantrappen G, et al. Improvement of gastric emptying in diabetic gastroparesis by erythromycin. Preliminary studies. N Engl J Med 1990; 322(15):1028–31.
34. Catnach SM, Fairclough PD. Erythromycin and the gut. Gut 1992;33(3):397–401.
35. Parkman HP, Pagano AP, Vozzelli MA, et al. Gastrokinetic effects of erythromycin: myogenic and neurogenic mechanisms of action in rabbit stomach. Am J Phys 1995;269(3 Pt 1):G418–26.
36. Hejazi RA, McCallum RW, Sarosiek I. Prokinetics in diabetic gastroparesis. Curr Gastroenterol Rep 2012;14(4):297–305.
37. Ray WA, Murray KT, Meredith S, et al. Oral erythromycin and the risk of sudden death from cardiac causes. N Engl J Med 2004;351(11):1089–96.
38. Larson JM, Tavakkoli A, Drane WE, et al. Advantages of azithromycin over erythromycin in improving the gastric emptying half-time in adult patients with gastroparesis. J Neurogastroenterol Motil 2010;16(4):407–13.
39. Bortolotti M, Mari C, Brunelli F, et al. Effect of intravenous clarithromycin on interdigestive gastroduodenal motility of patients with functional dyspepsia and Helicobacter pylori gastritis. Dig Dis Sci 1999;44(12):2439–42.
40. Manabe N, Wong BS, Camilleri M. New-generation 5-HT4 receptor agonists: potential for treatment of gastrointestinal motility disorders. Expert Opin Investig Drugs 2010;19(6):765–75.
41. Shin A, Acosta A, Camilleri M, et al. A randomized trial of 5-Hydroxytryptamine 4-receptor agonist, YKP10811, on colonic transit and bowel function in functional constipation. Clin Gastroenterol Hepatol 2014. [Epub ahead of print].
42. Bouras E, Camilleri M, Burton D, et al. Prucalopride accelerates gastrointestinal and colonic transit in patients with constipation without a rectal evacuation disorder. Gastroenterology 2001;120(2):354–60.
43. Bortolotti M, Cucchiara S, Sarti P, et al. Comparison between the effects of neostigmine and ranitidine on interdigestive gastroduodenal motility of patients with gastroparesis. Digestion 1995;56(2):96–9.
44. Lucey MA, Patil V, Girling K, et al. Does neostigmine increase gastric emptying in the critically ill?–results of a pilot study. Crit Care Resusc 2003;5(1):14–9.

45. Leming S, Broad J, Cozens SJ, et al. GSK962040: a small molecule motilin receptor agonist which increases gastrointestinal motility in conscious dogs. Neurogastroenterol Motil 2011;23(10):958–958.e410.
46. Broad J, Mukherjee S, Samadi M, et al. Regional- and agonist-dependent facilitation of human neurogastrointestinal functions by motilin receptor agonists. Br J Pharmacol 2012;167(4):763–74.
47. Sanger GJ, Westaway SM, Barnes AA, et al. GSK962040: a small molecule, selective motilin receptor agonist, effective as a stimulant of human and rabbit gastrointestinal motility. Neurogastroenterol Motil 2009;21(6):657–64 e30–1.
48. Trudel L, Tomasetto C, Rio MC, et al. Ghrelin/motilin-related peptide is a potent prokinetic to reverse gastric postoperative ileus in rat. Am J Physiol Gastrointest Liver Physiol 2002;282(6):G948–52.
49. Dass NB, Munonyara M, Bassil AK, et al. Growth hormone secretagogue receptors in rat and human gastrointestinal tract and the effects of ghrelin. Neuroscience 2003;120(2):443–53.
50. Tack J, Depoortere I, Bisschops R, et al. Influence of ghrelin on gastric emptying and meal-related symptoms in idiopathic gastroparesis. Aliment Pharmacol Ther 2005;22(9):847–53.
51. Murray CD, Martin NM, Patterson M, et al. Ghrelin enhances gastric emptying in diabetic gastroparesis: a double blind, placebo controlled, crossover study. Gut 2005;54(12):1693–8.
52. Camilleri M, Papathanasopoulos A, Odunsi ST. Actions and therapeutic pathways of ghrelin for gastrointestinal disorders. Nat Rev Gastroenterol Hepatol 2009;6(6): 343–52.
53. Shin A, Camilleri M, Busciglio I, et al. The ghrelin agonist RM-131 accelerates gastric emptying of solids and reduces symptoms in patients with type 1 diabetes mellitus. Clin Gastroenterol Hepatol 2013;11(11):1453–9.
54. Lembo A, Camilleri M, McCallum R, et al. A phase 2, randomized, double-blind, placebo-controlled study to evaluate the safety and efficacy of RM-131 in patients with diabetic gastroparesis. Gastroenterology 2014;146(Suppl 1): S158–9.
55. Ejskjaer N, Wo JM, Esfandyari T, et al. A phase 2a, randomized, double-blind 28-day study of TZP-102 a ghrelin receptor agonist for diabetic gastroparesis. Neurogastroenterol Motil 2013;25(2):e140–50.
56. Longstreth GF, Malagelada JR, Kelly KA. Metoclopramide stimulation of gastric motility and emptying in diabetic gastroparesis. Ann Intern Med 1977;86(2):195–6.
57. Loo FD, Palmer DW, Soergel KH, et al. Gastric emptying in patients with diabetes mellitus. Gastroenterology 1984;86(3):485–94.
58. Watts GF, Armitage M, Sinclair J, et al. Treatment of diabetic gastroparesis with oral domperidone. Diabet Med 1985;2(6):491–2.
59. Soykan I, Sarosiek I, Shifflett J, et al. Effect of chronic oral domperidone therapy on gastrointestinal symptoms and gastric emptying in patients with Parkinson's disease. Mov Disord 1997;12(6):952–7.
60. Kozarek R. Domperidone for symptomatic management of diabetic gastroparesis in metoclopramide treatment failures. Adv Ther 1990;7:61–8.
61. Koch KL, Stern RM, Stewart WR, et al. Gastric emptying and gastric myoelectrical activity in patients with diabetic gastroparesis: effect of long-term domperidone treatment. Am J Gastroenterol 1989;84(9):1069–75.
62. Horowitz M, Harding PE, Chatterton BE, et al. Acute and chronic effects of domperidone on gastric emptying in diabetic autonomic neuropathy. Dig Dis Sci 1985;30(1):1–9.

63. Silvers D, Kipnes M, Broadstone V, et al. Domperidone in the management of symptoms of diabetic gastroparesis: efficacy, tolerability, and quality-of-life outcomes in a multicenter controlled trial. DOM-USA-5 Study Group. Clin Ther 1998;20(3):438–53.

64. Braun AP. Domperidone in the treatment of symptoms of delayed gastric emptying in diabetic patients. Adv Ther 1989;6:51–62.

65. Heer M, Muller-Duysing W, Benes I, et al. Diabetic gastroparesis: treatment with domperidone–a double-blind, placebo-controlled trial. Digestion 1983;27(4): 214–7.

66. Nagler J, Miskovitz P. Clinical evaluation of domperidone in the treatment of chronic postprandial idiopathic upper gastrointestinal distress. Am J Gastroenterol 1981;76(6):495–9.

67. Franzese A, Borrelli O, Corrado G, et al. Domperidone is more effective than cisapride in children with diabetic gastroparesis. Aliment Pharmacol Ther 2002; 16(5):951–7.

Nutritional Considerations in the Patient with Gastroparesis

Carol Rees Parrish, MS, RD

KEYWORDS

• Diet • Nutrition • Nutritional assessment • Enteral • Nutritional support

KEY POINTS

• Patients with gastroparesis (GP) are at high risk for nutritional compromise, not only because of chronic nausea and vomiting, which can result in poor intake, but also because of potential anatomic changes such as gastric resection or bypass.

• Target weight should be set for patient and intervention provided before a patient becomes severely malnourished.

• Use of parenteral nutrition (PN) should be reserved only for those patients who fail enteral feedings.

INTRODUCTION

A 57-year-old woman presents to the gastrointestinal (GI) clinic with myositis, poorly controlled diabetes mellitus (DM), nausea, vomiting, dehydration, and a 10-lb (4.5-kg) unintentional weight loss. GP is confirmed by gastric emptying study. Oral diet modification failed with continued nausea, vomiting, further weight loss, and aggravated glycemic control due to steroid therapy. On her third admission and a weight loss of 30 lb (210 to 180 lb [95.3 to 81.6 kg]), the decision was made to place a percutaneous endoscopic gastrostomy (PEG) with a jejunal extension (PEG/J) for enteral nutrition (EN), hydration, and medication delivery. Feedings went well initially in the hospital, but the patient continued to eat and drink after discharge when she felt better, resulting in 2 more admissions due to failed therapy and poor glycemic control. In an effort to give her some relief and keep her hospital free, the patient was strongly encouraged to stop eating and drinking anything other than a few ice chips, and she was miserable enough that she agreed. Tube feeding goals were met nocturnally, glycemic control improved, and she was discharged without readmission. She then followed up in GI nutrition clinic to ensure nutritional goals continued to be met.

This article originally appeared in Gastroenterology Clinics, Volume 44, Issue 1, March 2015.
Department of Nutrition Services, University of Virginia Health System, PO Box 800673, Charlottesville, VA 22908-0673, USA
E-mail address: crp3a@virginia.edu

Clinics Collections 7 (2015) 317–329
http://dx.doi.org/10.1016/j.ccol.2015.06.022

Gastroparesis

GP, defined as delayed gastric emptying for greater than 3 months, is documented by a delayed gastric emptying study in a patient devoid of mechanical or functional obstruction, can be profoundly incapacitating. This debilitating process alters one's ability to work, attend school, or carry out other normal daily activities. GP can affect the patient's emotional, mental, and social well-being, as well as the body's ability to function normally; basically, it compromises life.[1] Eating becomes a chore and is not pleasurable, and as a result, weight loss and compromised nutritional status are common in moderate to severe cases. Furthermore, in those with DM, glycemic control can become difficult.[2] The following outlines a practical approach to nutritional care of the patient with GP from nutritional assessment and oral dietary intervention to, finally, nutritional support.

NUTRITIONAL ASSESSMENT

Initial and ongoing nutritional assessment and intervention are critical aspects of care of the patient with GP.[3,4] Thorough assessment distinguishes those patients who need simple dietary changes from those who are so malnourished that nutritional support is justified. For example, a patient who develops nausea while eating the usual 3 large meals per day may not require supplemental calories, but rather smaller, more frequent meals. In contrast, the patient with severe GP who has significant vomiting after intake of clear liquids may require gastric decompression and jejunal feeding to provide not only nutrients, fluids, and medications but also symptom relief.

Unintentional Weight Loss

Unintentional weight loss over time is one of the most basic yet undeniable indicators that a patient's nutritional status is in trouble.[5] Comparing a current weight (once the patient has been rehydrated) with the patient's usual weight and documenting the percentage of total weight loss over time can stratify the degree of nutritional risk and help guide therapy. Use of an ideal body weight instead of a patient's actual weight is not recommended, as it may overestimate or underestimate the degree of nutritional risk.

Glycemic Control

In patients with DM, it is often difficult to sort out which came first, poor glucose control or GP. Regardless, good glycemic control (especially any wide swings in glucose control) is necessary for improving gastric emptying, nutrient utilization, and preventing catabolism.[6] In addition, out-of-control DM may be the primary reason the patient is losing weight. Glycemic control can be monitored by patient glycemic records and periodic measurement of glycosylated hemoglobin (HbA1C) level.

Bowel Habits

Constipation can worsen the symptoms of GP, and chronic constipation may be a sign of a more generalized intestinal dysmotility.[7] When practitioners justifiably pay so much attention to the upper gut in patients with chronic nausea and vomiting, they sometimes tend to overlook the lower tract; in fact, this author's experience is that while the gastroenterologist focuses on the GP, the primary care physician is taking care of the bowels, and sometimes their interventions are at odds with one another. For example, the addition of fiber bulking agents to help with constipation only exacerbates delayed gastric emptying. Identifying normal bowel habits is also important, particularly with inpatients who are on bed rest and perhaps pain medications, because during a hospitalization, physicians often prescribe nightly docusate to the patient who normally uses Miralax (polyethylene glycol 3350) twice a day at home.

NUTRITIONAL INTERVENTION—ORAL DIET

Prospective controlled trials regarding dietary contributions in this patient population are near nonexistent; hence, diet therapy has been devised based on known emptying characteristics of protein, fat, and carbohydrate and emptying of liquid foods versus solids.[6,8] Other than 2 small studies evaluating large versus small food particle size and symptom response in patients with insulin-treated DM, single-meal trials in heterogeneous populations with GP or normal volunteers and patient surveys are all that has been published to date.[8,9] Diet therapy and nutritional supplementation therefore must be individualized, taking into consideration the underlying cause of the GP such as postsurgical process versus underlying chronic disease course. See Appendix 1 for one institution's sample diet for GP (more complete and other versions available at www.ginutrition.virginia.edu under patient education materials).

Smaller, More Frequent Meals

The larger the volume of food ingested, the slower the emptying, and both caloric density and bulk (fiber) contribute to this.[10] Early satiety is a frequent complaint; hence, smaller amounts of food at frequent intervals during the day is the first nutritional intervention that should be implemented. Six or more small meals/snacks during the course of the day may be needed for patients to take in enough food to meet their nutritional needs.

Fat

Physiologically, it is well known that fat slows gastric emptying, and patients with GP are therefore often advised to restrict fat in their diet. However, eliminating fat also removes a significant calorie source and requires patients to eat larger volumes of food if they are to meet nutrient needs and stop weight loss. It may be that solid foods high in fat are the culprit; clinically, this author has found that fat-containing liquids are often well tolerated and can be a valuable source of nutrition for the patient with GP.

Decreasing Fiber

High-fiber foods and stool-bulking agents delay gastric emptying, leading to early satiety and symptom exacerbation in those with GP. Some patients may even present with a gastric bezoar as the first indication that they have GP. Small-bowel bacterial overgrowth (SBBO) is a known risk factor in those with dysmotility disorders, and frequent use of proton pump inhibitors, which is not uncommon in this population, further aggravates the problem. Consuming a high-fiber diet, or using a fiber-containing tube feeding formula in those requiring enteral nutritional support, can intensify abdominal distension, gas, bloating, reflux, and diarrhea. For those patients who have formed a bezoar, fiber avoidance is especially important.[11]

Another dietary intervention under investigation in dysmotility disorders is the avoidance of FODMAPs, or fermentable oligo-di-monosaccharides and polyols.[12,13] FODMAPs are highly fermentable by gut bacteria, as well as highly osmotic, and they too can further accentuate symptoms in those with GP. They are not only found in certain foods but are also added to some enteral formulas (fructooligosaccharides [FOS] are one of them) in addition to many liquid medications for flavorings, including sugar alcohols such as sorbitol and xylitol.[14] Their effect can be additive, so that a patient on enteral feedings with a fiber-containing formula and liquid medications may seem intolerant to the tube feeding, when in fact the problem is purely the FODMAP/fiber load they are receiving.[15]

Liquids Versus Solids

As liquid emptying is usually preserved in patients with GP, transitioning to more liquid calories in the diet may help patients meet their nutritional needs, especially during exacerbations. It may help in some patients to have them start the day with some solid food but then consume more liquid-type meals as the day progresses and the feeling of fullness increases. As mentioned earlier, fat-containing nutritional drinks are often well tolerated.

Particle Size

In the normal setting, a major function of the stomach is to grind food into smaller particles (trituration) initiating digestion. This function may be impaired or lost in the patient with GP, so a focus on chewing foods well may help to compensate and aid in this process to improve emptying. Two small studies[9,16] have demonstrated symptom improvement when ground foods versus solid food meals were provided. It should be noted that with good dentition, grinding food before ingesting would seem unnecessary, yet good dental care can be difficult for these patients. Not only can frequent vomiting alter enamel and weaken teeth but also when just getting off the couch is a chore, it can be hard enough just to make it to physician appointments and easy to delay dental treatment. Although pureed foods have not been studied, if grinding food into smaller particles has been shown to decrease symptoms, pureeing food may be an option for patients having difficulty tolerating even ground foods. With a good blender, anything can be pulverized if adequate liquid is added.

Patient Positioning

Positioning or use of gravity may also play a role in helping patients tolerate an oral diet. If turning on one's right side is necessary to undergo a barium swallow, then patients may get some relief by sitting upright for 1 to 2 hours after a meal or by even going for a gentle walk.

SPECIAL CONSIDERATION—VITAMINS AND MINERALS

Patients who have had prolonged nausea and vomiting leading to poor nutritional intake are at risk for multiple nutrient deficiencies. In a large multicenter study evaluating food frequency questionnaires, patients with GP from idiopathic or DM cause were found to have diets deficient in calories and numerous vitamins and minerals.[17] When eating nearly ceases, taking vitamins and minerals generally does too. Patients with GP due to a previous gastric surgery are at even greater risk for nutrient deficiencies because of anatomic changes and alterations in nutrient utilization.[18] For example, patients with a subtotal gastrectomy are more at risk for iron and vitamins B_{12}, D, and E deficiencies; gastric bypass surgery, a procedure that creates malabsorption, significantly increases the risk for an even wider range of nutrient deficiencies.[19] See **Box 1** for those nutrients that may warrant particular attention, although any patient with significant and unintentional weight loss is at risk for pan-nutrient deficiencies.

It may be prudent to provide supplements to patients with malnutrition or known poor nutritional intake with a therapeutic vitamin and mineral supplement for an empiric length of time (~4 weeks) until they are eating normally again, or, if requiring enteral feedings, until goal delivery rate is achieved. Chewable or liquid supplements may be better tolerated in some than the tablet form; for others, a smaller dose (such as one-half tablet, twice a day) may work better; remember, any is better than none in

---

Box 1
Nutrients that may warrant particular attention in the patient with gastroparesis

- Vitamin D (25-OH vitamin D)

- Serum vitamin B_{12}/methylmalonic acid (methylmalonic acid In those at high risk for small bowel bacterial overgrowth (SBBO), as vitamin B_{12} can be converted to biologically inactive form in the gut before absorption)

- Iron/ferritin (in non–acute phase setting)

- Folate: elevated serum folate level may be suggestive (but not diagnostic) of SBBO in patients with a dysmotility disorder. Bacteria in the small bowel synthesize folate, which is then absorbed into the bloodstream, resulting in elevated serum levels.[20]

- Vitamin E (gastric resection 2 years post-op)

- Thiamine: gastric bypass or others with vomiting greater than 3 weeks[19]

From University of Virginia Health System, Nutrition Support Traineeship Syllabus. Charlottesville (VA): University of Virginia; 2013; with permission.

---

those who need it. Avoid giving multiple, individual supplements, as this not only gets costly but is also time consuming and compliance may decrease.

NUTRITIONAL SUPPORT

Patients unable to maintain a healthy weight despite oral diet modifications are candidates for specialized nutritional support. A defined target weight should be set with the patient; if a patient is unable to achieve this or drops below this weight, nutritional support should be initiated. Indications for enteral access and nutritional support include the following[3]:

- Unintentional weight loss of greater than 5% to 10% over 3 to 6 months
- Inability to meet weight goals
- Weight falls to less than what was agreed on by patient and physician as time for intervention
- Need for gastric decompression
- Frequent hospitalizations, with or without weight loss
  - Dehydration
  - Diabetic ketoacidosis
  - Refractory nausea/vomiting
  - Requiring access for consistent delivery of medications, hydration, and nutrition
- Overall quality of life is unsustainable or plain failure to thrive

Enteral Nutrition

In patients who cannot consistently meet their nutritional requirements or regain the much needed lost weight, EN support is recommended. EN is associated with fewer infections and complications, is less expensive, and is less labor intensive for nursing staff and caregivers compared with PN. The selection of the best enteral access device varies between health care institutions and continues to be a source of debate owing to the lack of prospective trials evaluating the various approaches. Vented and nonvented options are available. For those with uncontrolled vomiting, a venting port indicates that there is a separate gastric port to drain off gastric secretions in an effort to give the patient relief from ongoing vomiting,[21] although careful monitoring is needed if this route is chosen because of the potential risk for hypochloremic metabolic alkalosis.[22] Nonvented tubes do not offer such an option. See **Box 2** for enteral access options. A more in-depth discussion on various enteral access techniques is available elsewhere.[3,6] Regardless of the type of access chosen, jejunal feeding has been shown to improve symptoms, glycemic control and reduce the need for hospitalization.[23–25]

The enteral feeding regimen

A standard, polymeric formula should be well tolerated by the vast majority of patients. Although a significant number of those with GP have DM, specialized formulas for those with DM have not demonstrated an outcome benefit to date, are considerably more expensive, and contain fiber as well as FOS, a FODMAP.[15,26] Fiber-containing formulas may cause abdominal discomfort in patients with GP and intestinal dysmotility (see section on fiber in the oral diet section earlier in the discussion). To avoid blaming unsuccessful enteral feeding on what might be exacerbation of SBBO due to fiber and FODMAP formulas, a nonfiber, non-FOS formula is recommended at the initiation of enteral feeding. Once a patient is well established and tolerating the regimen, different formulas can be trialed if desired.

To prevent clouding the issue of enteral tolerance versus persistent oral food intolerance, a strict period of withholding oral food should be enlisted for at least 48 hours during EN initiation or until the patient is clearly tolerating EN well. This method avoids blaming persistent symptoms of GP on enteral feeding intolerance, when it is the oral intake that is responsible. If a patient is to be cycled to either nocturnal or daytime feedings, this should be initiated at the outset, especially in those with insulin-dependent DM. Otherwise, the whole process of achieving glycemic control has to be undertaken twice: first on continuous feeding, then again when changing the patient to nocturnal feeding, resulting in a delay in discharge. Discharging a patient home on continuous EN, unless absolutely necessary, should be avoided. Continuous EN does not allow freedom from the pump or the return of a patient's quality of life. In those having to remain on continuous EN, an enteral backpack should be obtained for the patient before discharge; if the home care company says they do not have them, then another home care company should be chosen for the patient. For patients who require insulin and are going to be put on nocturnal EN delivery, blood glucose monitoring and short-acting insulin coverage should be done every 4 hours during EN infusion for the first 48 hours or until longer-acting insulin needs can be determined to maximize glycemic control. This procedure ensures nutrient repletion and also prevents further alteration to gastric emptying due to poor control. More in-depth discussion and trouble-shooting enteral feeding tolerance is available elsewhere.[3,8]

Parenteral Nutrition

The use of PN should be the exception in the patient with GP unless the patient suffers from a dysmotility that extends beyond the stomach into the small bowel or colon or has a pandysmotility disorder such as chronic intestinal pseudo-obstruction. In those patients with significant malnutrition, peripheral PN may be used short term as a bridge until enteral access is achieved, although some might argue that dextrose added to standing intravenous fluids can be an effective way to initiate the refeeding process. Transition to EN should be pursued when clinically feasible.

SUMMARY

GP potentially compromises not only one's nutritional status but also all aspects of life. Nutritional assessment and timely nutritional support are an important aspect of care in this patient population. Good glycemic control not only is essential for maximizing

Box 2
Enteral access options: short term and long term

Nonvented Tubes

- Gastric tube or percutaneous endoscopic gastrostomy (PEG): typically not done in a patient with severe GP given the delayed gastric emptying. In milder cases, because liquids empty differently than solids, gastric delivery may be acceptable.

- Nasogastric, nasoduodenal, or nasojejunal: tends to migrate back into stomach with persistent vomiting; not a long-term option.

- Direct percutaneous endoscopic jejunostomy: difficult to place; not commonly placed in most institutions.

- Surgical or laparoscopic jejunal tube: common to many facilities.

- Interventional radiologically (IR) placed: largest tube that can be placed is an 18F catheter; unless facility has investigated and chosen specific tubes meant for long term, many tubes placed are not meant to be used long term or be exposed to gastric acid for long. In addition, many IR departments may place feeding tubes but have nothing set up to prepare the patient for home in terms of teaching the patient how to care for the tube, how to use the tube for enteral feeding, equipment and formula needed, as well as set the patient up with home care; all of this is left up to the referring physician, and if the referring physician is not aware he/she needs to do this, the patient suffers in the mayhem that follows (this author has seen this happen numerous times at outside facilities).

Vented Tubes

- Separate G and J tubes: gastric venting may be improved as there is no internal J tube taking up lumen space within the larger tube to impair venting; 2 separate tube sites to care for, with potential infection and leakage issues, not to mention the cosmetic aspects.

- PEG with a jejunal extension (often called Jet-PEG): abdominal placement is important; author's experience, to the right of the spine, lower antrum (not too close to the pylorus), facing the pylorus, easier to place j-arm with less stomach to traverse, hence less "play" on the j-arm by movement of spine, decreasing migration of j-arm back into the stomach. Smaller j-arms are more prone to clogging; advise 12F j-arm with goal to put feeding ports past ligament of Treitz. Education about medications via j-arm is crucial. If j-arm clogs, gets kinked, cannot be repaired, then patient only needs a new j-arm.

- Long-term G-J tubes: one tube that has a gastric tube housing a smaller tube within. The outer gastric tube is smaller, hence the internal jejunal tube is too. These tubes may not vent as well and clog more often as a result. Tube failure means the tube needs replacing.

- Nasogastric-jejunal tube: these tubes are meant to be used short term; because the larger gastric tube needs to handle gastric decompression, it is made of harder plastic, and therefore comfort is an issue for patients. The jejunal tube within is also of small diameter (8–10F), hence the clog potential as well as kinking is high. Placement of these tubes often requires fluoroscopy, unless the endoscopist is experienced, as these tubes often come back up into the proximal small bowel or stomach when the endoscope is removed.

  o Examples include the following:

  ■ Dobbhoff Naso-Jejunal Feeding and Gastric Decompression Tube, Covidien (Mansfield, MA) (16F)

  • www.kendallpatientcare.com/pageBuilder.aspx?webPageID=0&topicID=72623&xsl=xsl/productPagePrint.xsl

  ■ Compat Stay-Put Nasojejunal Feeding Tube, Nestle (Nestle HealthCare Nutrition, Inc., Florham Park, NJ)

  • www.nestlehealthscience.us/products/compat-stay-put%E2%84%A2-nasojejunal-feeding-tube

■ Jejunal Feeding/Gastric Decompression Tube, Bard (Bard Access Systems, Inc., Salt Lake City, UT)

  • www.bardaccess.com/feed-jejunal.php

■ Silicone Gastro-Duodenal Levin Tube, Vygon (Vygon Sa, Lansdale, PA), Alibaba, 3T-Medical

  • www.hellotrade.com/vygon-sa/silicone-gastro-duodenal-tube.html

From University of Virginia Health System, Nutrition Support Traineeship Syllabus; Charlottesville, VA; 2013; with permission.

nutrient utilization in those with DM but is also critical for removing delayed gastric emptying from hyperglycemia. Nutritional intervention can decrease symptoms, replenish nutrient stores, reduced hospitalizations, and improve an individual's overall quality of life. See **Box 3** for further resources.

Box 3
Resources for physicians and for patients with gastroparesis

• University of Virginia Health System, GI Nutrition Web site www.ginutrition.virginia.edu links to

  ○ Patient education materials

    ■ Several diets for gastroparesis and low FODMAPs

      • Short version

      • Long version

      • Renal

      • Diabetes

      • Low FODMAP

  ○ Nutrition Articles in Practical Gastroenterology

    ■ Parrish CR, McCray S. Gastroparesis & nutrition: the art. Pract Gastroenterol 2011;XXXV(9):26.

    ■ Parrish CR, Yoshida C. Nutrition intervention for the patient with gastroparesis: an update. Pract Gastroenterol 2005;XXIX(8):29.

• Association of Gastrointestinal Motility Disorders, Inc

  www.agmd-gimotility.org

• Cyclic Vomiting Association

  www.cvsaonline.org/

• International Foundation for Functional Gastrointestinal Disorders

  www.iffgd.org/

• Gastroparesis Dysmotility Association

  www.digestivedistress.com

REFERENCES

1. Camilleri M, Bharucha AE, Farrugia G. Epidemiology, mechanisms, and management of diabetic gastroparesis. Clin Gastroenterol Hepatol 2011;9(1):5–12.
2. Uppalapati SS, Ramzan Z, Fisher RS, et al. Factors contributing to hospitalization for gastroparesis exacerbations. Dig Dis Sci 2009;54:2404–9.
3. Parrish CR, Yoshida C. Nutrition intervention for the patient with gastroparesis: an update. Pract Gastroenterol 2005;XXIX(8):29. Available at: www.ginutrition. virginia.edu.
4. Abell TL, Bernstein RK, Cutts T, et al. Treatment of gastroparesis: a multidisciplinary clinical review. Neurogastroenterol Motil 2006;18:263–83.
5. Jensen GL, Hsiao PY, Wheeler D. Nutrition screening and assessment. In: Mueller CM, editor. The A.S.P.E.N. adult nutrition support core curriculum. 2nd edition. Silver Spring (MD): American Society for Parenteral and Enteral Nutrition; 2012. p. 155–69.
6. Camilleri M, Parkman HP, Shafi MA, et al. Clinical guideline: management of gastroparesis. Am J Gastroenterol 2013;108(1):18–37.
7. Schiller LR. Nutrients and constipation: cause or cure? Pract Gastroenterol 2008; XXXII(4):43. Available at: www.ginutrition.virginia.edu.
8. Parrish CR, McCray S. Gastroparesis & nutrition: the art. Pract Gastroenterol 2011;XXXV(9):26. Available at: www.ginutrition.virginia.edu.
9. Olausson EA, Störsrud S, Grundin H, et al. A small particle size diet reduces upper gastrointestinal symptoms in patients with diabetic gastroparesis: a randomized controlled trial. Am J Gastroenterol 2014;109(3):375–85.
10. Camilleri M. Integrated upper gastrointestinal response to food intake. Gastroenterology 2006;131:640–58.
11. Sanders MK. Bezoars: from mystical charms to medical and nutritional management. Pract Gastroenterol 2004;XXVIII(1):37. Available at: www.ginutrition. virginia.edu.
12. Barrett JS. Extending our knowledge of fermentable, short-chain carbohydrates for managing gastrointestinal symptoms. Nutr Clin Pract 2013;28(3):300–6.
13. Gibson PR, Shepherd SJ. Evidence-based dietary management of functional gastrointestinal symptoms: the FODMAP approach. J Gastroenterol Hepatol 2010;25(2):252–8.
14. Wolever TM, Piekarz A, Hollads M, et al. Sugar alcohols and diabetes: a review. Can J Diabetes 2002;26(4):356–62.
15. Halmos EP. Role of FODMAP content in enteral nutrition-associated diarrhea. J Gastroenterol Hepatol 2013;28(Suppl 4):25–8.
16. Olausson EA, Alpsten M, Larsson A, et al. Small particle size of a solid meal increases gastric emptying and late postprandial glycaemic response in diabetic subjects with gastroparesis. Diabetes Res Clin Pract 2008;80:231–7.
17. Parkman HP, Yates KP, Hasler WL, et al. Dietary intake and nutritional deficiencies in patients with diabetic or idiopathic gastroparesis. Gastroenterology 2011; 141(2):486–98.
18. Radigan A. Post-gastrectomy: Managing the nutrition fall-out. Pract Gastroenterol 2004;XXVIII(6):63. Available at: www.ginutrition.virginia.edu.
19. O'Donnell K. Severe micronutrient deficiencies in RYGB patients: rare but potentially devastating. Pract Gastroenterol 2011;XXXV(11):13. Available at: www. ginutrition.virginia.edu.
20. Hoffbrand AV, Tabaqchali S, Mollin DL, et al. High serum folate levels in intestinal blind-loop syndrome. Lancet 1966;1(7451):1339–42.

21. Kim CH, Nelson DK. Venting percutaneous gastrostomy in the treatment of refractory idiopathic gastroparesis. Gastrointest Endosc 1998;47:67–70.
22. Parrish CR, Quatrara B. Reinfusion of intestinal secretions: a viable option for select patients. Pract Gastroenterol 2010;XXXIV(4):26. Available at: www.ginutrition.virginia.edu.
23. Fontana RJ, Barnett JL. Jejunostomy tube placement in refractory diabetic gastroparesis: a retrospective review. Am J Gastroenterol 1996;91(10):2174–8.
24. Maple JT, Petersen BT, Baron TH, et al. Direct percutaneous endoscopic jejunostomy: outcomes in 307 consecutive attempts. Am J Gastroenterol 2005;100(12):2681–8.
25. Parkman HP, Hasler WL, Fisher RS. American Gastroenterological Association technical review on the diagnosis and treatment of gastroparesis. Gastroenterology 2004;127:1592–622.
26. Hise ME, Fuhrman MP. The effect of diabetic-specific formulae on clinical and glycemic indicators. Pract Gastroenterol 2009;XXXIII(5):20–36. Available at: www.ginutrition.virginia.edu.

APPENDIX 1: GASTROPARESIS DIET TIPS
Introduction

Gastroparesis means stomach (*gastro*) paralysis (*paresis*). In gastroparesis, the stomach empties too slowly. Gastroparesis can have many causes, so symptoms range from mild (but annoying) to severe and week-to-week or even day-to-day.

This handout is designed to give some suggestions for diet changes in the hope that symptoms will improve or even stop. Very few research studies have been done to guide one as to which foods are better tolerated by patients with gastroparesis. The suggestions are mostly based on experience and the understanding of how the stomach and different foods normally empty. Anyone with gastroparesis should see a doctor and a Registered Dietitian for advice on how to maximize their nutritional status.

The Basics

Volume
The larger the meal, the slower the stomach empties. It is important to decrease the amount of food eaten at a meal, so one has to eat more often. Smaller meals more often (6–8 or more if needed) may allow one to eat enough.

Liquids versus Solids
If decreasing the meal size and increasing the number of meals does not work, the next step is to switch to more liquid-type foods. Liquids empty the stomach more easily than solids do. Pureed foods may also be better.

Fiber
Fiber (found in many fruits, vegetables, and grains) may slow stomach emptying and fill the stomach up too fast; this does not leave room for foods that may be easier tolerated. A *bezoar* is a mixture of food fibers that may get stuck in the stomach and not empty well, like a hairball in a cat. For patients who have had a bezoar, fiber restriction is important. This restriction includes avoiding over-the-counter fiber/bulking medicines like Metamucil (psyllium husk) and others.

Fat
Fat may slow stomach emptying in some patients, but many can easily consume fat in beverages. Experience at the University of Virginia Health System is that fat in liquid forms, such as whole milk, milk shakes, and nutritional supplements, is often well tolerated. Unless a fat-containing food or fluid clearly causes worse symptoms, fat

should not be limited, because people with gastroparesis often need all the calories they can get, as eating enough may be very hard to do. Liquid fat is often well tolerated, pleasurable, and provides a great source of calories in smaller amounts.

Medications

There are a few medications that can slow stomach emptying. Patients should ask their doctor if any of the medicines they are taking could be slowing down stomach emptying.

Getting Started

- Set a goal weight you want to meet.
- Avoid large meals.
- Eat enough to meet your goal weight. It may be 4 to 8 smaller meals and snacks.
- Avoid solid foods that are high in fat, and avoid adding too much fat to foods. High-fat drinks are usually okay; try them and see.
- Eat nutritious foods first before filling up on empty calories such as candy, cakes, and sodas.
- Chew foods well, especially meats. Meats may be easier to eat if ground or puréed.
- Avoid high-fiber foods because they may be harder for your stomach to empty.
- Sit up while eating, and stay upright for at least 1 hour after you finish. Try taking a nice walk after meals.
- If you have diabetes, keep your blood sugar under control. Let your doctor know if your blood sugar runs greater than 200 mg/dL on a regular basis.

Getting your Calories

When getting enough calories is a daily struggle, make everything you eat and drink count:

- Take medications with calorie-containing beverages such as milk, juice, and sweet tea instead of water or diet drinks.
- High-calorie drinks are better than water because they provide calories and fluid. Use peach, pear, or papaya nectar; fruit juices and drinks; Hawaiian Punch; Hi C; lemonade; Kool-Aid; sweet tea; even soda.
- Fortify milk by adding dry milk powder: add 1 cup powdered milk to 1 quart milk.
- Drink whole milk if tolerated instead of skim or 2%. Use whole, condensed, or evaporated milk when preparing cream-based soups, custards, puddings, and hot cereals, smoothies, and milkshakes.
- Add Carnation Instant Breakfast, protein powder, dry milk powder, or other flavored powders or flavored syrups to whole milk or juices.
- Make custards and puddings with eggs or egg substitutes such as Eggbeaters.
- Try adding ice cream, sherbet, and sorbet to ready-made supplements such as Nutra-shakes, Ensure, or Boost. Peanut butter, chocolate syrup, or caramel sauce is also great in these.

Suggested Foods for Gastroparesis

Starches

Breads: white bread and "light" whole wheat bread (no nuts, seeds), including French/Italian, bagels (plain or egg), English muffin, plain roll, pita bread, tortilla (flour or corn), pancake, waffle, naan, and flat bread

Cereals: quick oats (plain), grits, cream of wheat, cream of rice, and puffed wheat and rice cereals, such as Cheerios, Sugar Pops, Kix, Rice Krispies, Fruit Loops, Special K, and Cocoa Crispies

Grains/potatoes: rice (plain), pasta, macaroni (plain), bulgur wheat (couscous), barley, sweet and white potatoes (no skin, plain), yams, French fries (baked)

Crackers/chips: arrowroot, breadsticks, matzoh, melba toast, oyster, saltines, soda, zwieback, water crackers, baked potato chips, pretzels

Meats, Fish, and Poultry, Ground or Pureed

Beef: baby beef, chipped beef, flank steak, tenderloin, plate skirt steak, round (bottom or top), rump

Veal: leg, loin, rib, shank, shoulder

Pork: lean pork, tenderloin, pork chops, ham

Poultry (skinless): chicken, turkey

Wild game (no skin): venison, rabbit, squirrel, pheasant, duck, goose

Fish/shellfish (fresh or frozen, plain, no breading): crab, lobster, shrimp, clams, scallops, oysters, tuna (in water)

Cheese: cottage cheese, grated parmesan

Other: eggs (no creamed or fried), egg white, egg substitute; tofu, strained baby meats (all)

Vegetables (cooked, and if necessary, blenderized/strained)

Beets, tomato sauce, tomato juice, tomato paste or purée, carrots, strained baby vegetables (all), mushrooms, vegetable juice

Fruits and Juices (cooked and, if necessary, blenderized/strained)

Fruits, applesauce, banana, peaches (canned), pears (canned), strained baby fruits (all), juices (all), fruit drinks, fruit flavored beverages

Milk Products (if tolerated)

Milk, any as tolerated, chocolate, buttermilk, yogurt (without fruit pieces), frozen yogurt, kefir (liquid yogurt), evaporated milk, condensed milk, milk powder, custard/pudding

Soups

Broth, bouillon, strained creamed soups (with milk or water)

Beverages

Hot cocoa (made with water or milk), Kool-Aid, lemonade, Tang, and similar powdered products, Gatorade or Powerade, soft drinks, coffee/coffee drinks, tea/chai

Seasonings/Gravies

Cranberry sauce (smooth), fat-free gravies, Molly McButter, Butter Buds

Mustard, ketchup, vegetable oil spray, soy sauce, teriyaki sauce, tabasco sauce, vanilla and other flavoring extracts, vinegar

Desserts/Sweets

Angel food cake, animal crackers, gelatin, ginger snaps, graham crackers, popsicles, plain sherbet, vanilla wafers, gum, gum drops, hard candy

Jelly beans, lemon drops, rolled candy (such as Lifesavers), marshmallows

Seedless jams and jellies

The following foods have been associated with bezoar formation and may need to be avoided (see Fiber section).

Apples, berries, coconut, figs, oranges, persimmons, brussels sprouts
Green beans, legumes, potato peels, sauerkraut

When Solids Do Not Seem to Be Working, Try Blenderized Food

Any food can be blenderized, but solid foods need to be thinned down with some type of liquid.

- If you do not have a blender, strained baby foods may be used and can be thinned down as needed with milk, soy or rice milk, water, or broth.
- Always clean the blender well. Any food left in the blender for more than 1 to 2 hours could cause food poisoning.
- Meats, fish, poultry, and ham: blend with broths, water, milk, vegetable or V-8 juice, tomato sauce, or gravies.
- Vegetables: blend with water, tomato juice, broth, strained baby vegetables.
- Starches: potatoes, pasta, rice: blend with soups, broth, milk, water, or gravies; add strained baby meats to add protein if needed. Consider using hot cereals, such as cream of wheat or rice, grits, as your starch at lunch and dinner.
- Fruits: blend with their own juices, other fruit juices, water, strained baby fruits.
- Cereals: make with caloric beverage such as whole milk (or even evaporated/condensed milk), soy or rice milk, juice, Ensure, Boost, or store brand equivalent, instead of water. Add sugars, honey, molasses, syrups, or other flavorings and butter or vegetable oil for extra calories.
- Mixed dishes: lasagna, macaroni and cheese, spaghetti, chili, chop suey: add adequate liquid of your choice, blend well, and strain.

From University of Virginia Health System, Digestive Health Center, Charlottesville, VA; 2014; with permission.

Approach to Patients with Esophageal Dysphagia

Udayakumar Navaneethan, MD, Steve Eubanks, MD*

KEYWORDS

* Dysphagia * Endoscopy * Manometry

KEY POINTS

* Patients present to a physician with complaints of difficulty swallowing, and the approach to evaluating these problems can be challenging for those who do not manage this complaint regularly.
* Dysphagia refers to difficulty with swallowing where there are problems with the transit of food from the mouth to the hypopharynx or through the esophagus.
* The most important step in assessing dysphagia is to determine whether it is oropharyngeal or esophageal in origin; potential causes and subsequent investigation and management can differ greatly.
* Numerous tools are available to aid with the determination of the cause of dysphagia and assist with the formulation of a logical treatment algorithm.

INTRODUCTION

Dysphagia refers to difficulty with swallowing where there are problems with the transit of food from the mouth to the hypopharynx or through the esophagus. Dysphagia can be classified based on the location and by the physiologic circumstances in which it occurs. Dysphagia is classified as oropharyngeal or esophageal dysphagia based on location.[1] In terms of physiology, dysphagia can be classified based on the transport of an ingested bolus. The transport depends on the consistency and size of the bolus, the caliber of the lumen, the integrity of peristaltic contraction, and whether there is deglutitive inhibition of both the upper and lower esophageal sphincter (LES). Structural dysphagia is caused by an oversized bolus or a narrow lumen; motor

This article originally appeared in Surgical Clinics, Volume 95, Issue 3, June 2015.

Grant Support: None.

Conflict of Interest: None of the authors declared financial conflict of interest.

Center for Interventional Endoscopy, Florida Hospital Institute for Minimally Invasive Therapy, 601 E. Rollins Street, Orlando, FL 32803, USA

* Corresponding author. Institute for Surgical Advancement, Florida Hospital, 2415 North Orange Avenue, Suite 401, Orlando, FL 32804.

E-mail address: steve.eubanks.MD@flhosp.org

Clinics Collections 7 (2015) 331–337

http://dx.doi.org/10.1016/j.ccol.2015.06.023

Abbreviations	
CT	Computed tomography
EGD	Esophagogastroduodenoscopy
EUS	Endoscopic ultrasound
HRM	High-resolution manometry
LES	Lower esophageal sphincter

dysphagia is secondary to abnormalities of peristalsis or impaired deglutitive inhibition of the sphincters. The most important initial step in assessing dysphagia is to determine whether it is oropharyngeal or esophageal in origin, because their potential causes and subsequent investigation and management can differ greatly. Patients with oropharyngeal dysphagia present with symptoms of cough after swallowing and nasopharyngeal regurgitation.[1] It is seen commonly in patients with a history of head and neck surgery or radiation treatment, stroke, and other neurologic conditions, such as Parkinson's disease and motor neuron disease. This article provides an outline for approaching patients with esophageal dysphagia in terms of etiologies and clinical evaluation. The article discusses initially the physiology of esophageal swallowing, followed by pathophysiology and clinical evaluation of patients with various etiologies of esophageal dysphagia.

PHYSIOLOGY OF ESOPHAGEAL SWALLOWING

Swallowing begins with a voluntary (oral) phase that includes preparation during which food is masticated and mixed with saliva. Once the food is transferred to the esophagus through a complex physiologic transfer and relaxation of the upper esophageal sphincter, peristaltic contractions propel the food through the esophagus. The LES relaxes as the food enters the esophagus and remains relaxed until the peristaltic contraction has delivered the bolus into the stomach.[2] Peristaltic contractions elicited in response to a swallow are called primary peristalsis and involve sequenced inhibition followed by contraction of the musculature along the entire length of the esophagus. Local distention of the esophagus anywhere along its length activates secondary peristalsis that begins at the point of distention and proceeds distally. Tertiary esophageal contractions are nonperistaltic, disordered esophageal contractions. The distal esophagus and LES are composed of smooth muscle and are controlled by excitatory and inhibitory neurons within the esophageal myenteric plexus.[2] Peristalsis results from the patterned activation of inhibitory followed by excitatory ganglionic neurons, with progressive dominance of the inhibitory neurons distally. The function of the LES is supplemented by the right diaphragmatic crus, which acts as an external sphincter during inspiration, cough, or abdominal straining.[2]

PATHOPHYSIOLOGY AND ETIOLOGIES OF ESOPHAGEAL DYSPHAGIA

Solid food esophageal dysphagia becomes apparent when the esophageal lumen is narrowed to less than 13 mm; the normal diameter of the lumen varies from 2 to 3 cm. However, dysphagia can occur even with larger diameters when patients have motility disorders. The most common structural causes of dysphagia are Schatzki's rings, eosinophilic esophagitis, and peptic strictures. Disorders of motility could be secondary to abnormalities of peristalsis and/or deglutitive inhibition. In general, the etiologies of esophageal dysphagia can be divided broadly into either mechanical or dysmotility (**Box 1**). However, in a number of conditions, dysphagia could be mediated by both mechanical and dysmotility mechanisms.

Box 1
Etiologies of esophageal dysphagia

Mechanical causes

Benign strictures

- Peptic stricture
- Schatzki's ring
- Esophageal webs
- Anastomotic stricture
- Eosinophilic esophagitis
- Post fundoplication
- Radiation-induced strictures
- Postendoscopic mucosal resection
- Extrinsic compression from vascular compression (dysphagia lusorio)
- Extrinsic compression from benign lymph nodes or enlarged left atrium

Malignant strictures

- Esophageal adenocarcinoma
- Squamous cell cancer
- Extrinsic compression from malignant lymph nodes

Dysmotility

- Achalasia
- Hypotensive peristalsis
- Hypertensive peristalsis
- Nutcracker esophagus
- Diffuse esophageal spasm
- Functional obstruction

CLINICAL ASSESSMENT

The history and clinical assessment give clues to the etiologies of dysphagia and the evaluation required. Dysphagia to the type of food provides clues to the etiologies of dysphagia. Intermittent dysphagia that occurs only with solid food implies structural dysphagia, whereas constant dysphagia with both liquids and solids strongly suggests a motor abnormality.[2] Dysphagia that is progressive over the course of weeks to months raises concern for neoplasia. Episodic dysphagia to solids that is unchanged over years indicates a benign disease process such as a Schatzki's ring or eosinophilic esophagitis. Food impaction with a prolonged inability to pass an ingested bolus even with ingestion of liquid is typical of a structural dysphagia. Chest pain frequently accompanies dysphagia whether it is related to motor disorders, structural disorders, or reflux disease. A prolonged history of heartburn preceding the onset of dysphagia is suggestive of peptic stricture and, less commonly, esophageal adenocarcinoma. A history of head and neck surgery, ingestion of caustic agents or pills, previous radiation or chemotherapy, or associated mucocutaneous diseases may help to isolate the cause of dysphagia. With accompanying odynophagia, which usually is indicative of ulceration, infectious, or pill-induced esophagitis should be suspected. A strong history of allergy increases concerns for eosinophilic esophagitis.

CLINICAL INVESTIGATIONS

The initial clinical investigations depends on the suspected etiology. If mechanical causes, such as an obstructing mass lesion or stricture, are suspected, upper endoscopy is the initial investigation of choice. In contrast, if motility disorders such as achalasia are suspected, high-resolution manometry is the initial investigation. Radiographic evaluation with a barium swallow remains a useful investigation in some situations when upper endoscopy evaluation is normal.

Barium Swallow

The sensitivity of barium radiography for detecting esophageal strictures is greater than that of endoscopy, particularly for esophageal webs and rings, and remains the best initial evaluation strategy for dysphagia. The advantages are that it is noninvasive, can be done in patients who are poor candidates for endoscopic evaluation, and provides a good functional assessment of the esophagus. Barium swallow may also demonstrate anatomic abnormalities such as a stricture and Schatzki's ring.[3] The major drawback is that it is usually followed by endoscopic evaluation. A timed barium swallow is, however, used to follow up on treatment after achalasia as the height of the barium column at 1 minute after contrast ingestion 6 months after treatment was found to correlate with symptom scores.[3]

Upper Endoscopy

Upper esophagogastroduodenoscopy (EGD) is the first-choice investigation in patients with dysphagia, particularly with mechanical etiologies for dysphagia. It can diagnose intraluminal tumors, strictures and inflammatory disorders such as reflux disease, eosinophilic esophagitis, and pill-induced ulceration. In a systematic review of endoscopic findings in eosinophilic esophagitis, esophageal rings accounted for 44%; strictures, 21%; narrow-caliber esophagus, 9%; linear furrows, 48%; white plaques or exudates, 27%; pallor or decreased vasculature, 41%; and erosive esophagitis, 17%.[4] The endoscopic examination was normal in 17% of cases of eosinophilic esophagitis.[4] In patients who present for routine endoscopy for any indication, the prevalence of eosinophilic esophagitis is 6.5%, and in those undergoing an EGD for dysphagia, the prevalence is 10% to 15%.[5] In addition to the ability to take mucosal biopsies, EGD also has the opportunity of therapeutic potential with dilatation, which is useful for esophageal web, peptic stricture, anastomotic stricture, radiation-related stricture, and Schatzki's ring. In addition, it is a useful adjunct in the evaluation of underlying motility disorder. It may show the presence of a dilated esophagus, sigmoid esophagus with lack of contractions, and a tight LES, suggesting achalasia. Also, in evaluation of patients with achalasia, EGD is always performed to rule out pseudoachalasia secondary to tumors of the gastroesophageal junction and gastric cardia. Also, in achalasia patients who are unfit for surgical treatment, pneumatic balloon dilatation and botulinum toxin injection may offer alternative treatment. Recently, per oral endoscopic myotomy offers an exciting option in patients with achalasia.[6]

Manometry

Manometry is the most sensitive currently available technique to diagnose esophageal motility disorders.[7] High-resolution esophageal manometry (HRM) is a revolutionary step beyond conventional manometry, the traditional method of assessing esophageal motility. HRM has been developed with up to 36 recording points.[8] This enables pressure measurements of 1 cm or less apart along the entire esophagus. In HRM, the distal end of the catheter is passed into the gastric compartment below the LES and the catheter can provide recording from the stomach through the esophagus into the oropharynx.[8] During an HRM study, plots are generated, also known as "Clouse" plots. These plots are presented as a color spectrum on a plot of esophageal position (y-axis) against time (x-axis) produces a pressure topograph of swallowing generated by computer software during 10 wet (5 mL water) swallows.[8] HRM helps in the diagnosis of specific motility disorders; for example, the manometric finding of aperistalsis and incomplete LES relaxation without evidence of a mechanical obstruction solidifies the diagnosis of achalasia in the appropriate setting.[9]

Diagnostic Algorithm

In patients presenting with dysphagia, the initial evaluation includes EGD to rule out important etiologies such as cancer and stricture. In addition, evaluation for eosinophilic esophagitis needs to be performed with biopsies of the esophagus. Barium swallow evaluation can be performed in elderly patients who are not candidates for EGD. In patients with normal EGD and biopsies with dysphagia, HRM is required for evaluation.

Esophageal Cancer

The possibility of the cause for dysphagia being cancer of the esophagus is the greatest concern in the majority of patients who present with difficulty swallowing. In the United States, 18,000 people were diagnosed with esophageal cancer in 2014 and 15,000 patients died owing to esophageal cancer in the United States in 2014. The most common symptoms for patients who present with esophageal cancer are dysphagia (74%) and weight loss (57.3%).[10] The evaluation of the patient who is suspected or confirmed of having esophageal cancer can involve the following studies:

- Upper endoscopy
- Endoscopic biopsy
- Barium esophagram
- CT
- Endoscopic ultrasound (EUS)
- Bone scan
- Positron emission tomography

The patient with esophageal cancer presenting with dysphagia and weight loss usually describes difficulty swallowing solids, but often retains the ability to swallow liquids until the tumor is very advanced. The weight loss in esophageal cancer patients often exceeds what would be expected from the degree of dysphagia. Upper endoscopy is often the initial procedure or study performed in this patient population. Endoscopic evaluation allows direct visualization and simultaneous acquisition of tissue samples when indicated. The pattern of cell type of esophageal cancer is changing. In 2000, pathologic evaluation of esophageal cancers revealed squamous cell carcinoma in approximately 52% of patients and adenocarcinoma in 42% of patients.[10] Currently, The National Cancer Institute describes more than 50% of esophageal cancers as adenocarcinoma, primarily arising from Barrett's esophagus, and fewer than one-half of cancers as squamous cell carcinoma. The remaining tumors are usually sarcomas or small cell cancers. Benign gastrointestinal tumors such as gastrointestinal stromal tumors can be found within the esophagus. Endoscopy with biopsy is highly sensitive and specific for the diagnosis of esophageal cancer.

Box 2
Percentage of esophageal cancer patients by stage at time of diagnosis

Stage 1: 13.3%

Stage 2: 34.7%

Stage 3: 35.7%

Stage 4: 12.3%

Staging of esophageal cancer after establishing tissue diagnosis is necessary for planning treatment options and strategies. CT is used to evaluate the mass and involvement of surrounding structures. Additionally, CT can be very helpful in identifying metastatic tumors. EUS is being used with increasing frequency owing to the ability of this technology to define clearly the layers of the esophageal wall involved with the tumor. EUS is also highly sensitive in identifying adjacent nodal metastases and can guide needle biopsies of nodes suspected of containing metastatic disease. Positron emission tomography is used frequently to evaluate the patient for local and distant metastatic disease. Less frequently, nuclear medicine bone scans are used to evaluate the patient for bone metastases.

Esophageal cancer can be a highly lethal disease and the overall disease-free survival at 1 year after diagnosis is only 43%. Most patients are diagnosed with stage 2 (34.7%) or stage 3 (35.7%) disease (**Box 2**).[10]

SUMMARY

Patients frequently present to a physician with complaints of difficulty swallowing. The approach to evaluating systematically these problems can be challenging for those who do not manage this type of patient regularly. The potential for life-threatening malignancies is present and makes this evaluation a priority. Numerous excellent tools are available to aid with the determination of the cause of dysphagia and assist with the formulation of a logical treatment algorithm.

REFERENCES

1. Kuo P, Holloway RH, Nguyen NQ. Current and future techniques in the evaluation of dysphagia. J Gastroenterol Hepatol 2012;27(5):873–81.
2. Patel D, Vaezi MF. Normal esophageal physiology and laryngopharyngeal reflux. Otolaryngol Clin North Am 2013;46(6):1023–41.
3. Andersson M, Lundell L, Kostic S, et al. Evaluation of the response to treatment in patients with idiopathic achalasia by the timed barium esophagogram: results from a randomized clinical trial. Dis Esophagus 2009;22:264–73.
4. Kim HP, Vance RB, Shaheen NJ, et al. The prevalence and diagnostic utility of endoscopic features of eosinophilic esophagitis: a meta-analysis. Clin Gastroenterol Hepatol 2012;10(9):988–96.
5. Peery AF, Cao H, Dominik R, et al. Variable reliability of endoscopic findings with white-light and narrow-band imaging for patients with suspected eosinophilic esophagitis. Clin Gastroenterol Hepatol 2011;9:475–80.
6. Familiari P, Gigante G, Marchese M, et al. Peroral endoscopic myotomy for esophageal achalasia: outcomes of the first 100 patients with short-term follow-up. Ann Surg 2014. [Epub ahead of print].

7. Bogte A, Bredenoord AJ, Oors J, et al. Reproducibility of esophageal high-resolution manometry. Neurogastroenterol Motil 2011;23:e271–6.

8. Rice TW, Shay SS. A primer of high-resolution esophageal manometry. Semin Thorac Cardiovasc Surg 2011;23(3):181–90.

9. Vaezi MF, Pandolfino JE, Vela MF. ACG clinical guideline: diagnosis and management of achalasia. Am J Gastroenterol 2013;108(8):1238–49.

10. Daly JM, Fry WA, Little AG, et al. Esophageal cancer: results of an ACS patient care survey. J Am Coll Surg 2000;190(5):562–72.

Oropharyngeal Dysphagia in Children

Mechanism, Source, and Management

Venkata S.P.B. Durvasula, MD, FRCS ENT[a], Ashley C. O'Neill, MS[b],
Gresham T. Richter, MD[a],*

KEYWORDS

- Oropharyngeal dysphagia • Dysphagia • Pediatric dysphagia
- Swallowing disorders • Microaspiration • Aspiration • Children • Pharyngeal

KEY POINTS

- Oropharyngeal dysphagia (OPD) is the presence of laryngeal penetration or aspiration of food contents, predominately liquid, during oral ingestion.
- The incidence of OPD in children is on the rise due to increasing life expectancy of premature infants and children with complex medical conditions.
- Identification and resolution of OPD in children is best determined by the presence or absence of symptoms, including wet respirations and coughing and choking during drinking.
- An initial clinical evaluation of feeding and swallowing is instrumental in assessment of OPD in children whereas video fluoroscopic swallow studies (VFSSs) and fibreoptic endoscopic evaluations of swallowing (FEES) remain the best tools for confirming aspiration in infants and children.
- Persistent OPD in neurologically normal children demands careful evaluation for potential etiologies and is best managed by a dedicated multidisciplinary team.

INTRODUCTION

Swallowing disorders can be identified at all ages. Coughing, choking, and wet respirations with feeding are all evidence of feeding problems in newborns and children. When left undiscovered or untreated, recurrent cough, bronchiectasis, reactive airway

This article originally appeared in Otolaryngologic Clinics of North America, Volume 47, Issue 5, October 2014.

Disclosures: Nil.

Funding Sources: Nil.

[a] Department of Pediatric Otolaryngology and Head and Neck surgery, Arkansas Children's Hospital, 1 Children's Way, Slot #836, Little Rock, AR 72202, USA; [b] Department of Audiology and Speech Pathology, Arkansas Children's Hospital, 1 Children's Way, Slot #113, Little Rock, AR 72202, USA

* Corresponding author.

E-mail address: GTRichter@uams.edu

Clinics Collections 7 (2015) 339–368

http://dx.doi.org/10.1016/j.ccol.2015.06.024

disease, and pneumonias may ensue. The cycle of symptoms and sickness is frequently stressful to patients and their caretakers who simply want their child to eat normally. The duration of dysphagia and difficulty in identifying the source compounds this anxiety. Unfortunately, epidemiologic data and sound diagnostic and treatment protocols for dysphagia are not well established.

Swallowing disorders in infants and children are common, with 25% of the pediatric population reported to experience some type of nonspecific feeding difficulty.[1] OPD is the most commonly encountered feeding disorder and refers to the dysfunction of the oral and pharyngeal phase of swallowing that results in laryngeal penetration and aspiration of solid or liquid food. As expected, higher rates of OPD are discovered in children with prematurity, upper aerodigestive tract anomalies, central nervous system (CNS) malformations, neurodevelopmental delays, and craniofacial syndromes. OPD is rarely an isolated event, however, and occurs in both developmentally delayed and normal children.

Recent advances in neonatal medicine have improved the survival of premature infants (<37 weeks' gestation) and those with complex medical conditions, thereby increasing the number of children in the community with residual difficulties with feeding and OPD.[2,3] The correlation between prematurity, complex medical conditions and feeding disorders in children is well established.[4,5] Pediatricians and otolaryngologists now see a greater number of children with persistent OPD. This includes developmentally normal and neurologically intact children who, as demonstrated by Sheikh and colleagues,[6] can present with chronic aspiration. The impact of OPD on the health of developmentally normal children emphasizes the importance of an extensive work-up and effective algorithm for treatment. Subtle inflammatory and anatomic problems are frequently present in otherwise healthy children with OPD.

Delayed reflexes, hypotonia, and generalized discoordination complicate the control of normal swallowing function in neurologically or developmentally affected children. Alternative feeding options or modified diets help maintain nutrition in this population pending improvement in function and strength. Gastrostomy tubes are frequently necessary to achieve fluid and nutritional goals. Depending on the underlying neurologic condition, dysphagia may take many years to improve and may never reach a normal state. Nonetheless, inflammatory and anatomic conditions, such as reflux, generalized respiratory illness, and upper aerodigestive anatomic anomalies, need to be assessed for in neurologically affected children because they may exacerbate their OPD.

The psychological impact of OPD on the family complicates early intervention because significant dysfunctional interactions between mothers and their infants with feeding disorders have been found.[7,8] The chronic nature of OPD with associated complications and the strain on the child and the family requires a dedicated team that caters to the medical, social, and dietary needs of these patients. Such a multidisciplinary team should consist of, with varying degrees of involvement, a pediatric otolaryngologist, pulmonologist, gastroenterologist, pediatric surgeon, speech and language pathologist (SLP), radiologist, nutritionist, occupational therapist, psychologist, and social worker. The objective of this clinical review is to provide pediatricians and otolaryngologists a global understanding of the potential causes of dysphagia and to provide an algorithm for diagnosing and treating infants and children with complicated or persistent OPD.

MECHANISM OF NORMAL AND DYSFUNCTIONAL SWALLOWING

Normal swallowing is a complex process that involves both voluntary and involuntary mechanisms. It includes 4 phases: oral preparatory, oral transit, pharyngeal, and esophageal. The oral preparatory phase involves grinding or chewing the food and mixing with saliva, creating a food bolus of appropriate size and consistency. The food bolus is voluntarily pushed backwards into the oropharynx. The backward movement to the oropharynx triggers the reflex pharyngeal phase.

The pharyngeal phase of swallowing is reflex mediated by the stimulation of the afferent receptors along the anterior tonsillar pillars, base of tongue, and epiglottis. The resultant efferent motor muscular activity is mediated by the glossopharyngeal (cranial nerve [CN] IX) and vagus (CN X) nerves. This muscular activity is a complex and coordinated contraction involving a series of muscle groups to ensure quick bolus passage across the relaxed cricopharyngeal or upper esophageal sphincter (UES) while simultaneously protecting the airway. The bolus is directed posteriorly by the voluntary propulsion of the tongue and then by the sequential reflex contractions of pharyngeal constrictors. The soft palate moves against the posterior pharyngeal wall to close the nasopharyngeal port. At the same time, the hyoid is advanced anteriorly by contraction of the strap muscles while pulling the larynx anteriorly and superiorly. In the process, the epiglottis is retroflexed to cover the laryngeal introitus.

During the pharyngeal phase, various measures protect the airway to prevent aspiration. The pharyngoglottal closure reflex is initiated by the sensory and chemoreceptors in the pharynx and larynx and is mediated by the CN IX and CN X nerves. When stimulated, adduction of true vocal cords and approximation of arytenoid cartilages occurs by contraction of the thyroarytenoid and interarytenoid muscles, thereby closing the laryngeal inlet.[9,10]

The swallow center of the CNS is located in the medulla along the nucleus tractus solitarius and the nuclei of the reticular system of the fourth ventricle. The supranuclear connections are relayed from the swallow center via the hypothalamus to the cerebral cortex. The swallow center is the area for coordination of the afferent and efferent activity in swallowing and transmits inhibitory impulses to the adjacent respiratory center, located in the medulla, thus inhibiting respiration during swallowing. The afferent oropharyngeal, pharyngeal, and laryngeal receptors relay information via afferent nerves in CN IX and CN X and the efferent arm is relayed via the same nerves from nuclei located in the nucleus ambiguus (**Fig. 1**).

The laryngeal adductor reflex (LAR) is the second protective reflex that is more specific to the supraglottic portion of larynx. It is mediated by the internal sensory division of the superior laryngeal nerve (CN X) supplying the mucosal surface of the epiglottis, aryepiglottic folds, and posterior larynx above the vocal cords. The LAR coordinates the sensory input from these areas and relays them to the medulla. The efferent return through the recurrent laryngeal nerve (CN X) causes contraction of the thyroarytenoid and interarytenoid muscles, which results in reflex closure and protection of the airway.

The significance of normal laryngopharyngeal sensation is demonstrated by recent studies using FEES with sensory testing. Evidence suggests that laryngopharyngeal sensation is reduced or inhibiting in pediatric and adult patients with OPD.[11]

The stimulation of the swallow center in the medulla inhibits the adjacent respiratory center that results in a temporary cessation of respiration, which accompanies the laryngeal upward movement, the closure of epiglottis, and the reflex closure of the larynx during the process of deglutition. The temporal coordination of breathing and pharyngeal phase of swallow is critical. Unfortunately this process can be severely disrupted in children with neurologic conditions[12] and chronic lung disease associated with prematurity,[13] thus increasing the risk of aspiration in these groups.

The movement of the food bolus below the pharynx occurs with opening of the UES, primarily by reflex relaxation of the cricopharyngeus muscle, and aided by the upward

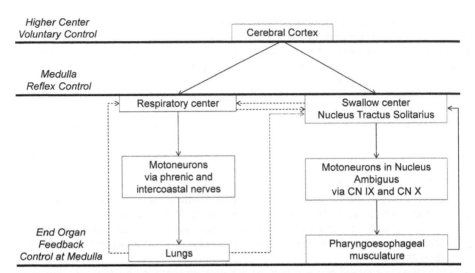

Fig. 1. The neural regulation of swallow. Cerebral cortex is involved in voluntary control of both respiratory and swallows centers located in the medulla. Dotted lines indicate inhibitory influence and continuous lines indicate stimulatory effect. Inflation of lungs inhibits both centers. Stimulation of pharyngoesophageal musculature stimulates deglutition. Both medullary centers have inhibitory influence on one another.

and anterior movement of larynx. This is followed by the esophageal phase of swallowing, which is reflex mediated under the influence of the autonomic nervous system of cervical and thoracic ganglia.

Age-Related Differences—Maturation of Swallow with Age

All the phases of swallowing are demonstrable in children, adolescents, and adults. There are some inherent differences, however, in swallowing between neonates, infants and adolescents. The oral phase in neonates and infants is a primitive sucking reflex. The buccal pads are prominent to aid sucking; the tongue protrudes whereas the perioral muscles, including the lips, cheeks, tongue, and palate act rhythmically and synergistically like a single organ to compress the nipple and express its contents. In the first 3 months, infants fail to differentiate consistency between solids and liquids and use the same suck reflex for both. Furthermore, the pharyngeal phase in infants lasts longer than in adults.[14] In spite of the longer duration of the pharyngeal phase in infants, no aspiration is noticed in a majority, possibly due to a more efficient laryngeal closure owing to the softer cartilaginous framework.[15,16]

The coordination between breathing and swallowing, as described previously in adults, translates into a coordinated suck-swallow-breathe sequence in infants, so that they can suck efficiently and swallow rapidly with minimal interruption in airflow. Poor coordination of this sequence is associated with prematurity[17] and patients with cerebral palsy (CP).[12] Upper airway obstruction in neonates and infants may interrupt this sequence mainly by breathlessness and prolonged sucking when infants are unable to generate a sufficient suction pressure in the presence of obstruction. This subtle discoordination between eating and breathing contributes to OPD in infants with upper airway obstruction.[18]

As an infant matures, the jaw grows and the buccal pads are absorbed to increase the intraoral space. The protrusion of tongue, which is an important component of suckling, is gradually lost by 6 months and replaced by raising and lowering of the tongue. This is coupled with increasing use of tongue intrinsic musculature, which is responsible for the development of propulsive action.[19] At this stage, the infants may be fed with solids as their voluntary swallow function starts to mature beyond the primitive suckling. The rhythmic biting in response to stimulation of the alveolar ridge gradually develops into mastication with the development of deciduous teeth. This stage represents a maturation of swallowing that may continue to 24 months of age.[20] These changes represent a continuum of development in response to stimulation in the form of changing oral feeding habits. Lack of development is often noticed in infants on gastrostomy feeds who develop oral aversion and OPD if oral stimulation is not attempted.[21]

ETIOLOGY OF OROPHARYNGEAL DYSPHAGIA

Efficient and effective swallowing relies on 2 important steps. The voluntary oral skills that involve preparation of the food bolus and the reflex patterned motor actions of swallowing. This combination results in the coordinated action and inhibition of the muscle groups located around the oropharynx and esophagus responsible for the passage of food into the stomach. As discussed previously, voluntary oral skills are not present until 6 months of age and may be a primary source of dysfunction in this age group. This is especially true if neonatal hospitalization and chronic illness prevents normal oral intake and stimulation at this key developmental age.

Frequently, OPD is multifactorial (**Box 1**). Developmental and neurologic delays can result in discoordination of swallow and contribute to OPD. Inflammatory, obstructive, and anatomic conditions may also be involved and are more frequently seen in developmentally normal individuals. Contributing factors may be grossly apparent at presentation or only through meticulous investigation. For example, prematurity and laryngomalacia can both independently contribute to OPD but premature patients have more prolonged symptoms than seen in those with laryngomalacia alone.[22] Contributing factors in children with OPD are outlined.

Prematurity

A functionally appropriate feeding pattern in neonates and young infants involves a coordinated suck-swallow-breathing rhythm so that an infant can suck efficiently and swallow rapidly with minimal airflow interruption. Due to neurologic immaturity, prematurity less than 34 weeks may be associated with poor coordination of this rhythm. Prematurity contributes to a delay in the pharyngeal phase of swallowing as demonstrated on high-resolution manometry studies of neurologically normal preterm infants at 31 to 32 weeks. Poor pharyngeal pressures coupled with poor coordination of pharyngeal propulsion and UES relaxation were found compared with term infants.[23] Weaker pharyngeal pressures were presumably related to neurologic immaturity in the premature infants.

Premature infants also have a weak suck reflex.[24] A sucking pattern consists of suckling bursts. An immature pattern may include a short burst of 4 to 6 sucks at 1 to 1.5 sucks/s and a mature pattern may consist of approximately 30 sucks at 2 sucks/s.[25] The number of sucking bursts gradually increases by term gestation.[26] These suckling bursts should be coordinated with breathing and swallowing. A poorly coordinated suck-swallow-breathe sequence is found in infants born before 34 weeks of gestation due to lack of myelination in the medulla.[27] A mature sucking pattern is characterized by prolonged suckling bursts of more than 10 sucks with suck-swallow-breathe in equal proportions with a ratio of 1:1:1. A delay in maturation of the swallow and sucking reflex is reported in patients born very early when sucking

Box 1
Common contributors to oropharyngeal dysphagia in infants and children

Neuromuscular
- Cerebral palsy (CP)
- Head trauma
- Mild developmental delays
- Hypoxic injury
- Arnold-Chiari malformations
- Muscular dystrophy
- Prematurity

Larynx and trachea-bronchial tree
- Vocal cord paralysis
- Glottic/subglottic stenosis
- Laryngeal cleft
- Tracheoesophageal fistula

Anatomic

Nasal and nasopharyngeal
- CHARGE[a] syndrome
- Narrow piriform aperture

Oral cavity and oropharynx
- Cleft lip and cleft palate
- Ranula, etc.
- Lymphatic malformations
- Down syndrome
- Beckwith-Wiedeman syndrome

Craniofacial syndromes
- Crouzon syndrome
- Treacher Collins syndrome
- Goldenhar syndrome
- Pierre Robin syndrome

Hypopharnyx/supraglottis
- Congenital cysts
- Laryngomalacia

Neoplastic

Benign
- Vascular malformations of aerodigestive tract
- Leiomyoma

Malignant
- Lymphoma
- Rhabdomyosarcoma

Esophagus
- Esophageal atresia
- Vascular rings/anomalies
- Achalasia

Physiologic
- Gastroesophageal reflux disease (GERD)/ Laryngopharyngeal reflux (LPR)
- Eosinophilic esophagitis (EoE)
- Sinonasal secretions

Postsurgical
- Strictures of esophagus
- Nerve injury
- Tracheostomy
- Laryngotracheal reconstruction

Acquired
- Foreign body
- Chemical injury—ingestion of alkali, acid, corrosive, etc
- Medication induced
- Adenotonsillar hypertrophy

Behavioral
- Poor conditioning
- Oral aversion
- Globus
- Solid food dysphagia

[a] CHARGE stands for coloboma of the eye, heart defects, atresia of the nasal choanae, retardation of growth and/or development, genital abnormalities, and ear abnormalities.

patterns were analyzed at a corrected age of 40 weeks. Extremely preterm infants born at 24 to 29 weeks' gestation generate significantly fewer bursts and sucks per burst than more mature preterm infants (30–32 weeks) and those born at term.[28] This causes preterm infants to have a tendency to aspirate easily and fatigue quickly. This can make breastfeeding difficult and accounts for more desaturations in preterm infants when feeding.[24]

Preterm infants are also more likely to suffer anoxia or hypoxia at birth. This can result in permanent, but sometimes subtle, neurologic damage, including dysfunctional feeding patterns. A higher incidence of CP is found in preterm infants with lower gestational age (24–26 weeks) compared with those born later.[29] These patients primarily suffer with poor and noncoordinated oral skills required for sucking. They also exhibit poor head control, uncoordinated tongue movements, impaired palatal function, poor gag reflex, and laryngopharyngeal hyposensitivity; all of which increase the risk of OPD and aspiration. Subtle and radiographically undetectable hypoxic injury to the swallowing and respiratory centers in premature infants may help explain the increased incidence of OPD in these children.

Intubation as a newborn can also contribute to OPD in this population. The presence of an endotracheal tube and the resultant remodeling of the soft palate can lead to palatopharyngeal incompetence, nasal reflux, or a defective integration of the suck-swallow mechanism.[30] On the other hand, the presence of a tracheostomy tube in a newborn can prevent the normal rise of subglottic pressure and laryngeal elevation necessary for an effective pharyngeal phase of swallowing.

Neurologic Disorders

The manifestation, course, and possible resolution of OPD in neurologically affected children are determined by the nature, site, and evolution of the CNS defect. The prognosis for recovery also is influenced strongly by whether the underlying neurologic condition is static or progressive. Static neurologic conditions include CP, cerebrovascular accident, Arnold-Chiari malformation, syringomyelia, congenital viral infections with varicella, cytomegalovirus, tumors, and injuries to the brainstem. Progressive neurologic disorders are not limited to but include myopathies, neuropathies, and metabolic disorders like mucopolysaccharidosis. Children with static neurologic diagnoses generally improve in their OPD with developmental progress. Children with progressive neurologic conditions demonstrate early improvement but eventually lose these skills.

The most common neurologic condition encountered in children with OPD is CP. CP affects volitional oral movements and the involuntary reflexes (LARs) and compromises the neurologically dependent reflexive pharyngeal swallow. The situation is worsened by poor coordination of the suck-swallow-breathe sequence as infants.[12] CP patients frequently have a weak gag reflex and are prone to silent aspiration.[31] Volitional movements are affected when there is cortical injury or periventricular leukomalacia whereas reflex inhibition suggests subcortical injury involving brainstem and basal ganglia. Although it is hard to predict the incidence of OPD in CP patients, 85% to 90% of patients with CP are affected by dysphagia.[2] Chronic aspiration may be further complicated by the presence of gastroesophageal reflux disease (GERD) and drooling, which are present in more than 50% of cases.[32,33] Drooling is secondary to impaired volitional movements whereas posterior salivation causes recurrent aspiration and subsequent pulmonary infections.[34]

Other common static conditions include Arnold-Chiari and central arteriovenous malformations, which may be present with only subtle clinical evidence of OPD. A high index of suspicion for OPD is necessary in these patients. Greenlee and colleagues[35] reported that children with a Chiari malformation type 1 (CM-I) were most likely to present with OPD under 3 years of age. After evaluating the signs and symptoms of CM-I in children younger than 6 years of age, Albert and colleagues[36] also determined that 77.8% presented with OPD between 0 and 2 years of age. Indirect neurologic signs, such as a hoarse cry, delayed milestones, unsteady gait, and worsening OPD on VFSS, also may be present and should prompt an early brain MR imaging or neurology consult. This approach has been recommended in neurologically intact children with worsening or persistent OPD after 2 years of age. In a child with new onset of OPD, CNS neoplasms should also be ruled out using MR imaging.

O'Neill and colleagues[37] demonstrated that more than 50% of children with Down syndrome had evidence of persistent OPD. The mean age at diagnosis of OPD was 1.6 years. Resolution rates of OPD were also poor (15%) in this population, especially in patients with significant neurologic delay and prior tracheostomies. They suspected that inherent hypotonia and poor pharyngeal reflexes in the Down syndrome children contributed to the swallowing results found in their study. Moreover, procedures aimed at reducing upper airway obstruction had no effect on the resolution rates of OPD in their study.

Anatomic Contributors to OPD

Poor coordination of the suck-swallow-breath sequence may be observed in infants with upper airway obstruction. Similarly, in older infants and children, upper airway obstruction complicates swallowing by limiting normal respiration; this is particularly true in patients when OPD is multifactorial. Conditions associated with airway obstruction may contribute to OPD and include both congenital and acquired entities (**Box 2**).

Nasal or nasopharyngeal obstruction in an infant can complicate coordination of the suck-swallow-breathing rhythm. This is because neonates up to 3 months of age are obligate nasal breathers. Bilateral choanal atresia often causes respiration difficulty and swallowing dysfunction. Choanal stenosis patients typically fatigue and take short breaks during feeding, making coordination difficult. In older infants and children, nasal obstruction may be a result of allergic rhinitis, turbinate hypertrophy, adenoid hypertrophy, sinusitis, pyriform aperture stenosis, or nasopharyngeal or nasal congenital masses, such as glioma, meningocele, and nasal dermoid. It is important to document an appropriate patency of the nasopharyngeal airway in the evaluation of OPD. This is

---

Box 2
Anatomic correlates contributing to OPD in infants and children

Infants	*Older children*
• Laryngomalacia	• Sinusitis
• Laryngeal cleft	• Allergic rhinitis
• Tracheoesophageal fistula	• Adenoidal hypertrophy
• Esophageal atresia	• Adenotonsillar hypertrophy
• Vascular rings	• Narrow piriform aperture
• Vocal cord paralysis	• Cricopharyngeal achalasia
• Bilateral choanal atresia	
• Gliomas/meneingocele	
• Cleft palate/cleft lip	
• Congenital cysts	

particularly relevant in late infancy and the early second year of life when adenoid hypertrophy is a primary source of obstruction. Anecdotal evidence suggests that chronic rhinitis and nasal obstruction affect VFSS results and complicate weaning off a modified diet in young children with OPD.

Development of normal oral and oropharyngeal anatomy is important for natural suckling in neonates and the preparatory phases of swallowing in children. Craniofacial dysmorphisms and cleft lip or cleft palate have an impact on normal oral intake. Some children, as seen in Beckwith-Wiedemann syndrome, have a disproportionately large tongue that interferes with early oral preparation and oropharyngeal function.

Laryngeal elevation propels the food bolus whereas protective reflexes in the hypopharynx and larynx aid in the coordination of breathing and swallowing and at the same time offer laryngeal protection. Anatomic abnormalities of the hyphopharynx and larynx can result in OPD. These include vocal fold paralysis, vallecular cysts, laryngotracheal clefts, glottic webs, laryngomalacia, and subglottic stenosis. Laryngotracheal reconstruction, with alteration of normal laryngeal anatomy, can contribute to temporary or long-term OPD.[38] Vocal fold paralysis with the loss of recurrent laryngeal nerve function increases the chance of aspiration owing to reduced vocal fold adduction, an open posterior glottis, and potentially the loss of sensation associated with superior laryngeal nerve weakness. Airway obstruction due to webs or subglottic stenosis with difficulties in ventilation cause early fatigue of respiration and swallowing, leading to OPD. Deep laryngeal clefts (Benjamin-Inglis types 2–4) allow for passage of food contents directly into the larynx below the level of the vocal folds. The diagnosis and management of the less obvious type 1 laryngeal clefts can be challenging with late diagnosis and persistent OPD. These laryngoesophageal defects may often be associated with esophageal dysmotility and complicated by GERD.

Laryngomalacia is the most common cause of stridor in newborns and infants due to redundancy and/or weakness of the supraglottic larynx. Airway symptoms are secondary to dynamic inspiratory collapse of the supraglottic structures and redundant mucosa. Laryngomalacia is associated with OPD in more than 50% of patients.[22] Airway obstruction may interfere with the suck-swallow-breathing rhythm pattern and increases dysphagla and GERD, which in turn can reduce laryngeal sensation and exacerbate laryngeal edema. Management of GERD can improve the respiratory pattern and dysphagia and result in improved weight gain in these patients.[39] Laryngomalacia is associated with reduced laryngeal sensitivity, which enhances the risk of silent aspiration.[40] Increased diameter and surface area of the nerve endings have been reported in supra-arytenoid specimens harvested from laryngomalacia patients that may represent an autocrine enhancement of dysfunctional nervous system due to laryngomalacia.[41]

Cervical and distal esophageal anatomic anomalies may also contribute to persistent OPD, including esophageal atresia, tracheoesophageal fistula (TEF), and cricopharyngeal achalasia.

Dysphagia can be a persistent issue after repair of both esophageal atresia and TEF owing to disrupted upper esophageal neuromuscular control and chronic GERD. Patients may be on a modified diet (liquid thickeners) for many years after the repair. It is important to rule out an associated laryngeal cleft because this may also be present in a significant number of patients with distal esophageal anatomic anomalies.

The cricopharyngeus muscle is a striated muscle that is contracted at rest, thus keeping the esophagus closed during respiration. Cricopharyngeal achalasia is thought to involve spasm or incomplete relaxation of the cricopharyngeus muscle. This is uncommon in children but can be diagnosed by identification of a prominent bar on VFSS, with OPD found in approximately 50% of cases. Increased pressures proximal to the muscle can also be demonstrated on manometry[42] and confirmed by electromyography.[43] Management with cricopharyngeus myotomy or dilatation has been reported useful in relieving symptoms of affected patients.[42,44,45]

Inflammatory Conditions

Gastroesophageal reflux (GER) is a normal physiologic phenomenon known to occur in all healthy infants. Actual repeated expulsion of gastroesophageal contents from the oral cavity in GER is reported to occur in approximately 40% of infants.[46] On the other hand, the prevalence of symptomatic or pathologic GER or GERD is estimated to occur in 10% to 20% of infants in North America.[47] Some children are at higher risk of GERD, including those with neurologic impairment, obesity, esophageal achalasia, hiatal hernia, prematurity, bronchopulmonary dyplasia, and esophageal atresia.[48] GERD can contribute to persistent OPD by reducing mucosal sensation and laryngeal reactivity (LAR) during the pharyngeal phase of swallowing owing to mucosal injury by caustic reflex contents. Reduced laryngeal sensation has been demonstrated in the setting of chronic reflux in both animals and infants.[49] In view of the prevalence of GERD, treatment has become an important part of OPD management in children.[50]

Eosinophilic esophagitis (EoE) is a chronic immune-mediated condition characterized by clinical symptoms secondary to esophageal dysfunction and histologically by eosinophilic infiltration of the esophagus.[51,52] Feeding difficulties are the most common symptoms in infants and toddlers, with vomiting and retrosternal pain in children and adolescents. The main histologic feature of EoE is striking eosinophilia of esophageal mucosa with microabcesses and basal zone hyperplasia. The relationship to EoE to OPD is unclear. EoE is associated, however, with GERD and food allergies, both of which are thought to contribute to chronic inflammation and reduced sensitivity of the larynx.[53,54] Such a reaction to cow milk protein has been described[55] and careful history with radioallergosorbent (RAST) testing may be useful to help identify the cause quickly.

Esophageal biopsies and histology usually confirms the diagnosis of EoE and the management consists of dietary modification and reflux therapy. Three diet forms are commonly prescribed: an elemental diet that is a liquid formula based on amino acids and free of all allergens,[56] a 6-food elimination diet that removes commonly identified allergens,[57] or a targeted elimination diet[58] that eliminates food identified as allergic to patient after testing. Swallowed corticosteroids are also effective in treating acute exacerbations of EoE but the disease often relapses after discontinuation.

EVALUATION OF PEDIATRIC OROPHARYNGEAL DYSPHAGIA
History and Physical Examination

Slow feeding, blue spells, frequent respiratory pauses, or wheeze and/or cough during the feed suggests OPD in an infant. Wet respirations (biphasic washing machine sound) with a wet cry or voice suggest silent aspiration and OPD in both infants and children. The importance of detecting a postprandial wet voice by itself is not considered diagnostic but is likely useful in identifying those with dysphagia related to laryngeal dysfunction.[59] Airway symptoms, such as breathlessness, stridor, and wheeze, may mask silent aspiration and a high index of suspicion for OPD in these patients is well served. Weight gain is an important predictor of health and nutrition in children with OPD and should be followed closely. Discussion of perinatal events and gestational age help tease out the cause of OPD in otherwise normal children. Parents should also be asked about potential neurologic, inflammatory, and anatomic sources of OPD (discussed previously). A history of recurrent and chronic lower respiratory tract infections, reactive airway disease, and pneumonia, especially if severe enough to warrant hospitalization, is an important symptom of pediatric OPD. In less severe cases, infants may sound congested due to chronic respiratory secretions and bronchitis from chronic microaspiration. Delays in speech and gait may also indicate subtle central pathology in older children.

A complete and thorough otolaryngology examination is essential in the diagnosis of OPD and exploration of potential etiology. Syndromic facial characteristics should be searched for. Auscultation for wheezing, course breath sounds, and wet voice/cry or respiration before and after eating is essential. This is best performed by an SLP who can observe subtle symptoms of OPD during oral intake and postprandially. Nasal patency and identification of upper aerodigestive tract obstruction are essential components of the examination.[50]

Flexible fiberoptic nasolaryngoscopy should be performed as routine part of the examination in patients with OPD. This provides anatomic detail of the nasal cavity, nasopharynx, oropharynx, hypopharynx, and larynx while identifying evidence of chronic mucosal inflammation of these sites, which may be secondary to rhinitis, postnasal drip, and GERD. Low lying tonsils, laryngomalacia, laryngeal clefts, and evidence of hypopharyngeal residue can be seen with this examination.

In all cases of suspected OPD it is important to involve SLP early in the process of evaluation. Clinical bedside evaluation or clinical feeding evaluation can be easily performed (**Box 3**). Evaluation using 3-oz water challenge[60] has been described. With this brief study, a child is observed during and after oral consumption of up to 3 oz of water. OPD can manifest with coughing, choking, or tearing occurring during or shortly after the test. Suiter and colleagues[61] reported their results in children between

---

Box 3
Clinical bedside evaluation for a patient with suspected oropharyngeal dysphagia

History

Medical history: obtain thorough medical history from caregivers about child

Feeding history: obtain past feeding history and current feeding schedule for child

Examination

Inspection: make observations regarding child's oral sensorimotor (OM) skills at rest, such as open-mouth posture, drooling, low tone, facial symmetry, etc.

Palpation: with babies, used gloved finger to feel inside child's mouth to assess tongue mobility, restrictive frenulum, status of palate

Observe feeding ability

1. Bottle—child's ability to latch on to bottle nipple, child's efficiency in expressing liquid from the bottle, anterior liquid loss

2. Sippy cup/straw drinking—OM skills

3. Spoon feeding—ability to close lips on spoon, remove bolus, etc.

4. Solid ingestion—ability to manipulate/chew solid prior to swallow

Observe for signs of aspiration

Distress/increased work of breathing/stridor/gagging/gulping/choking/coughing during feed. Increased congestion (nasal or chest) or wet vocal quality or wheezing during or directly after feed

2 and 18 years of age. Compared with FEES, the investigators concluded that the 3-oz challenge had high sensitivity but a low specificity, indicating a high false-positive rate, suggesting that normal children who cleared this test may be safely given thin liquids. It is not a good screening tool for children at high risk of aspiration, however, and is not a good indicator of silent aspiration.

Chest Radiograph

A chest radiograph (CXR) is a good initial screening tool in children with suspect OPD but is not necessary in all. In the setting of fever, a CXR may be useful to identify an active pulmonary process. CXRs in chronic cases of OPD show bronchial thickening, hyperinflation, and segmental or subsegmental infiltrates. The infiltrates in OPD follow discreet patterns and settle in dependent areas, such as the posterior aspects of the lower lobes. Unfortunately, CXR is largely insensitive to early pulmonary injury related to chronic microaspiration.[62]

High-Resolution CT Scan

High-resolution CT (HRCT) is recommended when CXRs show evidence of chronic aspiration–related pulmonary injury and in cases where the severity of injury is not known. HRCT is sensitive compared with a plain CXR in detecting and delineating aspiration-related parenchymal injury. HRCT can detect bronchiectasis, centrilobular opacities (tree-in-bud), air trapping, and bronchial thickening.[63] Although not specific to aspiration, these findings are consistent with chronic aspiration.

MR imaging Scan of Head and Cervical Spine

MR imaging scan of the head and cervical spine is recommended to delineate intracranial pathology in selected cases of OPD. A diagnosis of Chiari I malformation using MR imaging can be made easily in younger patients, even those with minimal or no neurologic symptoms.[64] MR imaging scan is not routinely performed in all cases of OPD but should be considered in cases associated with even mild developmental delays or neurologic deficits because they are identified with increasing age of the child. An infant or child with progressively worsening OPD should undergo early MR imaging because this may be a sign of a potential central cause. This is also true for the neurologically intact and developmentally normal children who continue to have OPD beyond the age of 2.5 years. MR imaging scan may help in detection of minor cerebellar infarcts, Chiari malformations, vascular anomalies, or tumors affecting the swallow center in the medulla.[36]

Lipid-Laden Macrophage Index

The lipid-laden macrophage index (LLMI) can be used to help diagnose aspiration. Gastric contents often contain lipid material that can be taken up by the pulmonary macrophages after aspiration. For the LLMI as described by Colombo and Hallberg,[65] the macrophages are graded 0–4 based on the amount of lipid in the cytoplasm of each macrophage. A total of 100 macrophages is usually studied; hence, indices could range between 0 and 400. Furuya and colleagues[66] studied 41 children with pulmonary pathology and suspicion of aspiration and reported that an LLMI greater than 165 had a 98.6% sensitivity, 78% specificity, and 87.8% overall accuracy as a diagnostic test for aspiration. Kieran and colleagues[67] reported significantly higher LLMI in patients undergoing surgery for type 1 and type 2 laryngeal clefts and proposed measuring LLMI in cleft patients as an indicator of pulmonary injury. Although the LLMI may be increased in aspiration, it is not very specific. Other comorbidities seen in aspirators, such as asthma, GERD, and recurrent pneumonia, may also contribute to LLMI elevation.[68] Thus, LLMI is not routinely performed to assess aspiration, but it may be helpful in cases like chronic cough, where no other reason is found.

Microlaryngobronchoscopy and Esophagoscopy

A complete microlaryngobronchoscopy (MLB) is performed in cases of suspected anatomic sources of OPD, for example, a patient with history suggesting a laryngeal cleft or subglottic pathology. MLB should also be considered in a normal child with more than 2 years of age, who has objective evidence (VFSS/FEES) of aspiration, to rule out undetected laryngotracheal anomalies contributing to OPD. MLB may be also be required when office based flexible provides evidence of laryngeal anomalies contributing to OPD (laryngomalacia most commonly) that may require surgical management. MLB should be performed with patients breathing spontaneously to observe laryngeal function. Palpation is the best way to identify a type 1 cleft that may otherwise be missed. MLB is often performed with a planned esophagoscopy or vice versa. Esophagoscopy allows assessment and, if necessary, biopsies to identify GERD and EoE. The number of esophageal biopsies required remains unclear; however, 2 biopsies at the proximal, mid, and distal esphagous should be able to capture evidence of inflammation if present.

Instrumental Evaluations of Swallowing

VFSSs and FEES are the most commonly used tests in the evaluation of aspiration in infants and children. FEES may also be used with sensitivity testing. Both techniques have advantages and disadvantages, as outlined in **Table 1**, but are extremely useful in providing objective evidence of OPD. Although considered gold standard, these tests are confounded by a poor intrarater and inter-rater reliability because normative data for standardization are not available.[69]

Table 1
VFSS and FEES comparison

VFSS	FEES
Allows real-time view of oral preparatory; oral, pharyngeal, and cervical esophageal phases of swallow; and how structures interact during bolus transit	Oral phase is not visible; only before and after the swallow can be viewed; view is obstructed during the swallow by epiglottic inversion
Swallowing structures are visible only via videofluoroscopy	The anatomy of the nasopharynx, the supraglottic structures, and the true vocal cords are visible
Detects aspiration	Trace aspiration may be missed
Radiation exposure	No radiation exposure
Sample of swallows may be small due to time constraints and to attempts to limit radiation exposure	Multiple swallows of different consistencies may be viewed
Expensive procedure and requires appointment in radiology department	May be performed during outpatient clinic visit with otolaryngologist and SLP
Requires patient participation	Nasopharyngoscope may be invasive/ uncomfortable for patient and thus lead to decreased cooperation
Study must be performed in radiology suite and patient must sit in swallow study chair	FEES can be performed at beside; may be more appropriate for medically complex children who are not mobile

Videofluoroscopic swallow study

The VFSS is the primary tool for formal dysphagia evaluation. The VFSS is performed by a team of professionals, including a radiologist and an SLP with extensive training in feeding and swallowing assessment and management.[70] In some institutions, an OT along with a radiologist may evaluate a child's swallowing function. VFSS may be warranted if a child demonstrates consistent signs and symptoms of aspiration during or immediately after a feeding. Other symptoms may include increased feeding times and poor weight gain. Prior to scheduling a swallow study, a child should be clinically evaluated by a physician and an SLP. During the clinical evaluation, the SLP obtains the child's pertinent medical history and observes the child clinically during a feeding.[71] In situations where a child's feeding cannot be observed by the SLP prior to the study, a thorough medical and feeding history for the child should be obtained.

For the study, the infant or younger child sits in a booster or tumbleform seat (Ability One Company, Bolingbrook, IL, USA) in the swallow study chair. Videofluoroscopy is used to capture the various stages of the swallow in real time. The lateral view is most common, although, in some cases, anterior-posterior view may be useful if asymmetry is suspected. Preferably, the caregiver stands in front of the child and helps the child during the feeding. The SLP, however, may also perform the feeding.[71] The initial consistency and manner of intake chosen depends on what liquids/solids the child is currently taking by mouth, the medical history of the child, and what information the SLP expects to gain from the study.

Information about the oral preparatory and oral, pharyngeal, and esophageal phases of the swallow may be obtained during VFSS. During the study, the SLP monitors a child's feeding. Reduced oral motor skills may be observed for several reasons, including prematurity, developmental delay, upper airway obstruction, and neurologic impairment.[72]

Delayed initiation of the swallow may lead to pooling of the barium in the valleculae or pyriform sinuses. Supraglottic penetration may be documented during the study, including a description of when, how deep, and how often these penetrations occur (**Fig. 2**). Shallow or midlevel penetration may be viewed without the presence of other swallowing dysfunction. Frequent, deep penetration, however, is often an indicator that the child is at a higher risk of aspiration with that consistency, flow, and manner of intake.[73] Transglottic aspiration may occur before, during, or after the swallow.

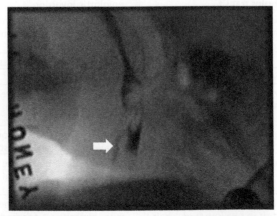

Fig. 2. VFSS image showing aspiration during the pharyngeal phase of swallow in a child. The aspirate is denoted by arrow.

Aspiration before the swallow indicates delayed initiation of the pharyngeal swallow. Aspiration during the swallow indicates incompetent or delayed pharyngoglottal reflex or true vocal cord dysfunction, and aspiration after the swallow occurs with pharyngeal residue. The SLP should note whether or not the child had any response to the aspiration event (absent cough, immediate cough, and delayed cough). Silent aspiration is frequently noted on VFSS in neurologically impaired children, children with developmental delays, and premature infants.[74,75] If pharyngeal residue is observed after the swallow, the amount and location of the residue should be noted. Pharyngeal residue may indicate reduced tongue base retraction and/or reduced pharyngeal contraction.[71]

The cause of a child's dysphagia may be better understood after VFSS if there is an adequate sample obtained and if the child participated well. Results of the study and feeding recommendations for the child are then made to the caregivers. Recommendations may include position changes during feeding, altering the flow of the liquid with a slower manner of intake, or thickening of feeds to aid in oral and/or pharyngeal control of the bolus. These recommendations, especially regarding thickening of liquids, should be approved by a child's managing physician.

Fibreoptic endoscopic evaluation of swallowing

The FEES was initially described in adults but is now commonly used in infants and children to further assess swallowing patterns.[76,77] Although initially not widely used for dysphagia assessment,[62] the practice of FEES has gained acceptance as a useful diagnostic and therapeutic tool for pediatric dysphagia assessment and management.[78,79] FEES may be indicated if the child is not appropriate for an initial or follow-up VFSS or if further evaluation of the anatomic structures of swallowing is warranted. FEES provides the SLP more opportunities to view various consistencies and compensatory swallowing strategies during feeding without detrimental radiation exposure. For a child who is not an oral feeder, information may be gained by observing the child's management of secretions, sometimes with the use of dye.[79]

FEES is usually performed together by an otolaryngologist and SLP. The flexible nasolaryngoscope is positioned by the physician as the SLP administers feeding. Interpretation of the examination is performed by both team members. A qualified SLP[80] can also place the scope but requires another participant to assist with feeding. A nurse is often required to help hold a young child undergoing the examination. During FEES, the nasopharynx, oropharynx, hypopharynx, supraglottis, and true vocal folds are visible. Food contents in this study do not have to be mixed with barium. Food dye may be necessary, however, to provide better visualization of the bolus during transit. Epiglottic inversion, as a result of pharyngeal constriction and hypolaryngeal excursion, prevents viewing of bolus transit during part of the pharyngeal phase. Delayed initiation of the swallow, supraglottic penetration, frank aspiration, and/or pharyngeal residue, however, after the swallow are best determined by FEES.

In studies comparing adult VFSS and FEES results, FEES has been noted as sensitive in the detection of delayed initiation of the swallow, penetration, aspiration, and pharyngeal residue.[76,81] In the pediatric population, a study by Leder and Karas[79] in 2000 reported 100% agreement in 7 patients who underwent both VFSS and FEES in recognition of penetration and aspiration occurrence. Research continues regarding the sensitivity and specificity of FEES in the pediatric population.

Deciding which instrumental examination is most appropriate for a child depends on several factors. For some children, obtaining both VFSS and FEES is ideal to obtain a more comprehensive picture of the anatomy and swallowing mechanism. FEES provides for a detailed anatomic assessment of the pharynx and larynx along with swallowing function data. VFSS shows all phases of the swallow, which is helpful in some children. Children between ages 1.5 years and 4 years have difficulty participating in FEES and following directions. Thus, FEES is more commonly used in infants and older children after a previous VFSS to follow their OPD course without radiation.

MANAGEMENT OF PEDIATRIC OROPHARYNGEAL DYSPHAGIA

Once identified, OPD in children follows a protracted course compared with other medical issues treated by an otolaryngologist. Fortunately, nutrition for most infants and children with OPD can be maintained using a modified feeding program with liquid thickeners. Early and open discussions with the family regarding the duration from diagnosis to final OPD resolution should occur at the time of diagnosis. Evidence suggests that infants diagnosed with OPD may take 2 to 3 years to be ultimately weaned from their diet modification to normal thin consistencies.[82] This delay is related to both the interval between the diagnosis and identification of the cause and the weaning period to safely graduate to each subsequent thinner consistency. Currently, a well-established management protocol for OPD does not exist. A multidisciplinary effort is necessary to help identify the source and optimize gastrointestinal and pulmonary health. Periodic visits, endoscopies, surgical procedures, and instrumental evaluations of swallowing are required during the course of pediatric OPD management.

Initial Management

When OPD is suspected, the initial physician visit consists of establishing the diagnosis, exploring potential contributors, and determining the patient's safe alimentation. A stepwise algorithm, used by the authors' institution, is provided (**Fig. 3**) on the first physician visit. Early SLP consultation provides detailed information regarding feeding habits, overall safety, and need of a VFSS or FEES (see **Box 3**). The families' working relationship with the SLP is fundamental in establishing an appropriate feeding paradigm for the child.

Important information gathered for infants with suspected OPD includes nipple flow, length of feeding time, and signs/symptoms of aspiration during or after a feed. From this information, early interventions (**Box 4**) may be a change to slower flow nipples, implementation of pacing during the feed, and altering a child's feeding position. These early interventions should always be practiced prior to introducing a thickening agent. Empiric thickening of liquid intake, however, may also help slow flow and reduce GERD. This can enhance laryngeal protection until a formal instrumental evaluation can take place. Other compensatory feeding strategies include small volumes, reducing the interval between feeds, and changing the formula or bottles used. For babies with reflux-associated OPD, empiric thickening with rice cereal may control mild symptoms and the patient can be followed in clinic periodically for signs of improvement. Many of these children have subtle evidence of mild laryngomalacia (periodic stridor with feeds and shortened aryepiglottic folds). Breastfed children in this scenario may continue their diet, with reflux precautions, because breast milk is not caustic to the pulmonary system. If an infant continues to have feeding difficulties and associated respiratory illnesses, a formal swallowing evaluation is warranted. Patients with severe GERD with regurgitation should be referred for gastroenterology evaluation.

Pulmonary consultation should be performed in cases in which pulmonary medical therapy (inhaled steroids) is required, patients with moderate to severe aspiration, and patients with unusually persistent OPD. These include infants with OPD requiring

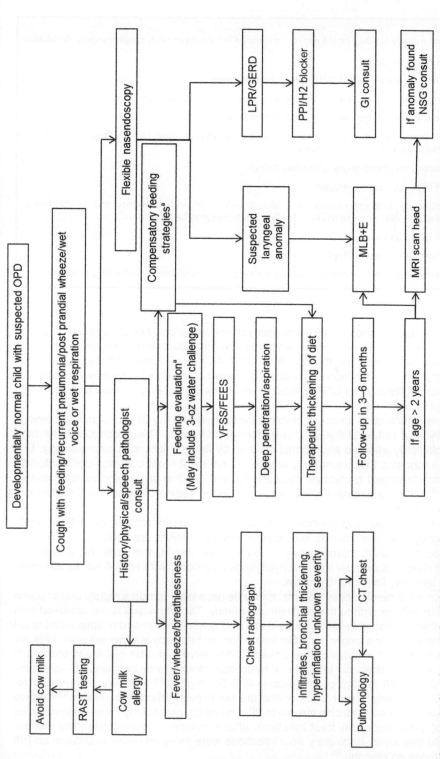

Fig. 3. Initial evaluation of a child with OPD. [a] Some patients with OPD may need just a bedside evaluation with compensatory feeding strategies without thickening of feed. Although SLP do not routinely include 3-oz water challenge, it may be used as a screening tool (for pros are cons please refer to the text). GI, gastroenterologist; H2 blocker, histamine H2 receptor antagonist; MLB+/−E, MLB with or without esophagoscopy; NSG, neuro surgery; RAST, radio allergo sorbent test.

Box 4
Compensatory feeding strategies recommended for a patient with oropharyngeal dysphagia

With bottle feeding

1. Change nipple shape and/or change flow of nipple

2. Implement external pacing to help with suck-swallow-breathe coordination

3. Feed in semiupright position or possibly side-lying position

4. Thicken liquids, if in spite of above measures patient continues to have feeding difficulties and is not efficient during feed

5. Patient may need ongoing feeding therapy

With sippy cup/open cup/straw

1. Introduce different manner of intake to help child with efficiency and safety during feeding—may need to thicken, feeding treatment may be helpful

With spoon and solids

1. Work on lip closure (feeding therapy)

2. Work on oral sensorimotor skills and learning to manipulate/chew (feeding therapy)

thickener greater than honey consistency or children older than 2.5 year still requiring honey-thick consistency. Instrumental swallowing evaluation may be necessary in this setting to help determine the severity of OPD. A CXR is valuable in the early investigation of pulmonary function and status. A CT scan of the chest is reserved for cases of concerning findings on CXR or those in which the impact of OPD on a patient's lungs cannot be assessed.

Investigation of an anatomic problem associated with the OPD or significant laryngopharyngeal reflux (LPR)/GERD is performed in infants. This is conducted for both neurologically affected and normal children by flexible fiberoptic laryngoscopy. Evidence suggests that prematurity and GERD are the 2 most common contributors to reduced laryngeal protective mechanisms and OPD in a developmentally normal child.[83] LPR management is recommended in the setting of signs and symptoms of reflux and OPD.

First-line therapy for LPR includes histamine H2 receptor antagonists (HRAs) at 6 to 10 mg/kg. The peak plasma level concentrations of HRAs are achieved at 2.5 hours and continue until approximately 6 hours. They should, therefore, be provided in 2 to 3 divided doses per day. Tachyphylaxis may occur with HRA 6 weeks after initiation and may limit long-term use.

In cases of persistent symptoms, it may be necessary to add a nightly proton pump inhibitor (PPI) or shift to this regimen completely. Tachyphalaxis is not observed with PPIs that are also able to inhibit meal-induced acid secretion and maintain gastric pH greater than 4 for a longer period of time. Maximum efficacy is achieved when PPIs are administered 30 minutes before a feed.[84] PPIs have a shorter half-life in children.[85] Thus, a higher dose per kilogram or twice-daily dosing is recommended—lansoprazole (0.73–1.66 mg/kg) or omeprazole (0.3–3.5 mg/kg).[86] PPIs are recommend for GERD in patients 1 year or older and are not proved effective in infants.[87] Caution has been advised regarding the use of PPIs in infants, particularly those with increased risk of lower respiratory tract infections, after a multicentric randomized trial demonstrated that lower respiratory tract infections were more common in children on PPI than those on placebo.[88]

Infants and children with suspected or confirmed OPD are followed every 1 to 3 months after the initial visit depending on the severity of dysphagia and LPR. Observation for and early control of inflammatory mediators of OPD and periodic assessment of developmental milestones and subtle delays are important components of clinical follow-up. When obvious laryngeal or other anatomic anomalies are detected (laryngeal cleft or severe laryngomalacia), an MLB is warranted for early corrective surgery and airway surveillance. Esophagoscopy with biopsies can be added to provide complete assessment of the entire aerodigestive tract under the same anesthetic.

Introducing Safe Alimentation

Safe alimentation entails a diet that can be negotiated during the pharyngeal phase with minimum risk of laryngeal penetration and aspiration into the trachea. This requires the use of an agent that is safe for dietary consumption and adequately thickens liquids to slow the pace at which they pass through the UES. The resultant and subtle delay during the pharyngeal phase of swallowing allows time for laryngeal closure and the LAR to protect the airway. In essence, the thicker the consistency, the more time (in milliseconds) available for the afferent-efferent reflex loop to complete laryngeal closure.[89]

The diet is therapeutically thickened to a consistency based on the findings on VFSS or FEES. Because these results are only a brief picture of a child's swallowing efficiency, they must be interpreted in the context of clinical data. A patient's clinical response and symptoms with a particular consistency take precedence in determining the appropriate degree of thickening. It is also important that the multidisciplinary members, including otolaryngologist, pulmonologist, gastroenterologist, dietician, and SLP, confer on the modified feeding regimen. Each discipline perceives the relative safety of the diet from a unique perspective.

In the absence of a multidisciplinary team, the general rule for a safe thickened diet is one level higher than the consistency deeply penetrating the larynx or aspirated. As long as this is tolerated, patients can be maintained on this consistency until symptoms resolve, they are asymptomatic during a clinical feeding evaluation, or an instrumental evaluation demonstrates safety (no aspiration) at lower levels of thickener. A weaning process from the thickener is then used (discussed later).

By increasing the viscosity of a child's liquid alimentation, the slower flowing fluid provides more time for oral and pharyngeal control of the bolus.[89] Various consistency levels are referred to when discussing swallowing dysfunction. Unthickened formulas, liquids, and breast milk are considered thin liquids. Nectar and honey refer to the degree of consistency obtained with specific recipes using thickening agents. These 2 consistencies can be further divided into thin or stiff (ie, thin nectar and stiff honey), demarcating a one-half step change in the degree of thickener. Dysphagia severity is often determined based on the results of a formal VFSS or FEES and the recommended feeding regimen. Penetration of thin liquids may be classified as mild pharyngeal dysphagia whereas transglottic aspiration of liquids may translate to moderate or severe dysphagia. This depends on the circumstances of the aspiration and a child's overall swallowing function.

Various commercial, artificial thickening agents exist for thickening liquids, like SimplyThick (SimplyThick, St Louis, MO, USA) and Thick-It (Kent Precision Foods Group, St Louis, MO, USA). Caution should be exercised when recommending use of thickening agents, especially in children with a history of prematurity, because thickening products may cause adverse gastrointestinal issues or exacerbate feeding difficulties. Infants and children need to be monitored for constipation or diarrhea secondary to thickener use. If present, consultation with gastroenterology is warranted.

Other patients may have prolonged feeding times and, in turn, poor oral intake, if feeding fatigue or incomplete intake results when a thickener is introduced.[90,91] Nutritional experts and speech therapy should assist when these issues arise. Currently, SimplyThick, whose product contains xanthan gum, does not recommend use of SimplyThick thickener in term or preterm infants 12 months and under. This warning extends to children under the age of 12 years with a history of necrotizing enterocolitis (http://www.simplythick.com/). Only gum-based thickening agents have been shown to successfully thicken expressed breast milk (EBM) and for the EBM to maintain this thicker consistency. EBM cannot maintain a thicker consistency when rice cereal or corn starch-based thickening agents are used, because inherent enzymes (amylase) denude rice and cornstarch.[92,93] EBM is, however, relatively safe to the pediatric pulmonary tree. Thus, an infant drinking EBM may continue in the presence of OPD when strict compensatory feeding strategies to reduce aspiration risk are also implemented.

OPD Follow-Up

The first follow-up visit for OPD, after compensatory feeding strategies with or without therapeutic thickener have been used, should be after 4 to 6 weeks. New feeding concerns, reflux control, pulmonary status, and gastrointestinal complaints secondary to a thickener agent, uncontrolled OPD or airway symptoms, and compliance should be addressed. An instrumental evaluation may be scheduled at this time if not previously performed. For stable infants with mild OPD (laryngeal penetration on nectar consistency), a 3 to 4 months' follow-up is often adequate. Once a safe and tolerable feeding regimen is implemented and confirmed, then periodic visits from 3 to 6 months should be sufficient, especially in those requiring higher levels of consistency. Children who are initiated on a thickened diet honey-thick or of greater thickness, frequently take months to years to improve. Periodic monitoring for weight gain, lower respiratory tract infections, developmental milestones, or worsening symptoms is also important.

Fortunately, in the majority of infants and children who are neurologically normal, OPD is associated with prematurity or LPR/GERD. These patients tend to improve or resolve their OPD by 2 to 3 years of age if no other new contributors arise.[94] Most patients improve with observation as neuromuscular maturity occurs and reflux subsides with increasing age. Severe dysphagia (requiring stiff honey), worsening symptoms, or failed improvement should prompt further investigation and testing of inflammatory, anatomic, and subtle neurologic contributors. In the setting of gradually worsening symptoms and poor achievement of physical milestones, including a newly weak or hoarse cry or gait instability, a neurology consult and MR imaging of the head is recommended to rule out CNS or dynamic neuromuscular causes.

Follow-up visits should include a thorough clinical history and examination and possible beside speech evaluation. Repeat flexible nasolaryngoscopy may be required in an older child with persistent OPD in which a FEES examination can also be conducted. It is the author's experience that once children are diagnosed and treated for OPD, they are more sensitive to the multiple anatomic and inflammatory factors that may contribute to the condition. For example, a reflux-associated OPD infant who persists into childhood may not resolve until intervention for cow's milk protein allergy, low-riding tonsillar hypertrophy, a shallow laryngeal cleft, or subtle cricopharyngeal achalasia.

A revised algorithm for management of this type of patient is provided in **Fig. 4**. In essence, potentially subtle sources of OPD need to be explored.[50] These include the use of a head MR imaging scan to rule out CM-I (or other CNS causes) and MLB with esophagoscopy for laryngeal sources (late-onset/persistent laryngomalacia and type 1 laryngeal clefts) and inflammatory contributors (EoE and GERD) to OPD. These

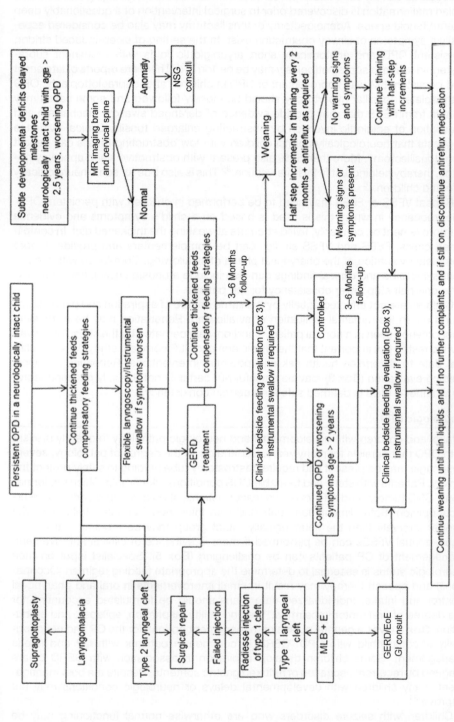

Fig. 4. Management algorithm for persistent OPD in neurologically normal child. Weaning priniciples. GI, gastroenterologist; MLB+E, MLB with or without esophagoscopy.

procedures can be used under the same anesthetic as the MR imaging first so that a Chiari malformation is discovered prior to surgical intervention of a questionably deep interarytenoid space. Adenoidectomy or tonsillectomy may also be considered especially if symptoms of airway obstruction exist. In the setting of sleep-induced stridor, persistent OPD and anatomically short aryepiglottic folds with prominent supra-arytenoid tissue, a supraglottoplasty may be performed. There are reports of late onset and persistent LM with improvement of OPD in children after supraglottoplasty. OPD with isolated tonsillar hypertrophy should be closely followed and some cases may benefit from FEES that may provide evidence of deranged swallow mechanism and prevention of epiglottic inversion by obstructing enlarged tonsils. Clinical evidence suggests that neurologically normal children with low obstructing tonsils can benefit from tonsillectomy. More than 50% also present with obstructive sleep apnea symptoms, thereby helping justify this intervention.[95] This is also true for some neurologically affected children.[18]

Repeat VFSS or FEES may need to be performed in children with persistent OPD. The frequency in which this is used is based on a child's symptoms and evidence of improvement or, contrarily, failed attempts at weaning the thickened diet. In complicated cases, FEES and VFSS studies can be complementary and provide a more complete evaluation of the pharyngeal phase of swallowing. Correlation with the patient symptoms and clinical findings can also include a bedside evaluation with thins (or a one-half step lower consistency for the patient).

Children are not affected equally by the same degree of aspiration and penetration[7] found on an instrumental evaluation of swallowing. Penetration may be a transient phenomenon seen in a normal patient[96] and only exacerbated by the stress of a swallowing test.[50] It is important that the physicians and SLP correlate study data and clinical data to determine health risk and potential interventions. Repeating a clinical feeding evaluation (**Box 3**) may be a useful but certainly not the only deciding factor on whether a child is deemed safe for a certain consistency.

Neurologic OPD

Infants and children with developmental and neurologic pathology frequently present with OPD that persists for many years. Depending on the degree of pathology, severe dysphagia may be present and require gastrostomy tube feeding to safely protect the airway. Patients with static and treatable CNS conditions, like Arnold-Chiari malformations, CNS tumors, and arteriovenous malformations, should undergo early neurosurgical opinion. Safe alimentation controlled with thickened feeds and follow-up with shorter intervals than the neurologically intact group may be required. As a child ages, annual VFSSs can be performed if there is evidence of clinical improvement. Management of CP patients can be challenging (**Box 5**). Specialist input on their neurologic status is essential to determine the appropriate feeding regimen. Occupational and speech therapy may result in small improvements in oral and pharyngeal control and intake. Individualized care plans should be formulated accounting for the degree of oral motor impairment, feeding ability, aspiration, epilepsy, and ambulation. **Box 5** gives a general outline of management options for the CP and neurologically affected child with OPD. GERD is common in patients with CP and needs management. Some children develop aspiration in association with GERD or are plagued by recurrent aspiration of refluxed gastric contents. Despite the best management many children with developmental delays or neurologic conditions may not improve.[37]

Children with seizure disorders who are otherwise normal functioning may be affected by OPD. Subtle disturbances in neuromuscular control and consciousness

---

Box 5

Assessment and management of oropharyngeal dysphagia in patients with neurologic pathology

History

Oral hygiene; occlusion; and assess drooling, gag reflex, ensure seizure control; rule out side effects of antiepileptic drugs

Volitional control of oral phase: sucking as neonate, oral-feeding habits

Developmental milestones, speech

History regarding aspiration: choking, postprandial tachypnea, wet voice, wet breathing

Examination

Rule out airway obstruction, dental examination

Oral sensorimotor examination (tongue lateralization, sensation, tone, strength, pathologic reactions)

Oropharyngeal stage of swallowing during eating and drinking (swallow on demand, oral control, frequency/efficiency/safety), 3-oz water challenge, VFSS

Speech (dysarthria/dyspraxia) and communication skills

Chest: assess for aspiration CXR—pulmonary consult

Assess: dental opinion/neurology opinion/physiotherapy/occupational therapy

Management

Thickener: as appropriate

GER: antireflux medication

Drooling: consider drooling treatment glycopyrrolate oral suspension (40–100 µg/kg/d with a maximum of 175 µg/kg/d), dosage given once daily

If no response, consider intense behavior therapy/surgical management: consider gastrostomy tube if failure to thrive, poor feeding with weight loss, recurrent pneumonias despite thickener, lack of progress and development

Speech pathologist

   Objective: modify food bolus, such as consistency, size, and texture; positioning of the patient; examining compensatory swallow maneuvers; posture and head control; mouth closure; lip seal; oral sensorimotor therapy for drooling

---

can affect normal swallowing by disrupting central midbrain processes. Some antiepileptics and neuroleptic drugs can contribute to neural blunting and subsequent OPD.

After excision of CNS neoplasms, patients may show improvement in dysphagia. Arnold-Chiari type 1–associated OPD usually resolves completely after posterior fossa decompression.[36] Those with progressive neurologic disorders, like mucopolysacharidoses and muscular dystrophy, show normal development initially but deteriorate rapidly and may need support for feeding and ventilation in later stages. Patients with CP show variable progress with some showing no improvement and others showing improving skills.

Clinical Course

Dysphagia in a neurologically normal child associated with prematurity and LPR tends to improve with time. This improvement is gradual with advanced neuromuscular coordination with age. These children can be managed expectantly with the diet that is deemed safe. Parents should be made aware of the need for watchfulness, however, regarding worsening symptoms.

Sheikh and colleagues[6] reported on a group of neurologically intact infants born at term without GER who had chronic aspiration due to dysphagia that resolved within 3 to 9 months. Research suggests that the average time to return to normal diet in the developmentally normal child with OPD is 3.2 years. In patients with an obvious laryngeal anomaly, the associated symptoms improve more quickly, but dysphagia improves slowly and gradually. Richter and colleagues[97] have noted a median interval of 3.8 months between supraglottoplasty for laryngomalacia and improvement of aspiration in infants. Durvasula and colleagues[22] reported 93.4% improvement of dysphagia at 6 months after supraglottoplasty in a cohort of 136 patients with laryngomalacia with no associated comorbidities. Preterm infants with gestation age less than 32 weeks at birth and laryngomalacia, however, had significantly high rates with 50% of patients still showing evidence of dysphagia 6 months after supraglottoplasty. The investigators thus concluded that prematurity has an independent role to play in dysphagia.

Similarly, Bakthavachalam and colleagues[98] reported in a case series of type 1 laryngeal clefts that the average time to resolution of aspiration was 7.8 months for the group managed surgically and 13.6 months for the nonsurgical group. They also reported that the average age of resolution of aspiration in patients with laryngeal cleft diagnosed before 2 years was significantly better than those who were diagnosed after 2 years. Repair of type 1 and type 2 clefts should be reserved for patients with persistent aspiration that is not improving with age, infants with cleft and recurrent pneumonia, those with worsening pulmonary status, and those with other severe comorbidities contributing to dysphagia. Endoscopic surgical repair is usually curative, but recently, augmentation of the cleft by injection of Radiesse (Merz Aesthetics, Franksville, WI, USA) in the interarytenoid notch has been reported with complete resolution of symptoms in 56%[99] and 72%.[100] Although concerns regarding long-term results of interarytenoid injection exist, it is prudent to try injection as a first step and reserving endoscopic repair for failures and relapses.

Weaning and Precautions

Signs and symptoms are the best predictors of successful weaning and return to normal swallowing. Dietary weaning is proposed when the signs and symptoms have improved for at least 6 months or when evident on VFSS or FEES. For example, improvement is declared in a patient who was aspirating honey but now only aspirates nectar. Despite VFSS evidence of improvement, weaning the thickener is recommended in a gradual manner with thinning trials of half-step increments in consistency. A patient on honey may be weaned to stiff nectar and observed for at least 2 to 3 months before proceeding to nectar consistency. Such a gradual approach is usually more successful and less stressful for the parent. The parents should be warned, however, that the original consistency should be on standby in case any signs and symptoms should recur or OPD should worsen. A comfortably feeding child is a good sign, but watering eyes, tachypnea, and wet respiration suggest poor swallow and silent aspiration. Bronchopulmonary events, like worsening asthma, increased need for respiratory medications, and lower respiratory tract infections, indicate aspiration. Parents should also be warned about transient worsening of swallowing, especially when there is an upper respiratory tract infection or fever that may improve once the acute condition has subsided. At this stage, the patient may be followed up once in 4 to 6 months. Medication for GERD should continue until the patient is on near-normal consistency.

Repeat VFSS is often performed in OPD cases once in 10 to 12 months. A repeat VFSS is not necessary, however, in cases showing clinical improvement and/or a VFSS showing no deep penetration or aspiration, unless symptoms worsen. In an infant, a repeat VFSS may be performed sooner due to the relatively quicker dynamic growth and functional improvement of the infant (ie, 6 months). Patients treated for laryngeal anomalies should have a repeat VFSS at 4 months after surgery to confirm their OPD status before weaning. Aspiration of thin fluids has shown increased risk of pneumonia, although similar risk was not noted on aspiration with puree consistency.[75,101] More caution should be in place, however, while introducing thinner consistencies.

There is variation in approach among physicians regarding interpretation of deep penetration on VFSS. Although some practitioners manage deep penetration as normal, others tend to be more careful and may continue a thickened diet. Friedman and Frazier in 2000[73] studied a group of 125 patients with dysphagia and reported that 85% of children with deep laryngeal penetration aspirated and suggested a strong correlation between the two. Emphasis on clinical history in such cases is important. Deep penetration in patients with recurrent pneumonias or neurologically impaired children should be considered higher risk and be treated like aspiration. A modified approach to radiation exposure has been used by the authors' team: the use of VFSSs is curtailed in infants and children who do not aspirate on prior studies and monitoring clinical symptoms during weaning proceeds.

SUMMARY

The incidence of OPD is on the rise due to increased awareness in neurologically normal children and increasing life expectancy of infants with prematurity and complex medical issues. Although a 3-oz water challenge test is a good clinical test for diagnosing OPD, VFSSs and FEES remain gold standard tests for diagnosing aspiration. Management is best accomplished by a multidisciplinary team with experience and training in pediatric OPD. Identification of subtle pathologies that can contribute to persistent OPD and appropriate medical and/or surgical management may expedite improvement in some patients. Most patients require modification of diet and medical management of GER. Repeat clinic assessment and slow weaning strategies are required, because neuromuscular control of the pharyngeal phase of swallowing requires time to improve.

REFERENCES

1. Miller CK, Willging JP. Advances in the evaluation and management of pediatric dysphagia. Curr Opin Otolaryngol Head Neck Surg 2003;11(6):442-6.
2. Lefton-Greif MA, Arvedson JC. Schoolchildren with dysphagia associated with medically complex conditions. Lang Speech Hear Serv Sch 2008;39(2):237-48.
3. Martin JA, Hamilton BE, Ventura SJ, et al. Births: final data for 2009. Natl Vital Stat Rep 2011;60(1):1-70.
4. Rommel N, De Meyer AM, Feenstra L, et al. The complexity of feeding problems in 700 infants and young children presenting to a tertiary care institution. J Pediatr Gastroenterol Nutr 2003;37(1):75-84.
5. Seddon PC, Khan Y. Respiratory problems in children with neurological impairment. Arch Dis Child 2003;88(1):75-8.
6. Sheikh S, Allen E, Shell R, et al. Chronic aspiration without gastroesophageal reflux as a cause of chronic respiratory symptoms in neurologically normal infants. Chest 2001;120(4):1190-5.

7. Hewetson R, Singh S. The lived experience of mothers of children with chronic feeding and/or swallowing difficulties. Dysphagia 2009;24(3):322–32.
8. Sleigh G. Mothers' voice: a qualitative study on feeding children with cerebral palsy. Child Care Health Dev 2005;31(4):373–83.
9. Jadcherla SR, Gupta A, Wang M, et al. Definition and implications of novel pharyngo-glottal reflex in human infants using concurrent manometry ultrasonography. Am J Gastroenterol 2009;104(10):2572–82.
10. Pereira NA, Motta AR, Vicente LC. Swallowing reflex: analysis of the efficiency of different stimuli on healthy young individuals. Pro Fono 2008;20(3):159–64.
11. Ulualp S, Brown A, Sanghavi R, et al. Assessment of laryngopharyngeal sensation in children with dysphagia. Laryngoscope 2013;123(9):2291–5.
12. Rempel G, Moussavi Z. The effect of viscosity on the breath-swallow pattern of young people with cerebral palsy. Dysphagia 2005;20(2):108–12.
13. Timms BJ, DiFiore JM, Martin RJ, et al. Increased respiratory drive as an inhibitor of oral feeding of preterm infants. J Pediatr 1993;123(1):127–31.
14. Kramer SS. Special swallowing problems in children. Gastrointest Radiol 1985; 10(3):241–50.
15. Harding R. Perinatal development of laryngeal function. J Dev Physiol 1984;6(3): 249–58.
16. Harding R. Function of the larynx in the fetus and newborn. Annu Rev Physiol 1984;46:645–59.
17. Lau C, Smith EO, Schanler RJ. Coordination of suck-swallow and swallow respiration in preterm infants. Acta Paediatr 2003;92(6):721–7.
18. Conley SF, Beecher RB, Delaney AL, et al. Outcomes of tonsillectomy in neurologically impaired children. Laryngoscope 2009;119(11):2231–41.
19. Sheppard JJ, Mysak ED. Ontogeny of infantile oral reflexes and emerging chewing. Child Dev 1984;55(3):831–43.
20. Stolovitz P, Gisel EG. Circumoral movements in response to three different food textures in children 6 months to 2 years of age. Dysphagia 1991;6(1):17–25.
21. Byars KC, Burklow KA, Ferguson K, et al. A multicomponent behavioral program for oral aversion in children dependent on gastrostomy feedings. J Pediatr Gastroenterol Nutr 2003;37(4):473–80.
22. Durvasula VS, Lawson BR, Bower CM, et al. Supraglottoplasty in premature infants with laryngomalacia: does gestation age at birth influence outcomes? Otolaryngol Head Neck Surg 2014;150(2):292–9.
23. Rommel N, van Wijk M, Boets B, et al. Development of pharyngo-esophageal physiology during swallowing in the preterm infant. Neurogastroenterol Motil 2011;23(10):e401–8.
24. Uhm KE, Yi SH, Chang HJ, et al. Videofluoroscopic swallowing study findings in full-term and preterm infants with Dysphagia. Ann Rehabil Med 2013;37(2): 175–82.
25. Derkay CS, Schechter GL. Anatomy and physiology of pediatric swallowing disorders. Otolaryngol Clin North Am 1998;31(3):397–404.
26. Medoff-Cooper B, McGrath JM, Bilker W. Nutritive sucking and neurobehavioral development in preterm infants from 34 weeks PCA to term. MCN Am J Matern Child Nurs 2000;25:64–70.
27. Hack M, Estabrook MM, Robertson SS. Development of sucking rhythm in preterm infants. Early Hum Dev 1985;11:133–40.
28. Medoff-Cooper B, McGrath JM, Shults J. Feeding patterns of full-term and preterm infants at forty weeks postconceptional age. J Dev Behav Pediatr 2002;23:231–6.

29. Ancel PY, Livinec F, Larroque B, et al. Cerebral palsy among very preterm children in relation to gestational age and neonatal ultrasound abnormalities: the EPIPAGE cohort study. Pediatrics 2006;117(3):828–35.
30. Rotschild A, Dison PJ, Chitayat D, et al. Mid-facial hypoplasia associated with long-term intubation for bronchopulmonary dysplasia. Am J Dis Child 1990; 144:1302–6.
31. Rogers B, Arvedson J, Buck G, et al. Characteristics of dysphagia in children with cerebral palsy. Dysphagia 1994;9(1):69–73.
32. Spiroglou K, Xinias I, Karatzas N, et al. Gastric emptying in children with cerebral palsy and gastroesophageal reflux. Pediatr Neurol 2004;31(3):177–82.
33. Tahmassebi JF, Curzon ME. Prevalence of drooling in children with cerebral palsy attending special schools. Dev Med Child Neurol 2003;45(9):613–7.
34. Tahmassebi JF, Curzon ME. The cause of drooling in children with cerebral palsy - hypersalivation or swallowing defect? Dev Med Child Neurol 1993; 35(4):285–97.
35. Greenlee JD, Donovan KA, Hasan DM, et al. Chiari I malformation in the very young child: the spectrum of presentations and experience in 31 children under age 6 years. Pediatrics 2002;110(6):1212–9.
36. Albert GW, Menezes AH, Hansen DR, et al. Chiari malformation Type I in children younger than age 6 years: presentation and surgical outcome. J Neurosurg Pediatr 2010;5(6):554–61.
37. O'Neill AC, Richter GT. Pharyngeal dysphagia in children with Down syndrome. Otolaryngol Head Neck Surg 2013;149(1):146–50.
38. Smith ME, Mortelliti AJ, Cotton RT, et al. Phonation and swallowing considerations in pediatric laryngotracheal reconstruction. Ann Otol Rhinol Laryngol 1992;101(9):731–8.
39. Thompson DM. Abnormal sensorimotor integrative function of the larynx in congenital laryngomalacia: a new theory of etiology. Laryngoscope 2007; 117(6 Pt 2 Suppl 114):1–33.
40. Link DT, Willging JP, Miller CK, et al. Pediatric laryngopharyngeal sensory testing during flexible endoscopic evaluation of swallowing: feasible and correlative. Head Neck Surg 2013;149(1):146–50.
41. Munson PD, Saad AG, El-Jamal SM, et al. Submucosal nerve hypertrophy in congenital laryngomalacia. Laryngoscope 2011;121:627–9.
42. Goyal RK, Martin SB, Shapiro J, et al. The role of cricopharyngeus muscle in pharyngoesophageal disorders. Dysphagia 1993;8(3):252–8.
43. Elidan J, Shochina M, Gonen B, et al. Electromyography of the inferior constrictor and cricopharyngeal muscles during swallowing. Ann Otol Rhinol Laryngol 1990;99(6 Pt 1):466–9.
44. Chun R, Sitton M, Tipnis NA, et al. Endoscopic cricopharyngeal myotomy for management of cricopharyngeal achalasia (CA) in an 18-month-old child. Laryngoscope 2013;123(3):797–800.
45. Dinari G, Danziger Y, Mimouni M, et al. Cricopharyngeal dysfunction in childhood: treatment by dilatations. J Pediatr Gastroenterol Nutr 1987;6(2): 212–6.
46. Dent J, El-Serag HB, Wallander MA, et al. Epidemiology of gastro-oesophageal reflux disease: a systematic review. Gut 2005;54(5):710–7.
47. Martin AJ, Pratt N, Kennedy JD, et al. Natural history and familial relationships of infant spilling to 9 years of age. Pediatrics 2002;109(6):1061–7.
48. Hassall E. Endoscopy in children with GERD: "the way we were" and the way we should be. Am J Gastroenterol 2002;97(7):1583–6.

49. Aviv JE, Liu H, Parides M, et al. Laryngopharyngeal sensory deficits in patients with laryngopharyngeal reflux and dysphagia. Ann Otol Rhinol Laryngol 2000; 109(11):1000–6.

50. Richter GT. Management of oropharyngeal dysphagia in the neurologically intact and developmentally normal child. Curr Opin Otolaryngol Head Neck Surg 2010;18(6):554–63.

51. Liacouras CA, Furuta GT, Hirano I, et al. Eosinophilic esophagitis: updated consensus recommendations for children and adults. J Allergy Clin Immunol 2011;128(1):3–20.

52. Dellon ES, Gonsalves N, Hirano I, et al, American College of Gastroenterology. ACG clinical guideline: evidenced based approach to the diagnosis and management of esophageal eosinophilia and eosinophilic esophagitis (EoE). Am J Gastroenterol 2013;108(5):679–92.

53. Dauer EH, Freese DK, El-Youssef M, et al. Clinical characteristics of eosinophilic esophagitis in children. Ann Otol Rhinol Laryngol 2005;114(11):827–33.

54. Dauer EH, Ponikau JU, Smyrk TC, et al. Airway manifestations of pediatric eosinophilic esophagitis: a clinical and histopathologic report of an emerging association. Ann Otol Rhinol Laryngol 2006;115(7):507–17.

55. Garcia-Careaga M Jr, Kerner JA Jr. Gastrointestinal manifestations of food allergies in pediatric patients. Nutr Clin Pract 2005;20(5):526–35.

56. Markowitz JE, Spergel JM, Ruchelli E, et al. Elemental diet is an effective treatment for eosinophilic esophagitis in children and adolescents. Am J Gastroenterol 2003;98(4):777–82.

57. Kagalwalla AF, Sentongo TA, Ritz S, et al. Effect of six-food elimination diet on clinical and histologic outcomes in eosinophilic esophagitis. Clin Gastroenterol Hepatol 2006;4(9):1097–102.

58. Furuta GT, Liacouras CA, Collins MH, et al, First International Gastrointestinal Eosinophil Research Symposium (FIGERS) Subcommittees. Eosinophilic esophagitis in children and adults: a systematic review and consensus recommendations for diagnosis and treatment. Gastroenterology 2007;133(4):1342–63.

59. Warms T, Richards J. "Wet Voice" as a predictor of penetration and aspiration in oropharyngeal dysphagia. Dysphagia 2000;15(2):84–8.

60. De Pippo KL, Holas MA, Reding MJ. Validation of the 3-ounce water swallow test for aspiration. Arch Neurol 1992;49(12):1259–61.

61. Suiter DM, Leder SB, Karas DB. The 3-ounce (90-cc) water swallow challenge: a screening test for children with suspected oropharyngeal dysphagia. Otolaryngol Head Neck Surg 2009;140(2):187–90.

62. Boesch RP, Daines C, Wilging JP, et al. Advances in the diagnosis and management of chronic pulmonary aspiration in children. Eur Respir J 2006;28(4):847–61.

63. de Benedictis FM, Carnielli VP, de Benedictis D. Aspiration lung disease. Pediatr Clin North Am 2009;56(1):173–90.

64. Steinbok P. Clinical features of Chiari I malformations. Childs Nerv Syst 2004; 20(5):329–31.

65. Colombo JL, Hallberg TK. Recurrent aspiration in children: lipid-laden alveolar macrophage quantitation. Pediatr Pulmonol 1987;3(2):86–9.

66. Furuya ME, Moreno-Cordova V, Ramirez-Figueroa JL, et al. Cutoff value of lipid-laden alveolar macrophages for diagnosing aspiration in infants and children. Pediatr Pulmonol 2007;42(5):452–7.

67. Kieran SM, Katz E, Rosen R, et al. The lipid laden macrophage index as a marker of aspiration in patients with type I and II laryngeal clefts. Int J Pediatr Otorhinolaryngol 2010;74(7):743–6.

68. Knauer-Fischer S, Ratjen F. Lipid-laden macrophages in bronchoalveolar lavage fluid as a marker for pulmonary aspiration. Pediatr Pulmonol 1999; 27(6):419–22.
69. Stoeckli SJ, Huisman TA, Seifert B, et al. Interrater reliability of videofluoroscopic swallow evaluation. Dysphagia 2003;18(1):53–7.
70. Logemann JA. The role of the speech language pathologist in the management of dysphagia. Otolaryngol Clin North Am 1988;21(4):783–8.
71. Arvedson JC. Assessment of pediatric dysphagia and feeding disorders: clinical and instrumental approaches. Dev Disabil Res Rev 2008;14(2):118–27.
72. Miller CK, Willging JP. The implications of upper airway obstruction on successful infant feeding. Semin Speech Lang 2007;28(3):190–203.
73. Friedman B, Frazier JB. Deep laryngeal penetration as a predictor of aspiration. Dysphagia 2000;15:153–8.
74. Newman LA, Keckley C, Petersen MC, et al. Swallowing function and medical diagnoses in infants suspected of dysphagia. Pediatrics 2001;108:E106.
75. Weir KA, McMahon S, Taylor S, et al. Oropharyngeal aspiration and silent aspiration in children. Chest 2011;140:589–97.
76. Langmore SE, Schatz K, Olsen N. Fiberoptic endoscopic examination of swallowing safety: a new procedure. Dysphagia 1988;2:216–9.
77. Willging JP. Endoscopic evaluation of swallowing in children. Int J Pediatr Otorhinolaryngol 1995;32(Suppl):S107–8.
78. Hartnick C, Hartley BE, Miller C, et al. Pediatric fiberoptic endoscopic evaluation of swallowing. Ann Otol Rhinol Laryngol 2000;109:996–9.
79. Leder SB, Karas DE. Fiberoptic endoscopic evaluation of swallowing in the pediatric population. Laryngoscope 2000;110:1132–6.
80. American Speech-Language-Hearing Association. Role of the speech-language pathologist in the performance and interpretation of endoscopic evaluation of swallowing. ASHA Position Statement. 2005. http://dx.doi.org/10.1044/policy. PS2005-00112. Available at: www.ASHA.org.
81. Miller CK, Willging JP, Strife JL, et al. Fiberoptic endoscopic examination of swallowing in infants and children with feeding disorders. Dysphagia 1994;9:266.
82. Lefton-Greif MA, Carroll JL, Loughlin GM. Long-term follow-up of oropharyngeal dysphagia in children without apparent risk factors. Pediatr Pulmonol 2006; 41(11):1040–8.
83. Giambra BK, Meinzen-Derr J. Exploration of the relationships among medical health history variables and aspiration. Int J Pediatr Otorhinolaryngol 2010; 74(4):387–92.
84. Rudolph CD, Mazur LJ, Liptak GS, et al, North American Society for Pediatric Gastroenterology and Nutrition. Guidelines for evaluation and treatment of gastroesophageal reflux in infants and children: recommendations of the North American Society for Pediatric Gastroenterology and Nutrition. J Pediatr Gastroenterol Nutr 2001;32(Suppl 2):S1–31.
85. Litalien C, Theoret Y, Faure C. Pharmacokinetics of proton pump inhibitors in children. Clin Pharmacokinet 2005;44(5):441–66.
86. Gibbons TE, Gold BD. The use of proton pump inhibitors in children: a comprehensive review. Paediatr Drugs 2003;5(1):25–40.
87. van der Pol RJ, Smits MJ, van Wijk MP, et al. Efficacy of proton-pump inhibitors in children with gastroesophageal reflux disease: a systematic review. Pediatrics 2011;127(5):925–35.
88. Orenstein SR, Hassall E, Furmaga-Jablonska W, et al. Multicenter, double-blind, randomized, placebo-controlled trial assessing the efficacy and safety of proton

pump inhibitor lansoprazole in infants with symptoms of gastroesophageal reflux disease. J Pediatr 2009;154(4):514–20.e4.

89. Miller CK. Aspiration and swallowing dysfunction in pediatric patients. Infant Child Adolesc Nutr 2011;3:336–43.

90. Gosa MS, Schooling T, Coleman J. Thickened liquids as a treatment for children with dysphagia and associated adverse effects: a systematic review. Infant Child Adolesc Nutr 2011;3:344–50.

91. McCallum S. Addressing nutrient density in the context of the use of thickened liquids in dysphagia treatment. Infant Child Adolesc Nutr 2011;3:351–60.

92. Cichero JA, Nicholson TM, September C. Thickened milk for the management of feeding and swallowing issues in infants: a call for interdisciplinary professional guidelines. J Hum Lact 2013;29(2):132–5.

93. Almeida MB, Almeida JA, Moreira ME, et al. Adequacy of human milk viscosity to respond to infants with dysphagia: experimental study. J Appl Oral Sci 2011; 19(6):554–9.

94. Montero M, Bower CM, Richter GT. Oropharyngeal dysphagia in neurologically normal children. Chicago: American Society of Pediatric Otolaryngology; 2011.

95. Friedman AB, O'Neill AC, Bower CM, et al. Impact of tonsillectomy on aspiration in neurologically normal children. Presented at Society of Ear Nose and Throat Advancement in Children Meeting. Kansas City, December 4–5, 2011.

96. Allen JE, White CJ, Leonard RJ, et al. Prevalence of penetration and aspiration on videofluoroscopy in normal individuals without dysphagia. Otolaryngol Head Neck Surg 2010;142(2):208–13.

97. Richter GT, Wootten CT, Rutter MJ, et al. Impact of supraglottoplasty on aspiration in severe laryngomalacia. Ann Otol Rhinol Laryngol 2009;118:259–66.

98. Bakthavachalam S, Schroeder JW Jr, Holinger LD. Diagnosis and management of type I posterior laryngeal clefts. Ann Otol Rhinol Laryngol 2010;119(4): 239–48.

99. Cohen MS, Zhuang L, Simons JP, et al. Injection laryngoplasty for type 1 laryngeal cleft in children. Otolaryngol Head Neck Surg 2011;144(5):789–93.

100. Mangat HS, El-Hakim H. Injection augmentation of type I laryngeal clefts. Otolaryngol Head Neck Surg 2012;146(5):764–8.

101. Weir K, McMahon S, Barry L, et al. Oropharyngeal aspiration and pneumonia in children. Pediatr Pulmonol 2007;42(11):1024–31.

Dysphagia in the Elderly

Abraham Khan, MD[a], Richard Carmona, BA[b],
Morris Traube, MD, JD[a],*

KEYWORDS

- Dysphagia • Oropharyngeal • Esophageal • Swallowing • Motility

KEY POINTS

- Dysphagia, or difficulty swallowing, is a common problem in the elderly and can cause malnutrition and significant morbidity.
- Key findings on clinical history and physical examination can suggest whether the patient has either predominantly oropharyngeal or esophageal dysphagia and guide the appropriate workup and treatment of these patients.
- The most common causes of oropharyngeal dysphagia are of neurologic origin and can be managed in conjunction with a clinical swallow specialist.
- Esophageal dysphagia may result from structural or functional disorders, and a video barium esophagram is a good initial test in the workup of these patients. Often a gastroenterologist will be consulted for evaluation, endoscopy, or manometry, followed by appropriate treatment.

INTRODUCTION

Dysphagia, or difficulty swallowing, is a common problem in the elderly. For example, nearly 50% of all patients residing in nursing homes suffer from a swallowing disorder.[1] One study found that 63% of elderly patients who denied any history of swallowing difficulties had abnormal swallowing parameters on radiologic swallow studies.[2]

The problem will certainly become more widespread. From 2010 to 2030, the elderly population is expected to increase from 39 million to 69 million Americans.[3] In 2050, elderly Americans, defined as those at least 65 years old, are expected to make up 20% of the total population, a substantial increase from 13% in 2010.[4] In addition to the discomfort that patients have from dysphagia, the complications associated with swallowing difficulty are substantial. Elderly patients with dysphagia have a significantly elevated risk of malnutrition and aspiration pneumonia. This risk is particularly

This article originally appeared in Clinics in Geriatric Medicine, Volume 30, Issue 1, February 2014.

[a] Division of Gastroenterology, Department of Medicine and Center for Esophageal Disease, NYU School of Medicine, 530 First Avenue, SKR 9N, New York, NY 10016, USA; [b] NYU School of Medicine, 550 First Avenue, New York, NY 10016, USA

* Corresponding author.

E-mail address: Morris.Traube@nyumc.org

true in the subpopulation with oropharyngeal dysphagia of neurologic origin, that is, cerebrovascular disease, brain injury, or neurodegenerative disease.

A study using the Subjective Global Assessment (SGA) to assess nutritional status found that 16% of patients with dysphagia related to nonprogressive brain disorders had concomitant malnutrition, whereas malnutrition was noted in 22% of patients whose dysphagia stemmed from neurodegenerative disease.[5] Elderly patients with malnutrition resulting from dysphagia show increased morbidity and mortality from several factors, including, but not limited to, a lowered immune response, decreased ability to recover from illness and heal wounds, and weakened respiratory drive/muscle strength.[6,7] Because of the likelihood of choking and aspirating with a swallowing disorder, which can aid in bacterial colonization, aspiration pneumonia is also common in patients with dysphagia. Up to 50% of patients with oropharyngeal dysphagia in nursing homes have aspiration pneumonia within 1 year, and the mortality rate approaches 45%.[5]

ANATOMY AND PHYSIOLOGY OF SWALLOWING

Before reviewing the specific swallowing disorders and the relevant approach to diagnosis, a basic understanding of the anatomy and physiology of swallowing is essential.[8] Typically, the process of swallowing is broken down into 3 primary phases: oral, pharyngeal, and esophageal. The oral phase, the only voluntary phase of swallowing, is often divided again into 2 subphases: the preparatory and transport phases.

During the oral preparatory phase, food enters into the oral cavity to be chewed and formed into an appropriate bolus for swallowing. This phase is dependent on voluntary action of chewing and swallowing the meal for nutrition. The coordinated manipulation and mastication of the food depends on several facial muscles and their cranial nerve signals, whereas chemoreceptors and mechanoreceptors are responsible for the stimulation of salivary glands. When the food has been adequately manipulated by means of mastication and salivary coating, the oral transport phase occurs. During this phase, the tongue moves the bolus posteriorly toward the oropharynx for swallowing.

During the pharyngeal phase, the velopharyngeal muscles mediate the closure of the nasopharynx to avoid nasal regurgitation. Preventing food from entering into the airway is one of the most important aspects of swallowing and requires the coordinated effort of the epiglottis, the vocal cords, and the larynx. The first step of this process is the closure of the true vocal cords, which is the most reliable protection against aspiration. This is followed by closure of the false vocal cords and superior displacement of the larynx. The superior and anterior placement of the larynx inverts the epiglottis so that it can further protect against aspiration. The other major function of the retroverted epiglottis is to route the bolus to the pyriform sinuses located on opposite sides of the pharynx. From the pyriform sinuses, the superior, middle, and inferior constrictor muscles contract respectively and are responsible for pharyngeal peristalsis. Mechanoreceptors are then continuously stimulated to promote the contraction of pharyngeal muscles until the bolus has completely passed into the esophagus. The pharyngeal phase of swallowing terminates when the bolus passes through the upper esophageal sphincter (UES), which is composed mostly of the cricopharyngeus muscle and fibers from the inferior pharyngeal constrictor.

After the bolus passes the UES, the esophageal phase of swallowing begins, and is entirely under involuntary control. The esophagus has 2 muscle layers, an inner circular muscle layer and an outer longitudinal muscle layer. Both central and peripheral neuromuscular control are necessary to pass the bolus from the striated muscle portion of the upper esophagus to the smooth muscle portion of the more distal esophagus and ultimately through the smooth muscle lower esophageal sphincter

(LES). The food bolus normally passes through the esophagus and into the stomach in 8 to 10 seconds. This coordinated series of contractions is referred to as *esophageal peristalsis*. Once the swallow is initiated, the LES relaxes. This relaxation is mediated by the vagus nerve and persists until the food bolus enters the stomach.[9]

PATHOPHYSIOLOGY OF DEGLUTITION IN THE ELDERLY

Two major types of dysphagia are used to describe abnormal swallowing. Patients can have oropharyngeal dysphagia, esophageal dysphagia, or a combination of both. Oropharyngeal dysphagia results from dysfunction in the swallowing process before food enters into the esophagus. Several changes in the elderly may predispose to dysphagia. Loss of jaw strength, salivary production, and dentition, as well as increased connective and fatty tissue in the tongue can affect the oral phase of swallowing.[10,11] However, typically, age-related changes to this phase of swallowing do not result in dysphagia. In the pharyngeal phase, the threshold needed for laryngeal elevation is increased and the elevation is less marked. After the age of 60, pharyngeal swallowing is significantly longer, sometimes requires multiple swallows per bolus, and can greatly increase the risk of aspiration.[12] The initiation of the esophageal phase can also be delayed in the elderly, resulting from a loss of UES elasticity or compliance.[11]

Along with these age-related changes, some neurologic disorders are much more common in the elderly and contribute to the increased prevalence of dysphagia. These disorders include transient ischemic attacks, strokes, and neurodegenerative diseases, such as Parkinson's disease. Other causes of dysphagia that are increased in the elderly include Zenker's diverticulum, achalasia, and esophageal tumors. These disorders are discussed below.

APPROACH TO DIAGNOSIS
History and Physical Examination

Taking a careful history and performing a physical examination is of extreme importance and is the first step in the diagnosis of dysphagia (**Box 1**). Three common related symptoms of dysphagia in the elderly include eating meals more slowly; choking, coughing, or throat-clearing either during or after meals; and feeling as if food is stuck

---

Box 1
Dysphagia: key associated findings

Historical Findings

- Choking, coughing, or throat clearing during or after meals
- Food stuck in throat or mid-chest
- Frequent pulmonary infections
- Weight loss, change in diet or consistency of food
- Neurologic changes

Physical Examination Findings

- Loss of dentition
- Abnormal lip closure or tongue range of motion
- Vocal changes
- Neurologic deficits

in the throat.[13] The patient should also be asked about any weight loss, general changes in diet or consistency of food, or neurologic changes. A history of smoking and alcohol abuse should raise concern of malignancy in both oropharyngeal and esophageal dysphagia.[1]

Certainly, dysphagia can be of acute onset as seen in a stroke; however, more often, dysphagia is of slow onset and only slowly progressive. Because of this insidious nature, patients often change the consistency of their food to avoid symptoms. Detail of the food consistencies that cause difficulty may also help discover the cause of dysphagia. Often, patients who struggle to swallow more with solid foods suffer from an obstruction, such as a stricture, ring, or web, whereas those who struggle with liquids are more likely to have dysphagia of neurologic origin. Furthermore, a history of frequent pulmonary infections may suggest that the patient is suffering from dysphagia and recurrent aspiration.

On physical examination, the oral cavity should be examined for loss of dentition, abnormal lip closure and strength of closure, and tongue range of motion. Voice quality should also be assessed, with careful attention paid to either dysarthria or a wet quality to the voice, which may indicate a laryngeal and neurologic condition, respectively. A neurologic examination should be performed to assess general evidence of neurologic dysfunction.

Testing and Referral

The relevant findings on history and physical examination will direct the appropriate testing or referrals for each patient with dysphagia (**Fig. 1**).

To determine the necessary steps in defining and treating each patient with dysphagia, it is important to decipher whether the complaints are consistent with supraesophageal symptoms. If the patient has signs of aspiration, especially with swallowing, or nasopharyngeal regurgitation, oropharyngeal dysphagia is suggested.

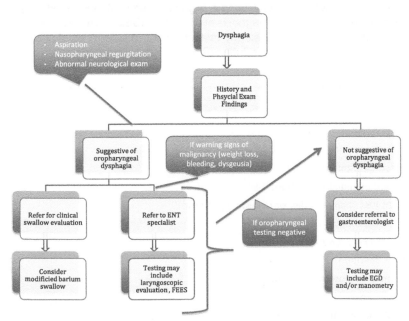

Fig. 1. Referrals and testing for dysphagia.

In this case, an appropriate initial test may be a clinical swallow evaluation, which typically is performed by a speech pathologist. During the examination, patients are given boluses of varying size and complexity.[14] Studies have found that such assessments can miss up to 50% of significant aspiration that is seen on videofluroroscopy.[15] Therefore, patients also generally undergo a modified barium swallow, which is a radiographic examination during which the patient is given foods of varying consistencies to assess dysphagia and aspiration.

Potential warning signs of malignancy, such as sudden weight loss, dysgeusia, or bleeding seen in a patient with oropharyngeal dysphagia, should lead to a referral to an ENT specialist. Besides a through head and neck evaluation, the ENT physician will also perform a laryngoscopic evaluation of the pharynx and larynx to look for tumors or other anatomic changes in the oropharynx, such as Zenker's diverticulum. Furthermore, the ENT physician may also perform a fiber optic endoscopic evaluation of swallowing (FEES), during which the patient is fed foods of varying consistencies, which are often colored for the purpose of visualization to assess swallowing function.[16] This evaluation is followed by endoscopic evaluation to check for food residue and entry of food particles into the larynx. If warning signs are present, computerized tomography may also be performed to rule out malignancy.

If the patient does not present with supraesophageal symptoms or if modified barium swallow/FEES study is negative, a barium video esophagram and gastroenterology referral should be considered. In some practices, a barium esophagram focuses primarily on the esophagus, although, in others, detailed attention is appropriately given to oropharyngeal swallowing. Appropriate esophageal radiography should include evaluation of not only the anatomy but also motility and function of the esophagus. In conjunction with fluoroscopic imaging, the patient swallows a barium suspension, which allows for visualization. It is often helpful to administer a solid bolus or barium tablet to assess for localized narrowing and temporal association of symptoms and holdup. Obstructions, such as esophageal strictures and tumors, can be seen, and even motility disorders such as achalasia can be suggested.[17] Because of its relatively low cost and simplicity, a barium esophagram is often recommended as the first-line test in a patient with likely esophageal dysphagia.[18]

As mentioned, referral to a gastroenterologist is appropriate if a patient has symptoms implying esophageal dysphagia. The specialist can perform an esophago-gastroduodenoscopy (EGD) or esophageal manometry, as indicated. An EGD is an endoscopic direct examination of the esophagus, stomach, and duodenum and can diagnose esophagitis, rings, webs, strictures, and tumors. If the patient's symptoms, such as long-term, chronic dysphagia, suggest esophageal dysmotility, esophageal manometry can be performed to help diagnose achalasia.[18] This procedure is performed by placing a thin catheter through the nose into the esophagus and assessing peristalsis in response to sips of water.

SPECIFIC DISORDERS

It is beyond the scope of this article to discuss every entity that causes dysphagia, but we discuss some of the most common disorders, especially those that disproportionately affect the elderly.

Oropharyngeal Dysphagia

Neuromuscular disorders

The most common causes of oropharyngeal dysphagia are of neurologic origin (Box 2).[19] Although an exact diagnosis can occasionally be made, this is not typically

---

Box 2
Disorders causing oropharyngeal dysphagia

Neuromuscular Causes

- Stroke
- Myasthenia gravis
- Parkinson's disease
- Amyotrophic lateral sclerosis (ALS)
- Multiple sclerosis (MS)
- Huntington's disease
- UES dysfunction
- Muscular dystrophy
- Other disorders of striated muscle

Structural Causes

- Head and neck tumors
- Zenker's diverticulum
- Cricopharyngeal bar/cricopharyngeal achalasia
- Osteophytes and other extrinsic causes

---

so. Furthermore, even if a neurologic disorder is diagnosed, often there is no specific treatment. However, certain disorders do lend themselves to a specific treatment; for example, anticholinesterase inhibitors are helpful in myasthenia gravis. Hence, if identified, it is important to treat the underlying neurologic disorder to improve dysphagia.[10]

Stroke is a common cause of dysphagia in the elderly. Importantly, each stroke patient should be clinically evaluated for signs of dysphagia and aspiration. Such swallowing dysfunction causes substantial morbidity and mortality, as it is estimated that approximately 50,000 stroke victims die each year in the United States from aspiration pneumonia related to dysphagia.[19] Studies show that more than 50% of all stroke patients will show clinical and fluoroscopic signs of dysphagia.[20] However, most stroke patients will regain healthy swallowing function within 1 or 2 weeks after infarction.[19]

Neurodegenerative diseases also play a large role in the increased frequency of dysphagia in the elderly population. Parkinson's disease, a disorder related to the degeneration of cells responsible for dopamine synthesis, causes widespread motor difficulties and tremor.[21] As symptoms of Parkinson's disease worsen, the risk of aspiration increases as a result of increased oropharyngeal transit time, among other factors.[22] Typically, the motor symptoms in Parkinson's disease are treated with the dopamine precursor L-DOPA, but the medication does not have the same efficacy in eliminating dysphagia. Other neuromuscular diseases that can cause dysphagia are listed in **Box 2**.

In most cases of neuromuscular-related oropharyngeal dysphagia, referral to a speech therapist is extremely helpful.[23] After appropriate clinical evaluation and examination, including either modified barium swallow or FEES study, the speech therapist will develop a treatment plan specific to the patient. Certain food consistencies can be eliminated from the diet, meal and bolus size can be adjusted, and swallowing techniques like the chin-tuck, head-turn, and supraglottic maneuvers can be used to avoid aspiration, enabling the patient to eat more comfortably and safely.[24,25] Dysphagia rehabilitation can also involve strengthening and coordinating muscles involved in swallowing using techniques such as the basic hard swallow, the Mendelsohn maneuver, and the Shaker head lift.[26] In the Mendelsohn maneuver, when a patient initiates a swallow, he holds the larynx at its highest point. This maneuver can increase muscle strength, swallow effort, and endurance. In the Shaker head lift, the patient is instructed to lie supine and lift the head up to look at the feet, holding this position for 1 minute. This exercise, in conjunction with sets of rapid head lifts, is performed over a 6-week period and has been found to significantly decrease aspiration. Of course, in some patients, no therapy can stop aspiration. In these unfortunate cases, artificial feeding, such as a gastrostomy tube, is considered as a last resort.

Structural disorders

Oropharyngeal structural disorders represent other causes of dysphagia in the elderly. These abnormalities, including Zenker's diverticulum, cricopharyngeal bar and achalasia, and tumors require specific treatment, but patients may also benefit from dysphagia rehabilitation guided by a speech pathologist.

Zenker's diverticula are increased in the elderly. They occur at Killian's triangle, which is located posteriorly in the pharynx between the inferior constrictor and cricopharyngeus muscles. These diverticula are typically diagnosed by esophagram. The precise cause of Zenker's diverticulum is still a subject of debate, but one prominent theory posits that it is caused by incomplete relaxation of the UES.[27] Indeed, the surgical treatment is primarily cricopharyngeal myotomy, currently typically performed through the oral route. Larger diverticula may also require diverticulopexy or, rarely, resection. Patients with mild symptoms or substantial comorbid conditions may benefit from dilation of the sphincter, foregoing surgery.[28] Sometimes, a radiologic cricopharyngeal bar, representing a poorly opening UES, may cause symptoms even in the absence of a Zenker's diverticulum. Such patients may also benefit from endoscopic dilation.

Head and neck tumors are a common structural cause of solid food dysphagia in the elderly. Patients with these tumors often have a notable history of smoking and alcohol use and are typically treated by an otolaryngologist, oncologist, and radiation oncologist. Dysphagia can lead to malnutrition and decreased quality of life in these patients, which both contribute to a poorer prognosis.[29] Dysphagia is often not relieved by surgical excision of the tumor, radiation therapy, or chemotherapy. Approximately 50% of patients still suffer from long-term oropharyngeal dysphagia after these treatments.[30] Swallow rehabilitation is important in these patients, because their dysphagia is often long lasting.

Esophageal Dysphagia

Structural disorders

Esophageal webs and rings are benign esophageal narrowings that may cause dysphagia (**Box 3**). An esophageal web is a mucosal and submucosal folding that causes obstruction and may rarely be associated with iron deficiency, as seen in Plummer-Vinson syndrome.[31] Esophageal rings are smooth mucosal constrictions that are seen on either esophagram or endoscopy. When located at the gastroesophageal junction, they are referred to as Schatzki rings, a very common cause of intermittent solid food dysphagia.[32] If multiple rings are seen, eosinophilic esophagitis should be considered. Vascular compression of the esophagus, including dysphagia lusoria and dysphagia aortica, also causes dysphagia.[33]

A peptic stricture is another benign esophageal narrowing that causes dysphagia and is common in the geriatric population. These strictures most often result from

> **Box 3**
> **Disorders causing esophageal dysphagia**
>
> *Structural Causes*
>
> - Esophageal webs
> - Esophageal rings, including Schatzki rings
> - Peptic and other strictures
> - Esophageal malignancies
> - Vascular compression and other extrinsic causes
>
> *Functional Causes*
>
> - Inflammatory disorders including erosive esophagitis
> - Eosinophilic esophagitis (EoE)
> - Achalasia
> - DES
> - Nutcracker esophagus
> - Hypertensive LES
> - Ineffective esophageal motility
> - Scleroderma and other rheumatologic disorders

chronic inflammation from prolonged acid reflux. Heller myotomy for treatment of achalasia, prolonged nasogastric tube placement, and scleroderma increase the risk of peptic stricture formation. With a mild stricture, patients typically have difficulty only with solid foods. As the stricture progresses, patients begin to have difficulty with softer foods and even with liquids. Appropriate treatment involves controlling the patient's reflux and endoscopic esophageal dilation.[34]

Esophageal malignancies are more common in the elderly, and patients often present with rapidly progressive dysphagia. Typically, the prognosis is poor if the diagnosis of cancer is made after the manifestation of dysphagia, because the cancer has already progressed.[35] Malignancies leading to esophageal dysphagia include primary esophageal adenocarcinoma, squamous cell carcinoma, and adenocarcinoma of the gastroesophageal junction/cardia. Esophageal adenocarcinoma often occurs in patients with longstanding gastroesophageal reflux disease (GERD) via development of Barrett's metaplasia and dysplasia.[36,37] Esophageal squamous cell carcinoma typically occurs in patients with a significant smoking and alcohol history. These patients' treatments are typically coordinated by a gastroenterologist, surgeon, and medical and radiation oncologists.[38]

Functional disorders

Esophageal inflammation is a common cause of dysphagia. Inflammatory complications arising from GERD, including erosive esophagitis, are a common cause of dysphagia in this subgroup.[39] If the patient's dysphagia is reflux related, treating the reflux itself can often improve the symptoms. Eosinophilic esophagitis is an inflammatory cause of dysphagia that is becoming increasingly prevalent.[40] It is present in patients of all ages and can be responsible for dysphagia in an elderly patient.[41] Eosinophilic esophagitis often results in food impaction.[42] Other inflammatory causes of esophageal dysphagia include infection, caustic ingestion, radiation, and pill esophagitis.

Several esophageal motility disorders lead to dysphagia, with achalasia being the best-described condition. These motility disorders are best diagnosed by esophageal manometry but are often initially suggested by esophageal imaging studies. Achalasia is defined as incomplete LES relaxation combined with a lack of peristalsis.[43] Patients have difficulty swallowing both liquid and solid foods; they often have concurrent chest pain and weight loss. Achalasia is prevalent in about 1 in 10,000, but it is important to identify and treat appropriately. The 2 primary treatment modalities for achalasia are endoscopic pneumatic balloon dilation and myotomy.[44] However, in the elderly with comorbid conditions, it is often most appropriate to forego such risky procedures and perform only botulinum toxin injection or mild endoscopic dilation.

Many other motility disorders cause dysphagia.[45] Diffuse esophageal spasm (DES) is a disorder with intermingled normal peristalsis and simultaneous contractions. DES can result in chest pain and intermittent dysphagia; it may be primary or secondary to reflux. Nutcracker esophagus is characterized by high amplitude peristaltic contractions in the distal esophagus, and hypertensive LES is characterized by a high resting LES pressure. Both of these motility disorders also may present with chest pain and dysphagia. Ineffective esophageal motility disorder is a manometric diagnosis of low-amplitude peristaltic contractions and can also cause dysphagia; the etiology is typically reflux. Finally, scleroderma can cause aperistalsis or low-amplitude esophageal contractions as well as a hypotensive LES. Both solid and liquid food dysphagia are seen in these patients, and many scleroderma patients have strictures secondary to reflux.[46]

SUMMARY

Dysphagia, or difficulty with the normal swallowing process, is a common problem in the elderly. Patients with dysphagia can have predominantly oropharyngeal symptoms, esophageal symptoms, or a combination of both. A good clinical history and physical examination can suggest the need for further testing in each particular patient with dysphagia. The most common causes of oropharyngeal dysphagia are of neurologic origin, and clinical swallow examinations, in conjunction with an ENT specialist if warning signs imply malignancy, are important in the workup and treatment decisions for these patients. If a patient has likely esophageal dysphagia, a barium esophagram is often the initial appropriate test, but referral to a gastrointestinal specialist for opinion, endoscopy, or manometry is often required.

REFERENCES

1. Reynolds J, George B. Dysphagia. In: Pitchumoni CS, Dharmarajan TS, editors. Geriatric gastroenterology. New York: Springer; 2012. p. 293–300.
2. Ekberg O, Feinberg MJ. Altered swallowing function in elderly patients without dysphagia: radiologic findings in 56 cases. Am J Roentgenol 1991;156(6):1181–4.
3. Day JC. Population projections of the United States by age, sex, race, and Hispanic origin: 1995 to 2050, U.S. Bureau of the Census, Current Population Reports. Washington, DC: U.S. Government Printing Office; 1996. p. 25–1130. Available at: http://www.census.gov/prod/1/pop/p25-1130/p251130.pdf.
4. US Census Bureau. The older population in the United States: 2010 to 2050. Available at: http://www.census.gov/prod/2010pubs/p25-1138.pdf. Accessed August, 2013.
5. Carrión S, Verin E, Clavé P, et al. Complications of oropharyngeal dysphagia: malnutrition and aspiration pneumonia. In: Ekberg O, editor. Dysphagia. Berlin, New York: Springer; 2012. p. 575–99.

6. Norman K, Pichard C, Lochs H, et al. Prognostic impact of disease-related malnutrition. Clin Nutr 2008;27(1):5–15.

7. Persson MD, Brismar KE, Katzarski KS, et al. Nutritional status using mini nutritional assessment and subjective global assessment predict mortality in geriatric patients. J Am Geriatr Soc 2002;50(12):1996–2002.

8. Schindler JS, Kelly JH. Swallowing disorders in the elderly. Laryngoscope 2002; 112(4):589–602.

9. Furness JB. The enteric nervous system and neurogastroenterology. Nature reviews. Gastroenterol Hepatol 2012;9(5):286–94.

10. Sura L, Madhavan A, Carnaby G, et al. Dysphagia in the elderly: management and nutritional considerations. Clin Interv Aging 2012;7:287–98.

11. Cook IJ. Oropharyngeal dysphagia. Gastroenterol Clin North Am 2009;38(3):411–31.

12. Aviv JE, Martin JH, Jones ME, et al. Age-related changes in pharyngeal and supraglottic sensation. Ann Otol Rhinol Laryngol 1994;103(10):749–52.

13. Roy N, Stemple J, Merrill RM, et al. Dysphagia in the elderly: preliminary evidence of prevalence, risk factors, and socioemotional effects. Ann Otol Rhinol Laryngol 2007;116(11):858–65.

14. Marques CH, de Rosso AL, Andre C. Bedside assessment of swallowing in stroke: water tests are not enough. Top Stroke Rehabil 2008;15(4):378–83.

15. Splaingard ML, Hutchins B, Sulton LD, et al. Aspiration in rehabilitation patients: videofluoroscopy vs bedside clinical assessment. Arch Phys Med Rehabil 1988; 69(8):637–40.

16. Umay EK, Unlu E, Saylam GK, et al. Evaluation of dysphagia in early stroke patients by bedside, endoscopic, and electrophysiological methods. Dysphagia 2013;28(3):395–403.

17. Cho YK, Choi MG, Oh SN, et al. Comparison of bolus transit patterns identified by esophageal impedance to barium esophagram in patients with dysphagia. Dis Esophagus 2012;25(1):17–25.

18. Spieker MR. Evaluating dysphagia. Am Fam Physician 2000;61(12):3639–48.

19. Dray TG, Hillel AD, Miller RM. Dysphagia caused by neurologic deficits. Otolaryngol Clin North Am 1998;31(3):507–24.

20. Mann G, Hankey GJ, Cameron D. Swallowing function after stroke: prognosis and prognostic factors at 6 months. Stroke 1999;30(4):744–8.

21. Shulman JM, De Jager PL, Feany MB. Parkinson's disease: genetics and pathogenesis. Annu Rev Pathol 2011;6:193–222.

22. Nagaya M, Kachi T, Yamada T, et al. Videofluorographic study of swallowing in Parkinson's disease. Dysphagia 1998;13(2):95–100.

23. Rosenvinge SK, Starke ID. Improving care for patients with dysphagia. Age Ageing 2005;34(6):587–93.

24. Smith SK, Roddam H, Sheldrick H. Rehabilitation or compensation: time for a fresh perspective on speech and language therapy for dysphagia and Parkinson's disease? Int J Lang Commun Disord 2012;47(4):351–64.

25. Boden K, Hallgren A, Witt Hedstrom H. Effects of three different swallow maneuvers analyzed by videomanometry. Acta Radiol 2006;47(7):628–33.

26. Burkhead LM, Sapienza CM, Rosenbek JC. Strength-training exercise in dysphagia rehabilitation: principles, procedures, and directions for future research. Dysphagia 2007;22(3):251–65.

27. Watemberg S, Landau O, Avrahami R. Zenker's diverticulum: reappraisal. Am J Gastroenterol 1996;91(8):1494–8.

28. Veenker EA, Andersen PE, Cohen JI. Cricopharyngeal spasm and Zenker's diverticulum. Head Neck 2003;25(8):681–94.

29. Grobbelaar EJ, Owen S, Torrance AD, et al. Nutritional challenges in head and neck cancer. Clin Otolaryngol Allied Sci 2004;29(4):307–13.
30. Garcia-Peris P, Paron L, Velasco C, et al. Long-term prevalence of oropharyngeal dysphagia in head and neck cancer patients: impact on quality of life. Clin Nutr 2007;26(6):710–7.
31. Hoffman RM, Jaffe PE. Plummer-Vinson syndrome. A case report and literature review. Arch Intern Med 1995;155(18):2008–11.
32. Jalil S, Castell DO. Schatzki's ring: a benign cause of dysphagia in adults. J Clin Gastroenterol 2002;35(4):295–8.
33. Janssen M, Baggen MG, Veen HF, et al. Dysphagia lusoria: clinical aspects, manometric findings, diagnosis, and therapy. Am J Gastroenterol 2000;95(6): 1411–6.
34. Siersema PD, de Wijkerslooth LR. Dilation of refractory benign esophageal strictures. Gastrointest Endosc 2009;70(5):1000–12.
35. Villaflor VM, Allaix ME, Minsky B, et al. Multidisciplinary approach for patients with esophageal cancer. World J Gastroenterol 2012;18(46):6737–46.
36. Lieberman DA, Oehlke M, Helfand M. Risk factors for Barrett's esophagus in community-based practice. GORGE consortium. Gastroenterology Outcomes Research Group in Endoscopy. Am J Gastroenterol 1997;92(8):1293–7.
37. Pera M, Cameron AJ, Trastek VF, et al. Increasing incidence of adenocarcinoma of the esophagus and esophagogastric junction. Gastroenterology 1993;104(2): 510–3.
38. Sgourakis G, Gockel I, Lang H. Endoscopic and surgical resection of T1a/T1b esophageal neoplasms: a systematic review. World J Gastroenterol 2013;19(9): 1424–37.
39. Triadafilopoulos G. Nonobstructive dysphagia in reflux esophagitis. Am J Gastroenterol 1989;84(6):614–8.
40. Dellon ES, Gonsalves N, Hirano I, et al. ACG clinical guideline: evidenced based approach to the diagnosis and management of esophageal eosinophilia and eosinophilic esophagitis (EoE). Am J Gastroenterol 2013;108(5):679–92 [quiz: 693].
41. Prasad GA, Talley NJ, Romero Y, et al. Prevalence and predictive factors of eosinophilic esophagitis in patients presenting with dysphagia: a prospective study. Am J Gastroenterol 2007;102(12):2627–32.
42. Straumann A, Bussmann C, Zuber M, et al. Eosinophilic esophagitis: analysis of food impaction and perforation in 251 adolescent and adult patients. Clin Gastroenterol Hepatol 2008;6(5):598–600.
43. Michael FV, John EP, Marcelo FV. ACG clinical guideline: diagnosis and management of achalasia. Am J Gastroenterol 2013;108(8):1238–49.
44. Stavropoulos SN, Friedel D, Modayil R, et al. Endoscopic approaches to treatment of achalasia. Therap Adv Gastroenterol 2013;6(2):115–35.
45. Lacy BE, Weiser K. Esophageal motility disorders: medical therapy. J Clin Gastroenterol 2008;42(5):652–8.
46. Ntoumazios SK, Voulgari PV, Potsis K, et al. Esophageal involvement in scleroderma: gastroesophageal reflux, the common problem. Semin Arthritis Rheum 2006;36(3):173–81.

Uses of Esophageal Function Testing: Dysphagia

Etsuro Yazaki, PhD, MAGIP[a,b], Philip Woodland, MBBS, PhD[a,b], Daniel Sifrim, MD, PhD[a,b],*

KEYWORDS

- Dysphagia • Esophageal motility • High-resolution manometry
- Impedance planimetry

KEY POINTS

- Esophageal function testing should be used for differential diagnosis of dysphagia after exclusion of structural causes.
- High-resolution manometry increases diagnostic yield and can predict treatment outcomes in achalasia.
- Impedance planimetry can help to identify abnormalities in esophagogastric junction distensibility in achalasia and eosinophilic esophagitis.

INTRODUCTION

Dysphagia is defined as a difficulty (or a sensation of difficulty) of food passage, which may be difficulty with initiating a swallow (oropharyngeal dysphagia) or the sensation that foods and/or liquids are hindered in their passage from the mouth to the stomach (esophageal dysphagia).[1] This distinction can be made from a careful medical history (oropharyngeal vs esophageal) in about 80% to 85% of cases.[2] This article discusses the use of esophageal function testing in the context of esophageal dysphagia.

Esophageal dysphagia may have structural/obstructive causes, secondary to motility disorders, or may be predominantly sensory. In a patient presenting with dysphagia the priority is to exclude a structural cause such as an esophageal malignancy. Hence, if the history is suggestive, the first clinical assessments for dysphagia should be endoscopy and/or barium swallow. At endoscopy, eosinophilic esophagitis can also be diagnosed or excluded by way of esophageal biopsy. **Box 1** summarizes common causes of dysphagia that should be excluded before esophageal function testing. There are other

This article originally appeared in Gastrointestinal Endoscopy Clinics, Volume 24, Issue 4, October 2014.

[a] Centre for Digestive Diseases, Barts and The London School of Medicine and Dentistry, Queen Mary University of London, London, UK; [b] Gastrointestinal Physiology Unit, Barts Health NHS Trust, Royal London Hospital, London, UK
* Corresponding author. Wingate Institute of Neurogastroenterology, 26 Ashfield Street, London E12AJ, United Kingdom.
E-mail address: d.sifrim@qmul.ac.uk

> **Box 1**
> **Causes of dysphagia that should be excluded before esophageal function testing**
>
> Tumors (esophageal, lung, lymphoma)
>
> Vascular compression (aortic, auricular)
>
> Esophageal rings and webs
>
> Chemical or radiation injury
>
> Peptic stricture
>
> Infectious esophagitis (herpes virus, *Candida albicans*)
>
> Eosinophilic esophagitis

rare causes of structural esophageal dysphagia such as lymphocytic esophagitis, esophageal compression by cardiovascular abnormalities, or esophageal involvement of Crohn disease, which can be considered if medical history is suggestive.

After exclusion of structural causes for dysphagia, esophageal function testing is used to assess motility disorders. Dysphagia can be the consequence of hypermotility or hypomotility of the circular and/or longitudinal muscle layers of the esophagus. It has recently been shown that decreased esophageal or esophagogastric junction (EGJ) distensibility can provoke dysphagia. The most well-established esophageal dysmotility is achalasia. Other motility disorders, including diffuse esophageal spasm, hypercontractile esophagus, and severe hypomotility can also cause dysphagia.[3] High-resolution manometry (HRM) is currently regarded as the gold standard investigation to identify and classify esophageal motility disorders. Simultaneous measurement of HRM and intraluminal impedance (high-resolution impedance manometry [HRIM]) can be useful to assess both motility and bolus transit.[4] Impedance planimetry (EndoFlip) has recently been introduced to measure distensibility of the esophageal body and EGJ in patients with achalasia and eosinophilic esophagitis.[5,6] This article discusses the use of esophageal function testing in patients with esophageal dysphagia after exclusion of structural abnormalities by normal endoscopy and or radiological examination.

DYSPHAGIA ASSOCIATED WITH ESOPHAGEAL MOTILITY DISORDERS DEFINED IN THE CHICAGO CLASSIFICATION
Achalasia

The most established esophageal dysmotility is achalasia. At endoscopy, achalasia can be suggested by esophageal food residue, appearance of esophageal body, and tightness of the lower esophageal sphincter (LES). HRM should be used to confirm diagnosis of achalasia and to identify the subtype of achalasia.

The Chicago Classification criteria of esophageal motility disorders are currently the standard reference for HRM classification.[7] According to this classification, 3 achalasia subtypes (shown in **Fig. 1**) are defined. As expected in achalasia, each is characterized by a failed relaxation of the lower esophageal sphincter during swallows (as determined on HRM by an LES integrated relaxation pressure [IRP], of >15 mm Hg), and by an absence of ordered peristalsis. In type I (classic) achalasia the IRP greater than or equal to 15 mm Hg is associated with a complete absence of esophageal pressure: 100% failed peristalsis. In type II (achalasia with esophageal compression) there is an IRP greater than or equal to 15 mm Hg and at least 20% of wet swallows associated with columns of panesophageal pressurization with greater than 30 mm Hg Type III (spastic achalasia) is defined as an IRP greater than or equal to 15 mm Hg with at least

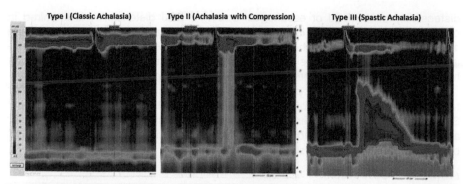

Fig. 1. Three subtypes of achalasia defined by HRM. Type II is considered the phenotype with best prognosis.

20% of wet swallows associated with either a preserved fragment of distal peristalsis or a premature (spastic, distal latency <4.5 seconds) contraction.[7]

As well as providing an excellent means of diagnosis, HRM can help predict outcome and guide choice of clinical intervention in achalasia. It has been shown that type II achalasia has the best outcome to treatment, followed by type I, then type III.[8] A study by Boeckxstaens and colleagues[9] showed that for type II and I achalasia outcomes were similar for pneumatic dilatation and surgical myotomy (although young men tend to do better with myotomy). In type III achalasia, outcomes are better with myotomy. Data regarding subtype outcomes from peroral endoscopic myotomy (POEM) are awaited.

Persistent Dysphagia After Treatment in Achalasia

A significant group of patients with achalasia present with recurrent dysphagia months or several years after successful initial treatment. It is common to perform esophageal function testing on these patients. The most useful tests in this situation (again, after excluding a structural cause) are HRM and a timed barium esophagram. Perhaps the most important question is whether there is residual increased pressure at the EGJ. Patients may have persistent increased resistance at the EGJ either because of increased residual EGJ pressures or decreased distensibility resulting in bolus retention. It is expected that peristaltic activity is still not present. The timed barium esophagogram (TBE) is a simple fluoroscopic evaluation of bolus clearance of esophagus, and is often a useful adjunct to HRM.[10] It involves taking multiple sequential films at predefined time intervals after swallowing a fixed volume of a barium solution of a specific density. After swallowing, upright radiographs are usually taken at 1, 3, and 5 minutes to assess barium clearance.

The patient with dysphagia after treatment of achalasia with a moderate to high IRP and a retained barium column on TBE requires retreatment. Barium column stasis on TBE predicts recurrent symptoms in patients with long-standing achalasia.[11]

Esophageal impedance can also give an idea of the level of liquid retention. Cho and colleagues[12] recently reported an excellent agreement between TBE and HRIM for assessing bolus retention at 5 minutes. As more data and confidence in the technique are gained it is possible that HRIM will be used as a single test to assess bolus retention and motor function in the management of treated achalasia.

The functional lumen imaging probe (EndoFLIP) uses impedance planimetry to calculate luminal diameters and, together with intraluminal pressure measurements, can be used to calculate distensibiltiy.[13] EndoFLIP has been used to measure distensibility of the EGJ or esophageal body.[6,14] EGJ distensibility is impaired in patients with achalasia, and is associated with the degree of esophageal emptying and clinical response. As such, it can be used to evaluate treatment efficacy in achalasia.[15] At present, impedance planimetry is only available in a few centers, but it may have the potential to guide therapy in the future if outcome studies are performed.

In summary, evaluation of patients with achalasia and recurrent symptoms after treatment can be widely performed using TBE and HRM with or without impedance. Symptomatic patients with persistent retention on TBE should be retreated. Whether asymptomatic patients with abnormal TBE, detected during routine follow-up, should be treated remains controversial.

EGJ Outflow Obstruction

Some patients with dysphagia without initial endoscopic or radiologic evidence of structural obstruction display increased IRP (as in achalasia) and normal peristalsis (therefore excluding a diagnosis of achalasia) during HRM. This pattern is classified as EGJ outflow obstruction.[7] A study reported that among 1000 consecutive HRM studies, 16 patients fulfilled the criteria characterized by impaired EGJ relaxation, often accompanied by increased intrabolus pressure, and intact peristalsis.[16]

In some patients the cause of EGJ outflow obstruction is mechanical obstruction (Box 2). It is recommended that patients with this motility pattern have endoscopic examination (if not already performed) and computed tomography (CT) or endoscopic ultrasonography evaluation of the EGJ. Note that patients with hiatal hernias are within this group because it has been shown that sliding hiatus hernias alter the pressure dynamics through the EGJ.[17] Patients with an EGJ outflow obstruction after surgical fundoplication are discussed later.

In the remainder of patients the failed relaxation of the EGJ is not mechanical, and the nature of this phenotype is the subject of some debate. It has been postulated that it represents an incomplete expression of achalasia (although this has not yet been shown histopathologically).[18] If mechanical obstruction (including sliding hiatal hernia) is excluded, it is considered a reasonable approach to dilate as in achalasia (although myotomy is less often practiced in this scenario).

Distal Esophageal Spasm

Distal esophageal spasm (DES) is an uncommon motility disorder often associated with dysphagia. As technology has evolved, so has the definition of esophageal spasm. With conventional manometry the diagnosis was defined by the presence of simultaneous contractions as well as preserved peristalsis, and was called diffuse esophageal spasm.[19] The greater resolution of HRM has led to a definition that takes into account

---

Box 2
Mechanical causes of EGJ outflow obstruction

EGJ mucosal/submucosal neoplasm

Fibrotic stenosis (eg, after inflammation/radiotherapy)

Eosinophilic esophagitis

Obstructing esophageal varices

Sliding hiatus hernia

After fundoplication[a]

[a] Postsurgical obstruction is not covered by the Chicago Classification.

the absence of adequate peristaltic inhibition. The key to the diagnosis is now measurement of the distal latency (the time between onset of the swallow and the deceleration point of the esophageal contraction, which cannot be measured on conventional manometry). The Chicago Classification diagnostic criteria for DES include a normal IRP and greater than or equal to 20% premature contractions (ie, distal latency <4.5 seconds).[7]

The difference between DES and type III achalasia is in the adequate or inadequate relaxation of the EGJ. In achalasia there can be significant esophageal shortening leading to pseudorelaxation of the EGJ. HRM does not have this limitation, and is therefore the investigation of choice in making this diagnostic distinction (**Fig. 2**).

If symptoms of pain or dysphagia are associated with DES then treatment is indicated. First it is sensible to rule out gastroesophageal reflux with reflux testing or empirical proton pump inhibitor treatment because DES and reflux frequently coexist (although the pathophysiologic relationship is not well defined). Other medical therapies are designed to relax smooth muscle or overcome the defective inhibitory neural function. Smooth muscle relaxants such as nitrates[20] and calcium channel antagonists[21] are often used, but controlled trials are lacking. The phosphodiesterase-5 inhibitor sildenafil blocks degradation of NO, resulting in a more prolonged smooth muscle relaxation and seems effective in relieving symptoms and improving manometric findings in spasm.[22] In addition, endoscopically injected botulinum toxin has been shown to have some benefit in terms of pain and dysphagia.[23] A future possibility for therapy is POEM, in which a long proximal myotomy has theoretic potential. There are preliminary reports suggesting some benefit.[24]

Hypercontractile Esophagus

Hypercontractile esophagus or hypertensive esophageal peristalsis used to refer to so-called nutcracker esophagus using conventional manometry.[19] The clinical relevance of nutcracker esophagus seems variable because its presence may or may not be associated with dysphagia. Tutuian and Castell[4] reported that 97% of patients with nutcracker esophagus had complete bolus transit assessed by combined multichannel intraluminal impedance and manometry. In the Chicago Classification, the distal contractile integral (DCI; an integral that takes into account the amplitude, length, and duration of contraction) is used to diagnose nutcracker esophagus, in which a

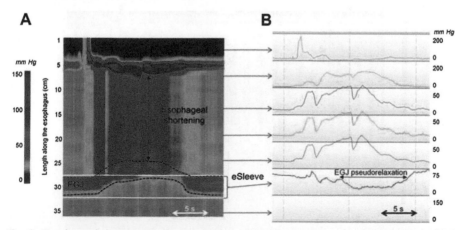

Fig. 2. Esophageal shortening observed using HRM (*A*) can cause pseudorelaxation of EGJ on conventional manometry (*B*). (*From* Roman S, Kahrilas P. Distal esophageal spasm. Dysphagia 2012;27:115–23; with permission.)

mean value of 5000 to 8000 mm Hg/s/cm is found. The classification also now defines hypercontractile esophagus, in which at least 1 wet-swallow DCI is greater than 8000 mm Hg·s·cm (a value not seen in any asymptomatic individual) with single or multiple peaks (jackhammer esophagus) in a context of normal EGJ relaxation.[7] Hypercontractile esophagus can be associated with dysphagia or chest pain.[25] Jackhammer esophagus (**Fig. 3**) is most likely to be accompanied by dysphagia.[26] Hypercontractility can be secondary to other underlying disorders such as EGJ outflow obstruction, so it is important to ensure that the IRP is normal before making the diagnosis. Treatment options are largely as described earlier for spasm.

Esophageal Hypomotility

One of the important roles of esophageal function testing is to evaluate unexplained dysphagia. Esophageal dysmotility patterns described so far are of major motor disorders associated with dysphagia. With the introduction of HRM, more detailed assessment of peristaltic integrity became possible, which brought the new manometric classifications of esophageal hypomotility (ie, weak peristalsis with small/large peristaltic defects or frequent failed peristalsis).[7]

At the extreme of esophageal hypomotility, HRM findings of 100% failed peristalsis with normal EGJ relaxation is defined as absent peristalsis.[7] Symptoms can be dysphagia and/or gastroesophageal reflux, and absent peristalsis can be a presentation of esophageal involvement in connective tissue disease (scleroderma; **Fig. 4**), which should be actively investigated.

Lesser degrees of esophageal hypomotility can be associated with dysphagia (although less reliably) and failure of esophageal bolus transit. Roman and colleagues[27] reported that weak peristalsis, but not failed peristalsis, occurred significantly more frequently in patients with unexplained dysphagia than in control subjects. The clinical relevance of esophageal hypomotility (particularly with small peristaltic defects) is not clear, especially because not all patients with weak peristalsis complain of dysphagia. Evaluation of bolus transit may give a clearer indication of clinical relevance. Kahrilas and colleagues[28] reported that incomplete bolus transit frequently occurred in the distal esophagus when contraction amplitude was less than 20 mm Hg. Esophageal pressure topography plots with breaks greater than 5 cm in

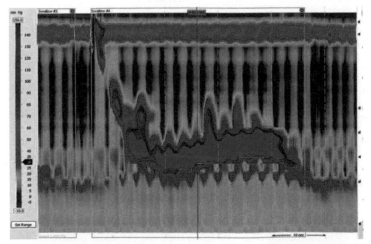

Fig. 3. Jackhammer esophagus: this type of hypermotility can be associated with dysphagia and/or chest pain.

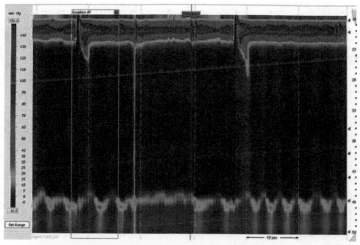

Fig. 4. Absent peristalsis in a patient with confirmed scleroderma.

20 mm Hg isobaric contour were closely associated with incomplete bolus transit.[27] HRIM is useful to investigate this patient group by measuring esophageal motility and bolus transport simultaneously.[4,27] Using impedance channels, it is possible to evaluate whether hypomotility is associated with incomplete bolus transit, and whether this corresponds with symptoms of dysphagia. A common treatment approach to patients with hypomotility and dysphagia is to use prokinetic therapy. Motilin agonists such as erythromycin, and dopamine antagonists such as metoclopramide, have been used, but a clinical benefit is not established.

INVESTIGATION OF DYSPHAGIA RESULTING FROM OTHER CAUSES
Dysphagia with Normal Esophageal Peristalsis on Wet Swallows

There is a patient group with dysphagia, especially with intermittent dysphagia for solids, whose HRM seems to be normal using the Chicago Classification. The limitation of diagnostic yield at HRM is that normal values are obtained from 10 wet swallows of 5 mL of water. Provocative swallows such as larger volume of water or solid swallowing at HRM might reproduce dysphagia in such a patient group and increase a diagnostic yield.

Sweis and colleagues[29,30] described use of standardized solid food and showed that abnormal pressure events at HRM were associated with dysphagia. **Fig. 5** shows

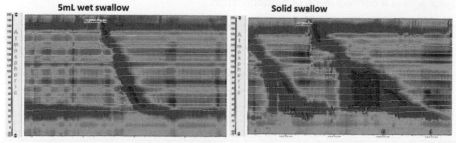

Fig. 5. This patient presented with dysphagia and chest pain during meals. Peristalsis was weak during liquid swallows (*left*). However, bread swallows (*right*) induced esophageal segmental pressurization associated with typical symptoms.

Wet swallow   **Solid swallow**

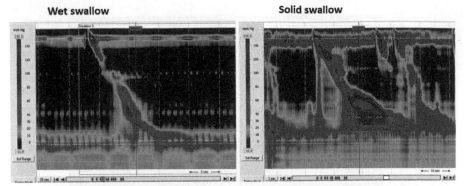

Fig. 6. This patient presented with dysphagia after Nissen fundoplication. Peristalsis and IRP were normal during wet swallows (*left*). However, bread swallows (*right*) induced esophageal segmental pressurization within the double high-pressure zone (*dotted area*) associated with typical symptoms.

an example of solid swallowing for one of our patients with solid dysphagia with and without retrosternal pain/pressure. Use of solid swallowing at HRM may be a helpful provocative test to diagnose abnormal pressure events not produced with standard 5-mL wet swallows. A standard classification is lacking, but it may be useful when careful consideration is given to the association of pressure events and symptoms.

Dysphagia Following Antireflux Surgery

Dysphagia is a recognized complication of fundoplication, and patients with dysphagia after antireflux surgery are often evaluated by HRM. In contrast with the preoperative state, normal values of the IRP are not described after antireflux surgery. A high IRP (in association with a high intrabolus pressure) may be a sign of EGJ outflow obstruction secondary to a too-tight fundoplication. Recent studies using HRM have reported that a dual high-pressure zone (HPZ) at the EGJ is a sign of failed or disrupted fundoplication.[31] The dual HPZ is caused by either slipped wrap or intrathoracic fundoplication.

A small series of postfundoplication patients with dysphagia and a double HPZ were studied with HRM at our unit. IRP did not reveal abnormal EGJ dynamics on wet swallows, and rapid swallow provocation tests provoked no obvious changes in pressure tomography at EGJ. An increased pressure within the dual HPZ during solid swallows was the only significant change and this could be an objective parameter to assess postfundoplication patients with dysphagia (**Fig. 6**). **Table 1** summarizes our preliminary findings. Redo fundoplication and dilatation are therapeutic options when dysphagia is a consequence of fundoplication.

Table 1
IRP and pressure within dual high-pressure zone (DHPZ) during different types of swallows

	IRP (mm Hg)	Pressure in DHPZ (mm Hg)
WS	8.65 ± 6.17	7.01 ± 4.42
MRS	5.75 ± 5.15	7.12 ± 5.96
200RS	4.62 ± 4.56	6.17 ± 7.75
SS	10.12 ± 2.92	25.41 ± 17.87[a]

[a] $P = .003$ against WS.

Abbreviations: MRS, multiple rapid swallows; WS, wet swallows; SS, solid swallows; 200RS, 200ml rapid swallows.

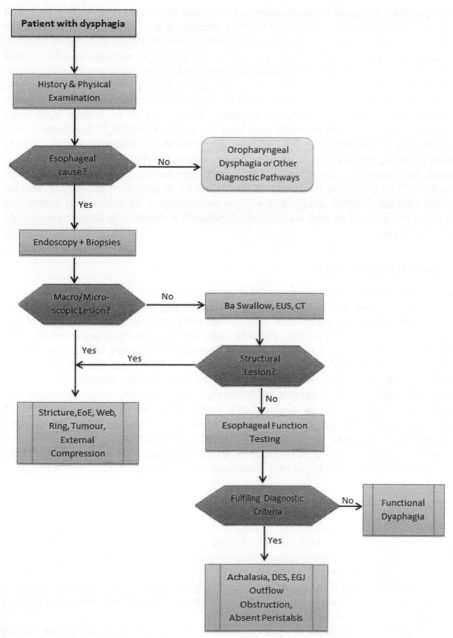

Fig. 7. Diagnosis and management of esophageal dysphagia. EoE, eosinophilic esophagitis; EUS, endoscopic ultrasonography.

Functional Dysphagia

Patients with dysphagia without any abnormalities at endoscopy or esophageal function testing can be classified as functional dysphagia. The Rome III diagnostic criteria for functional dysphagia are (1) a sense of solid and/or liquid food sticking, lodging, or passing abnormally through the esophagus; (2) absence of evidence that gastroesophageal reflux disease is the cause of the symptom; (3) absence of histopathology-based esophageal motility disorders and all 3 criteria fulfilled for the past 3 months with symptom onset at least 6 months before diagnosis. In order to confirm functional dysphagia, presence of dysphagic symptoms with normal bolus transit through the esophagus should be shown using esophagogram or HRIM. The mechanism of functional dysphagia is poorly understood. Peristaltic dysfunction not elicited by HRM (which is poor at assessing longitudinal muscle contraction, for example) may be present. Symptoms of functional dysphagia can be induced by intraluminal acid and balloon distention,[32] suggesting that esophageal hypersensitivity or reduced perception of mechanical stimuli may have a pathophysiologic role. Psychological stress maybe important in some patients, because this can affect both sensory perception and esophageal motor function.[33] As such, the fundamental mechanisms of symptom production remain poorly defined. Further application of new technologies for measuring motor and sensory physiology as well as CNS modulation[34] is needed to further investigate this condition.

DIAGNOSTIC FLOWCHART

A diagnostic flowchart of patients with dysphagia is shown in **Fig. 7**. First, accurate medical history needs to be taken. When symptoms suggest a nonesophageal cause, the patient requires investigations along other pathways such as neurologic or ear, nose, and throat investigations. Patients with esophageal dysphagia should have endoscopy with biopsy. If macroscopic/microscopic lesions are found from endoscopy, patients are treated accordingly. If endoscopy is normal, barium swallow or other diagnostic imaging investigations can be considered, especially for elderly patients. Once structural causes of dysphagia are ruled out, esophageal function testing is useful to diagnose possible dysmotility. HRM with or without impedance is an ideal option to diagnose primary esophageal dysmotility defined by the Chicago Classification. EndoFlip or TBE can be useful to further evaluate postoperative dysphagia such as after fundoplication or treated achalasia. If no esophageal motor disorders were diagnosed, the term functional dysphagia can be applied.

REFERENCES

1. Malagelada JR, Bazzoli F, Elewaut A, et al. WGO practice guideline - dysphagia: WGO. 2007. WGO Global Guideline. Available at: http://www. worldgastroenterology.org/assets/downloads/en/pdf/guidelines/08_dysphagia. pdf. Accessed May 23, 2014.
2. Chang YC, Chen SY, Lui LT, et al. Dysphagia in patients with nasopharyngeal cancer after radiation therapy: a videofluoroscopic swallowing study. Dysphagia 2003;18(2):135–43.
3. Pandolfino JE, Kahrilas PJ, Association AG. AGA technical review on the clinical use of esophageal manometry. Gastroenterology 2005;128(1):209–24.
4. Tutuian R, Castell DO. Combined multichannel intraluminal impedance and manometry clarifies esophageal function abnormalities: study in 350 patients. Am J Gastroenterol 2004;99(6):1011–9.
5. Massey BT. EndoFLIP assessment of achalasia therapy: interpreting the distensibility data is a bit of a stretch. Gastroenterology 2013;144(4):e17–8.
6. Kwiatek MA, Hirano I, Kahrilas PJ, et al. Mechanical properties of the esophagus in eosinophilic esophagitis. Gastroenterology 2011;140(1):82–90.

7. Bredenoord AJ, Fox M, Kahrilas PJ, et al. Chicago classification criteria of esophageal motility disorders defined in high resolution esophageal pressure topography. Neurogastroenterol Motil 2012;24(Suppl 1):57–65.

8. Pandolfino JE, Kwiatek MA, Nealis T. Achalasia: a new clinically relevant classification by high-resolution manometry. Gastroenterology 2008;135(5): 1526–33.

9. Boeckxstaens GE, Annese V, des Varannes SB, et al. Pneumatic dilation versus laparoscopic Heller's myotomy for idiopathic achalasia. N Engl J Med 2011; 364(19):1807–16.

10. Kostic SV, Rice TW, Baker ME, et al. Timed barium esophagogram: a simple physiologic assessment for achalasia. J Thorac Cardiovasc Surg 2000;120(5): 935–43.

11. Rohof WO, Lei A, Boeckxstaens GE. Esophageal stasis on a timed barium esophagogram predicts recurrent symptoms in patients with long-standing achalasia. Am J Gastroenterol 2013;108(1):49–55.

12. Cho YK, Lipowska AM, Nicodème F, et al. Assessing bolus retention in achalasia using high-resolution manometry with impedance: a comparator study with timed barium esophagram. Am J Gastroenterol 2014;109(6):829–35.

13. McMahon BP, Frøkjaer JB, Kunwald P, et al. The functional lumen imaging probe (FLIP) for evaluation of the esophagogastric junction. Am J Physiol Gastrointest Liver Physiol 2007;292(1):G377–84.

14. Kwiatek MA, Pandolfino JE, Hirano I, et al. Esophagogastric junction distensibility assessed with an endoscopic functional luminal imaging probe (EndoFLIP). Gastrointest Endosc 2010;72(2):272–8.

15. Rohof WO, Hirsch DP, Kessing BF, et al. Efficacy of treatment for patients with achalasia depends on the distensibility of the esophagogastric junction. Gastroenterology 2012;143(2):328–35.

16. Scherer JR, Kwiatek MA, Soper NJ, et al. Functional esophagogastric junction obstruction with intact peristalsis: a heterogeneous syndrome sometimes akin to achalasia. J Gastrointest Surg 2009;13(12):2219–25.

17. Pandolfino JE, Kwiatek MA, Ho K, et al. Unique features of esophagogastric junction pressure topography in hiatus hernia patients with dysphagia. Surgery 2010; 147(1):57–64.

18. Roman S, Kahrilas PJ. Challenges in the swallowing mechanism: nonobstructive dysphagia in the era of high-resolution manometry and impedance. Gastroenterol Clin North Am 2011;40(4):823–35, ix–x.

19. Spechler SJ, Castell DO. Classification of oesophageal motility abnormalities. Gut 2001;49(1):145–51.

20. Swamy N. Esophageal spasm: clinical and manometric response to nitroglycerine and long acting nitrites. Gastroenterology 1977;72(1):23–7.

21. Baunack AR, Weihrauch TR. Clinical efficacy of nifedipine and other calcium antagonists in patients with primary esophageal motor dysfunctions. Arzneimittelforschung 1991;41(6):595–602.

22. Eherer AJ, Schwetz I, Hammer HF, et al. Effect of sildenafil on oesophageal motor function in healthy subjects and patients with oesophageal motor disorders. Gut 2002;50(6):758–64.

23. Storr M, Allescher HD, Rösch T, et al. Treatment of symptomatic diffuse esophageal spasm by endoscopic injection of botulinum toxin: a prospective study with long term follow-up. Gastrointest Endosc 2001;54(6):18A.

24. Minami H, Isomoto H, Yamaguchi N, et al. Peroral endoscopic myotomy (POEM) for diffuse esophageal spasm. Endoscopy 2014;46(Suppl 1 UCTN):E79–81.

25. Ghosh S, Pandolfino J, Rice J, et al. Impaired deglutitive EGJ relaxation in clinical esophageal manometry: a quantitative analysis of 400 patients and 75 controls. Am J Physiol Gastrointest Liver Physiol 2007;293(4):G878–85.
26. Roman S, Pandolfino JE, Chen J, et al. Phenotypes and clinical context of hyper-contractility in high-resolution esophageal pressure topography (EPT). Am J Gastroenterol 2012;107(1):37–45.
27. Roman S, Lin Z, Kwiatek MA, et al. Weak peristalsis in esophageal pressure topography: classification and association with dysphagia. Am J Gastroenterol 2011;106(2):349–56.
28. Kahrilas P, Dodds W, Hogan W. Effect of peristaltic dysfunction on esophageal volume clearance. Gastroenterology 1988;94(1):73–80.
29. Sweis R, Anggiansah A, Wong T, et al. Normative values and inter-observer agreement for liquid and solid bolus swallows in upright and supine positions as assessed by esophageal high-resolution manometry. Neurogastroenterol Motil 2011;23(6):509.e198.
30. Sweis R, Anggiansah A, Wong T, et al. Assessment of esophageal dysfunction and symptoms during and after a standardized test meal: development and clinical validation of a new methodology utilizing high-resolution manometry. Neurogastroenterol Motil 2014;26(2):215–28.
31. Hoshino M, Srinivasan A, Mittal SK. High-resolution manometry patterns of lower esophageal sphincter complex in symptomatic post-fundoplication patients. J Gastrointest Surg 2012;16(4):705–14.
32. Deschner WK, Maher KA, Cattau EL, et al. Manometric responses to balloon distention in patients with nonobstructive dysphagia. Gastroenterology 1989; 97(5):1181–5.
33. Drossman DA, Corazziari E, Delvaux M, et al. ROME III: the functional gastrointestinal disorders. 3rd edition. Yale University Section of Digestive Disease. MacLean, VA: Degnon Associates; 2006.
34. Suntrup S, Teismann I, Wollbrink A, et al. Altered cortical swallowing processing in patients with functional dysphagia: a preliminary study. PLoS One 2014;9(2): e89665.

Benign Esophageal Tumors

Cindy Ha, MD[a], James Regan, MD[a], Ibrahim Bulent Cetindag, MD[a], Aman Ali, MD[b], John D. Mellinger, MD[a],*

KEYWORDS

- Leiomyoma • Gastrointestinal stromal tumor • Mediastinal cyst

KEY POINTS

- Endoscopic evaluation including endoscopic ultrasonography is foundational to the evaluation of benign and indeterminate esophageal pathology.
- Leiomyomas have distinctive distributions, behavior, and entailed therapeutic significance in pediatric patients.
- Immunohistochemical analysis is an important adjunctive diagnostic tool in distinguishing noncarcinomatous tumors of the esophagus.
- Symptomatic lesions and those with rapid change in size dictate surgical management.
- Endoscopic, thoracoscopic, and laparoscopic techniques including enucleation are widely used in the management of benign tumors of the esophagus.

INTRODUCTION

Unlike esophageal carcinoma, benign esophageal tumors and cysts are rare. Multiple autopsy series have been performed in the past, and although the specific results vary, the overall incidence is less than 1%. In addition, benign tumors account for less than 5% of all surgically resected esophageal tumors.[1] Nevertheless, the past century has shown an increasing trend in the incidence of these lesions, most likely a reflection of improving diagnostic methods,[2] and continued advancements in the understanding of their natural history and management. Benign esophageal tumors are often asymptomatic and typically require only close surveillance. If surgery is indicated because of symptoms or diagnostic uncertainty, many of these tumors can be successfully resected with excellent long-term outcomes. Because these lesions are rare, the general or gastrointestinal (GI) surgeon should have a strong foundation in their diagnosis and treatment.

This article originally appeared in Surgical Clinics, Volume 95, Issue 3, June 2015.

[a] Department of Surgery, Division of General Surgery at SIU, Southern Illinois University School of Medicine, 701 North First Street, Springfield, IL 62794, USA; [b] Department of Internal Medicine, Division of Gastroenterology, Southern Illinois University School of Medicine, 701 North First Street, Springfield, IL 62794, USA
* Corresponding author. PO Box 19638, 701 North First Street, Springfield, IL 62794.
E-mail address: jmellinger@siumed.edu

Clinics Collections 7 (2015) 393–416
http://dx.doi.org/10.1016/j.ccol.2015.06.027
2352-7986/15/$ – see front matter © 2015 Elsevier Inc. All rights reserved.

HISTORY

The first documented record of a benign esophageal tumor was in 1559 by Sussius. The tumor was discovered on autopsy, located in the distal esophagus, and has been cited as a leiomyoma, although histologic confirmation is lacking.[3] In 1763, Dallas-Monro performed one of the first treatments of a benign esophageal tumor when he excised a pedunculated esophageal mass using a snare from a 64-year-old man who had regurgitated the mass into his mouth. The first successful surgical treatment of a benign esophageal tumor is generally credited to Sauerbach, who performed a partial esophagectomy with esophagogastrostomy in 1932 for a myoma, most likely a leiomyoma. One year later, Oshawa performed the first open enucleation of an esophageal leiomyoma, and in 1937, Churchill performed the first open enucleation of a benign esophageal tumor in the United States for what was initially described as a neurofibroma but later reclassified as a leiomyoma.

According to Storey and Adams[4] in their case report and review of leiomyoma of the esophagus, only 16 documented surgical cases were found up until 1948, but between then and time of their publication in 1956, they found an additional 94 cases described, including 4 cases of their own. Since then, there have been many more recorded surgeries for benign esophageal tumors, and within the past 2 decades, there has been a shift toward minimally invasive approaches, specifically via thoracoscopy and endoscopy.

INCIDENCE

Several autopsy series and medical literature reviews have been performed in the past, searching for the true incidence of benign esophageal neoplasms. In 1932, Patterson[5] reported a total of 62 benign esophageal tumors during a 215-year period from 1717 to 1932. In 1944, Moersch[6] found 44 benign tumors and cysts in 7459 autopsy examinations, for an incidence of 0.59%. Plachta[7] in 1962 reviewed 19,982 postmortem examinations and found a total of 505 esophageal neoplasms, 90 of which were benign, resulting in an overall incidence of 0.45% with approximately 18% of all esophageal tumors being benign. In 1968, Attah and Hajdu[8] found 26 benign tumors among 15,454 autopsies during a 30-year period, for an incidence of 0.16%. Allowing for some variation among these studies, the overall incidence is cumulatively documented as less than 1%.[1] By way of comparison, malignant esophageal carcinoma is approximately 50 times more common.[9] The mean age of presentation for benign lesions is between the third and fifth decade of life, much younger than the mean age of presentation for esophageal carcinoma, and studies suggest a slight male predominance with an average ratio of 2:1.[1]

Unlike other benign tumors, esophageal duplications and cysts are more common in children. Accordingly, although such lesions are estimated to comprise only 0.5% to 3.3% of all benign esophageal masses in adults, they account for approximately 12% of all mediastinal tumors in the pediatric population. Between 25% and 35% of all esophageal duplications first become manifest in adults, and of these, most present in adults younger than 50 years.[10]

CLINICAL FEATURES

Benign esophageal tumors are generally slow-growing masses, and they may remain stable without any change in size for many years. At least 50% of benign esophageal masses are asymptomatic,[7] and they are frequently diagnosed incidentally on imaging or endoscopy performed for other reasons.[2] Choong and Meyers[1] broadly categorized the clinical presentations of benign esophageal neoplasms into 5 groups: asymptomatic, obstruction from intraluminal growth, compression of adjacent tissue by extraluminal tumor, regurgitation of a pedunculated tumor, and ulceration with bleeding.

The most common presenting symptom is dysphagia, and the degree of severity varies between patients. Because of the compliance of the esophagus, symptoms often occur late in the disease process as the lesions grow enough to cause luminal obstruction or compression. Typically, a size of 5 cm or more correlates with the likelihood of such symptoms developing.

The next most common symptoms are pain, usually retrosternal or epigastric in location, and pyrosis. Obstructive symptoms more commonly occur with intraluminal tumors,[1] and rarely, these tumors can present with ulceration,[11] bleeding, or regurgitation. Circumferential or annular involvement has been described, causing luminal narrowing and obstruction,[11] but this is an uncommon presentation.[1]

Respiratory symptoms may occur as well. Storey and Adams[4] found that 10 of the 110 reviewed patients presented with predominately respiratory symptoms, which were thought to be the result of tracheal or bronchial compression by the tumor. Presenting respiratory complaints are more common in the pediatric population.

In contrast to patients with malignant esophageal carcinomas, patients with benign tumors often present with multiple symptoms of long duration. Seremetis and colleagues[12] in their analysis of 838 cases of esophageal leiomyoma found that 30% of symptomatic patients reported a symptom duration of more than 5 years; another 30%, 2 to 5 years; and the remaining 40%, an average of 11 months.

DIAGNOSIS

Frequently, the diagnosis of a benign esophageal tumor or cyst is made incidentally on imaging or endoscopy performed for other indications. A plain chest radiograph may reveal a posterior and/or middle mediastinal, paraesophageal mass. However, the sensitivity and specificity of a plain radiograph is low, and the mass must reach a significant size before it becomes apparent on a chest radiograph.[4]

A contrast swallow study is most likely the best initial test to obtain in the evaluation of a symptomatic patient. Esophagography is usually performed in a biphasic manner with upright double-contrast views with high-density barium suspension and prone single-contrast views with low-density barium suspension. The former allows for evaluation of the mucosa, and the latter facilitates evaluation of any areas of luminal narrowing. Benign esophageal tumors usually are manifest as mobile lesions with smooth contours. Occasionally, altered peristalsis is seen with intraluminal tumors.[13]

Computed tomography (CT) of the chest is helpful in the evaluation of extraesophageal tumors and exclusion of other mediastinal masses that could lead to similar clinical presentations. The relationships between the esophageal tumor and surrounding tissues are also better defined with CT, which may be invaluable in preoperative planning when indicated by symptoms or diagnostic uncertainty.[14]

Endoscopy and endoscopic ultrasound (EUS) imaging are mandatory in the evaluation of a symptomatic esophageal tumor. In addition to excluding malignant carcinomas, endoscopy allows for visualization of the mucosa and biopsy of intraluminal and submucosal tumors. Although intramural tumors are not visualized on endoscopy, it is essential to confirm an intact mucosa if an intramural tumor is suspected. EUS imaging provides visualization of the esophageal layers and defines which layers are involved with the tumor, which is invaluable in perioperative planning and surveillance. In addition, EUS imaging can reveal certain unique sonographic characteristics that can aid in the diagnosis of the tumor. Lack of enlarged lymph nodes, smaller size, homogeneous echo pattern, and smooth borders favor a benign lesion on EUS imaging.[2] EUS imaging also allows needle biopsy of these lesions and any associated pathology including lymph nodes, which is more often diagnostic than simple endoluminal biopsy for lesions beyond the confines of the mucosa.[14]

MANAGEMENT

In the past, surgical resection was recommended for most esophageal neoplasms, including benign ones. However, recent advances have shown that most benign esophageal tumors are slow growing,[15] and with the exception of esophageal gastrointestinal stromal tumors (GISTs) and adenomas, malignant transformation is rare.[16] Accordingly, many of these lesions can be followed with serial studies if asymptomatic.[14] Historically, if surgery was indicated, an open approach was advocated. However, in the past 2 decades there has been an increasing shift toward minimally invasive techniques with endoscopic, laparoscopic, or thoracoscopic resections.[17] These methods are discussed in greater detail as they apply to each individual type of lesion in the following sections.

CLASSIFICATION

Benign esophageal tumors can be classified in several ways, and various classification schemes have been proposed in the past based on esophageal layer of origin, histologic cell type, and location as well as clinical appearance. Many of the histologic tumor types can occur in multiple and varying layers of the wall. Rice[2] described the 5 discrete esophageal layers seen on EUS imaging, specifically the superficial mucosa, deep mucosa, submucosa, muscularis propria, and paraesophageal tissue. As a way of characterizing layer of origin and relationship to adjacent structures, EUS imaging has become a practically essential tool in the diagnosis and characterization of these benign esophageal tumors. Having weighed all these variables, classification by location is probably the most practical method, primarily because it dictates the treatment strategy. A summary of a location-based classification scheme is given in **Box 1**.

Box 1
Classification of benign esophageal tumors

Intramural

Leiomyoma

Gastrointestinal stromal tumor

Schwannoma

Intraluminal

Epithelial polyps (adenomatous and inflammatory)

Lipomatous polyps

Fibrovascular polyps

Papilloma

Hemangioma

Granular cell tumor

Extraesophageal

Duplications and cysts

INTRAMURAL TUMORS
Leiomyoma

Leiomyoma is a benign smooth muscle tumor found throughout the GI tract, and although only 10% of all GI leiomyomas are located in the esophagus,[11] they are the most common benign esophageal masses, accounting for approximately two-thirds of all benign esophageal tumors.[14] Morgagni provided the first description of a GI leiomyoma in 1761.[4]

Many autopsy reviews have been performed to assess the incidence of benign esophageal tumors as documented earlier, and in regards to leiomyomas specifically, the general incidence ranges from 0.006% to 0.1%.[9] The incidence of clinically significant leiomyomas is much lower, as at least half of these lesions are asymptomatic and diagnosed incidentally. There has been an increase in incidence during the past few decades because of improved and more widespread use of endoscopy.[2]

Leiomyomas can arise from smooth muscle in the muscularis propria or muscularis mucosae, but the latter is much less commonly encountered, presenting as an intraluminal polypoid lesion in 7% of documented cases based on a review by Hatch and colleagues.[15] Most lesions arise from the muscularis propria, with 80% being found in intramural and 7% in extraesophageal positions. Most are solitary and involve a localized area of the esophageal wall. Less than 2.4% of documented cases reported multiple tumors, and 10% to 13% were annular with circumferential involvement.[14]

Anatomically, leiomyoma is found most often in the middle and distal thirds of the esophagus, which reflects the increasing proportion of smooth muscle as opposed to striated muscle within the esophageal wall. In their review of 838 cases, Seremetis and colleagues[12] found that 56% were found in the distal third, 33% in the middle third, and 11% in the upper third. Furthermore, approximately 6.8% also involved the gastroesophageal junction and/or proximal stomach.

These benign esophageal smooth muscle tumors can occur at any age, but more than 80% are found between the second and sixth decades, with the peak time of presentation between ages 30 and 50 years. It is also more commonly seen in adult men, with an overall 2:1 male to female ratio.[14] The natural history of the esophageal leiomyoma reflects an overall slow, indolent progression, and malignant transformation is extremely rare. There have only been 4 documented cases in the past of progression to leiomyosarcoma, and each case was heralded by a preceding change in size.[12,14,15]

Esophageal leiomyoma has rarely been found in the pediatric population.[11] In contradistinction to adults, leiomyomas in the pediatric population are twice as common in girls. Furthermore, 91% of cases show multiple tumors and/or diffuse involvement, with 35% involving the entire length of the esophagus. Individuals with this more diffuse form of involvement typically require more aggressive surgical management strategies, as outlined further in the discussion.[18]

Leiomyoma has been associated with a variety of other benign esophageal conditions such as achalasia, other dysmotility disorders, esophageal diverticulum, and gastroesophageal reflux. The most commonly associated condition is hiatal hernia, found in 4.5% to 23% of patients with leiomyoma.[14]

In the past, leiomyoma was considered apart of a spectrum of mesenchymal tumors, which also included GISTs. However, studies have shown that these 2 tumors are distinct entities in regards to ultrastructure, histology, and genetic and immunohistochemical markers.[16,19]

In regards to gross appearance, leiomyomas are firm, rubbery, well-encapsulated masses with smooth surfaces. They range from white, gray, tan, or yellow in color and often have a whorled appearance on cut section.[12] Although shapes vary, smaller ones tend to be oval or spherical and larger ones, horseshoe or dumbbell-like in shape. Most are small in size as well, likely reflecting the more slow-growing natural history, with approximately 50% less than 5 cm and 93% less than 15 cm.[14] On histologic examination, leiomyomas are characteristically composed of uniform spindle cells arranged in fascicles or whorls with eosinophilic cytoplasm and surrounding hypovascular connective tissue, few to no mitotic figures, bland cigar-ended nuclei, minimal to no cellular atypia, and overall hypocellularity.[12,14,16]

The description of GISTs in regards to gross, histologic, and immunohistochemical characteristics are discussed in more detail in a separate section, but in brief comparison for the sake of review of leiomyomas, GISTs grossly appear soft with fish flesh–like consistency and histologically appear overall basophilic with high cellularity and increased mitotic figures and cellular atypia. The histologic features in turn reflect the higher malignant potential and more aggressive nature of GISTs vis-à-vis leiomyomas.[16,19]

Although gross appearance and histology can help differentiate leiomyoma from GIST, the definitive foundation for distinguishing between these 2 entities lies in 4 immunohistochemical markers. Leiomyoma is typically positive for desmin and smooth muscle antigen (SMA) and negative for CD117 and CD34. By way of contrast, GISTs are uniformly positive for CD117 and almost uniformly positive for CD34, and usually negative for desmin and SMA. The most specific of these markers is CD117, which corresponds to the c-kit protein.[16]

These histopathologic and immunohistochemical characteristics are essential to differentiate leiomyoma from GIST, which in turn becomes important in defining management and surveillance strategies.

Approximately 50% of leiomyomas are asymptomatic and incidentally diagnosed, which likely reflects the smaller average size of these masses. Although not absolute, the presence of symptoms seems to trend directly with the increase in size, with symptoms usually presenting once the leiomyoma reaches a dimension of 5 cm.[1] Overall, symptoms tend to be vague and nonspecific in nature and develop over a longer duration than in the case of malignant esophageal lesions. Seremetis and colleagues[12] found that 30% of reviewed cases reported symptoms for more than 5 years and another 30% for 2 to 5 years; of the remaining 40%, the average length of symptom duration was 11 months. In addition, most present with multiple symptoms rather than 1 predominant one.[3]

The most common initial symptoms are dysphagia and/or chest pain. The pain is located usually in the epigastrium and/or retrosternal region and described as a pressurelike pain. The level of the dysphagia and pain vary widely, but in general, these symptoms are less severe and present less acutely compared with esophageal carcinomas.[15] Other frequently encountered symptoms include pyrosis, mild and gradual weight loss (rarely more than 20 lb [9.1 kg]), and nausea.[12] Respiratory symptoms such as dyspnea, recurrent respiratory infections, and cough can occur as well but are uncommon, occurring in approximately 10% of cases.[3] Hemorrhage and ulceration rarely occur with esophageal leiomyomas and constitute an indication for removal.[15]

In regards to the pediatric population, esophageal leiomyomas are more often symptomatic in contrast to adults. In addition, although dysphagia is still the most common presenting symptom in children, unlike in adults, the second most common symptom in pediatric patients is dyspnea, with respiratory symptoms in general being more often encountered.[18]

It is important to distinguish leiomyoma from leiomyomatosis, a benign condition characterized by diffuse smooth muscle proliferation. In leiomyomatosis, there is typically involvement of muscularis propria and muscularis mucosae along the entire length of the esophagus. Most patients, approximately 95%, are symptomatic, and it is often associated with Alport syndrome or other smooth muscle hypertrophy disorders affecting multiple organs.[20]

Although not particularly sensitive or specific, plain chest radiographs are often the first diagnostic modalities to suggest the presence of leiomyoma, leading to its incidental diagnosis. These lesions can be missed if they are small, but if large enough, an esophageal leiomyoma may appear as a smooth, round hyperdense mass in the posterior mediastinum.[3]

Because of its high sensitivity and noninvasive nature, barium swallow study is the best initial diagnostic test. Leiomyoma classically is seen as a smooth, well-defined filling defect with approximately half of the submucosal mass protruding into the lumen as a convex mass and the other half within the esophageal wall. It is often half-moon or crescent shaped and characteristically forms right or slight obtuse angles with the adjacent esophageal wall when seen on lateral view. The mass is usually mobile and nonobstructing, rarely presenting with proximal esophageal dilatation. Over the mass itself, flattened mucosal folds are classically described.[14]

In addition to barium swallow, endoscopic evaluation is mandatory (**Fig. 1**). Although leiomyomas, in the absence of ulceration, would be characterized by normal overlying mucosa and as such would not be well visualized by endoscopy, it is necessary to rule out mucosal abnormalities, which would point toward another cause. The presence and location of the tumor should also be identified.[12] The 4 characteristic endoscopic findings of leiomyoma according to Postlethwait are (1) intact, normal overlying mucosa; (2) tumor projecting into the lumen at varying degrees; (3) tumor mobility with overlying mucosa sliding easily over the mass itself; and (4) possible luminal narrowing but rarely any findings of stenosis or obstruction.[21]

If leiomyoma is suspected, blind endoscopic biopsy is not recommended as it increases the risk for perioperative complications and rarely obtains adequate tissue for diagnosis because of the submucosal location. In regards to the former, endoscopic biopsies increase the risk for adhesions to the mucosa during healing and as a result may complicate surgical enucleation, increasing the risk for violation of the mucosa at the time of resection via that technique.[22]

EUS imaging is emerging as an essential test in the diagnosis and management of leiomyoma. Although esophagoscopy is limited to partial mucosal visualization, EUS imaging allows evaluation of all esophageal layers. As described by Rice[2] and

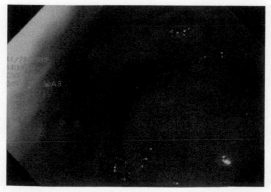

Fig. 1. Endoluminal endoscopic view of leiomyoma.

mentioned earlier, there are 5 alternating hyperechoic and hypoechoic layers visualized on EUS imaging, which in turn represent the mucosal, deep mucosal, submucosal, muscularis propria, and surrounding connective tissue layers, respectively. In the evaluation of an esophageal mass, EUS imaging provides the ability to determine the layer of origin as well as the ability to evaluate for other features such as size, borders, regional lymphadenopathy, echoic pattern, and local invasion.

On EUS imaging, leiomyoma appears as a well-circumscribed, homogenous, hypoechoic mass with smooth borders, arising from the third submucosal layer. There is no regional lymphadenopathy. Findings of size greater than 4 cm, irregular borders, invasion into other layers, and/or regional lymphadenopathy are atypical[14] and would require further workup to rule out malignancy, such as endoscopic biopsy,[22] fine-needle aspiration (FNA) via EUS imaging, and/or surgical enucleation or resection to rule out other causes.[14]

EUS-FNA may be used in conjunction with EUS imaging to obtain cytology and possibly more definitive diagnosis of leiomyoma (**Fig. 2**).[14] Cytology would allow for immunohistochemical analysis as well, which as described earlier, would help differentiate leiomyoma from GIST and leiomyosarcoma. Although EUS-FNA has not been proved more accurate than EUS imaging alone in terms of esophageal submucosal tumors specifically, it has been proved to improve diagnostic accuracy for similar gastric and duodenal tumors, and, accordingly, is worthy of consideration if more definitive diagnosis is needed.[23]

CT may also be performed to evaluate a possible esophageal leiomyoma with an estimated sensitivity of 91%. It is most helpful in evaluating for invasion, the presence of extrinsic compression, and anatomic relationships to nearby structures.[14] Leiomyoma classically appears as a smooth, well-demarcated, round or lobulated mass with homogenously low or isoattenuation. CT scanning does not typically differentiate cystic from solid masses and is therefore limited in its utility for evaluation of intramural pathology.[13]

The treatment of symptomatic leiomyoma is surgical enucleation, either via an open or a thoracoscopic approach (**Fig. 3**) or via laparoscopy for lesions in the distal esophagus or gastroesophageal junction area.[22] The management of asymptomatic leiomyoma, however, is more debatable as suggested by the natural history studies outlined earlier. In the past, the recommendation was to excise every esophageal leiomyoma diagnosed.[3,15] However, it has been demonstrated that leiomyoma rarely progresses to malignant leiomyosarcoma and often remains stable in size for years.[1]

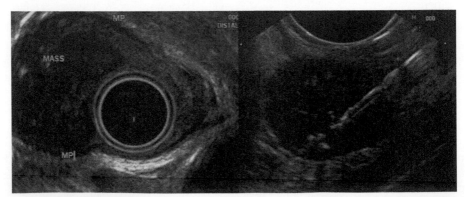

Fig. 2. EUS view of leiomyoma (*left*) and FNA needle in same under EUS guidance (*right*).

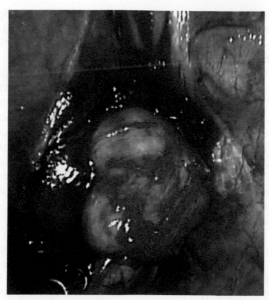

Fig. 3. Esophageal leiomyoma undergoing thoracoscopic enucleation. (*Courtesy of* Stephen R. Hazelrigg, MD, Department of Surgery, Southern Illinois University School of Medicine, IL.)

In general, the indications for surgery for leiomyoma is the presence of symptoms; size greater than 4 cm[14]; atypical findings on studies concerning for malignancy such as the presence of irregular borders, regional lymphadenopathy, heterogenous echoic pattern, or mucosal abnormalities; ulceration; and increase in size.[22] If the leiomyoma is small and asymptomatic, it may be followed with surveillance endoscopy and EUS imaging with or without chest CT every 6 to 12 months and perhaps at longer intervals if stability is demonstrated over time along with continuing asymptomatic clinical status.[14]

The technique for surgical removal of leiomyoma is enucleation via an open or a minimally invasive approach. In the past, thoracotomy or laparotomy was the standard approach.[9] The first documented thoracoscopic enucleation was by Everitt in 1992,[22] and since then, there has been a shift toward minimally invasive techniques. Multiple studies have been performed comparing open and minimally invasive approaches, and the overall mortality is not significantly different between the 2 approaches.[24–26] Minimally invasive techniques are associated with decreased postoperative respiratory complications, shorter hospital stays, and improved postoperative pain control and hence have become more standard as skills and instrumentation appropriate for such strategies have evolved.[25,26]

For the open technique, the approach depends on the location of the tumor. A right thoracotomy would be indicated to reach tumors of the upper two-thirds of the esophagus and left thoracotomy for those of the lower one-third and of intrathoracic location. For tumors of the intra-abdominal portion of the esophagus, including those involving the gastroesophageal junction, laparoscopy or laparotomy may be indicated. Intraoperative endoscopy and ultrasonography can be used to facilitate identification of the tumor and also to evaluate for possible intraoperative mucosal injury.[17]

The specific techniques in regards to right or left thoracoscopy or laparoscopy are generally the same with minimally invasive techniques. The placement of the trocars depends on the location of the lesion, and as in most minimally invasive strategies, the lesion should be in the base of a baseball diamond trocar configuration with the camera on the opposite corner of the diamond and working ports at the other angles of the same. Single lung ventilation is crucial for exposure of the mediastinum if a thoracoscopic approach is used.[25,26]

Regardless of open or minimally invasive technique, the key principles regarding the surgical enucleation of leiomyoma are largely the same. A longitudinal myotomy is created just over the tumor itself, taking care to stay over its apex, and after splitting the muscular coat, the tumor is visualized, often as a well-circumscribed, avascular mass. Blunt dissection is used to separate the tumor from the mucosa, often with the placement of a traction suture in the mass to facilitate the process, with the goal of avoiding violation of the mucosa itself.[22] This procedure can usually be accomplished without difficulty, noting that the risk of mucosal injury may be increased if preoperative endoscopic biopsy was performed.[17] If there are dense adhesions between the tumor and mucosa, possible malignancy must be considered as well, in which case frozen section may be indicated, recognizing that it may or may not be conclusive.[27]

After completing enucleation of the tumor, the presence of mucosal injuries can be evaluated with the use of intraoperative endoscopy and insufflation, and any injuries should be repaired with interrupted absorbable sutures.[17] Finally, it is recommended to reapproximate the myotomy muscle edges at the end to avoid possible postoperative mucosal bulging, diverticulum formation, and associated dysphagia and/or gastroesophageal reflux disease (GERD) symptoms.[9,17,22,24,25]

Variations of surgical enucleation include the balloon push-out method, a thoracoscopic approach with assistance of a balloon-mounted endoscope to promote intraluminal expulsion of the tumor from the esophageal wall,[14] and robotic-assisted thoracoscopic enucleation.[27,28]

Up to 10% of esophageal leiomyomas may require esophagectomy. In general, the indications for esophagectomy are size greater than 8 to 10 cm, annular morphology, multiple or diffuse involvement, extensive damage and/or ulceration to the mucosa, or presence of or suspicion for leiomyosarcoma.[12] Esophagectomy is more commonly required in the pediatric population because of the increased incidence of multiple tumors and diffuse esophageal involvement as detailed earlier.[18]

The mortality associated with open esophagectomy is 10.5% in adults[22] and up to 21% in children[18] and is primarily related to the risk of anastomotic leak and associated sepsis as well as pulmonary complications. The mortality of open enucleation is approximately 1.3%. There have been no reported deaths with patients treated with minimally invasive enucleation.[22]

Most patients treated with enucleation report complete resolution of their symptoms. According to a retrospective review by Jiang and colleagues[24] of 40 cases of thoracoscopic enucleation of leiomyoma, all patients had complete resolution of their symptoms at a mean follow-up of 27 months. In addition, there have been no documented cases of recurrence of leiomyoma after surgical removal. Postoperative complications are uncommon but include esophageal leak due to mucosal injury and GERD. The development of postoperative GERD is most likely due to a disturbance of esophageal motility or lower esophageal sphincter function and may require future fundoplication; however, it is overall uncommon and, as such, routine fundoplication with enucleation is not recommended.[17]

Endoscopic excision of leiomyoma is possible. This strategy may be especially appropriate for the occasional leiomyoma of muscularis mucosal origin with an intraluminal or polypoid growth pattern. In general, pedunculated lesions of this type are removed via endoscopic snare techniques. Endoscopic mucosal resection (EMR) has also become more popular in recent years for a variety of mucosal and submucosal pathologic conditions. As pertains to leiomyomas, submucosal saline injection followed by cap-fitted endoscopic snaring typical of EMR methodology has been described for more wide-based yet smaller lesions up to 2 cm in size. Ethanol injection also has been used as a tool for facilitating lesion necrosis and involution, yet the experience in the United States is limited.[9,14] Finally, endoscopic submucosal dissection (ESD) techniques continue to evolve and may become a more prevalent option for enucleation via an endoluminal approach in years to come, particularly again for lesions originating from the muscularis mucosa.

Gastrointestinal Stromal Tumor

The second most common esophageal mesenchymal tumor is the GIST. Even though these lesions have malignant potential, many behave in a benign manner, and these lesions are thought to be worthy of discussion for several reasons, including their similarities to other mesenchymal benign tumors, as well as the fact that GISTs must be distinguished from other lesions to make appropriate treatment decisions. Less than 5% of GISTs are found in the esophagus compared with 60% in the stomach and 30% in the small intestine.[19]

Based on the finding of shared expression of CD117 and CD34, GISTs are thought to arise from the interstitial cells of Cajal, also known as the GI pacemaker cells, and/or the intestinal mesenchymal precursor cells.

Most of these tumors present between the fifth and seventh decades of life. In a review of 17 esophageal GISTs by Miettinen and colleagues, the median age of presentation was 63 years, with a range from 49 to 75 years.[19] These tumors are rarely found before the age of 40 years, and the diagnosis of a GIST in a younger patient may suggest a lesion of particularly malignant potential. Like leiomyomas, approximately half are asymptomatic. Of the remaining, the most common presenting symptom is dysphagia followed by chest discomfort. Other less common symptoms include cough, gradual mild weight loss, and GI bleeding.

Similar to most other benign esophageal tumors, GISTs of the esophagus are most often located in the distal third and may extend to involve the gastroesophageal junction.[16,27] Sizes are widely variable. In a series by Miettinen of 17 esophageal GISTs, most were less than 10 cm, with a median size of 8 cm and range from 2.6 to 25 cm.[19]

The characteristic histologic findings include overall basophilic appearance with high cellularity and mild-to-no nuclear pleomorphism on hematoxylin-eosin staining. Like gastric GISTs, approximately 70% to 80% of esophageal GISTs are spindle cell tumors and the rest, predominately epithelioid tumors. The spindle cell form can present histologically with growth of tumors cells in solid sheets or in myxoid, pseudo-organoid, palisading, or perivascular collar patterns. Coagulation necrosis may be seen as well, but lymphatic or vascular or diffuse mucosal invasion is uncommon. Mitotic figures are more often found in GISTs than in leiomyomas, where they are quite rare. However, mitotic activity can still vary widely among GISTs and plays a key role in predicting malignant potential, as described in more detail later in discussion.[16]

As mentioned in the leiomyoma section, GISTs previously were classified alongside leiomyoma, schwannoma, and other mesenchymal tumors, but recent studies and discoveries have shown GISTs to be distinct from these other mesenchymal tumors. Although gross and histologic features may help differentiate GISTs from other similar tumors, the best method of distinction is immunohistochemical testing. The most reliable marker is the expression of c-kit protein, CD117, which is uniformly seen in GISTs. In addition, the vast majority also express CD34. In turn, GISTs are almost never positive for desmin, and most do not stain positive for α-smooth muscle actin

(SMA) either. Most studies show an approximately 20% to 40% frequency of SMA positivity in all GISTs throughout the GI tract, and the expression is usually partial and focal in comparison with the diffuse reactivity seen in leiomyomas.[16] Furthermore, GISTs are negative for S-100 as well in comparison with schwannomas.[19] These markers are invaluable in distinguishing these lesions and guiding decisions regarding management that are linked to underlying histology and the associated potential for future malignant behavior, which is significantly higher for GISTs.[16]

Because GISTs are also intramural esophageal tumors, the diagnostic workup is similar to that of leiomyoma. Typical workup includes a contrast swallow study, EGD, and EUS imaging, and findings are usually similar to leiomyoma, which makes distinguishing between the 2 tumors difficult based solely on such criteria.

Overall, approximately 70% of all GISTs are benign. In the past, these tumors were classified as benign or malignant based on mitotic activity and size, but studies have shown that prediction and classification of GISTs into those with benign versus malignant behavior can be challenging.[29] As a result, the National Institutes of Health (NIH) developed a classification scheme for GISTs in general, categorizing these tumors into 4 categories of risk for recurrence and metastasis, specifically very low risk, low risk, intermediate risk, and high risk, based on mitotic activity and size (**Table 1**).[30]

Although the NIH classification can provide some guidance in distinguishing low- and high-risk GISTs in regards to malignant potential, small size and/or low mitotic activity does not guarantee benign behavior. Other favorable prognostic factors include gastric location, low proliferation index, absence of infiltration to adjacent organs, DNA diploidy in G2 peak on flow cytometry, and possibly female gender and younger age.[19] In regards to esophageal GISTs in particular, mitotic index and size are not proven prognostic factors, possibly in part due to the low incidence.[31] Esophageal GISTs are more commonly aggressive and malignant histologically. Miettinen and colleagues reported in their series of 17 esophageal GISTs a mortality rate of 59% with a median survival of 27 months. One disease-associated death occurred in a patient with a mitotic rate less than 5 mitoses per 50 high-power field (HPF), again underlining the inconsistent relationship between malignant behavior and mitotic rate.[17]

Although it is important to differentiate GIST from leiomyoma for the reasons outlined, it is often difficult because the findings of the typical diagnostic studies of contrast swallow, EGD, and EUS imaging frequently overlap between the 2 entities. Occasionally, mucosal changes may be seen with GISTs in a manner less common with leiomyomas, which rarely are associated with such findings as mentioned previously. The appearance of ulceration, Barrett esophagus, and/or esophagitis accordingly calls for further investigation to rule out GIST as well as other possible malignant tumors such as carcinoma. However, mucosal changes are still uncommon.

Table 1	
Risk classification for GIST tumors	
Classification	**Size and/or Mitotic Activity**
Very low risk	<2 cm and <5 mitoses/50 HPF
Low risk	2–5 cm and <5 mitoses/50 HPF
Intermediate risk	<5 cm and 6–10 mitoses/50 HPF 5–10 cm and <5 mitoses/50 HPF
High risk	>5 cm and >5 mitoses/50 HPF >10 cm and mitotic rate any size and >10 mitoses/50 HPF

Abbreviation: HPF, high-power field.

Consequently, the addition of a PET scan[29] and/or FNA via EUS imaging may provide further assistance in distinguishing between GISTs and leiomyomas.[31]

GISTs are PET-avid, especially malignant GISTs, in comparison with leiomyomas.[29] Furthermore, FNA may be performed under EUS guidance and provide adequate tissue for immunohistochemical testing for CD117, CD34, and other markers. Blum and colleagues[27] recommended addition of EUS-FNA for any intramural esophageal tumor larger than 2 cm, demonstrating positive growth on serial surveillance examination and/or manifesting increased PET scan activity.

Although initially small GISTs may be observed with serial examinations similar to leiomyoma, once the actual diagnosis of GIST has been made, the management changes and usually entails a combination of medical and surgical treatments, specifically with complete resection of the mass.[23]

The management of GISTs has significantly changed in recent years because of introduction of imatinib, a monoclonal antibody inhibiting the tyrosine-kinase c-kit protein. Imatinib use is indicated for unresectable, recurrent, or residual GISTs and, in turn, can be used as primary, adjuvant, or neoadjuvant treatment. Its addition has led to a significant increase in median survival of patients with advanced GIST from approximately 20 to 60 months. Adjuvant imatinib is recommended for most patients for 2 years, including those with residual disease after resection or larger primary tumors. Serial CT and/or PET scans can help track disease response, which may be manifest as a decrease in tumor attenuation more so than size and decrease in maximum standard uptake value on PET.[32]

Along with the use of imatinib, complete surgical excision is recommended whenever possible and is still associated with the best chance for survival. Although the standard of surgical treatment is complete excision,[23,27,32] the optimal extent of surgery with regards to margin sizes and approaches has not yet been well defined[23]; however, negative margins without lymphadenectomy is generally considered an adequate resection.[27] Enucleation may be performed via open or minimally invasive approaches for smaller tumors of low malignant potential.[23] In general, an open approach may be preferred in the setting of known preoperative diagnosis of GIST because of the poor integrity of the tumor and high frequency of adhesions to the mucosa or submucosa,[27] but personal surgical experience may also play a role in determining the approach in such settings.

For larger tumors, esophagectomy with gastric tube reconstruction is recommended. The specific size threshold for enucleation versus esophagectomy has also not been well established. Blum and colleagues[27] recommended esophagectomy for GISTs greater than 2 cm, whereas Lee and colleagues[23] reported safe excision via enucleation of tumors up to 5 cm in size. The concurrent findings of mucosal and/or muscular invasion, involvement of the gastroesophageal junction, and other features relating to risk of malignant behavior as outlined play a role in determining the best approach and extent of resection. The techniques of enucleation and esophagectomy otherwise are similar to those described for leiomyomas. In comparison with leiomyoma, it is frequently difficult to assess adequacy of the resection intraoperatively because of the occasional presence of adhesions to surrounding layers blurring anatomic planes and the unreliability of frozen section to assess adequate margins. The adequacy of resection can only be assessed with immunohistochemical staining, which determines the presence or absence of tumors cells along the excised borders.

In the past, esophageal GISTs have been associated with poor prognosis with high mortality and recurrence rates. Blum and colleagues[27] cited only a 14% 5-year survival rate, but the addition of imatinib has significantly changed the outcomes and prognoses. Shingare and colleagues[33] in a series of 7 patients, all treated with imatinib and 3 with surgical excision, found no disease progression or metastasis in all patients at the end of mean follow-up of 26 months. The availability of newer-generation tyrosine kinase inhibitors for patients not responding to imatinib, such as gefitinib, erlotinib, and sunitinib, offers hope for alternative therapies focused on underlying tumor biology with these lesions.

Schwannoma

Schwannoma is the least common esophageal mesenchymal tumor. In general, they are uncommonly found in the GI tract, and of these, most occur in the stomach.[33] Esophageal schwannoma is extremely rare, with less than 30 reported cases in the literature.[34]

These submucosal tumors arise from the Schwann cells of the neural plexus within the GI tract wall, and although they can occur at any age, they most commonly present during middle age, between 50 and 60 years.[35] In a literature review of 19 reported cases, Murase and colleagues[37] reported a median age of 54 years, with a range from 10 to 79 years. In addition, there is a mild female predominance, with reported male to female ratios ranging from 1:1.6 and 1:2.8.

Unlike other benign esophageal tumors, schwannomas are located most frequently in the upper esophagus, specifically the cervical and upper thoracic regions. Size varies widely, ranging from less than 0.5 cm to up to 15 to 16 cm. Similar to leiomyoma and GIST, schwannoma is often asymptomatic, and if symptomatic, the most common presenting symptoms are dysphagia and chest discomfort.[36]

Grossly, these tumors are yellow-white to tan and appear rubbery and/or firm with glistening, smooth surfaces. They may appear trabeculated without necrosis or hemorrhage on cut surface. Histologically, schwannomas feature peripheral lymphoid cuffs composed of lymphoid follicles, moderate cellularity, and broad bundles, interlacing fascicles, or whorls of elongated cells.[37] Additional histologic characteristics also include nuclear palisading, intermixing collagen fibers, nuclear pleomorphism with evenly distributed chromatin, and inflammatory cell infiltrates composed of plasma cells and lymphocytes. The presence of the distinctive peripheral lymphoid cuff ranges from complete to partial between tumors, and may be missed depending on sectioning, but when seen, is pathognomonic for schwannoma.[36,37]

The diagnostic workup for schwannoma is similar to that of leiomyoma and GIST, consisting of contrast swallow study, EGD, and EUS imaging. CT and PET scans can also be added for further details, as mentioned previously.[36] Schwannomas characteristically appear homogenous on postenhanced CT images.[34] However, the findings from these diagnostic tests for schwannoma usually overlap with those of other submucosal tumors, including GIST, and immunohistochemical testing is required for definitive diagnosis. Adding EUS-FNA or proceeding to surgical excision may provide adequate tissue for such testing, and schwannomas characteristically express S-100 protein as well as vimentin and glial fibrillary acidic protein. On the other hand, they are negative for CD117, CD34, desmin, and SMA, thus allowing for differentiation from GISTs and leiomyomas.[16,38,39]

The management of schwannomas is similar to that of leiomyomas. Smaller, asymptomatic ones may be observed with serial examinations.[38] Indications for excision include larger size (generally >2 cm), the presence of symptoms, and/or the findings of growth on serial examinations. Schwannomas less than 2 cm may be safely excised endoscopically.[36] Larger ones may be enucleated through thoracotomy or thoracoscopy.[34,35,39]

There is a malignant potential associated with schwannomas as well with 3 to 4 reported cases of malignant schwannoma in the literature. The malignancy criteria are histologic and based on mitotic activity, cellularity, nuclear atypia, and presence of tumor necrosis. Of these, mitotic rate is the most reliable. The presence of 5 or more mitotic figures per 50 HPF correlates most strongly with malignancy. In the setting of malignant disease, complete surgical excision is necessary, and although some studies suggest enucleation may be adequate for smaller tumors with intact mucosa and absent local invasion, the standard is still esophagectomy.[39]

Granular Cell Tumor

Granular cell tumors (GCTs), historically known as granular cell myoblastomas, were first described by Abrikossoff in the 1920s. They are soft-tissue neoplasms that have a neural origin located in the submucosa. The exact cell type that they originate from is thought to be a Schwann cell because of staining characteristics; however, there is still some debate.

GCTs are mostly benign, but it is reported that 1% to 2% of cases are malignant.[40] GCTs are found in many different tissues, with approximately 1% to 8% located in the GI tract and around one-third of these localized to the esophagus.[41–43] Most of these are found in the distal esophagus.

GCTs are usually asymptomatic and found incidentally during radiological evaluation or endoscopy. When symptomatic they tend to be larger.[44] GCTs present similar to leiomyomas. The most common symptom accordingly is dysphagia; however, they may present with chest pain, cough, nausea, or gastroesophageal reflux. GCTs are often found on contrast radiography or during endoscopy. On endoscopy they appear as pale yellow wide-based polypoid lesions with intact thin mucosa protruding into the lumen. EUS imaging is useful in that it can help determine the size, location, and invading layer of the tumor. The tumor looks hypoechoic and is surrounded with hypoechoic mucosa. Definitive diagnosis can be difficult, and tissue is typically required. Tissue is usually obtained during endoscopy with multiple biopsies taken from the same site to reach the submucosal position. Histologic evaluation and immunostaining are performed to help differentiate malignant from benign tumors.

At present, there is no consensus on the treatment. But if the tumor is determined as benign, there are no instances of malignant transformation reported. However, there is 1% to 3% malignancy rate, and if the malignancy is suspected, resection is indicated. It has been suggested that symptomatic tumors, tumors larger then 10 mm, rapidly growing lesions, and those with histologic features concerning for malignancy be resected.[44,45] Conversely, small, asymptomatic tumors may be biopsied and followed up.[46,47] Historically, surgical treatment when dictated has been a transthoracic approach. However, EMR (**Fig. 4**) has been successful for lesions that do not extend beyond the submuscosal layer.[48–56]

Inflammatory Pseudotumor

Inflammatory pseudotumors are generally localized masses found in the distal esophagus. They arise from the mucosal layer and often appear as pedunculated lesions. It is thought that they originate from underlying injury such as mechanical injury or from ulceration as a result of chronic reflux. Infection with Epstein-Barr virus has been suggested as a cause, as has autoimmune disorders. These lesions can be mistaken for malignancy, so it is important to biopsy them when found for histologic characterization.

Histology of inflammatory pseudotumors show inflammatory changes and are composed of mostly fibroblasts, inflammatory cells, and blood vessels. Once these lesions are determined to not be a malignancy or other pathology mandating other

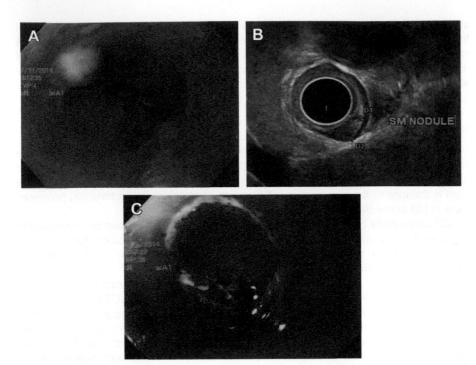

Fig. 4. Granular cell tumor of distal esophagus. (*A*) Endoscopic appearance (*upper left panel*); (*B*) EUS appearance (*upper right panel*); (*C*) after EMR using cap fitted endoscopic band and snare technique (*lower left panel*).

intervention, no specific treatment is required. If chronic reflux is suspected as the cause, treatment of reflux is suggested.

Hemangioma

Hemangiomas are benign vascular tumors that arise from the submucosal layer in the esophagus as a localized hypertrophy of blood vessels. They are benign tumors and represent approximately 3% of all benign tumors of the esophagus.[7] Given their rarity there are no data regarding their demographics. They can be found in the distal esophagus and can present as a solitary lesion or as multiple lesions in association with Rendu-Osler-Weber syndrome. As with other benign tumors of the esophagus, they are often asymptomatic. When symptomatic, their most common symptoms are dysphagia and hematemesis. Hematemesis is often the result of mucosal ulceration overlying the lesion and, given the vascular nature of the lesion, can be minimal or life threatening.

These tumors can be evaluated by several different techniques. On barium esophagography they appear as well-defined submucosal lesions. Endoscopy is often used, and they appear as bluish, polypoid submucosal lesions that are compressible. As opposed to some of the other submucosal lesions mentioned earlier, CT with contrast is particularly useful in confirming a diagnosis and delineating further characteristics.[57] MRI as well as radionuclide study or angiography may also be useful. EUS imaging has started to play an increasing role as it provides further characterization of the lesion including confirming the absence of continuity with major blood vessels.[58,59] Finally, a tissue biopsy may allow a tissue diagnosis; however, this should generally be avoided because of concern for inducing hemorrhage. If a bluish submucosal lesion is found on endoscopy, contrast-enhanced CT scan, radionuclide study, or angiography can establish the diagnosis. Generally, observation of asymptomatic lesions with no occult blood loss is an acceptable option, and signs of ongoing active or otherwise unexplained occult blood loss dictates intervention.

For symptomatic lesions several options have been reported. More recently, hemangiomas have been treated with endoscopic resection, sclerotherapy, radiation, laser fulguration, and video-assisted thoracoscopic resection.[60–63] However, both esophagectomy and tumor enucleation have been performed as well. Given their rarity and an increasing number of options described in their management, a multidisciplinary treatment discussion for symptomatic or bleeding lesions would seem appropriate.

Adenoma

Adenomatous polyps of the esophagus are the result of a benign neoplastic proliferation of columnar cells. They often occur in the distal esophagus and may share the same dysplastic characteristics as colonic adenomas. In the esophagus they have also been found to be associated with Barrett esophagus.[64,65] These polyps may harbor high-grade dysplasia or carcinoma or progress into the same over time. As such, it is recommended that they be removed endoscopically or rigorously sampled and ablated if documented as benign. If high-grade dysplasia or cancer is found, then aggressive surgical resection has historically been advised. EMR may be used for smaller lesions, recognizing that increasingly large lesions are being approached with techniques such as EMR and ESD after careful histologic and EUS evaluation, when appropriate. For sessile or wide-based lesions, aggressive sampling and excisional therapy treatment is indicated, with surgical resection still representing an appropriate consideration for patients of acceptable risk status who exhibit foci of invasive disease or high-grade dysplasia. When associated with Barrett esophagus, focal lesional treatment endoscopically with management of underlying GERD is appropriate, but presence of dysplasia or high-risk markers dictates mucosal ablative therapy.

Papilloma

Squamous papillomas of the esophagus are extremely rare. Their incidence was found to be 0.01% on an autopsy series and 0.07% in an endoscopy series.[66,67] They are more common in older individuals. The exact cause is unknown; however, it is thought that their development is related to chronic gastroesophageal reflux or infection with human papilloma virus or possibly a combination of the two. These lesions tend to be small and solitary and are found most often in the distal esophagus.[66] Rarely, multiple papillomas can be found, which may be associated with a rare condition known as esophageal papillomatosis.[68]

The lesions are generally asymptomatic and identified incidentally on endoscopy. Rarely, they may cause dysphagia. They are generally small, less than 1 cm, solitary, sessile projections that are generally pink and appear fleshy on endoscopy. Often they can be confused with squamous carcinoma, so it is imperative that they be biopsied. EUS imaging may be performed to determine the noninvasive nature of the lesion, but once diagnosed by biopsy, further workup is not indicated. There has only been one case of malignant transformation of an esophageal papilloma.[69] Resection of a papilloma is indicated if it is symptomatic due to obstruction, if it has atypical histologic features, or if malignancy cannot be ruled out. Endoscopic resection (EMR) is the treatment of choice. However, if this is not possible or cancer is still a concern after resection, then an esophagotomy with local resection can be performed.

Fibrovascular Polyp

Fibrovascular polyps are the most common benign intraluminal tumor of the esophagus. They are mostly located in the upper esophagus, generally located distal to the cricopharyngeus in the posterior midline above the confluence of the longitudinal layer of esophageal muscle called Lamier triangle. These lesions are the product of submucosal thickening that progresses to polypoid formation. They can be long because of peristalsis and its effect on the lesion once it develops.[70] They may have spectacular presentations, such as regurgitation from the mouth or even causing sudden death due to asphyxia.[11] It is most likely the aforementioned first case of resection of an esophageal tumor by Dallas-Monro was of this type, since the description was of a regurgitated, pedunculated tumor.

Contrast esophagography shows a large sausagelike elongated tumor.[11] CT and MRI may demonstrate heterogenous attenuation based on the relative amount of adipose and fibrous tissue.[71] Endoscopy demonstrates a fleshy, sausagelike elongated lesion typically arising from the postcricopharyngeal, posterior location outlined earlier.[70]

Once diagnosed, removal is recommended because of the risk for fatal airway complications. The resection planning is developed by information obtained by endoscopy and EUS imaging. The vascularity of the stalk, location, and size dictate the method of resection.[52] Smaller lesions are easily removed endoscopically with either direct snare or EMR techniques. It is recommended to have airway control during endoscopic procedures performed for this pathologic condition to minimize the risk of airway complications during the procedure. Larger lesions or those with abundant blood flow in the stalk demonstrated on EUS imaging require longitudinal esophagotomy on the opposite side of the tumor origin. The tumor stalk is ligated and resected, followed by 2-layer closure of the esophagotomy.[72]

EXTRAESOPHAGEAL TUMORS
Cysts and Duplications

Cysts and duplications are not neoplasms but malformations of the esophagus. They can cause symptoms similar to those of the lesions already discussed by creating mass effects and collectively constitute the second most common tumorlike condition of the esophagus. They can originate not only from the foregut itself but also from developmental aberrations of the trachea that may manifest with dysphagia, hemorrhage, and infection. Other cystic lesions besides congenital developmental cysts and duplications can include inclusion and neuroenteric cysts.

Histologically, esophageal duplication cysts have muscular and epithelial layers and an intramural component. Bronchogenic cysts originate from lung primordia and typically have cartilage in them. Inclusion cysts conversely have similar epithelial lining as esophageal duplications, yet there is no muscle or cartilage. The neuroenteric cysts are malformations resulting from aberrant separation of the foregut from the primitive spinal column. They are posterior in location and often associated with other spinal abnormalities such as spina bifida.[10]

Presenting symptoms in younger patients can include dysphagia or airway symptoms such as wheezing and stridor. In older patients, these lesions may present with infection, dysphagia, chest pain, hemorrhage, fistulization, and malignant transformation.[70]

Diagnosis is made by a combination of esophagography (**Fig. 5**), endoscopy and EUS imaging, and CT (**Fig. 6**) or MRI. These lesions are generally not biopsied because the resulting scar tissue from these biopsies may make future resection more challenging. If a smooth lesion is seen on endoscopy and EUS imaging documents the fluid-filled nature of the lesion (**Fig. 7**), a cross-sectional imaging study is typically obtained next to

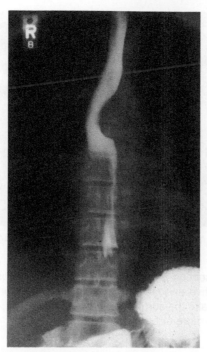

Fig. 5. Extrinsic compression of esophagus due to adjacent cystic lesion on barium study. (*Courtesy of* Stephen R. Hazelrigg, MD, Department of Surgery, Southern Illinois University School of Medicine, IL.)

further delineate the characteristics and extent of the pathology for operative planning purposes. On cross-sectional imaging, the fluid-filled nature of the lesion is typically confirmed, although previous infections can make this determination difficult because the attenuation of the fluid is thicker in such cysts. In those situations, the findings on EUS imaging are used in a complimentary manner for establishing the diagnosis. As for all posterior mediastinal tumors, if the cyst appears to be neuroenteric, an MRI and neurosurgical consultation may be appropriate in preoperative planning.

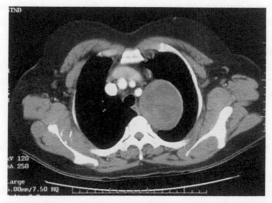

Fig. 6. Posterior mediastinal cyst compressing esophagus. (*Courtesy of* Stephen R. Hazelrigg, MD, Department of Surgery, Southern Illinois University School of Medicine, IL.)

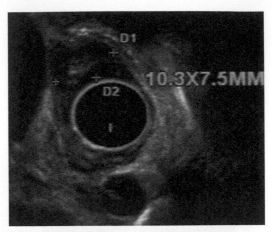

Fig. 7. Radial EUS image of intramural duplication cyst of esophagus.

Once diagnosed, resection is recommended, and thoracoscopy is typically successful with intraoperative endoscopic assistance.[73] A history of previous biopsies and/or infection may make the surgical resection challenging, and in such instances, thoracotomy should be more strongly considered.

SUMMARY

Given the rarity of benign esophageal tumors, the clinician must have a thorough grasp of their causes, behaviors, and respective management strategies. Many of these lesions may be safely observed if they are asymptomatic and stable on serial assessment. Symptomatic and larger or growing lesions require more careful characterization by EUS imaging, FNA, and cross-sectional imaging to guide therapeutic decision making. A familiarity with related medical conditions such as GERD and Barrett esophagus, with the distinctive patterns of disease characterizing pediatric and adult patient groups, and with the biologic complexities characterizing behavior and treatment of pathologies such as GISTs, is a requisite cognitive skill set for the managing provider. Removal of symptomatic lesions can be approached increasingly by minimally invasive methods and with some pathologies with advancing endoluminal resective techniques. Surgeons managing these patients should either have the current skills necessary for their management, including skills in minimally invasive thoracoscopic and laparoscopic surgery as well as therapeutic endoscopy and EUS imaging, or participate in multidisciplinary treatment teams that include individuals with these skills. With appropriate characterization of the pathologic condition, these lesions are increasingly able to be appropriately managed with techniques that can optimize outcomes and limit both short- and long-term morbidity and risk for the patient.

REFERENCES

1. Choong CK, Meyers BF. Benign esophageal tumors: introduction, incidence, classification, and clinical features. Semin Thorac Cardiovasc Surg 2003;15: 3–8 No. 1. WB Saunders.
2. Rice TW. Benign esophageal tumors: esophagoscopy and endoscopic esophageal ultrasound. Semin Thorac Cardiovasc Surg 2003;15:20–6 No. 1. WB Saunders.

3. Watson RR, O'Connor TM, Weisel W. Solid benign tumors of the esophagus. Ann Thorac Surg 1967;4(1):80–91.
4. Storey CF, Adams WC Jr. Leiomyoma of the esophagus: a report of four cases and review of the surgical literature. Am J Surg 1956;91(1):3–23.
5. Patterson EJ. Benign neoplasms of the esophagus: report of a case of myxofibroma. Ann Otol Rhinol Laryngol 1932;41(3):942–50.
6. Moersch HJ. Benign tumor of the esophagus. Ann Otol Rhinol Laryngol 1944;53: 800–17.
7. Plachta A. Benign tumors of the esophagus. Review of literature and report of 99 cases. Am J Gastroenterol 1962;38:639–52.
8. Attah EB, Hajdu SI. Benign and malignant tumors of the esophagus at autopsy. J Thorac Cardiovasc Surg 1968;55(3):396.
9. Mutrie CJ, Donahue DM, Wain JC, et al. Esophageal leiomyoma: a 40-year experience. Ann Thorac Surg 2005;79(4):1122–5.
10. Arbona JL, Fazzi JG, Mayoral J. Congenital esophageal cysts: case report and review of literature. Am J Gastroenterol 1984;79(3):177–82.
11. Levine MS, Buck JL, Pantongrag-Brown L, et al. Fibrovascular polyps of the esophagus: clinical, radiographic, and pathologic findings in 16 patients. AJR Am J Roentgenol 1996;166:781–7.
12. Seremetis MG, Lyons WS, deGuzman VC, et al. Leiomyomata of the esophagus. An analysis of 838 cases. Cancer 1976;38:2166–77.
13. Levine MS. Benign tumors of the esophagus: radiologic evaluation. Semin Thorac Cardiovasc Surg 2003;15:9–19 No. 1. WB Saunders.
14. Lee LS, Singhal S, Brinster CJ, et al. Current management of esophageal leiomyoma. J Am Coll Surg 2004;198:136–46.
15. Hatch GF III, George F, Hatch KF, et al. Tumors of the esophagus. World J Surg 2000;24:401–11.
16. Miettinen M, Sarlomo-Rikala M, Sobin LH, et al. Esophageal stromal tumors: a clinicopathologic, immunohistochemical, and molecular genetic study of 17 cases and comparison with esophageal leiomyomas and leiomyosarcomas. Am J Surg Pathol 2000;24:211–22.
17. Kent M, d'Amato T, Nordman C, et al. Minimally invasive resection of benign esophageal tumors. J Thorac Cardiovasc Surg 2007;134:176–81.
18. Bourque MD, Spigland N, Bensoussan AL, et al. Esophageal leiomyoma in children: two case reports and review of the literature. J Pediatr Surg 1989;24: 1103–7.
19. Miettinen M, Lasota J. Gastrointestinal stromal tumors–definition, clinical, histological, immunohistochemical, and molecular genetic features and differential diagnosis. Virchows Arch 2001;438:1–12.
20. Calabrese C, Fabbri A, Fusaroli P, et al. Diffuse esophageal leiomyomatosis: case report and review. Gastrointest Endosc 2002;55:590–3.
21. Postlethwait RW. Benign tumors and cysts of the esophagus. Surg Clin North Am 1983;63:925–31.
22. Samphire J, Nafteux P, Luketich J. Minimally invasive techniques for resection of benign esophageal tumors. Semin Thorac Cardiovasc Surg 2003;15:35–43 No. 1. WB Saunders.
23. Lee HJ, Park SI, Kim DK, et al. Surgical resection of esophageal gastrointestinal stromal tumors. Ann Thorac Surg 2009;87:1569–71.
24. Jiang G, Zhao H, Yang F, et al. Thoracoscopic enucleation of esophageal leiomyoma: a retrospective study on 40 cases. Dis Esophagus 2009;22: 279–83.

25. Von Rahden BH, Stein HJ, Feussner H, et al. Enucleation of submucosal tumors of the esophagus: minimally invasive versus open approach. Surg Endosc 2004;18: 924–30.
26. Zaninotto G, Portale G, Costantini M, et al. Minimally invasive enucleation of esophageal leiomyoma. Surg Endosc 2006;20:1904–8.
27. Blum MG, Bilimoria KY, Wayne JD, et al. Surgical considerations for the management and resection of esophageal gastrointestinal stromal tumors. Ann Thorac Surg 2007;84:1717–23.
28. Bodner JC, Zitt M, Ott H, et al. Robotic-assisted thoracoscopic surgery (RATS) for benign and malignant esophageal tumors. Ann Thorac Surg 2005;80:1202–6.
29. Chang WC, Tzao C, Shen DH, et al. Gastrointestinal stromal tumor (GIST) of the esophagus detected by positron emission tomography/computed tomography. Dig Dis Sci 2005;50:1315–8.
30. Joensuu H. Risk stratification of patients diagnosed with gastrointestinal stromal tumor. Hum Pathol 2008;39:1411–9.
31. Emory TS, Sobin LH, Lukes L, et al. Prognosis of gastrointestinal smooth-muscle (stromal) tumors: dependence on anatomic site. Am J Surg Pathol 1999;23: 82–7.
32. Portale G, Zaninotto G, Costantini M, et al. Esophageal GIST: case report of surgical enucleation and update on current diagnostic and therapeutic options. Int J Surg Pathol 2007;15:393–6.
33. Shinagare AB, Zukotynski KA, Krajewski KM, et al. Esophageal gastrointestinal stromal tumor: report of 7 patients. Cancer Imaging 2012;12:100–8.
34. Kwon MS, Lee SS, Ahn GH. Schwannomas of the gastrointestinal tract: clinicopathological features of 12 cases including a case of esophageal tumor compared with those of gastrointestinal stromal tumors and leiomyomas of the gastrointestinal tract. Pathol Res Pract 2002;198:605–13.
35. Yoon HY, Kim CB, Lee YH, et al. An obstructing large schwannoma in the esophagus. J Gastrointest Surg 2008;12:761–3.
36. Kobayashi N, Kikuchi S, Shimao H, et al. Benign esophageal schwannoma: report of a case. Surg Today 2000;30:526–9.
37. Murase K, Hino A, Ozeki Y, et al. Malignant schwannoma of the esophagus with lymph node metastasis: literature review of schwannoma of the esophagus. J Gastroenterol 2001;36:772–7.
38. Iwata H, Kataoka M, Yamakawa Y, et al. Esophageal schwannoma. Ann Thorac Surg 1993;56:376–7.
39. Hou YY, Tan YS, Xu JF, et al. Schwannoma of the gastrointestinal tract: a clinicopathological, immunohistochemical and ultrastructural study of 33 cases. Histopathology 2006;48:536–45.
40. Fanburg-smith JC, Meis-Kindblom JM, Fante R, et al. Malignant granular cell tumor of soft tissue: diagnostic criteria and clinicopathologic correlation. Am J Surg Pathol 1998;22:779–94.
41. Lack EE, Worsham GF, Callihan MD, et al. Granular cell tumor: a clinicopathlogic study of 110 patients. J Surg Oncol 1980;13:301–16.
42. McSwain GR, Colpitt R, Kreutner A, et al. Granular cell myoblastoma. Surg Gynecol Obstet 1980;150:703–10.
43. Johnston J, Helwig EB. Granular cell tumors of the gastrointestinal tract and perineal region: a study of 74 cases. Dig Dis Sci 1981;26:807–16.
44. Coutinho DS, Soga J, Yoshikawa T, et al. Granular cell tumors or the esophagus: a report of two cases and review of the literature. Am J Gastroenterol 1985;80:758.

45. Percinel S, Savas B, Yilmaz G, et al. Granular cell tumor of the esophagus: report of 5 cases and review of diagnostic and therapeutic techniques. Dis Esophagus 2007;20:435–43.
46. Voskuil J, Van Dijk MM, Wagenaar SS, et al. Occurrence of esophageal granular cell tumors in the Netherlands between 1988 and 1994. Dig Dis Sci 2001;24: 1610–4.
47. Mineo TC, Biancari F, Francioni, et al. Conservative approach to granular cell tumor of the esophagus: three case reports. Scand Cardiovasc J 1995;29:141–4.
48. Hyun JH, Jeen YT, Chu HJ, et al. Endoscopic resection of submucosal tumor of the esophagus: result in 62 patients. Endoscopy 1997;29:165–70.
49. Fujiwara Y, Watanabe T, Hamasaki N, et al. Endoscopic resection of two granular cell tumours of the oesophagus. Eur J Gastroenterol Hepatol 1999;11:1413–6.
50. Fotiadis C, Manolis EN, Troupis TG, et al. Endoscopic resection of a large granular cell tumor of the esophagus. J Surg Oncol 2000;75:277–9.
51. van der Peet DL, Berends FJ, Klinkengerg-Knol EC, et al. Endoscopic treatment of benign esophageal tumors: case report of three patients. Surg Endosc 2001; 15:1489.
52. Kinney T, Waxman I. Treatment of benign esophageal tumors by endoscopic techniques. Semin Thorac Cardiovasc Surg 2003;15:27–34.
53. Wehrmann T, Martchenko K, Nakamura M, et al. Endoscopic resection of submucosal esophageal tumors: a prospective case series. Endoscopy 2004;36:802–7.
54. Bataglia G, Rampado S, Bocus P, et al. Single-band mucosectomy of granular cell tumor of the esophagus: safe and easy technique. Surg Endosc 2006;20: 1296–8.
55. Zhong N, Katzka DA, Smyrk TC, et al. Endoscopic diagnosis and resection of esophageal granular cell tumors. Dis Esophagus 2011;24:438–543.
56. Kahng DH, Kim GH, Park DY, et al. Endoscopic resection of granular cell tumors in the gastrointestinal tract: a single center experience. Surg Endosc 2013;27: 3228–36.
57. Taylor FH, Fowler FC, Betsill WL, et al. Hemangioma of the esophagus. Ann Thorac Surg 1996;61:726.
58. Tominaga K, Arakawa T, Ando K, et al. Oesophageal cavernous haemangioma diagnosed histologically, not by endoscopic procedures. J Gastroenterol Hepatol 2000;15:215–9.
59. Cantero D, Yoshida T, Ito M, et al. Esophageal hemangioma:endoscopic diagnosis and treatment. Endoscopy 1994;26:250–3.
60. Yoshikane H, Suzuki T, Yoshioka N, et al. Hemangioma of the esophagus. Endoscopic imaging and endoscopic resection. Endoscopy 1995;27:267.
61. Shigemitsu K, Naomoto Y, Yamatsuji T, et al. Esophageal hemangioma successfully treated by fulguration using potassium titanyl phosphate/yttrium aluminum garnet (KTP/YAG) laser: a case report. Dis Esophagus 2000;13:161.
62. Aoki T, Okagawa K, Uemura Y, et al. Successful treatment of an esophageal hemangioma by endoscopic injection sclerotherapy: report of a case. Surg Today 1997;27:450.
63. Ramo OJ, Salo JA, Bardini R, et al. Treatment of a submucosal hemangioma of the esophagus using simultaneous video-assisted thoracoscopy and esophagoscopy: Description of a new minimally invasive technique. Endoscopy 1997;29: S27–8.
64. Lee RG. Adenomas arising in Barrett's esophagus. Am J Clin Pathol 1986;85:629–32.
65. McDonald GB, Brand DL, Thorning DR. Multiple adenomatous neoplasms arising in columnar-lined (Barrett's) esophagus. Gastroenterology 1977;72:1317–21.

66. Weitzer S, Hentel W. Squamous papilloma of esophagus. Case report and review of the literature. Am J Gastroenterol 1968;50:391.
67. Mosca S, Manes G, Onaco R, et al. Squamous papilloma of the esophagus: long-term follow up. J Gastroenterol Hepatol 2001;16:857–61.
68. Sandvik AK, Aase S, Kvberg KH, et al. Papillomatosis of the esophagus. J Clin Gastroenterol 1996;22:35–7.
69. Van Cutsem E, Geboes K, Vantrappen G, et al. Malignant degeneration of esophageal squamous papilloma associated with the human papillomavirus. Gastroenterology 1992;103:1119.
70. Pitichote H, Ferguson MK. Minimally invasive treatment of benign esophageal tumors. Surgical management of benign esophageal disorders. Springer-Verlag; 2014. p. 181–99.
71. Ascenti G, Racchiusa S, Mazziotti S, et al. Giant fibrovascular polyp of the esophagus: CT and MR findings. Abdom Imaging 1999;24(2):109–10.
72. Solerio D, Gasparri G, Ruffini E, et al. Giant fibrovascular polyp of the esophagus. Dis Esophagus 2005;18(6):410–2.
73. Hirose S, Clifton MS, Bratton B, et al. Thoracoscopic resection of foregut duplication cysts. J Laparoendosc Adv Surg Tech A 2006;16(5):526–9.

Colonic Polyps
Are We Ready to Resect and Discard?

Cesare Hassan, MD[a],*, Alessandro Repici, MD[a], Angelo Zullo, MD[a], Vijay Kanakadandi, MD[b], Prateek Sharma, MD[b]

KEYWORDS

- Electronic chromoendoscopy • Colonoscopy • Polypectomy
- Narrow-band imaging
- Preservation and incorporation of valuable endoscopic innovations

KEY POINTS

- The very low prevalence of advanced neoplasia in diminutive lesions supports the safety of resect and discard or discard policies.
- Although dye-chromoendoscopy or electronic chromoendoscopy at high magnification seem accurate for in vivo polyp prediction, they seem unfeasible in Western countries. Low-magnification electronic chromoendoscopy seems simple to be implemented in these countries, and an adequate, albeit variable, accuracy has been shown.
- The ability of low-magnification electronic chromoendoscopy in meeting American Society for Gastrointestinal Endoscopy thresholds is uncertain, depending on disease prevalence, technical accuracy, and the surveillance interval adopted for low-risk adenomas.

INTRODUCTION

Colorectal cancer (CRC) represents a major cause of morbidity and mortality in Western countries.[1-3] Endoscopic screening has been shown to be effective in reducing CRC incidence and/or mortality,[4-6] and population-based screening is widely recommended in the United States and Europe.[7,8] It has been estimated that greater than 60% of the eligible American population underwent CRC screening, with colonoscopy as the dominating test.[3] Despite that colonoscopy screening has been shown to be cost-effective or cost-saving in the long term,[9,10] screening costs, as well as exploitation of medical and technological resources, mainly incurs in the short term, while the benefits tend

This article originally appeared in Gastrointestinal Endoscopy Clinics, Volume 23, Issue 3, July 2013.

No funding was obtained.

a Digestive Endoscopy Unit, IRCCS Istituto Clinico Humanitas, Via Manzoni 56, Rozzano, Milan 20089, Italy; b Division of Gastroenterology and Hepatology, Veterans Affairs Medical Center, University of Kansas School of Medicine, 4801 East Linwood Boulevard, Kansas City, MO 64128-2295, USA

* Corresponding author. Digestive Endoscopy Unit, IRCCS Istituto Clinico Humanitas, Via Manzoni 56, Rozzano, Milan 20089, Italy.

E-mail address: cesareh@hotmail.com

Clinics Collections 7 (2015) 417–432
http://dx.doi.org/10.1016/j.ccol.2015.06.028
2352-7986/15/$ – see front matter © 2015 Elsevier Inc. All rights reserved.

to appear only after several years. An annual volume of approximately 14 million colonoscopies has been estimated in the United States, representing a substantial economic and financial burden to the society.[11]

A major determinant of the cost of colonoscopy is represented by polypectomy,[12] seemingly related to the high prevalence of polypoid (or nonpolypoid) lesions in the general population. It has been recently estimated in published US series that up to 42% of subjects will present with at least one polyp at screening colonoscopy; this rate is likely to increase with the widespread implementation of high-definition endoscopy and quality assurance programs for screening colonoscopy.[13,14] Polypectomy costs are partially related to the cost of pathologic examination. When considering diminutive polyps (≤ 5 mm in size), which represent more than 60% of all polyps detected by colonoscopy during average-risk screening,[13] the additional cost of postpolypectomy pathologic examination is mainly justified by the necessity to differentiate between precancerous adenomatous and hyperplastic polyps—which may require different policies of postpolypectomy follow-up because of the low prevalence of advanced neoplasia.[15,16]

WHAT IS RESECT AND DISCARD STRATEGY?

Despite being proposed and used by Japanese endoscopists since the early 1990s,[17] in vivo characterization of polyp histology with standard chromoendoscopy failed to gain popularity in Western countries. This failure to gain popularity has been related to several reasons, including the need of dye-spraying, which may be tedious and time-consuming. The advent of electronic chromoendoscopy (EC), preserving the benefits of chromoendoscopy without the disadvantages of dye-spraying, opened the door for optical prediction of polyp histology in Western countries. In preliminary studies, EC has been shown to be able to differentiate between adenomatous and hyperplastic histology of diminutive or small polyps with an adequate degree of accuracy, also predicting the correct interval of postpolypectomy surveillance.[18–20] For these reasons, it has been proposed that EC may prevent the need for standard histologic assessment of diminutive lesions, with future management decisions being driven only by the in vivo endoscopic prediction, also named resect and discard policy.[18,21] It has also been suggested that diminutive hyperplastic polyps in the distal colon may be left in situ after characterization (ie, a discard [without resection] policy).[18,21] When considering the high prevalence of such lesions in the general population, these strategies/policies may be expected to result in substantial savings when applied to a program of colonoscopy screening.[12,22] However, an inappropriate application of resect and discard or discard policies could also result in incorrect surveillance timings or in the nonremoval of serious lesions, causing undesired outcomes and risk of medical litigations.[12,22] For this reason, the American Society for Gastrointestinal Endoscopy recently published a white paper providing specific thresholds and criteria to be met before the clinical implementation of such practices.[23]

DISTRIBUTION OF HISTOLOGY WITHIN DIMINUTIVE AND SMALL POLYPS AND NATURAL HISTORY

The clinical application of a resect and discard strategy strictly depends on the histologic distribution among diminutive polyps. Irrespectively of the EC accuracy in polyp characterization, the relative distribution between hyperplastic and adenomatous histotypes would intrinsically affect the chances of false-positive or false-negative results within these lesions. A very high prevalence of hyperplastic lesions may be expected to marginalize the risk of a false-negative result by increasing the negative predictive value at a certain level of sensitivity, but it would also increase the possibility of false-positive results by reducing the positive predictive value, irrespective of the level of specificity. Second, an excessively high prevalence of advanced histology (ie, high-grade dysplasia, villous histology, or invasive cancer) would prevent the application of a resect and discard policy, because of the inability of EC in differentiating between nonadvanced and advanced adenomas. The clinical outcome of the discard strategy would also be affected by the natural history of unresected diminutive lesions. Although there is a general agreement on the lack of malignant potential of diminutive hyperplastic lesions in the distal colon, any false-negative result of polyp characterization would result in the nonremoval of a diminutive adenoma. A less aggressive natural history of such lesion would lead to a "safer" discard policy. Third, the association between some types of serrated lesions and a higher risk of CRC would not support a discard policy for proximal lesions,[24] unless in vivo characterization of polyp histology could reliably predict such a diagnosis.

Distribution of (Advanced) Adenomatous and Hyperplastic Histotypes Within Subcentimetric Lesions

Table 1 lists the available screening series providing estimates on the frequency of adenomatous lesions among subcentimetric lesions collected from a cumulative population of 18,549 subjects.[25–28] In detail, among 15,128 diminutive polyps, 51% were adenomatous, the remaining being nonadenomatous (mostly hyperplastic). It is however possible that these estimates are an overestimation when limiting the analysis to the distal colon, because of the well-known high prevalence of tiny hyperplastic lesions in this location. For instance, in a consecutive series of 235 distal polyps, including 220 polyps ≤5 mm lesions, only 38 were actually adenomatous, corresponding to a 16% overall frequency of adenomatous type.[29] Compared with diminutive polyps, the rate of adenomatous component seemed to be substantially higher in small (6–9 mm) polyps, corresponding to 64% among the identified 3197 small (6–9 mm) lesions (see **Table 1**).[25–28]

Regarding the relative prevalence of advanced neoplasia in subcentimetric lesions, in a previous systematic review including 20,562 subjects who underwent screening colonoscopy, fewer than 1% (0.8%) of patients with diminutive-only lesions had an advanced adenoma, whereas less than 5% (4.9%) of patients with small-only lesions had an advanced adenoma.[13] When restricting this analysis to invasive cancer, less than 0.1% of patients with a subcentimeter polyp as the largest lesion were affected, corresponding to a 0.04% (1:2726) and 0.07% (1:1488) risk for invasive cancer in diminutive and small polyps, respectively. These findings have been confirmed

Table 1
Relative prevalence of adenomatous histotype among diminutive and small lesions in large cohorts of subjects undertaking endoscopic or CTC screening

Series	≤5 mm		6–9 mm	
	No.	Rate Adenomatous	No.	Rate Adenomatous
Pickhardt et al,[25,a] 2003	966	64%	262	61%
Lieberman et al,[26,b] 2008	3744	50%	1198	68%
Rex et al,[27,a] 2009	8798	49%	1282	59%
Gupta et al,[28,a] 2012	1620	60%	455	71%
Total	15,128	51%	3197	64%

[a] Per polyp analysis.
[b] Per patient analysis.

recently by a retrospective analysis of 3 screening studies, including 2361 polyps, showing a 0.5% and 1.5% prevalence of advanced neoplasia within diminutive and small polyps, respectively.[28] Similarly, a retrospective analysis on 5124 asymptomatic subjects confirmed a very low risk of advanced neoplasia and invasive cancer in 464 patients with 6- to 9-mm polyps as the largest lesion, corresponding to a 3.9% and 0% risk, respectively.[30] Of note, the prevalence of sessile or traditional serrated adenoma was also shown to be very low in subcentimetric lesions, being cumulatively present in 0.3% to 0.5% and 0.8% to 1.3% of diminutive and small lesions, respectively.[26,28]

All these data would indicate that in the screening setting less than half of all diminutive lesions (<5 mm) will be adenomatous, whereas the risk of advanced neoplasia is extremely low. These probabilities are probably much less in the rectosigmoid colon. On the other hand, nearly 2 of 3 small lesions (6–9 mm) will be adenomatous, and the risk of advanced neoplasia ranges between 1.5% and 5%.

Natural History of Unresected Subcentimetric Lesions

In 2 prospective Northern European endoscopic studies, Hoff and colleagues[31] and Hofstad and colleagues[32] followed up 194 diminutive polyps and 253 polyps ≤10 mm detected for 3 and 2 years, respectively. No diminutive polyp reached a >5 mm size and only 0.5% of ≤10 mm polyps eclipsed the 10-mm threshold after a 1-year time interval; no case of high-grade dysplasia or carcinoma was registered.[31,32] Pickhardt and colleagues[33] followed 128 computed tomographic colonoscopy (CTC)-detected 6- to 9-mm polyps by repeating CTC after 2 years, recommending polypectomy for those polyps with interval growth. Overall, 116 small polyps did not show significant growth at a second CTC, whereas 12 (9.3%) polyps showed an interval growth of 1 mm or more. At histology, all growing lesions were adenomatous, but no cancer was detected[33]; this was recently confirmed by a Japanese study, in which only 2.9% of 408 subcentimetric lesions followed up for 43.1 months reached a size of ≥10 mm, without the occurrence of any invasive cancer.[34] Overall, these studies indicate that, at least in the short term, most of the ≤10-mm polyps do not present any relevant growth and do not progress to invasive cancer. This statement may be reassuring, when considering the (extremely) low risk of discarding an (advanced) adenoma in the distal colon (see later discussion). Natural history of sessile serrated lesions has been only marginally addressed. In a large series, it has been shown that only the presence of a proximal or ≥10-mm sessile serrated lesion is associated with an increased risk of metachronous neoplasia.[24]

METHODS FOR POLYPS CHARACTERIZATION: ADVANCED ENDOSCOPIC IMAGING
White Light

Despite that an in vivo prediction of polyp histology may be to some extent feasible at white-light (WL) endoscopy,[35,36] a WL-based resect and discard policy has never been formally implemented, presumably related to several reasons. First, WL accuracy in polyp characterization has been shown to be suboptimal and consistently inferior to that of more advanced endoscopic techniques.[18,35,36] Second, no clear classification criteria for WL in vivo polyp characterization have been proposed, preventing a clear assessment of interobserver/intra-observer variability.[18,35,36] Third, no formal training has been tested in a controlled environment. Fourth, high-definition WL endoscopy has been shown to be inferior to chromoendoscopy techniques in predicting polyp histology.[37] Fifth, although mucosal or vascular characteristics of some lesions may already be depicted at WL, this is usually more feasible for large rather than for diminutive lesions (ie, those amenable to a resect and discard policy). These limitations overall explain why a systematic policy of postpolypectomy pathologic referral has been universally implemented, at least in Western countries.[38]

(Dye-)Chromoendoscopy

The field of advanced endoscopic imaging, aiming to predict histology of (non-) polypoid colorectal lesions based on endoscopic features reliably, began in the early 1990s, when Japanese endoscopists showed the possibility of accurately discriminating between nonneoplastic and neoplastic histotype by depicting various pit patterns of colorectal lesions after staining with nonabsorbable or absorbable dyes.[17,39,40] Pit pattern–based classification at magnifying endoscopy has since been extensively validated, showing a high accuracy for differentiating between non-neoplastic (pit pattern I-II) and neoplastic lesions (pit pattern III-V), and, among those neoplastic, between precancerous and malignant phenotypes.[41] An adequate level of interobserver and intra-observer agreement was also shown, assuring the reproducibility of the technique.[17,39,40,42] For these reasons, chromoendoscopy gained immediate acceptance among Japanese endoscopists, allowing an early implementation of optical-based endoscopic policies in that country.[34,41,43] Despite all these favorable characteristics, however, chromoendoscopy unexpectedly failed to be implemented in Western countries. Albeit unclear, such failure may be explained by several reasons. First, high-magnification colonoscopes were not readily available in Europe and the United States. Second, chromoendoscopy requires a long learning curve with at least 200 to 300 procedures.[17,35] Third, the technique seems inconvenient to several Western endoscopists, because of the time required for dye spraying and zoom interpretation. Fourth, the excessive staining in the area surrounding the targeted lesion may mask a serious lesion. Fifth, chromoendoscopy has been generally perceived as a technique to differentiate between noninvasive and invasive lesions rather than to discriminate between nonneoplastic and neoplastic features.

High-magnification and Low-magnification Electronic Chromoendoscopy

The development of electronic or virtual chromoendoscopy (EC) revitalized the interest for advanced endoscopic imaging in Western countries. The main advantages of EC are the simple and immediate activation and the wide availability on the new generations of endoscopes. To differentiate between neoplastic (adenomatous) and nonneoplastic (hyperplastic) lesions, EC also exploits the neo-angiogenesis of neoplastic lesions rather than only the mucosal pit pattern. Narrow-band imaging (NBI; Olympus Inc, Shinjuku-Ku, Japan) is based on the modification of the spectral features with an optical color separation filter narrowing the bandwidth of spectral transmittance. In this system, the center wavelengths of the dedicated trichromatic optical filters are 540 and 415 nm, with bandwidths of 30 nm, to optimize hemoglobin light absorption.[44] By use of this narrow spectrum, the contrast of the superficial capillary pattern in the superficial layer is markedly increased, and thus clear visualization of vascular structures may be achieved during endoscopy.[44] The electronic button on the control section of the colonoscope allows switching between WL and NBI views. Differently from the optical-based NBI, flexible spectral imaging color enhancement (FICE) and I-Scan achieve a similar effect with a software-based postprocessing of the endoscopic image.[45,46]

EC had been initially applied in the setting of high-optical magnification (HM-EC) to predict polyp histology. HM-EC allowed the identification of the honeycomb microvascular pattern around the single glands, leading to a "capillary" or vascular pattern classification.[47] Such classification had been shown to have an adequate degree of accuracy for differentiating between adenomatous and hyperplastic lesions.[35,36,44,45,48–61] As shown in **Table 2**, sensitivity and specificity of HM-EC ranged

Table 2
Studies reporting accuracy of EC in differentiating between adenomatous and hyperplastic lesions at high-magnification colonoscopy

Author	Country	No. of Patients	No. of Polyps	Adenomatous Prevalence	Endoscopist	EC-pit Pattern	EC-vascular Pattern	EC-sensitivity	EC-specificity
Machida et al,[44] 2004	Japan	34	43	79%	—	Yes	Yes	100%	75%
Chiu et al,[36] 2007	Taiwan	133	180	78%	Experienced	No	Yes	91%	80%
Su et al,[35] 2006	Taiwan	78	110	59%	Experienced	No	Yes	96%	88%
Hirata et al,[62] 2007	Japan	99	148	89%	—	Yes	No	99%	94%
East et al,[48] 2007	UK	20	31	64%	Experienced	Yes	Yes	77%	50%
Tischendorf et al,[49] 2007	Germany	52	100	63%	Experienced	Yes	Yes	90%	89%
East et al,[50] 2008	UK	62	116	43%	Experienced	Yes	Yes	98%	88%
Sano et al,[51] 2009	Japan	92	150	74%	Experienced	No	Yes	96%	92%
van den Broek et al,[52] 2009	The Netherlands	32	50	44%	Experienced and Inexperienced	Yes	No	88%	56%
van den Broek et al,[52] 2009	The Netherlands	32	50	44%	Experienced and Inexperienced	Yes	No	90%	55%
Wada et al,[53] 2009	Japan	495	617	95%	Experienced	No	Yes	91%	97%
Tischendorf et al,[55] 2010	Germany	131	100	58%	Experienced	No	Yes	92%	89%
Tischendorf et al,[54] 2010	Germany	223	209	77%	Experienced	No	Yes	94%	86%
Ignjatovic et al,[57] 2011	UK	—	80	50%	Experienced and Inexperienced	No	Yes	93%	59%
Ignjatovic et al,[57] 2011	UK	—	80	50%	Experienced and Inexperienced	No	Yes	90%	33%
Sato et al,[58] 2011	Japan	183	424	80%	Experienced and Inexperienced	No	Yes	91%	77%
Gross et al,[56] 2011	Germany	214	434	59%	Experienced and Inexperienced	No	Yes	93%	92%
Gross et al,[56] 2011	Germany	214	434	59%	Experienced and Inexperienced	No	Yes	86%	88%
Takemura et al,[61] 2012	Japan	—	371	87%	Experienced	Yes	Yes	98%	99%
Kuiper et al,[60] 2012	The Netherlands	64	154	37%	Experienced	Yes	No	81%	93%
Yoo et al,[59] 2011	Korea	68	107	93%	Experienced	Yes	No	89%	88%
Yoo et al,[59] 2011	Korea	68	107	93%	Experienced	No	Yes	92%	88%

between 77% and 100%, and 50% and 100%, respectively. HM-EC appeared also to be superior to WL and similar to (dye-)chromoendoscopy for in vivo polyp characterization.[35,36] In contrast to dye chromoendoscopy, the learning curve appeared to be short, and a high degree of reproducibility, at least among expert endoscopists, was shown.[50,54,57,58] The possibility of developing a reliable computer-aided system for predicting the histology of colorectal lesions by HM-NBI has also been shown.[56,61] However, HM-EC shared a major limitation with chromoendoscopy (ie, the nonavailability of HM-endoscopes in Western countries). For this reason, EC had been mainly implemented in association with low-optical magnification (LM-EC) endoscopy in Western countries,[63] also exploiting the higher resolution of high-definition endoscopes.[64]

Different from HM-EC, LM-EC has been relatively ineffective in depicting the microvascular patterns or pit patterns of many subcentimetric polyps.[36] To compensate for this deficiency, a different diagnostic approach has been introduced that mostly exploits a *gestalt* appreciation of the polyp surface, hue, and vascularization (**Fig. 1**).[37,63,65] In detail, adenomatous polyps mainly appear as dark or brown lesions, as an effect of the neoplastic neo-angiogenesis, whereas hyperplastic polyps are usually pale or at best showing isolated lacy vessels on the surface.[19,37,63,65] Second, LM-EC permits the use of a simplified pit pattern in adenomatous lesions, whereas hyperplastic polyps usually show a lack of any pit pattern.[19,37,63,65] However, in a head-to-head comparison, LM-EC was shown to be inferior to HM-EC,[36] and HM-EC has been consistently shown to be superior to either standard or high-definition LM-EC.[37,57,64] The accuracy of LM-EC has shown some variability in preliminary studies, with sensitivity and specificity ranging between 61% and 91%, and between 32% and 98%, respectively (**Table 3**).[18–20,29,37,55,57,63–65,67–74] This range may, at least in part, be explained by a high degree of heterogeneity in the methodology adopted across the studies. First, several studies did not restrict the analysis to diminutive or subcentimetric polyps, substantially changing the expected prevalence of disease.[18–20,29,37,55,57,63–65,67–74] Moreover, different EC-based classifications, based on either pit or vascular patterns, were adopted in these studies, preventing a clear comparison across the series (see **Table 3**),[18–20,29,37,55,57,63–65,67–74] and participating endoscopists already experienced in EC generally achieved better accuracies than less-trained endoscopists (see **Table 3**).[18–20,29,37,55,57,63–65,67–74] Finally, LM-EC has been shown to be largely unable to differentiate between hyperplastic and sessile serrated lesions or adenomas.[63]

To address such variability, a new classification system (NBI International Colorectal Endoscopic [NICE]) has been validated recently with an adequate interobserver and

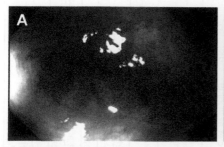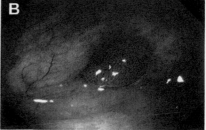

Fig. 1. Appearance of subcentimetric colorectal lesions at narrow-band imaging at low-optical magnification: (A) bland, featureless appearance, thin blood vessels coursing across the polyp surface and not surrounding pits (hyperplastic); (B) brown color, oval pits, short, thick blood vessels (adenomatous).

Table 3
Studies reporting the accuracy of EC in differentiating between adenomatous and hyperplastic lesions at low-magnification colonoscopy

Author	Country	Setting	No. of Polyps	Adenomatous Prevalence	Endoscopist	EC-pit Pattern	EC-vascular Pattern	EC-sensitivity	EC-specificity
Kuiper et al,[66] 2011	The Netherlands	High	238	49%	Experienced	Yes	No	87%	63%
Chiu et al,[36] 2007	Taiwan	Artificial	180	78%	Experienced	No	Yes	84%	71%
Rastogi et al,[63] 2008	USA	Screening/surveillance	123	59%	Experienced	Yes / No	No / Yes	97% / 86%	86% / 97%
Sikka et al,[37] 2008	USA	Artificial	80	61%	Inexperienced	Yes	Yes	95%	90%
Rogart et al,[65] 2008	USA	Unselected	265	49%	Inexperienced	Yes	Yes	80%	81%
Rex,[19] 2009	USA	Unselected	451	51%	Experienced	Yes	Yes	96%	92%
Tischendorf et al,[55] 2010	Germany	Artificial	100	63%	Experienced	No	Yes	92%	89%
Buchner et al,[67] 2010	USA	Unselected	119	68%	Experienced	—	—	77%	71%
Ignjatovic et al,[18] 2009	UK	High	278	71%	Experienced and Inexperienced	No	Yes	94%	89%
Henry et al,[68] 2010	USA	Unselected	126	53%	Experienced	No	Yes	93%	88%
Ignjatovic et al,[69] 2011	UK	Artificial	630	50%	Experienced and Inexperienced	Yes	Yes	87%	84%
Ignjatovic et al,[57,c] 2011	UK	Artificial	80	50%	Experienced. / Inexperienced	No / No	Yes / Yes	74% / 61%	56% / 32%
Rastogi et al,[70] 2011	USA	Screening/surveillance	—	—	Experienced	Yes	Yes	90%	68%
Gupta et al,[20] 2012	USA	Screening/surveillance	1254	64%	Experienced	Yes	Yes	94%	72%
Hewett et al,[71] 2012	USA	Unselected	236	63%	Experienced	Yes	Yes	98%	69%
Kuiper et al,[72] 2012	The Netherlands	Unselected	108	46%	Experienced	Yes	No	77%	79%
Hewett et al,[29] 2012	USA	Screening/surveillance	235	16%	Experienced	Yes	Yes	94%	98%
Paggi et al,[73] 2012	Italy	Unselected	511	69%	Experienced	Yes	Yes	95%	66%
Longcroft-Wheaton et al,[64] 2012	UK	Unselected	150	64%	Experienced	Yes	Yes	83% / 93%	82% / 81%
Ladabaum et al,[74] 2013	USA	Unselected	2596	65%	Inexperienced	Yes	Yes	91%	40%

intra-observer agreement among experienced and nonexperienced endoscopists (Table 4).[71] It has been shown that very short training sessions may be sufficient to reach an adequate EC accuracy, at least in an artificial setting.[75] In the NICE classification, the level of confidence of the endoscopist in in vivo histologic prediction has been introduced, showing a substantial deterioration of LM-EC accuracy when passing from high-level to low-level confidence of diagnosis.[71,74]

RESECT AND DISCARD STRATEGIES/POLICIES

The American Society for Gastrointestinal Endoscopy recently developed a Preservation and Incorporation of Valuable Endoscopic Innovations (PIVI) statement for real-time endoscopic assessment of the histology of diminutive colorectal polyps.[76] In detail, it was determined that:

1. For colorectal polyps ≤5 mm in size to be resected and discarded without pathologic assessment, endoscopic technology (when used with high confidence) used to determine histology of polyps ≤5 mm in size, when combined with histopathologic assessment of polyps >5 mm in size, should provide a ≥90% agreement in assignment of post-polypectomy surveillance intervals when compared with decisions based on pathology assessment of all identified polyps."
2. For a technology to be used to guide the decision to leave suspected rectosigmoid hyperplastic polyps ≤5 mm in size in place (without resection), the technology should provide ≥90% negative predictive value (when used with high confidence) for adenomatous histology."

Resect and Discard (1° PIVI)

Both statements show how the feasibility of in vivo prediction policies is a complex decision-making process that depends on multiple variables, including EC accuracy, level of diagnostic confidence, prevalence of disease, histology of nonassessable polyps, as well as the type of postpolypectomy guidelines adopted.[76] When further analyzing the first statement (ie, resect and discard strategy), the correspondence between the optical prediction and the assignment of postpolypectomy surveillance intervals is not only related to the interaction between EC accuracy and relative

Table 4
The NICE Classification[a] for differentiating between hyperplastic and adenomatous histology

NICE Criterion	Type 1	Type 2
Color	Same or lighter than background	Browner relative to background (verify color arises from vessels)
Vessels	None, or isolated lacy vessels coursing across the lesion	Brown vessels surrounding white structures[b]
Surface pattern	Dark or white spots of uniform size, or homogeneous absence of pattern	Oval, tubular, or branched white structures[b] surrounded by brown vessels
Most likely pathologic abnormality	Hyperplastic	Adenoma

[a] Can be applied using colonoscopes both with or without optical (zoom) magnification.
[b] These structures may represent the pits and the epithelium of the crypt opening.
 From Hewett DG, Kaltenbach T, Sano Y, et al. Validation of a simple classification system for endoscopic diagnosis of small colorectal polyps using narrow-band imaging. Gastroenterology 2012;143:599–607.e1; with permission.

prevalence of adenomatous polyps, but also to the recommendations adopted for the surveillance intervals. The recent update from the *US Multi-Society Task Force on Colorectal Cancer* indicates a 10-year interval for distal small (<10 mm) hyperplastic polyps and a 5- to 10-year interval for 1 to 2 tubular adenomas <10 mm, whereas a 3-year interval is recommended for those with advanced histology or ≥3 adenomas.[15] When considering the inability of EC in differentiating between adenomas with favorable or advanced histology, the first issue is whether EC-based recommendations may still achieve a 90% agreement based on the available evidence. Because of the very low prevalence of advanced neoplasia within diminutive lesions (0.8%, see discussion above), this may be reasonably excluded. The second issue is whether EC-based differentiation between nonadvanced adenomatous and hyperplastic lesions may provide a >90% agreement in the assignment of the surveillance intervals. This >90% agreement appears to depend mainly on a complex interaction between EC accuracy and on whether a 5-year or a 10-year schedule is chosen for subjects with 1 to 2 tubular adenomas <10 mm. If a 5-year schedule is adopted, the role of EC accuracy is important, because false-negative results would experience an inappropriate surveillance delay at 10 years, whereas those false positives would have a substantial anticipation of the examination at 5 years. When adopting these criteria, some series have reported favorable results (by experienced EC endoscopists) but the majority failed to match the 1° PIVI, especially when EC was performed by less dedicated endoscopists (**Table 5**). On the other hand, if a 10-year schedule is

Table 5
Studies reporting accuracy of EC in matching the desired thresholds for the 2 proposed PIVIs (see text)

Author	Country	No. of Patients	No. of Polyps	Experienced	High/low Confidence	1° PIVI	2° PIVI
Rex,[19] 2009	USA	136	451	Experienced	Yes	Yes	—
Ignjatovic et al,[18] 2009	UK	130	278	Experienced and Inexperienced	Yes	Yes	Yes
Rastogi et al,[70] 2011	USA	—	—	Experienced	No	No	No
Gupta et al,[20] 2012	USA	410	1254	Experienced	No	No/Yes	Yes
Hewett et al,[71] 2012	USA	108	236	Experienced	Yes	—	Yes
Kuiper et al,[72] 2012	The Netherlands	308	108	Inexperienced	Yes	No	—
Hewett et al,[29] 2012	US	31	235	Experienced	Yes	—	Yes
Paggi et al,[73] 2012	Italy	286	511	Experienced	Yes	No	—
Longcroft-Wheaton et al,[64] 2012	UK	51	150	Experienced	No	No/Yes	No
Longcroft-Wheaton et al,[64] 2012	UK	50	143	Experienced	No	Yes	No
Ladabaum et al,[74] 2013	USA	1673	2596	Inexperienced	Yes	No/Yes	Yes

recommended, as also supported by European guidelines,[16,77] the differentiation between ≤ 2 diminutive polyps between hyperplastic and adenomatous would become irrelevant in the assignment of the surveillance interval, marginalizing any possibility of error. When adopting these criteria, most of the studies succeeded in meeting the 1° PIVI.

Discard (2° PIVI)

The high prevalence of hyperplastic lesions in the rectosigmoid tract undermines the cost-effectiveness of polypectomy. For this reason, a discard (leave-in-place) policy would seem reasonable. This policy has been confirmed by 2 series that specifically applied EC predictions on rectosigmoid lesions (see **Table 5**).[29,74] The failure of meeting the 2° PIVI in other studies would seem to be related mainly to the fact that the analysis was not restricted to rectosigmoid lesions, thereby artificially inflating the relative prevalence of the adenomatous histotype (see **Table 5**). Moreover, the very low risk of neoplastic progression in the few false-negative cases would be marginalized by the favorable natural history (at least at 3–5 years) of unresected adenomas (see discussion above).

SUMMARY

The extremely low prevalence of advanced neoplasia in diminutive lesions, especially in the distal colon, would support the safety of resect and discard or discard policies. This safety is further increased by the low risk of metachronous advanced neoplasia in those with 1 to 2 tubular subcentimetric adenomas.[15] Based on the efficacy, characterization of colorectal lesions with dye-chromoendoscopy or EC at high-optical magnification would presumably assure the highest level of accuracy. On the other hand, high-definition low-magnification EC seems to be reasonably accurate in in vivo histologic prediction, although a high degree of variability has been shown among the available studies. Such an approach may be also expected to be generalizable and reproducible, because of the short-term training period required. When implementing low-magnification EC policies, a major determinant would be represented by the type of surveillance intervals adopted for 1 to 2 low-risk adenomas. If a 10-year interval is adopted, EC-based strategies may be expected to be implemented widely in Western countries, because of an extremely high risk/benefit profile. If, on the other hand, a 5-year interval is adopted, a high level of EC accuracy is required.

REFERENCES

1. Ferlay J, Autier P, Boniol M, et al. Estimates of the cancer incidence and mortality in Europe in 2006. Ann Oncol 2007;18:581–92.
2. Edwards BK, Ward E, Kohler BA, et al. Annual report to the nation on the status of cancer, 1975-2006, featuring colorectal cancer trends and impact of interventions (risk factors, screening, and treatment) to reduce future rates. Cancer 2010;116:544–73.
3. Joseph DA, King JB, Miller JW, et al. Prevalence of colorectal cancer screening among adults–Behavioral Risk Factor Surveillance System, United States, 2010. MMWR Morb Mortal Wkly Rep 2012;61(Suppl):51–6.
4. Winawer SJ, Zauber AG, Ho MN, et al. Prevention of colorectal cancer by colonoscopic polypectomy. The National Polyp Study Workgroup. N Engl J Med 1993;329:1977–81.
5. Atkin W, Kralj-Hans I, Wardle J, et al. Colorectal cancer screening. Randomised trials of flexible sigmoidoscopy. BMJ 2010;341:c4618.

6. Baxter NN, Goldwasser MA, Paszat LF, et al. Association of colonoscopy and death from colorectal cancer. Ann Intern Med 2009;150:1–8.

7. Levin B, Lieberman DA, McFarland B, et al. Screening and surveillance for the early detection of colorectal cancer and adenomatous polyps, 2008: a joint guideline from the American Cancer Society, the US Multi-Society Task Force on Colorectal Cancer, and the American College of Radiology. Gastroenterology 2008;134:1570–95.

8. Rex DK, Johnson DA, Anderson JC, et al. American College of Gastroenterology guidelines for colorectal cancer screening 2009 [corrected]. Am J Gastroenterol 2009;104:739–50.

9. Pignone M, Saha S, Hoerger T, et al. Cost-effectiveness analyses of colorectal cancer screening: a systematic review for the U.S. Preventive Services Task Force. Ann Intern Med 2002;137:96–104.

10. Lansdorp-Vogelaar I, van Ballegooijen M, Zauber AG, et al. Effect of rising chemotherapy costs on the cost savings of colorectal cancer screening. J Natl Cancer Inst 2009;101:1412–22.

11. Seeff LC, Richards TB, Shapiro JA, et al. How many endoscopies are performed for colorectal cancer screening? Results from CDC's survey of endoscopic capacity. Gastroenterology 2004;127:1670–7.

12. Hassan C, Pickhardt PJ, Rex DK. A resect and discard strategy would improve cost-effectiveness of colorectal cancer screening. Clin Gastroenterol Hepatol 2010;8:865–9, 869.e1–3.

13. Hassan C, Pickhardt PJ, Kim DH, et al. Systematic review: distribution of advanced neoplasia according to polyp size at screening colonoscopy. Aliment Pharmacol Ther 2010;31:210–7.

14. Rex DK, Bond JH, Winawer S, et al. Quality in the technical performance of colonoscopy and the continuous quality improvement process for colonoscopy: recommendations of the U.S. Multi-Society Task Force on Colorectal Cancer. Am J Gastroenterol 2002;97:1296–308.

15. Lieberman DA, Rex DK, Winawer S, et al. Guidelines for colonoscopy surveillance after screening and polypectomy: a consensus update by the US Multi-Society Task Force on Colorectal Cancer. Gastroenterology 2012;143:844–57.

16. Atkin WS, Valori R, Kuipers EJ, et al. European guidelines for quality assurance in colorectal cancer screening and diagnosis. First Edition–Colonoscopic surveillance following adenoma removal. Endoscopy 2012;44(Suppl 3):SE151–63.

17. Kudo S, Tamura S, Nakajima T, et al. Diagnosis of colorectal tumorous lesions by magnifying endoscopy. Gastrointest Endosc 1996;44:8–14.

18. Ignjatovic A, East JE, Suzuki N, et al. Optical diagnosis of small colorectal polyps at routine colonoscopy (Detect InSpect ChAracterise Resect and Discard; DISCARD trial): a prospective cohort study. Lancet Oncol 2009;10:1171–8.

19. Rex DK. Narrow-band imaging without optical magnification for histologic analysis of colorectal polyps. Gastroenterology 2009;136:1174–81.

20. Gupta N, Bansal A, Rao D, et al. Accuracy of in vivo optical diagnosis of colon polyp histology by narrow-band imaging in predicting colonoscopy surveillance intervals. Gastrointest Endosc 2012;75:494–502.

21. Rex DK. Reducing costs of colon polyp management. Lancet Oncol 2009;10:1135–6.

22. Kessler WR, Imperiale TF, Klein RW, et al. A quantitative assessment of the risks and cost savings of forgoing histologic examination of diminutive polyps. Endoscopy 2011;43:683–91.

23. Rex DK, Kahi C, O'Brien M, et al. The American Society for Gastrointestinal Endoscopy PIVI (Preservation and Incorporation of Valuable Endoscopic Innovations) on real-time endoscopic assessment of the histology of diminutive colorectal polyps. Gastrointest Endosc 2011;73:419–22.

24. Schreiner MA, Weiss DG, Lieberman DA. Proximal and large hyperplastic and nondysplastic serrated polyps detected by colonoscopy are associated with neoplasia. Gastroenterology 2010;139:1497–502.

25. Pickhardt PJ, Choi JR, Hwang I, et al. Computed tomographic virtual colonoscopy to screen for colorectal neoplasia in asymptomatic adults. N Engl J Med 2003;349:2191–200.

26. Lieberman D, Moravec M, Holub J, et al. Polyp size and advanced histology in patients undergoing colonoscopy screening: implications for CT colonography. Gastroenterology 2008;135:1100–5.

27. Rex DK, Overhiser AJ, Chen SC, et al. Estimation of impact of American College of Radiology recommendations on CT colonography reporting for resection of high-risk adenoma findings. Am J Gastroenterol 2009;104:149–53.

28. Gupta N, Bansal A, Rao D, et al. Prevalence of advanced histological features in diminutive and small colon polyps. Gastrointest Endosc 2012;75:1022–30.

29. Hewett DG, Huffman ME, Rex DK. Leaving distal colorectal hyperplastic polyps in place can be achieved with high accuracy by using narrow-band imaging: an observational study. Gastrointest Endosc 2012;76:374–80.

30. Pickhardt PJ, Hain KS, Kim DH, et al. Low rates of cancer or high-grade dysplasia in colorectal polyps collected from computed tomography colonography screening. Clin Gastroenterol Hepatol 2010;8:610–5.

31. Hoff G, Foerster A, Vatn MH, et al. Epidemiology of polyps in the rectum and colon. Recovery and evaluation of unresected polyps 2 years after detection. Scand J Gastroenterol 1986;21:853–62.

32. Hofstad B, Vatn MH, Andersen SN, et al. Growth of colorectal polyps: redetection and evaluation of unresected polyps for a period of three years. Gut 1996;39:449–56.

33. Pickhardt PJ, Kim DK, Cash BD, et al. The natural history of small polyps at CT colonography. Presented at the Annual meeting for the Society of Gastrointestinal Radiologists, Rancho Mirage, CA, Feb 17–22, 2008.

34. Hisabe T, Tsuda S, Matsui T, et al. Natural history of small colorectal protuberant adenomas. Dig Endosc 2010;22(Suppl 1):S43–6.

35. Su MY, Hsu CM, Ho YP, et al. Comparative study of conventional colonoscopy, chromoendoscopy, and narrow-band imaging systems in differential diagnosis of neoplastic and nonneoplastic colonic polyps. Am J Gastroenterol 2006;101:2711–6.

36. Chiu HM, Chang CY, Chen CC, et al. A prospective comparative study of narrow-band imaging, chromoendoscopy, and conventional colonoscopy in the diagnosis of colorectal neoplasia. Gut 2007;56:373–9.

37. Sikka S, Ringold DA, Jonnalagadda S, et al. Comparison of white light and narrow band high definition images in predicting colon polyp histology, using standard colonoscopes without optical magnification. Endoscopy 2008;40:818–22.

38. Winawer SJ, Zauber AG, Fletcher RH, et al. Guidelines for colonoscopy surveillance after polypectomy: a consensus update by the US Multi-Society Task Force on Colorectal Cancer and the American Cancer Society. CA Cancer J Clin 2006;56:143–59 [quiz: 184–5].

39. Kato S, Fujii T, Koba I, et al. Assessment of colorectal lesions using magnifying colonoscopy and mucosal dye spraying: can significant lesions be distinguished? Endoscopy 2001;33:306–10.

40. Fu KI, Sano Y, Kato S, et al. Chromoendoscopy using indigo carmine dye spraying with magnifying observation is the most reliable method for differential diagnosis between non-neoplastic and neoplastic colorectal lesions: a prospective study. Endoscopy 2004;36:1089–93.

41. Kudo S, Lambert R, Allen JI, et al. Nonpolypoid neoplastic lesions of the colorectal mucosa. Gastrointest Endosc 2008;68:S3–47.

42. Lambert R, Kudo SE, Vieth M, et al. Pragmatic classification of superficial neoplastic colorectal lesions. Gastrointest Endosc 2009;70:1182–99.

43. Hinoi T, Lucas PC, Kuick R, et al. CDX2 regulates liver intestine-cadherin expression in normal and malignant colon epithelium and intestinal metaplasia. Gastroenterology 2002;123:1565–77.

44. Machida H, Sano Y, Hamamoto Y, et al. Narrow-band imaging in the diagnosis of colorectal mucosal lesions: a pilot study. Endoscopy 2004;36:1094–8.

45. Pohl J, Nguyen-Tat M, Pecho O, et al. Computed virtual chromoendoscopy for classification of small colorectal lesions: a prospective comparative study. Am J Gastroenterol 2008;103:562–9.

46. Lee CK, Lee SH, Hwangbo Y. Narrow-band imaging versus I-Scan for the real-time histological prediction of diminutive colonic polyps: a prospective comparative study by using the simple unified endoscopic classification. Gastrointest Endosc 2011;74:603–9.

47. Konerding MA, Fait E, Gaumann A. 3D microvascular architecture of precancerous lesions and invasive carcinomas of the colon. Br J Cancer 2001; 84:1354–62.

48. East JE, Suzuki N, Saunders BP. Comparison of magnified pit pattern interpretation with narrow band imaging versus chromoendoscopy for diminutive colonic polyps: a pilot study. Gastrointest Endosc 2007;66:310–6.

49. Tischendorf JJ, Wasmuth HE, Koch A, et al. Value of magnifying chromoendoscopy and narrow band imaging (NBI) in classifying colorectal polyps: a prospective controlled study. Endoscopy 2007;39:1092–6.

50. East JE, Suzuki N, Basset P, et al. Narrow band imaging with magnification for the characterization of small and diminutive colonic polyps: pit pattern and vascular pattern intensity. Endoscopy 2008;40:811–7.

51. Sano Y, Ikematsu H, Fu KI, et al. Meshed capillary vessels by use of narrow-band imaging for differential diagnosis of small colorectal polyps. Gastrointest Endosc 2009;69:278–83.

52. van den Broek FJ, van Soest EJ, Naber AH, et al. Combining autofluorescence imaging and narrow-band imaging for the differentiation of adenomas from non-neoplastic colonic polyps among experienced and non-experienced endoscopists. Am J Gastroenterol 2009;104:1498–507.

53. Wada Y, Kudo SE, Kashida H, et al. Diagnosis of colorectal lesions with the magnifying narrow-band imaging system. Gastrointest Endosc 2009;70: 522–31.

54. Tischendorf JJ, Gross S, Winograd R, et al. Computer-aided classification of colorectal polyps based on vascular patterns: a pilot study. Endoscopy 2010; 42:203–7.

55. Tischendorf JJ, Schirin-Sokhan R, Steetz K, et al. Value of magnifying endoscopy in classifying colorectal polyps based on vascular pattern. Endoscopy 2010;42:22–7.

56. Gross S, Trautwein C, Behrens A, et al. Computer-based classification of small colorectal polyps by using narrow-band imaging with optical magnification. Gastrointest Endosc 2011;74:1354–9.

57. Ignjatovic A, East JE, Guenther T, et al. What is the most reliable imaging modality for small colonic polyp characterization? Study of white-light, autofluorescence, and narrow-band imaging. Endoscopy 2011;43:94–9.

58. Sato R, Fujiya M, Watari J, et al. The diagnostic accuracy of high-resolution endoscopy, autofluorescence imaging and narrow-band imaging for differentially diagnosing colon adenoma. Endoscopy 2011;43:862–8.

59. Yoo HY, Lee MS, Ko BM, et al. Correlation of narrow band imaging with magnifying colonoscopy and histology in colorectal tumors. Clin Endosc 2011;44:44–50.

60. Kuiper T, van den Broek FJ, van Eeden S, et al. Feasibility and accuracy of confocal endomicroscopy in comparison with narrow-band imaging and chromoendoscopy for the differentiation of colorectal lesions. Am J Gastroenterol 2012;107:543–50.

61. Takemura Y, Yoshida S, Tanaka S, et al. Computer-aided system for predicting the histology of colorectal tumors by using narrow-band imaging magnifying colonoscopy (with video). Gastrointest Endosc 2012;75:179–85.

62. Hirata M, Tanaka S, Oka S, et al. Magnifying endoscopy with narrow band imaging for diagnosis of colorectal tumors. Gastrointest Endosc 2007;65:988–95.

63. Rastogi A, Bansal A, Wani S, et al. Narrow-band imaging colonoscopy–a pilot feasibility study for the detection of polyps and correlation of surface patterns with polyp histologic diagnosis. Gastrointest Endosc 2008;67:280–6.

64. Longcroft-Wheaton G, Brown J, Cowlishaw D, et al. High-definition vs. standard-definition colonoscopy in the characterization of small colonic polyps: results from a randomized trial. Endoscopy 2012;44:905–10.

65. Rogart JN, Jain D, Siddiqui UD, et al. Narrow-band imaging without high magnification to differentiate polyps during real-time colonoscopy: improvement with experience. Gastrointest Endosc 2008;68:1136–45.

66. Kuiper T, van den Broek FJ, Naber AH, et al. Endoscopic trimodal imaging detects colonic neoplasia as well as standard video endoscopy. Gastroenterology 2011;140:1887–94.

67. Buchner AM, Shahid MW, Heckman MG, et al. Comparison of probe-based confocal laser endomicroscopy with virtual chromoendoscopy for classification of colon polyps. Gastroenterology 2010;138:834–42.

68. Henry ZH, Yeaton P, Shami VM, et al. Meshed capillary vessels found on narrow-band imaging without optical magnification effectively identifies colorectal neoplasia: a North American validation of the Japanese experience. Gastrointest Endosc 2010;72:118–26.

69. Ignjatovic A, Thomas-Gibson S, East JE, et al. Development and validation of a training module on the use of narrow-band imaging in differentiation of small adenomas from hyperplastic colorectal polyps. Gastrointest Endosc 2011;73:128–33.

70. Rastogi A, Early DS, Gupta N, et al. Randomized, controlled trial of standard-definition white-light, high-definition white-light, and narrow-band imaging colonoscopy for the detection of colon polyps and prediction of polyp histology. Gastrointest Endosc 2011;74:593–602.

71. Hewett DG, Kaltenbach T, Sano Y, et al. Validation of a simple classification system for endoscopic diagnosis of small colorectal polyps using narrow-band imaging. Gastroenterology 2012;143:599–607.e1.

72. Kuiper T, Marsman WA, Jansen JM, et al. Accuracy for optical diagnosis of small colorectal polyps in nonacademic settings. Clin Gastroenterol Hepatol 2012;10: 1016–20 [quiz: e79].

73. Paggi S, Rondonotti E, Amato A, et al. Resect and discard strategy in clinical practice: a prospective cohort study. Endoscopy 2012;44:899–904.

74. Ladabaum U, Fioritto A, Mittani A, et al. Real-time optical biopsy of colon polyps with narrow band imaging in community practice does not yet meet key thresholds for clinical decisions. Gastroenterology 2013;144(1):81–91.

75. Raghavendra M, Hewett DG, Rex DK. Differentiating adenomas from hyperplastic colorectal polyps: narrow-band imaging can be learned in 20 minutes. Gastrointest Endosc 2010;72:572–6.

76. Rex DK, Fennerty MB, Sharma P, et al. Bringing new endoscopic imaging technology into everyday practice: what is the role of professional GI societies? Polyp imaging as a template for moving endoscopic innovation forward to answer key clinical questions. Gastrointest Endosc 2010;71:142–6.

77. Denis B, Bottlaender J, Weiss AM, et al. Some diminutive colorectal polyps can be removed and discarded without pathological examination. Endoscopy 2011; 43:81–6.

Integrating Systemic and Surgical Approaches to Treating Metastatic Colorectal Cancer

Kaihong Mi, MD, PhD[a], Matthew F. Kalady, MD[a,b],
Cristiano Quintini, MD[c], Alok A. Khorana, MD[a,*]

KEYWORDS

- Colorectal cancer • Liver metastases • Liver-directed therapy
- Antiangiogenic therapy • Antineoplastic therapy

KEY POINTS

- Median survival has increased substantially in recent years to nearly 30 months in patients with metastatic colorectal cancer treated with contemporary regimens.
- All patients with metastatic disease should undergo evaluation for potential resectability and/or liver-directed therapy, which can significantly improve outcomes and potentially cure a minority of patients.
- Chemotherapy regimens in initial and subsequent settings should be accompanied by a targeted agent, unless specific contraindications exist.
- RAS status should be checked in all patients with metastatic colorectal cancer. Anti–epidermal growth factor receptor antibodies should be only used in patients with "extended" RAS wild-type tumors.

INTRODUCTION

Metastatic colorectal cancer is an important contributor to the public health burden of cancer-related mortality. An estimated 136,830 people in the United States will be diagnosed with colorectal cancer in 2014. Approximately one-fifth of these patients will have distant metastatic disease at the time of presentation.[1] The spread of primary colorectal cancer can occur by lymphatic and hematogenous dissemination, as well as by contiguous and transperitoneal routes. The presence of right upper quadrant

This article originally appeared in Surgical Oncology Clinics, Volume 24, Issue 1, January 2015.
Dr Khorana discloses consulting honoraria from Genentech, Inc.
[a] Taussig Cancer Institute, Department of Hematology and Oncology, Cleveland Clinic, 9500 Euclid Avenue, Cleveland, OH 44195, USA; [b] Digestive Disease Institute, Department of Colorectal Surgery, Cleveland Clinic, 9500 Euclid Avenue, Cleveland, OH 44195, USA; [c] Digestive Disease Institute, HPB and Liver Transplant Program, Cleveland Clinic, 9500 Euclid Avenue, Cleveland, OH 44195, USA
* Corresponding author. 9500 Euclid Avenue, R35, Cleveland, OH 44195.
E-mail address: Khorana@ccf.org

Clinics Collections 7 (2015) 433–448
http://dx.doi.org/10.1016/j.ccol.2015.06.029
2352-7986/15/$ – see front matter © 2015 Elsevier Inc. All rights reserved.

pain, abdominal distension, early satiety, supraclavicular adenopathy, or periumbilical nodules usually signals advanced metastatic disease. However, given extensive staging and surveillance protocols, it is also common to identify metastatic disease based on imaging studies. The first site of hematogenous dissemination is usually the liver, followed by the lungs and bone. An exception is rectal cancer, which may metastasize initially to the lung because the inferior rectal vein drains into the inferior vena cava rather than into the portal venous system.

Although the prognosis for patients with metastatic disease without specific treatment remains limited, multiple new treatment options developed during the past 2 decades are now available for the treatment of metastatic disease. As a result, median survival has increased to nearly 30 months in the latest large randomized study,[2] from approximately 6 months in the 1990s.[3] This improvement in survival has been driven not by a single "magic bullet" but by the sequential deployment of a variety of chemotherapy and so-called targeted therapy agents. This latter class includes monoclonal antibodies to vascular endothelial growth factor (VEGF) (bevacizumab) and epidermal growth factor receptor (EGFR) (cetuximab and panitumumab), aflibercept, a recombinant fusion protein also directed against VEGF, and regorafenib, an active inhibitor of multiple tyrosine kinases. Finally, a small but substantial minority of patients with isolated sites of metastases may potentially be curable with surgery and liver-directed therapies.

The availability of multiple therapeutic agents for the treatment of metastatic colorectal cancer therefore requires a strategic approach to maximize patient benefit, in terms of both life expectancy and quality of life. When determining initial treatment, the first step is to evaluate whether the patient is potentially curable by a surgical resection of metastases either at the time of diagnosis or after conversion therapy. This approach will guide the choice and timing of chemotherapy. Treatments with the potential highest response rates and the greatest potential to downsize metastasis are the most appropriate for potentially curable patients. If the patient does not seem curable, treatment regimens that offer the longest progression-free survival (PFS) and overall survival (OS) and that maintain quality of life as long as possible are to be preferred. This review focuses on describing systemic approaches to the treatment of patients with metastatic colorectal cancer, with notes on the incorporation of liver-directed and primary resection modalities in the appropriate context.

SYSTEMIC REGIMENS FOR METASTATIC COLORECTAL CANCER

In patients with unresectable metastatic colorectal cancer, who comprise most cases, systemic treatment is focused on tumor control, which is occasionally symptom-directed (palliative) and not curative. The treatment goals are to increase life expectancy while maintaining quality of life for as long as possible. In this context, the model of distinct lines of chemotherapy is being abandoned in favor of a continuum-of-care approach similar to that taken in other chronic illnesses.[4] Using currently available data, the authors propose an algorithm for treatment selection based on emerging clinical and molecular data (**Fig. 1**).

The 3 active conventional chemotherapy agents for metastatic colorectal cancer are fluoropyrimidines (including intravenous 5-fluorouracil or its oral prodrug equivalent, capecitabine), irinotecan, and oxaliplatin (**Table 1**). Patients clearly benefit from access to all active agents.[4,5] A variety of targeted therapy agents are also available (**Table 2**), which are incorporated into conventional chemotherapy regimens at various time points across the continuum of care.

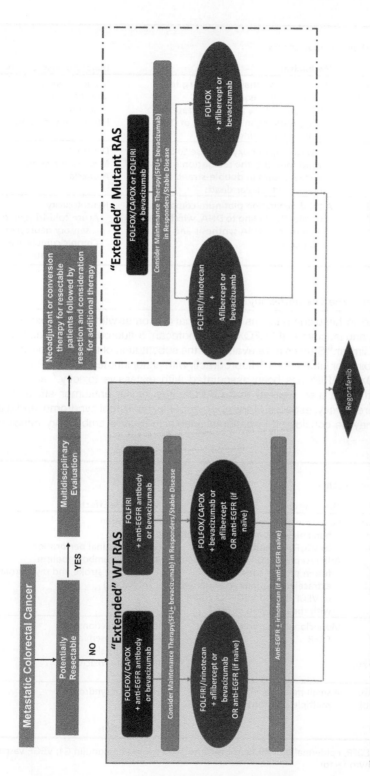

Fig. 1. A proposed algorithm for selection of systemic treatment and integration with surgical resection in patients with metastatic colorectal carcinoma, based on available clinical and molecular data. 5FU, 5-fluorouracil; CAPOX, capecitabine and oxaliplatin; FOLFIRI, irinotecan, 5-fluorouracil, and leucovorin; FOLFOX, oxaliplatin, 5-fluorouracil, and leucovorin; WT, wild-type.

Table 1
Conventional chemotherapy agents

Category	Mechanism	Major Adverse Effects
Fluoropyrimidines (5-fluorouracil/ capecitabine)	Thymidylate synthase inhibitors; the accumulated deoxyuridine monophosphate misincorporates into DNA, resulting in inhibition of DNA synthesis and function	Myelosuppression Mucositis and/or diarrhea Hand-foot syndrome
Irinotecan	Converted by carboxylesterase to SN38, which prevents the relegation of DNA and further results in double-strand DNA breaks and cellular death	Diarrhea Myelosuppression Alopecia
Oxaliplatin	A third-generation platinum compound, covalently binding to DNA, which results in inhibition of DNA synthesis and transcription	Neurotoxicity Acute cold-triggered sensory neuropathy Chronic cumulative sensory neuropathy

Initial Treatment: The Chemotherapy Backbone

Data from head-to-head comparisons suggest that outcomes with first-line oxaliplatin, 5-fluorouracil, and leucovorin (FOLFOX) and irinotecan, 5-fluorouracil, and leucovorin (FOLFIRI) are similar.[6] Studies have evaluated the substitution of the oral fluoropyrimidine capecitabine for intravenous 5-fluorouracil, with either irinotecan (CAPIRI) or oxaliplatin (CAPOX). CAPIRI has been associated with excessive toxicity,[7] and is not recommended. Data also suggest that CAPOX has similar antitumor efficacy but potentially more toxicity, especially thrombocytopenia, hand-foot syndrome, and diarrhea,[8,9] but may be considered in patients unable to receive ambulatory infusional

Table 2
Targeted therapy agents

Category	Mechanism	Major Side Effects
VEGF inhibitors (bevacizumab, aflibercept)	Bevacizumab: a recombinant humanized monoclonal antibody to VEGF-A receptors Aflibercept: a VEGF receptor decoy fusion protein consisting of extracellular domain components of VEGF-R1 and VEGF-R2 fused with the Fc region of IgG1	Hypertension Bleeding Gastrointestinal perforation Arterial thromboembolism (including stroke and myocardial infarction)
Anti-EGFR antibodies (cetuximab, panitumumab)	Monoclonal antibodies against EGFR	Infusion reactions Hypomagnesemia Pruritus/dry skin Pulmonary toxicity Diarrhea
Kinase inhibitor (regorafenib)	A small-molecule inhibitor of multiple cell-signaling kinases	Hand-foot syndrome Fatigue Diarrhea Hypertension

Abbreviations: EGFR, epidermal growth factor receptor; IgG1, immunoglobulin G1; VEGF, vascular endothelial growth factor.

therapy. Irinotecan and oxaliplatin (IROX) may be considered in a small proportion of patients who are intolerant of 5-fluorouracil.[10]

The choice between initial FOLFIRI and FOLFOX or CAPOX should be based on expected treatment-related toxicity in the context of coexisting comorbidities for any given patients. For instance, a patient with long-standing diabetes mellitus or pre-existing neuropathy may be recommended FOLFIRI rather than the neuropathy-inducing FOLFOX regimen. For patients who are not candidates for an intensive oxaliplatin-based or irinotecan-based regimen because of comorbidities, performance status, or personal preference, fluoropyrimidine therapy alone (with or without a targeted therapy agent) can be considered. In early studies, high rates of successful resection and favorable long-term survival rates for patients with initially unresectable liver metastases have been reported for a triplet regimen that combines all 3 classes of conventional chemotherapy (FOLFOXIRI),[11,12] and this regimen may be considered in highly select patients until additional randomized data are available.

For patients receiving a FOLFIRI-like regimen after progression on FOLFOX, expected response rates are between 4% and 20%, and PFS of 2.5 to 7.1 months, respectively.[13,14] On the other hand, studies of oxaliplatin-based therapy in patients failing an initial irinotecan-based regimen describe response rates around 10%, and median time to progression (TTP) of 4 to 5 months.[14,15] The current standard approach to metastatic colorectal cancer includes either oxaliplatin-based therapy after progression on a FOLFIRI-like regimen, or irinotecan-based therapy after progression on a FOLFOX-like regimen; most clinicians, including the authors, prefer an oxaliplatin-based regimen first, based on perceived higher response rate and slightly better toxicity profile, although neither of these perceptions has been substantially proved in head-to-head studies. FOLFIRI is preferred in patients with a history of adjuvant FOLFOX in the preceding 12 months.

The Chemotherapy Backbone: Bottom Line

- Either FOLFOX or FOLFIRI can be used in the first-line setting, depending on patient preferences and concerns about specific toxicities.
- Single-agent fluoropyrimidine may be used in settings where patients are unable or unwilling to receive combination therapy.
- FOLFOXIRI may be considered in highly select patients in whom a high response rate and aggressive approach are warranted.
- Targeted agents should be added to all chemotherapy backbones when possible.

Incorporating Anti–Vascular Endothelial Growth Factor Agents

The anti-VEGF monoclonal antibody, bevacizumab, does not have significant single-agent activity in metastatic colorectal cancer.[16] However, multiple clinical trials have shown that it adds benefits to first-line fluoropyrimidine-, oxaliplatin- and irinotecan-based regimens given across the continuum of care in patients with metastatic disease.[17–19] In the randomized TREE-2 trial, for instance, adding bevacizumab to oxaliplatin and 5-fluorouracil-containing regimens in previously untreated patients resulted in a median OS of 23.7 months versus 18.2 months for the combined non–bevacizumab-treated groups.[20] The addition of bevacizumab to oxaliplatin-based regimen in previously treated patients with metastatic colorectal cancer (with 5-fluorouracil or irinotecan) also led to improved PFS (7.3 vs 4.7 months) and median OS (12.9 vs 10.8 months) compared with FOLFOX alone in the ECOG 3200 trial conducted in the second-line setting.[16] Thus, the accepted consensus in the management of metastatic colorectal cancer is to add bevacizumab to the chemotherapy backbone chosen for the individual patient for initial or subsequent treatments. Bevacizumab is associated with increased rates of grade 3 or 4 hypertension, bowel perforation, impaired wound healing, arterial thromboembolism, and bleeding events.[21] Careful patient selection and monitoring for toxicity is important, as is timing of discontinuation of treatment if surgical intervention is to be considered. Given that the half-life of bevacizumab is approximately 3 weeks, the authors' general recommendation is to hold bevacizumab for a period of 4 to 6 weeks before and after surgery to avoid post-surgical complications such as wound dehiscence.

Traditional teaching with conventional treatments has been to discontinue all classes of drugs when patients progress. It is unclear, however, whether a similar strategy should be adopted with biological agents, particularly those with antiangiogenic activity. The efficacy of continuing bevacizumab beyond progression was tested in the ML18147 phase III trial, which demonstrated a significant improvement in PFS (5.7 vs 4.1 months) and OS (11.2 vs 9.8 months). Bevacizumab-related adverse events were not increased in comparison with historical data of first-line bevacizumab treatment.[22]

Aflibercept is a recombinant fusion protein that binds with higher affinity to VEGF-A than does bevacizumab in a cell-free system.[23] In the United States, aflibercept is approved for use in combination with FOLFIRI for the treatment of patients with metastatic colorectal cancer that is resistant to or has progressed following an oxaliplatin-containing regimen, based on the placebo-controlled VELOUR trial.[24] The median OS was significantly longer in patients treated with aflibercept (13.5 vs 12.1 months) as was median PFS (6.9 vs 4.7 months). Treatment benefit was similar regardless of prior bevacizumab exposure (about 30% of patients in the trial).[25] However, there are no head-to-head trials comparing continuation of bevacizumab beyond progression with switching to aflibercept in this setting; hence, either strategy is considered appropriate.

Incorporating Anti–Epidermal Growth Factor Receptor Agents: Role of Precision Therapy

Anti-EGFR agents can improve outcomes in metastatic disease, both as single agents and in combination regimens. Biomarker analysis is critical to patient selection for therapy with an EGFR inhibitor, a form of so-called precision or personalized medicine whereby tumor mutations in individual specimens are used to select systemic therapy. Activating mutations in KRAS, which result in constitutive activation of the RAS-RAF-ERK pathway, lead to resistance to anti-EGFR therapy.[26] In 2009, the American Society of Clinical Oncology recommended that all patients being considered for anti-EGFR therapy undergo KRAS mutation testing of their tumors, and that treatment with these agents be restricted to those with wild-type (WT) KRAS,[27] defined as an absence of mutations in exon 2 of KRAS gene by qualitative real-time polymerase chain reaction. Emerging data suggest that resistance to anti-EGFR therapies can also be mediated by lower-frequency mutations in KRAS outside of exon 2 and in NRAS.[28–31] In 2013, the PRIME study demonstrated that within the so-called classic WT KRAS population (without mutations in exon 2), patients with mutations in other KRAS exons (exons 3 and 4) or in NRAS (exons 2 and 3) did not benefit from the addition of panitumumab to FOLFOX. Of concern, such patients had a nonsignificantly worse PFS (7.3 vs 8.0 months, $P = .33$) and OS (hazard ratio 1.39, $P = .12$) with the addition of anti-EGFR therapy.[28] Furthermore, the addition of panitumumab to chemotherapy increased OS significantly in patients with so-called extended WT RAS (no mutations in exons 2, 3, and 4 of KRAS and NRAS).[28] Other analyses have confirmed these findings. The emerging consensus is that all patients with metastatic colorectal cancer should be tested for extended RAS mutations and that those with such mutations should not be recommended anti-EGFR therapy.

First-line cetuximab was explored in the CRYSTAL trial in previously untreated metastatic colorectal cancer; patients were randomly assigned to FOLFIRI with or without cetuximab. Among patients with WT KRAS, response rates were significantly higher in those who received cetuximab (57% vs 40%), as was median PFS and OS (23.5 vs 20 months).[32] The EPIC trial randomly assigned 1298 oxaliplatin-refractory patients to irinotecan with or without cetuximab. PFS was significantly higher with combined therapy (4 vs 2.6 months), as were rates of objective response (16% vs 4%) and overall disease control (61% vs 46%).[33] Increasing data also support the efficacy of first-, second-, and third-line panitumumab in combination with oxaliplatin-based or irinotecan-based regimens in patients with WT RAS tumors.[28,34–39] Cetuximab and panitumumab appear to have comparable efficacy when used as single agents for salvage therapy in patients with chemotherapy-refractory metastatic colorectal cancer,[40,41] and when used for initial or subsequent therapy for metastatic colorectal cancer in conjunction with an irinotecan-based chemotherapy regimen. The choice of anti-EGFR agent largely depends on provider comfort with specific agents, concerns regarding infusional reactions, and logistics (cetuximab is a weekly regimen whereas panitumumab is every other week).

Although response rates in individual studies were higher with the addition of cetuximab to chemotherapy than by adding bevacizumab in patients with WT KRAS status, the median survival benefit is similar.[16,20,32,33] Where there is likelihood of converting patients to resectable metastatic disease, the improved response rates support using anti-EGFR therapy in the first-line setting. Dual antibody therapy targeting both VEGF and EGFR has been tested and found to lead to worsened outcomes, and is therefore not recommended.[42,43]

Among patients with WT RAS, an important issue is whether to add bevacizumab or anti-EGFR therapy to the chemotherapy backbone as initial therapy. Two initial trials with small sample sizes suggested benefit for an "anti-EGFR first" approach.[30,31] However, definitive results from the largest such study, C80405, a US Intergroup study, were presented in 2014 and showed no survival difference for either cetuximab or bevacizumab when combined with a chemotherapy backbone in the initial treatment setting (29.9 vs 29 months, $P = .34$).[2] Therefore, either antibody can be used in the initial therapy setting, with choice driven again by toxicity, patient preference, and logistics. It should be noted that C80405 did include patients who may have had extended RAS mutations (only classic KRAS mutants were excluded); results of this subgroup analysis may alter the final conclusions in the future.

Regorafenib

Regorafenib targets a variety of kinases implicated in angiogenic and tumor growth-promoting pathways. Its activity in refractory metastatic colorectal cancer was demonstrated in the CORRECT trial.[44] Patients who had progressed after multiple standard therapies assigned to regorafenib had a modest though statistically significant improvement in median OS (6.4 vs 5 months), and PFS (1.9 months vs 1.7 months).[44] At present, regorafenib is reserved for patients whose cancers have progressed on the other standard chemotherapeutic and targeted therapy agents.

Targeted Therapy: Bottom Line

- All chemotherapy backbones in initial and subsequent settings should be accompanied by one targeted agent, unless specific contraindications exist.

- Anti-EGFR approaches should be used only in patients with extended RAS WT tumors.
- Bevacizumab or anti-EGFR therapy may be used in the initial setting in such extended RAS WT patients.
- Bevacizumab may be continued beyond progression with a change in chemotherapy backbone.
- Dual antibody therapy should be avoided.

MAINTENANCE REGIMENS

Approximately 75% of patients discontinue first-line chemotherapy in trials for reasons other than progressive disease, and face the question of whether to consider maintenance chemotherapy or take a chemotherapy break. The OPTIMOX trials showed that oxaliplatin can be safely stopped after 6 cycles in a FOLFOX regimen, and that complete discontinuation of chemotherapy had a negative impact on PFS compared with maintenance therapy with 5-fluorouracil.[45,46] Results from CAIRO-3 showed that maintenance therapy with bevacizumab plus capecitabine after 6 cycles of CAPOX plus bevacizumab was associated with a significant longer PFS (8.5 vs 4.1 months).[47] Decisions regarding maintenance therapy versus treatment breaks must also take into account patient preferences and cost.

POTENTIALLY CURABLE ADVANCED COLORECTAL CANCER

The liver is the first site of hematogenous dissemination in most patients with colorectal cancer. Approximately 10% of patients can live past 5 years even with metastatic disease.[48] The definition of resectable metastatic disease is evolving, and there is not an accepted standard: even bilobar metastases and extrahepatic disease are no longer considered contraindications. Decision-making in this setting requires multidisciplinary collaboration: a practical approach requires that patients should be medically fit for surgery, existing liver disease should be resectable with adequate liver remnant, and extrahepatic disease should be controlled. Surgical resection is the preferred treatment in patients with oligometastatic disease primarily in the liver, with 5-year survival rates of approximately 50% to 60% in patients with favorable prognostic features.[49,50] Approximately one-fifth of such patients survive beyond 10 years in some series,[51] and this applies also to nonhepatic disease in certain series. When the primary tumor site is controlled and the metastatic disease is limited in lungs without extrapulmonary location (except for resectable or resected hepatic lesion), resection of isolated pulmonary metastases can increase survival rates up to 40% at 5 years.[25,52]

Select patients with initially unresectable liver metastases may become eligible for resection if the response to chemotherapy is sufficient. This approach has been termed conversion therapy to distinguish it from neoadjuvant therapy. Conversion therapy allows 12% to 33% of initially unresectable or borderline resectable metastases to become eligible for metastasectomy.[11,12,53] Five-year survival rates average 30% to 35%, which is substantially better than expected with chemotherapy alone.

A regimen with a high likelihood of objective response is typically chosen because of the strong correlation with subsequent resection rates. However, the choice of regimen is not well established. The triplet chemotherapy regimen FOLFOXIRI with bevacizumab was associated with significantly higher response rates (65% vs 53%) and PFS (median 12.2 vs 9 months) in comparison with FOLFIRI plus bevacizumab in the phase III TRIBE trial.[11] However, FOLFOXIRI did not result in a significantly higher secondary complete (R0) liver resection rate (15% vs 12%), and was associated with greater adverse effects.[54] Combination of anti-EGFR inhibitor with either irinotecan-based or oxaliplatin-based regimens has shown modestly improved resection rates in patients with WT KRAS status.[55,56] The German multicenter randomized phase II trial (CELM study), by using FOLFOX plus cetuximab or FOLFIRI plus cetuximab, showed 62% tumor response in all patients with 70% in WT KRAS patients, but no OS and PFS improvement.[55] A promising recent phase II study reported a surgical R0 resection conversion rate of approximately 70% (14 of 20 patients) with FOLFOX with dose-escalating cetuximab in initially unresectable patients with WT KRAS status.[57] Hepatic intra-arterial chemotherapy either alone or in addition to systemic therapy also has the potential to downstage hepatic metastases.[58,59] However, there are no randomized trials comparing hepatic pumps with contemporary systemic chemotherapy alone, and this approach is not currently widely used in the United States.

For patients with initially resectable liver metastases, a common sequence (particularly for patients with synchronous metastatic disease) is initial systemic chemotherapy, mainly to obtain prognostic information, treat potentially disseminated micrometastases as early as possible, evaluate for emerging additional metastases, and test the chemosensitivity of the tumor. Upfront surgery is an appropriate option for patients with metachronous presentation of hepatic metastases. The European Organization for Research and Treatment of Cancer Intergroup trial 40983 enrolled 364 resectable patients with up to 4 metastases without prior exposure to oxaliplatin who were randomly assigned to liver resection with or without perioperative FOLFOX chemotherapy.[60] Initial chemotherapy improved patient selection for hepatic resection. The postoperative complication rate was significantly higher in the chemotherapy group (25% vs 16%). However, the postoperative mortality was not higher than surgery alone (1 vs 2 deaths). In the latest update, at a median follow-up of 8.5 years, there was a nonstatistically significant trend in 5-year PFS favoring chemotherapy (38% vs 33%), but 5-year OS was not significantly better in the chemotherapy group (51% vs 48%).[61] A recent retrospective study suggested that neoadjuvant therapy only benefits high-risk patients.[62] In patients with more than 2 risk factors, those who received neoadjuvant chemotherapy had improved median survival (38.9 vs 28.4 months). By contrast, for low-risk patients, survival outcomes were similar with or without neoadjuvant chemotherapy, median survival (60.0 vs 60.0 months) and 5-year OS (64% vs 57%, $P>.05$).[62]

Liver metastases recur in up to 80% of patients after liver resection, with approximately half being confined to the liver. In these patients, provided that the aforementioned resectability criteria are fulfilled, repeat liver resection is safe and can lead to survival rates that are equivalent to those reported for first hepatectomy.[63,64] It is therefore important to monitor patients carefully to detect hepatic recurrence at a resectable stage. Only limited evidence is available regarding the optimal follow-up strategy after liver resection for metastatic colorectal cancer.[65,66] The following surveillance strategy for patients with metastatic disease rendered disease-free is reasonable: carcinoembryonic antigen, liver function tests, and computed tomography scan of the chest, abdomen, and pelvis every 3 to 6 months for 2 years, then every 6 to 12 months for up to 5 years.

Other Liver-Directed Treatments

Several other regional therapies, including local tumor ablation, regional hepatic intra-arterial chemotherapy or chemoembolization, and stereotactic body radiation therapy, are options for patients with liver-isolated colorectal cancer metastases who are not candidates for surgery.[67,68] These therapies are often incorporated with initial hepatic resection or used as alternatives in patients who are not medically fit enough to undergo surgical resection. Although these methods can provide excellent local control, long-term survival outcomes are not well studied.

ROLE FOR RESECTION OF PRIMARY TUMOR

There are 2 broad indications for resection of the primary tumor in metastatic colorectal cancer: palliation of symptoms and intention cure. The approach therefore can be categorized according to symptoms of the primary tumor and resectability of the metastatic disease.

Symptomatic Primary Tumor with Unresectable Metastatic Disease

The most common symptoms requiring intervention of the primary tumor are obstruction, bleeding/anemia, and perforation. There is generally not time nor a role for neoadjuvant chemotherapy in this setting. The goal is to palliate symptoms and improve the quality of life. Although surgical oncology principles are encouraged, diffuse disease or carcinomatosis may not allow a proper oncologic operation. For example, a diverting stoma or bypass of an obstructing tumor may be performed to limit morbidity and facilitate quicker transition to systemic therapy.

Symptomatic Primary with Resectable Metastatic Disease

As already mentioned, treatment of symptomatic tumors requires timely intervention. However, if the metastatic disease is treatable surgically, a decision must be made as regards timing. The primary objective is to relieve the symptoms and approach the primary tumor with surgical oncologic principles such as high ligation of vessels, adequate lymph node harvest, minimal manipulation of the tumor, and achievement of adequate margins. If the symptom is acute obstruction or perforation and the patient requires emergent surgery, only the primary tumor should be approached. In the setting of an elective operation, the decision to resect liver metastases depends on the extent of disease and magnitude of surgery required. In general, if a simple wedge resection/metastasectomy is all that is required, the liver may be addressed at the same time as the colon resection. If more extensive liver resection is required, the primary tumor alone should be addressed with a plan for chemotherapy and staged liver resection.

Asymptomatic Primary Tumor with Unresectable Metastatic Disease

The role for resection of an asymptomatic primary tumor in the setting of unresectable distant disease is controversial. Although retrospective data suggest a survival benefit of resection and a prospective study showed that an unresected primary led to major morbidity in a subgroup of patients (n = 12 of 86),[69] the evidence is not definitive. Proponents of resection argue that patients may achieve a better response to chemotherapy with a lower tumor burden, and that it eliminates the risk of complications developing during chemotherapy such as obstruction or perforation. The argument against resection is based on the potential for postoperative complications that may delay or even prevent chemotherapy.[70] Factors associated with improved survival include age less than 70 years, no extrahepatic disease, good functional status, and liver burden less than 50%.[70]

Asymptomatic Primary Tumor with Resectable Metastatic Disease

Resecting the primary tumor remains the essential cornerstone of treatment in resectable metastatic disease. The timing of resection of the primary in relation to liver resection and chemotherapy remains an issue of debate, and multiple approaches show equipoise. The classic approach involves resection of the primary tumor, followed by adjuvant chemotherapy, then metastasectomy. Some groups champion neoadjuvant therapy to attack the systemic disease first, as distant diseases determine survival. This approach allows the tumor biology to declare itself through response to therapy. Patients who progress and become unresectable are saved from the morbidity of surgery on the primary. Patients who respond will go on to resection of the primary and liver lesions. Both synchronous resections and staged resections have been described. Some groups prefer a staged resection with a liver-first approach, but the success is variable.[71] Management of these cases is best served by discussion with a multidisciplinary team involving hepatobiliary surgeons, colorectal surgeons, and oncologists.

SUMMARY AND FUTURE DIRECTIONS

The past decade has seen an impressive improvement in outcomes for patients with metastatic colorectal cancer. Patients seen in the clinic today can have discussions about expected survival outcomes ranging in "years." Even the term "cure" is not out of place in a discussion in the metastatic setting. This remarkable improvement in outcomes has resulted not from a "magic bullet" but from a convergence of forces: new drugs and regimens that can be used sequentially to allow quality of life and extended life expectancy, improvement in surgical techniques, and data demonstrating the value of surgical resection and liver-directed therapy.

Integrating personalized medicine into the care of patients with colorectal cancer will be the next step forward. The development of biomarkers that predict response to anti-EGFR therapy is an example of how molecular profiling can significantly improve outcomes in patients with RAS WT tumors, and can spare patients with RAS mutant tumors both toxicity and cost. Commercial vendors are already offering next-generation genomic sequencing at the bedside. The authors and others are participating in novel trials that offer targeted agents based on mutations identified using genomic sequencing. As additional data become available, it is anticipated that far greater individualization of treatment will be possible. In a recent analysis of 1290 colorectal cancers using gene-expression profiling, 6 clinically different subtypes were identified, each showing different degrees of activation of Wnt signaling and "stemness," response to anti-EGFR and irinotecan-based therapy, and survival in the adjuvant and metastatic settings.[72] Further such research will accelerate novel drug development and testing, and allow clinicians to continually refine and individualize treatment. The successes of the past decade have raised hopes and expectations that the conversion of metastatic colorectal cancer from a lethal to a chronic illness, with durable remissions and even cures, can be a reality for most patients.

ACKNOWLEDGMENTS

Dr A.A. Khorana would like to acknowledge research support from the Sondra and Stephen Hardis Chair in Oncology Research and the Scott Hamilton CARES Initiative. Dr M.F. Kalady is the Krause-Lieberman Chair in Colorectal Surgery.

REFERENCES

1. Siegel R, Ma J, Zou Z, et al. Cancer statistics, 2014. CA Cancer J Clin 2014;64(1): 9–29.
2. Venook AP, Niedzwiecki D, Lenz HJ, et al. CALGB/SWOG 80405: phase III trial of irinotecan/5-FU/leucovorin (FOLFIRI) or oxaliplatin/5-FU/leucovorin (mFOLFOX6)

with bevacizumab (BV) or cetuximab (CET) for patients (pts) with KRAS wild-type (wt) untreated metastatic adenocarcinoma of the colon or rectum (MCRC). J Clin Oncol 2014;32:5s.

3. Scheithauer W, Rosen H, Kornek GV, et al. Randomised comparison of combination chemotherapy plus supportive care with supportive care alone in patients with metastatic colorectal cancer. BMJ 1993;306(6880):752–5.

4. Goldberg RM, Rothenberg ML, Van Cutsem E, et al. The continuum of care: a paradigm for the management of metastatic colorectal cancer. Oncologist 2007;12(1):38–50.

5. Grothey A, Sargent D. Overall survival of patients with advanced colorectal cancer correlates with availability of fluorouracil, irinotecan, and oxaliplatin regardless of whether doublet or single-agent therapy is used first line. J Clin Oncol 2005;23(36):9441–2.

6. Colucci G, Gebbia V, Paoletti G, et al. Phase III randomized trial of FOLFIRI versus FOLFOX4 in the treatment of advanced colorectal cancer: a multicenter study of the Gruppo Oncologico Dell'Italia Meridionale. J Clin Oncol 2005; 23(22):4866–75.

7. Patt YZ, Lee FC, Liebmann JE, et al. Capecitabine plus 3-weekly irinotecan (XELIRI regimen) as first-line chemotherapy for metastatic colorectal cancer: phase II trial results. Am J Clin Oncol 2007;30(4):350–7.

8. Diaz-Rubio E, Tabernero J, Gomez-Espana A, et al. Phase III study of capecitabine plus oxaliplatin compared with continuous-infusion fluorouracil plus oxaliplatin as first-line therapy in metastatic colorectal cancer: final report of the Spanish Cooperative Group for the treatment of digestive tumors trial. J Clin Oncol 2007; 25(27):4224–30.

9. Porschen R, Arkenau HT, Kubicka S, et al. Phase III study of capecitabine plus oxaliplatin compared with fluorouracil and leucovorin plus oxaliplatin in metastatic colorectal cancer: a final report of the AIO Colorectal Study Group. J Clin Oncol 2007;25(27):4217–23.

10. Sanoff HK, Sargent DJ, Campbell ME, et al. Five-year data and prognostic factor analysis of oxaliplatin and irinotecan combinations for advanced colorectal cancer: N9741. J Clin Oncol 2008;26(35):5721–7.

11. Falcone A, Ricci S, Brunetti I, et al. Phase III trial of infusional fluorouracil, leucovorin, oxaliplatin, and irinotecan (FOLFOXIRI) compared with infusional fluorouracil, leucovorin, and irinotecan (FOLFIRI) as first-line treatment for metastatic colorectal cancer: the Gruppo Oncologico Nord Ovest. J Clin Oncol 2007;25(13):1670–6.

12. Masi G, Loupakis F, Pollina L, et al. Long-term outcome of initially unresectable metastatic colorectal cancer patients treated with 5-fluorouracil/leucovorin, oxaliplatin, and irinotecan (FOLFOXIRI) followed by radical surgery of metastases. Ann Surg 2009;249(3):420–5.

13. Bidard FC, Tournigand C, Andre T, et al. Efficacy of FOLFIRI-3 (irinotecan D1,D3 combined with LV5-FU) or other irinotecan-based regimens in oxaliplatin-pretreated metastatic colorectal cancer in the GERCOR OPTIMOX1 study. Ann Oncol 2009;20(6):1042–7.

14. Tournigand C, Andre T, Achille E, et al. FOLFIRI followed by FOLFOX6 or the reverse sequence in advanced colorectal cancer: a randomized GERCOR study. J Clin Oncol 2004;22(2):229–37.

15. Rothenberg ML, Oza AM, Bigelow RH, et al. Superiority of oxaliplatin and fluorouracil-leucovorin compared with either therapy alone in patients with progressive colorectal cancer after irinotecan and fluorouracil-leucovorin: interim results of a phase III trial. J Clin Oncol 2003;21(11):2059–69.

16. Giantonio BJ, Catalano PJ, Meropol NJ, et al. Bevacizumab in combination with oxaliplatin, fluorouracil, and leucovorin (FOLFOX4) for previously treated metastatic colorectal cancer: results from the Eastern Cooperative Oncology Group Study E3200. J Clin Oncol 2007;25(12):1539–44.

17. Hurwitz HI, Fehrenbacher L, Hainsworth JD, et al. Bevacizumab in combination with fluorouracil and leucovorin: an active regimen for first-line metastatic colorectal cancer. J Clin Oncol 2005;23(15):3502–8.

18. Kabbinavar FF, Hambleton J, Mass RD, et al. Combined analysis of efficacy: the addition of bevacizumab to fluorouracil/leucovorin improves survival for patients with metastatic colorectal cancer. J Clin Oncol 2005;23(16):3706–12.

19. Vincenzi B, Santini D, Russo A, et al. Bevacizumab in association with de Gramont 5-fluorouracil/folinic acid in patients with oxaliplatin-, irinotecan-, and cetuximab-refractory colorectal cancer: a single-center phase 2 trial. Cancer 2009;115(20):4849–56.

20. Hochster HS, Hart LL, Ramanathan RK, et al. Safety and efficacy of oxaliplatin and fluoropyrimidine regimens with or without bevacizumab as first-line treatment of metastatic colorectal cancer: results of the TREE Study. J Clin Oncol 2008; 26(21):3523–9.

21. Scappaticci FA, Skillings JR, Holden SN, et al. Arterial thromboembolic events in patients with metastatic carcinoma treated with chemotherapy and bevacizumab. J Natl Cancer Inst 2007;99(16):1232–9.

22. Bennouna J, Sastre J, Arnold D, et al. Continuation of bevacizumab after first progression in metastatic colorectal cancer (ML18147): a randomised phase 3 trial. Lancet Oncol 2013;14(1):29–37.

23. Holash J, Davis S, Papadopoulos N, et al. VEGF-Trap: a VEGF blocker with potent antitumor effects. Proc Natl Acad Sci U S A 2002;99(17):11393–8.

24. Joulain F, Van Cutsem E, Iqbal SU, et al. Aflibercept versus placebo in combination with FOLFIRI in previously treated metastatic colorectal cancer (mCRC): mean overall survival (OS) estimation from a phase III trial (VELOUR). J Clin Oncol 2012;30(15). Abstract: 3602.

25. Allegra CJ, Lakomy R, Tabernero J, et al. Effects of prior bevacizumab (B) use on outcomes from the VELOUR study: a phase III study of aflibercept (Afl) and FOLFIRI in patients (pts) with metastatic colorectal cancer (mCRC) after failure of an oxaliplatin regimen. J Clin Oncol 2012;30(15). Abstract: 3505.

26. Dahabreh IJ, Terasawa T, Castaldi PJ, et al. Systematic review: anti-epidermal growth factor receptor treatment effect modification by KRAS mutations in advanced colorectal cancer. Ann Intern Med 2011;154(1):37–49.

27. Allegra CJ, Jessup JM, Somerfield MR, et al. American Society of Clinical Oncology provisional clinical opinion: testing for KRAS gene mutations in patients with metastatic colorectal carcinoma to predict response to anti-epidermal growth factor receptor monoclonal antibody therapy. J Clin Oncol 2009;27(12): 2091–6.

28. Douillard JY, Oliner KS, Siena S, et al. Panitumumab-FOLFOX4 treatment and RAS mutations in colorectal cancer. N Engl J Med 2013;369(11):1023–34.

29. Loupakis F, Ruzzo A, Cremolini C, et al. KRAS codon 61, 146 and BRAF mutations predict resistance to cetuximab plus irinotecan in KRAS codon 12 and 13 wild-type metastatic colorectal cancer. Br J Cancer 2009;101(4):715–21.

30. Schwartzberg LS, Rivera F, Karthaus M, et al. Analysis of KRAS/NRAS mutations in PEAK: A randomized phase II study of FOLFOX6 plus panitumumab (pmab) or bevacizumab (bev) as first-line treatment (tx) for wild-type (WT) KRAS (exon 2) metastatic colorectal cancer (mCRC). J Clin Oncol 2013;31(15). Abstract: 3631.

31. Stintzing S, Jung A, Rossius L, et al. Analysis of KRAS/NRAS and BRAF mutations in FIRE-3: a randomized phase III study of FOLFIRI plus cetuximab or bevacizumab as first-line treatment for wild-type (WT) KRAS (exon 2) metastatic colorectal cancer (mCRC) patients. Data presented at the 13th annual European Cancer Congress (ECC), Amsterdam, The Netherlands. September 28, 2013.

32. Van Cutsem E, Kohne CH, Lang I, et al. Cetuximab plus irinotecan, fluorouracil, and leucovorin as first-line treatment for metastatic colorectal cancer: updated analysis of overall survival according to tumor KRAS and BRAF mutation status. J Clin Oncol 2011;29(15):2011–9.

33. Sobrero AF, Maurel J, Fehrenbacher L, et al. EPIC: phase III trial of cetuximab plus irinotecan after fluoropyrimidine and oxaliplatin failure in patients with metastatic colorectal cancer. J Clin Oncol 2008;26(14):2311–9.

34. Andre T, Blons H, Mabro M, et al. Panitumumab combined with irinotecan for patients with KRAS wild-type metastatic colorectal cancer refractory to standard chemotherapy: a GERCOR efficacy, tolerance, and translational molecular study. Ann Oncol 2013;24(2):412–9.

35. Cohn AL, Shumaker GC, Khandelwal P, et al. An open-label, single-arm, phase 2 trial of panitumumab plus FOLFIRI as second-line therapy in patients with metastatic colorectal cancer. Clin Colorectal Cancer 2011;10(3):171–7.

36. Douillard JY, Siena S, Cassidy J, et al. Randomized, phase III trial of panitumumab with infusional fluorouracil, leucovorin, and oxaliplatin (FOLFOX4) versus FOLFOX4 alone as first-line treatment in patients with previously untreated metastatic colorectal cancer: the PRIME study. J Clin Oncol 2010;28(31):4697–705.

37. Kohne CH, Hofheinz R, Mineur L, et al. First-line panitumumab plus irinotecan/5-fluorouracil/leucovorin treatment in patients with metastatic colorectal cancer. J Cancer Res Clin Oncol 2012;138(1):65–72.

38. Peeters M, Price TJ, Cervantes A, et al. Final results from a randomized phase 3 study of FOLFIRI {+/-} panitumumab for second-line treatment of metastatic colorectal cancer. Ann Oncol 2014;25(1):107–16.

39. Seymour MT, Brown SR, Middleton G, et al. Panitumumab and irinotecan versus irinotecan alone for patients with KRAS wild-type, fluorouracil-resistant advanced colorectal cancer (PICCOLO): a prospectively stratified randomised trial. Lancet Oncol 2013;14(8):749–59.

40. Price T, Peeters M, Kim TW, et al. ASPECCT: a randomized, multicenter, open-label, phase 3 study of panitumumab (pmab) vs cetuximab (cmab) for previously treated wild-type (WT) KRAS metastatic colorectal cancer (mCRC). Data presented at the 2013 annual European Cancer Congress (ECC), Amsterdam, The Netherlands. September 29, 2013.

41. Van Cutsem E, Peeters M, Siena S, et al. Open-label phase III trial of panitumumab plus best supportive care compared with best supportive care alone in patients with chemotherapy-refractory metastatic colorectal cancer. J Clin Oncol 2007;25(13):1658–64.

42. Hecht JR, Mitchell E, Chidiac T, et al. A randomized phase IIIB trial of chemotherapy, bevacizumab, and panitumumab compared with chemotherapy and bevacizumab alone for metastatic colorectal cancer. J Clin Oncol 2009;27(5):672–80.

43. Tol J, Koopman M, Cats A, et al. Chemotherapy, bevacizumab, and cetuximab in metastatic colorectal cancer. N Engl J Med 2009;360(6):563–72.

44. Grothey A, Van Cutsem E, Sobrero A, et al. Regorafenib monotherapy for previously treated metastatic colorectal cancer (CORRECT): an international, multicentre, randomised, placebo-controlled, phase 3 trial. Lancet 2013;381(9863):303–12.

45. Chibaudel B, Maindrault-Goebel F, Lledo G, et al. Can chemotherapy be discontinued in unresectable metastatic colorectal cancer? The GERCOR OPTIMOX2 Study. J Clin Oncol 2009;27(34):5727–33.
46. Tournigand C, Cervantes A, Figer A, et al. OPTIMOX1: a randomized study of FOLFOX4 or FOLFOX7 with oxaliplatin in a stop-and-go fashion in advanced colorectal cancer–a GERCOR study. J Clin Oncol 2006;24(3):394–400.
47. Koopman M, Simkens L, May A, et al. Final results and subgroup analyses of the phase 3 CAIRO3 study: maintenance treatment with capecitabine and bevacizumab versus observation after induction treatment with chemotherapy and bevacizumab in metastatic colorectal cancer (mCRC). J Clin Oncol 2014;32(3). Abstract: LBA388.
48. Ferrarotto R, Pathak P, Maru D, et al. Durable complete responses in metastatic colorectal cancer treated with chemotherapy alone. Clin Colorectal Cancer 2011; 10(3):178–82.
49. Rees M, Tekkis PP, Welsh FK, et al. Evaluation of long-term survival after hepatic resection for metastatic colorectal cancer: a multifactorial model of 929 patients. Ann Surg 2008;247(1):125–35.
50. Fong Y, Fortner J, Sun RL, et al. Clinical score for predicting recurrence after hepatic resection for metastatic colorectal cancer: analysis of 1001 consecutive cases. Ann Surg 1999;230(3):309–18 [discussion: 318–21].
51. Tomlinson JS, Jarnagin WR, DeMatteo RP, et al. Actual 10-year survival after resection of colorectal liver metastases defines cure. J Clin Oncol 2007;25(29):4575–80.
52. Pfannschmidt J, Dienemann H, Hoffmann H. Surgical resection of pulmonary metastases from colorectal cancer: a systematic review of published series. Ann Thorac Surg 2007;84(1):324–38.
53. Adam R, Wicherts DA, de Haas RJ, et al. Patients with initially unresectable colorectal liver metastases: is there a possibility of cure? J Clin Oncol 2009;27(11): 1829–35.
54. Falcone A, Cremolini C, Masi G, et al. FOLFOXIRI/bevacizumab (bev) versus FOLFIRI/bev as first-line treatment in unresectable metastatic colorectal cancer (mCRC) patients (pts): results of the phase III TRIBE trial by GONO group. J Clin Oncol 2013;31(15). Abstract: 3505.
55. Folprecht G, Gruenberger T, Bechstein W, et al. Survival of patients with initially unresectable colorectal liver metastases treated with FOLFOX/cetuximab or FOLFIRI/cetuximab in a multidisciplinary concept (CELIM study). Ann Oncol 2014; 25(5):1018–25.
56. Ye LC, Liu TS, Ren L, et al. Randomized controlled trial of cetuximab plus chemotherapy for patients with KRAS wild-type unresectable colorectal liver-limited metastases. J Clin Oncol 2013;31(16):1931–8.
57. Wagman LD, Geller DA, Jacobs SA, et al. NSABP FC-6: phase II study to determine surgical conversion rate in patients (pts) receiving neoadjuvant (NA) mFOLFOX7 plus dose-escalating cetuximab (C) for unresectable K-RAS wild-type (WT) colorectal cancer with metastases (mCRC) confined to the liver. Ann Surg Oncol 2014;21:S13.
58. Goere D, Deshaies I, de Baere T, et al. Prolonged survival of initially unresectable hepatic colorectal cancer patients treated with hepatic arterial infusion of oxaliplatin followed by radical surgery of metastases. Ann Surg 2010;251(4):686–91.
59. Kemeny NE, Melendez FD, Capanu M, et al. Conversion to resectability using hepatic artery infusion plus systemic chemotherapy for the treatment of unresectable liver metastases from colorectal carcinoma. J Clin Oncol 2009;27(21): 3465–71.

60. Nordlinger B, Sorbye H, Glimelius B, et al. Perioperative chemotherapy with FOL-FOX4 and surgery versus surgery alone for resectable liver metastases from colorectal cancer (EORTC Intergroup trial 40983): a randomised controlled trial. Lancet 2008;371(9617):1007–16.
61. Nordlinger B, Sorbye H, Glimelius B, et al. Perioperative FOLFOX4 chemotherapy and surgery versus surgery alone for resectable liver metastases from colorectal cancer (EORTC 40983): long-term results of a randomised, controlled, phase 3 trial. Lancet Oncol 2013;14(12):1208–15.
62. Zhu D, Zhong Y, Wei Y, et al. Effect of neoadjuvant chemotherapy in patients with resectable colorectal liver metastases. PLoS One 2014;9(1):e86543.
63. Adam R, Bismuth H, Castaing D, et al. Repeat hepatectomy for colorectal liver metastases. Ann Surg 1997;225(1):51–60 [discussion: 60–2].
64. Kulik U, Bektas H, Klempnauer J, et al. Repeat liver resection for colorectal metastases. Br J Surg 2013;100(7):926–32.
65. Jones RP, Jackson R, Dunne DF, et al. Systematic review and meta-analysis of follow-up after hepatectomy for colorectal liver metastases. Br J Surg 2012; 99(4):477–86.
66. Verberne CJ, Wiggers T, Vermeulen KM, et al. Detection of recurrences during follow-up after liver surgery for colorectal metastases: both carcinoembryonic antigen (CEA) and imaging are important. Ann Surg Oncol 2013;20(2):457–63.
67. Fiorentini G, Aliberti C, Tilli M, et al. Intra-arterial infusion of irinotecan-loaded drug-eluting beads (DEBIRI) versus intravenous therapy (FOLFIRI) for hepatic metastases from colorectal cancer: final results of a phase III study. Anticancer Res 2012;32(4):1387–95.
68. Wong SL, Mangu PB, Choti MA, et al. American Society of Clinical Oncology 2009 clinical evidence review on radiofrequency ablation of hepatic metastases from colorectal cancer. J Clin Oncol 2010;28(3):493–508.
69. McCahill LE, Yothers G, Sharif S, et al. Primary mFOLFOX6 plus bevacizumab without resection of the primary tumor for patients presenting with surgically unresectable metastatic colon cancer and an intact asymptomatic colon cancer: definitive analysis of NSABP trial C-10. J Clin Oncol 2012;30(26):3223–8.
70. de Mestier L, Manceau G, Neuzillet C, et al. Primary tumor resection in colorectal cancer with unresectable synchronous metastases: a review. World J Gastrointest Oncol 2014;6(6):156–69.
71. Jegatheeswaran S, Mason JM, Hancock HC, et al. The liver-first approach to the management of colorectal cancer with synchronous hepatic metastases: a systematic review. JAMA Surg 2013;148(4):385–91.
72. Sadanandam A, Lyssiotis CA, Homicsko K, et al. A colorectal cancer classification system that associates cellular phenotype and responses to therapy. Nat Med 2013;19(5):619–25.

Constipation
Understanding Mechanisms and Management

Vanessa C. Costilla, MD[a], Amy E. Foxx-Orenstein, DO[b],*

KEYWORDS

- Chronic constipation • Constipation testing • Anorectal manometry
- Dyssynergic defecation • Pelvic floor dysfunction • Outlet dysfunction
- Slow transit constipation

KEY POINTS

- Patients usually have a broader definition of constipation than physicians that encompasses myriad symptoms, including hard stools, feeling of incomplete evacuation, abdominal discomfort, bloating and distension, and excessive straining.
- There are 3 primary types of constipation: functional, slow transit, and outlet dysfunction, and many secondary causes.
- Diagnostic testing is not routinely recommended in the initial evaluation of constipation in the absence of alarm signs and should be targeted at symptoms or signs elicited in the history or physical that suggest an organic process.
- Because sedentary lifestyle and low-fiber diets are associated with constipation, self-management strategies of lifestyle changes that include increased exercise, high-fiber diets, and toilet training are often effective first-line management.
- Fiber and fiber supplements can worsen symptoms in some types of constipation.
- A variety of over-the-counter and prescription medications with unique mechanisms of action are available to remedy constipation.

INTRODUCTION

Constipation is one of the most common gastrointestinal disorders seen by gastroenterologists and primary care physicians. Symptoms of constipation occur frequently, with the greatest prevalence in the elderly. The prevalence in adults older than 60 years is 33%, whereas the overall prevalence among adults of all ages is about 16%.[1] Constipation is found more frequently in women[2] and in lower socioeconomic populations.

This article originally appeared in Clinics in Geriatric Medicine, Volume 30, Issue 1, February 2014.
No funding.
No conflict of interest.
[a] Department of Internal Medicine, Mayo Clinic in Arizona, Scottsdale, AZ, USA; [b] Division of Gastroenterology, Mayo Clinic in Arizona, 13400 East Shea Boulevard, Scottsdale, AZ 85259, USA
* Corresponding author.
E-mail address: foxx-orenstein.amy@mayo.edu

Clinics Collections 7 (2015) 449–457
http://dx.doi.org/10.1016/j.ccol.2015.06.030
2352-7986/15/$ – see front matter Published by Elsevier Inc.

Constipation reduces quality of life and poses a large economic burden, with more than $820 million spent on laxatives each year.[3] Complications of constipation include hemorrhoids, fecal impaction, stercoral ulcers, fecal incontinence, rectal prolapse, volvulus, and excessive perineal or inadequate perineal descent. These complications often lead to emergency department visits and hospitalizations. The mechanisms and management of chronic constipation in the elderly are the focus of this article.

Chronic Constipation: Definitions

Physicians and patients often have different definitions of constipation. Physicians typically define chronic constipation as infrequent bowel movements, usually less than 3 per week, for at least 3 of the prior 12 months. Patients usually have a broader definition that encompasses myriad symptoms including hard stools, feeling of incomplete evacuation, abdominal discomfort, bloating and distension, excessive straining, sense of anorectal blockage during defecation, and the need for manual maneuvers.[1]

Primary Constipation

Chronic constipation can be divided into 2 main categories: primary and secondary. Primary constipation is further divided into 3 main types: functional, outlet dysfunction, and slow transit constipation. There can be overlap of primary types of constipation.

- Functional constipation is diagnosed using the Rome III criteria (**Box 1**). Functional idiopathic constipation is distinct from constipation-predominant irritable bowel syndrome (C-IBS) (**Box 2**), based on the severity of abdominal pain. C-IBS is characterized by abdominal pain or discomfort that improves with defecation.[4]
- Outlet dysfunction (also called *defecation disorders* and *pelvic floor dysfunction*) encompasses several defecation disorders in which the patient experiences difficult or unsatisfactory expulsion of stool from the rectum. Several causes exist, including presence of an anal fissure or stricture, hemorrhoids, rectocele, enterocele, impaired descent (excessive or inadequate), and dyssynergic defecation.[5] Dyssynergic defecation is the impaired relaxation and coordination of abdominal and pelvic floor muscles during evacuation.

Box 1
Functional constipation: Rome III criteria

1. Must include 2 or more of the following:
   a. Straining during at least 25% of defecations
   b. Lumpy or hard stools in at least 25% of defecations
   c. Sensation of incomplete evacuation for at least 25% of defecations
   d. Sensation of anorectal obstruction/blockage for at least 25% of defecations
   e. Manuel maneuvers to facilitate at least 25% of defecations (eg, digital evacuation, support of the pelvic floor)
   f. Fewer than 3 defecations per week
2. Loose stools are rarely present without the use of laxatives
3. Insufficient stools are rarely present without the use of laxatives
4. Criteria fulfilled for the last 3 months with symptom onset at least 6 months prior to diagnosis.[4]

> **Box 2**
> **Irritable bowel syndrome: constipation predominant**
>
> Recurrent abdominal pain or discomfort (uncomfortable sensation not described as pain) at least 3 days per month in the last 3 months associated with 2 or more of the following:
>
> 1. Improvement with defecation
> 2. Onset associated with a change in frequency of stool
> 3. Onset associated with a change in form (appearance) of stool
> 4. Less than 25% of bowel movements were loose stools
> 5. Criterion fulfilled for at least 6 months prior to diagnosis.[4]

- Slow-transit constipation (also called *delayed transit* and *colonoparesis*) is defined as prolonged stool transit (>3 days) through the colon.[6] Patients typically have prolonged time between bowel movements, experience lack of urge to defecate, abdominal distension, and worse symptoms with a high-fiber diet.

Secondary Constipation

Secondary constipation may be caused by diet, medications, and underlying medical conditions (**Table 1**). Diets low in fiber and low fluid intake are associated with increased constipation. Elderly patients who often have a decreased appetite or

Table 1
Secondary causes of constipation

Medications	Neurologic and Myopathic Disorders	Other Conditions Associated with Constipation
Analgesics: *opiates, nonsteroidal anti-inflammatory agents*	Diabetes mellitus	Anorexia
Anticholinergic agents: antihistamines, belladonna	Parkinson's disease	Hypothyroidism
Anticonvulsants: carbamazepine	Connective tissue disorders	Pregnancy
Antihypertensives: calcium channel blockers (verapamil), diuretics, central acting agents (clonidine), β-blockers	Central nervous system lesions (stroke, spinal or gangilion tumor)	Psychological and psychiatric disorders
Antiparkinsonian agents: dopamine agents, benztropine	Amyloidosis	Paraneoplastic syndromes
Antispasmodics	Hirschprung's disease	Pseudo-obstruction
Antidepressants: tricyclic agents, monoamine oxidase inhibitors	Autoimmune	—
Antipsychotics	Chagas disease	—
Metal ion containing agents: antacids, sucralfate, ferrous sulfate	—	—

medical conditions that cause them to have poor intake, such as Alzheimer's dementia, are at especially high risk for dehydration that can lead to constipation.

Several medications are associated with constipation, including anticholinergic drugs, opioids, calcium-channel blockers, and nonsteroidal anti-inflammatory drugs. Anticholinergic drugs can decrease intestinal smooth-muscle contractility.[7] Calcium-channel blockers, especially verapamil, are notorious for causing severe constipation by causing rectosigmoid dysmotility.[8] Elderly patients are often on several of these medications simultaneously.

Several diseases are associated with constipation, including hypothyroidism, diabetes mellitus, and Parkinson's. Rare causes of constipation include amyloidosis and paraneoplastic syndromes. Paraneoplastic syndromes can cause pseudo-obstruction in some patients.

CLINICAL EVALUATION

Evaluation of constipation begins with a detailed history and physical examination, including a visual and digital anal examination. This initial assessment will help identify primary and secondary causes of constipation and the presence of alarm symptoms (**Box 3**). A thorough visual inspection can identify excoriation, hemorrhoids, anal asymmetry, and anal halo, a circumferential thickening of the anus that occurs with rectal prolapse. When bearing down as if to evacuate, one can assess the degree of perineal descent and the presence of rectal prolapse. The digital rectal examination allows for recognition of anatomic abnormalities. Sharp knifelike pain during the digital rectal examination indicates active mucosal injury, such as acute or chronic fissure, ulcer, or inflammation. Fecal impaction, often masked by loose stool or overflow (paradoxic) incontinence, can also be recognized with the digital rectal examination.

Diagnostic Testing

Diagnostic testing for constipation is not routinely recommended early on in the absence of alarm signs. Also, a person's age, functional status, ability to perform testing, and whether results will alter the treatment are considered. A treat-and-test approach is practical and cost effective when testing can be pursued in patients refractory to conservative treatment. Diagnostic testing is often targeted at symptoms or signs elicited in the history or physical that suggest an organic process and should be used if the information gained is apt to alter treatment. Not all patients require the same diagnostic approach.

When alarm symptoms are present, a dedicated evaluation of the colon with colonoscopy, or in selected cases, computed tomographic colography or flexible

---

Box 3
Alarm signs and symptoms

Involuntary weight loss

Hematochezia

Family history of colon cancer or inflammatory bowel disease

Positive fecal occult blood testing

Iron deficiency anemia

Change in symptoms

Nocturnal symptoms

sigmoidoscopy, should be performed. Colonoscopy is indicated in all patients older than 50 years who have never had colorectal cancer screening. Colorectal cancer screening should cease when patients have less than a 10-year life expectancy.

- Anorectal manometry systems quantify internal and external anal sphincter function at rest and during defecatory maneuvers, rectal sensation, and compliance.[9] Anorectal manometry, along with the rectal balloon expulsion test should be performed in patients who do not respond to laxatives or empiric medical therapy for constipation.[1] It may also aid in assessing an objective response to biofeedback therapy or neuromuscular training in patients with dyssynergic defecation. The balloon expulsion test can help identify outlet obstruction but does not exclude a functional or slow transit disorder.
- A colonic transit study objectively measures the speed of stool movement through the colon. Methods to measure colonic transit are radiopaque markers (Sitzmarks), colonic scintigraphy, and wireless motility capsule. These tests are useful for objectively confirming a patients' subjective complaint of constipation or decreased bowel frequency, confirming slow transit, and for documentation of regional delays in transit.[10] The wireless motility capsule or SmartPill is a data recording device that provides information on intestinal pH and transit times of the stomach, small bowel, and colon, which can help exclude a more global gastrointestinal transit disorder.[11]
- Standard defecography provides dynamic evaluation of the pelvic floor and can indicate the presence of failed evacuation caused by various outlet disorders including dyssynergia, rectal prolapse, enterocele, rectocele, cystocele, and degree of perineal descent. Dynamic pelvic magnetic resonance imaging is the only imaging modality that can evaluate global pelvic floor anatomy and the anal sphincter without radiation exposure.[12]
- Colonic manometry can be considered in adults with refractory constipation unresponsive to conventional treatment.[13] Colonic manometry, available mostly in tertiary care centers, may help identify colonic neuropathy, myopathy, or normal colonic function before consideration of colectomy in patients with severe constipation.

NONPHARMACOLOGIC MANAGEMENT OF CONSTIPATION

Because sedentary lifestyle and low-fiber diets are associated with constipation, self-management strategies of lifestyle changes that include increased exercise, high-fiber diets, and toilet training are often effective first-line management. Patients should be instructed to recognize and respond to the urge to defecate, especially in the morning. A regimented daily routine that ends with an evening fiber supplement and begins with mild physical activity, a hot caffeinated beverage, and high-fiber breakfast within an hour of arising takes advantage of known factors that stimulate intestinal motility and the gastrocolic reflex to facilitate defecation.[6]

Dietary Changes

The recommended dose of fiber intake per day is 25 to 30 g; most Americans consume less than half of this amount. Increased fiber consumption and hydration is the first line of therapy for patients with chronic constipation. Patients should strive to increase their dietary fiber by incorporating foods such as prunes, bananas, kiwis, other fruits, vegetables, grains, and bran. Fiber serves to bulk and soften stool. When initiating fiber, it should be titrated up slowly as to not cause abdominal cramping and bloating. Patients may require fiber supplementation to reach the recommended

25 to 30 g daily. Patients with slow transit constipation or refractory pelvic floor dyssynergia do not respond well to high fiber, which should be minimized in this particular group.

Biofeedback

Biofeedback is an effective treatment option for patients with constipation caused by outlet obstruction, particularly dyssynergic defecation. During anorectal biofeedback, patients are trained to use breathing techniques with relaxation of the pelvic floor muscles to produce a propulsive force that facilitates effective evacuation.

PHARMACOLOGIC MANAGEMENT OF CONSTIPATION

When lifestyle, dietary changes, and nonpharmacologic interventions are not enough to ameliorate symptoms, a variety of over-the-counter and prescription medications are available to remedy constipation (**Table 2**).

Table 2
Pharmacologic agents for constipation

Class	Mechanism	Examples
Fiber	Increases the water absorbency properties of stool. Insoluble fiber resists bacterial degradation in the colon and can retain more water than soluble fiber	Bran, psyllium, inulin, methylcellulose, calcium polycarophil
Stimulant laxatives	Directly stimulate mucosa or myenteric plexus to trigger peristaltic contractions and inhibit water absorption	Senna, Bisacodyl, castor oil
Stool softeners	Enhance interaction of stool and water	Docusate
Osmotic laxatives	Create an osmotic gradient caused by poorly absorbed ions and molecules, drawing water into the intestinal lumen that results in soft stool and increased intestinal transit	Polyethylene glycol, lactulose Sorbitol, sodium phosphate, magnesium phosphate
Lubricants	Decrease water absorption and soften stool, allowing easier passage	Mineral oil
Chloride-channel activators	Selectively activate enterocyte type 2 chloride channels, resulting in chloride secretion into the intestinal lumen followed by passive diffusion of sodium and water	Lubiprostone
GC-C activators	Stimulate intestinal epithelial cell GC-C receptors, which increases chloride and bicarbonate secretion and fluid secretion and accelerates stool transit	Linaclotide
Serotonin agents	Stimulate intestinal secretion and motility through activation of 5-Hydroxytryptamine receptor 4 receptors of the enteric nervous system within the gastrointestinal tract	Cisapride, Tegaserod, prucalapride

Abbreviation: GC-C, guanylate cyclase C.

Bulk Fiber

Fiber and fiber supplements (eg, bran, psyllium, methylcellulose, inulin, calcium poly-carbophil) increase the water absorbency properties of stool, stool bulk, consistency, stool weight,[6] and intraluminal volume. Fiber is subject to bacterial fermentation that produces short-chain fatty acids that increase luminal osmolarity and water retention, potentiating the effect on laxation. Common side effects are bloating and flatulence. Fiber is not effective for everyone; it may worsen constipation symptoms in patients with slow transit constipation or refractory outlet dysfunction.

Stimulant Laxatives

Stimulant laxatives act by directly stimulating the mucosa or myenteric plexus on contact that triggers high-amplitude peristaltic contractions and by inhibiting water absorption to increase intestinal motility. Side effects include bothersome abdominal cramping and pain that limit their use and electrolyte abnormalities.

Stool Softeners

Stool softeners act as detergents to enhance interaction between stool and water, which promotes softer stool consistency and facilitates evacuation of hard stool.

Lubricants

Mineral oil is the most commonly used lubricant laxative. This agent decreases water absorption and will soften stool, allowing easier passage. Anal seepage of oily material is common, and lipoid pneumonia can occur if the material is aspirated.

Osmotic Laxatives

Osmotic agents, both saline and hyperosmotic types, create an osmotic gradient through the action of poorly absorbed ions and molecules that are not absorbed in the small bowel but metabolized in the colon. This results in luminal water retention and thus an increase in stool water content, which leads to softer stool and increased intestinal transit.[14] Side effects include abdominal bloating, flatulence, cramping, and distention. These agents are generally well tolerated for long-term use.[15]

Chloride-Channel Activator

Lubiprostone is the sole available agent in this class available by prescription. Chloride-channel activation selectively activates enterocyte type 2 chloride channels, resulting in chloride secretion into the intestinal lumen followed by passive diffusion of sodium and water. The sum effect is an increase in stool water, bowel distention, peristalsis, and laxation without a direct effect on smooth muscle.[16] Side effects are nausea (30%), headache, and diarrhea.[17] Subjects older than 65 experienced fewer and less-severe side effects with lubiprostone than did younger patients.[18]

Guanylate Cyclase C Activator

Linaclotide is the only available agent in this class available by prescription. Linaclotide selectively stimulates intestinal epithelial cell guanylate cyclase C (GC-C) receptors, resulting in an increase in intracellular and extracellular cyclic guanosine monophosphate (cGMP). The net luminal effect is increased chloride and bicarbonate secretion, increased fluid secretion, accelerated stool transit, and laxation.[19] Linaclotide also ameliorates visceral hypersensitivity through a mechanism believed to be dependent on GC-C/cGMP.[20] Evidence indicates that cGMP fluxes out of the epithelial cells into the serosal space to act on the submucosal afferent pain fibers to suppress the nerve firing rate.[21]

Serotonin Agonists

Serotonin agonists stimulate intestinal secretion and motility through activation of 5-hydroxytryptamine receptor 4 receptors of the enteric nervous system within the gastrointestinal tract. Some have been discontinued or restricted (cisapride, Tegaserod) because of potentially harmful cardiovascular side effects. Prucalapride is currently available in Europe and Canada.

SUMMARY

Constipation is a common disorder across all age groups encountered in clinical practice. The prevalence increases significantly with age. It reduces quality of life and imposes a large economic burden on individuals and the health system. As sedentary lifestyle and low-fiber diets contribute to constipation, treatment typically includes increased physical activity, high-fiber diets, and bowel management techniques to facilitate evacuation. However, fiber can worsen some types of chronic constipation. Limited testing will identify the specific type of constipation and could be used if the information gained is apt to alter treatment. Not all patients require the same diagnostic approach. A variety of medications with unique mechanisms of action are available to treat constipation.

REFERENCES

1. Bharucha AE, Dorn SD, Lembo A, et al. American Gastroenterological Association medical position statement on constipation. Gastroenterology 2013;144(1): 211–7.
2. Higgins PD, Johanson JF. Epidemiology of constipation in North America: a systematic review. Am J Gastroenterol 2004;99(4):750–9.
3. Dennison C, Prasad M, Lloyd A, et al. The health-related quality of life and economic burden of constipation. Pharmacoeconomics 2005;23(5):461–76.
4. Longstreth GF, Thompson WG, Chey WD, et al. Functional bowel disorders. Gastroenterology 2006;130(5):1480–91.
5. Foxx-Orenstein AE, McNally MA, Odunsi ST. Update on constipation: one treatment does not fit all. Cleve Clin J Med 2008;75(11):813–24.
6. Gallegos-Orozco JF, Foxx-Orenstein AE, Sterler SM, et al. Chronic constipation in the elderly. Am J Gastroenterol 2012;107(1):18–25 [quiz: 26].
7. Ness J, Hoth A, Barnett MJ, et al. Anticholinergic medications in community-dwelling older veterans: prevalence of anticholinergic symptoms, symptom burden, and adverse drug events. Am J Geriatr Pharmacother 2006;4(1):42–51.
8. Traube M, McCallum RW. Calcium-channel blockers and the gastrointestinal tract. American College of Gastroenterology's Committee on FDA related matters. Am J Gastroenterol 1984;79(11):892–6.
9. Rao SS, Singh S. Clinical utility of colonic and anorectal manometry in chronic constipation. J Clin Gastroenterol 2010;44(9):597–609.
10. Diamant NE, Kamm MA, Wald A, et al. AGA technical review on anorectal testing techniques. Gastroenterology 1999;116(3):735–60.
11. Saad RJ, Hasler WL. A technical review and clinical assessment of the wireless motility capsule. Gastroenterol Hepatol (N Y) 2011;7(12):795–804.
12. Fletcher JG, Busse RF, Riederer SJ, et al. Magnetic resonance imaging of anatomic and dynamic defects of the pelvic floor in defecatory disorders. Am J Gastroenterol 2003;98(2):399–411.

13. Bharucha AE, Pemberton JH, Locke GR 3rd, et al. Gastroenterological Association technical review on constipation. Gastroenterology 2013;144(1):218–38.
14. Xing JH, Soffer EE. Adverse effects of laxatives. Dis Colon Rectum 2001;44(8): 1201–9.
15. Ford AC, Suares NC. Effect of laxatives and pharmacological therapies in chronic idiopathic constipation: systematic review and meta-analysis. Gut 2011;60(2): 209–18.
16. Lacy BE, Levy LC. Lubiprostone: a novel treatment for chronic constipation. Clin Interv Aging 2008;3(2):357–64.
17. Lacy BE, Chey WD. Lubiprostone: chronic constipation and irritable bowel syndrome with constipation. Expert Opin Pharmacother 2009;10(1):143–52.
18. Barish CF, Drossman D, Johanson JF, et al. Efficacy and safety of lubiprostone in patients with chronic constipation. Dig Dis Sci 2010;55(4):1090–7.
19. Harris LA, Crowell MD. Linaclotide, a new direction in the treatment of irritable bowel syndrome and chronic constipation. Curr Opin Mol Ther 2007;9(4):403–10.
20. Johnston JM, Kurtz CB, Macdougall JE, et al. Linaclotide improves abdominal pain and bowel habits in a phase IIb study of patients with irritable bowel syndrome with constipation. Gastroenterology 2010;139(6):1877–86.e2.
21. Silos-Santiago I, Hannig G, Eutamene H, et al. Gastrointestinal pain: unraveling a novel endogenous pathway through uroguanylin/guanylate cyclase-C/cGMP activation. Pain 2013;154(9):1820–30.

The Genetic Predisposition and the Interplay of Host Genetics and Gut Microbiome in Crohn Disease

Hu Jianzhong, PhD

KEYWORDS

- Gut microbiome • Host genetics • Crohn disease

KEY POINTS

- Association between host genetics and Crohn disease.
- Association between gut microbiome and Crohn disease.
- Effect of Crohn disease–associated host genetics on gut microbiome.

HOST GENETICS AND CROHN DISEASE

Crohn disease (CD) is an inflammatory bowel disease (IBD) resulting from defects in the regulatory constraints on mucosal immune response to enteric bacteria, which arises in genetically predisposed individuals.[1,2] Common manifestations of CD include inflammation, diarrhea, and weight loss. According to a report by the US Centers for Disease Control and Prevention, CD may affect more than 700,000 individuals in the United States alone. Geographic statistics showed that the incidence and prevalence of CD also increase across time and in other countries around the world, indicating its emergence as a global disease.[3–5] CD has no gender preference and can occur at any age, but it is more prevalent among adolescents and young adults between the ages of 15 and 35 years.[6] Extensive genetic studies involving linkage analyses, candidate gene studies, and, most recently, genome-wide association studies (GWAS) with imputation and meta-analyses to combine the power of multiple individual GWAS have identified more than 140 loci predisposing to CD.[1,7,8] Emerging evidence from network analysis and biological function studies has shown that many major CD susceptibility loci encode genes involved in cross-talked complex pathways of host

This article originally appeared in Clinics in Laboratory Medicine, Volume 34, Issue 4, December 2014.

The authors declare that there are no conflicts of interest.

Department of Genetics and Genomic Sciences, Icahn School of Medicine at Mount Sinai, 1425 Madison Avenue, 14-70 Icahn Building, New York, NY 10029, USA

E-mail address: Jianzhong.hu@mssm.edu

immune responses. Jostins and colleagues[8] further grouped these genes into several major immunologic pathways, including:

- Genes involved in T-cell circulating, including many specific T-cell subsets, such as T-helper cells (TH17 cells) (*STAT3*), memory T cells (*SP110*), and regulatory T cells (*STAT5B*).
- Genes in recognition of microbial-associated molecular patterns, including bacterial or fungi sensors *NOD1*,[9] *CARD9*, *NOD2/CARD15*,[10–17] and toll-like receptors (*TLRs*).
- Genes involved in autophagy process, including *IRGM*, encoding an autophagy protein that plays an important role in innate immunity against intracellular pathogens and CD-associated adherent-invasive *Escherichia coli* bacteria[18–20]; *ATG16L1*, a key component of the autophagy complex that processes and kills intracellular microbes,[11,13,17,21] and *LRRK2*, encoding a complex protein with multiple functional domains, recently found to regulate autophagosome formation through a calcium-dependent pathway.[22]
- Genes involved in maintenance of epithelial barrier integrity, including *DLG5*, encoding a member of the family of disks large (DLG) homologs with proposed function in the transmission of extracellular signals to the cytoskeleton and in the maintenance of epithelial cell structure[23]; fucosyltransferase 2 (*FUT2*) encoding an enzyme to synthesize the H antigen in body fluids and on the intestinal mucosa. A recent study suggested its role in CD pathogenesis by reprogramming the gut microbiome energy metabolism[24]; and other genes, including *BPI*, *DMBT1*, *IBD5*, *ITLN1*, *MUC1*, *MUC19*, *NKX2-3*, *SLC22A5*, *PTGER4*, *XBP1*, *ZNF365*.[8]
- Genes in regulation of cytokine production, specifically interferon-γ, interleukin 12 (IL-12), tumor necrosis factor α, IL-10 signaling, *IL17*, *IL18RAP*, *CCR6*, and so forth.
- Genes with proposed function in other immunologic processes.

MICROBIOME AND CROHN DISEASE

Although CD has a strong genetic predisposition, overall, only ~14% total phenotypic variances of CD can be explained by risk loci.[8] Epidemiologic studies suggest that environmental factors are also essential contributors to the CD pathogenesis. For instance, smoking has been shown to be a risk factor for CD.[25] Many other environmental factors for IBD, including diet, infectious agents, medicine, stress, and social factors have been investigated. Those environmental factors may act independently or synergistically with genetic factors on the CD pathogenesis.

Recently, many studies have found that the identity and relative abundance of members of human-associated microbial communities are associated with different states of CD.[26,27] Microbes that live on and inside the human body (microbiota) consist of more than 100 trillion microbial cells and outnumber the quantity of the host cells by a factor of 10:1.[28] Commensal bacteria provide a wide range of metabolic functions that the human body lacks. They facilitate diverse processes such as digestion, absorption, and storage of nutrients, as well as protection against pathogen colonization through competition for nutrients, secretion of antimicrobial substances, and microniche exclusion.[29] Commensal bacteria also promote angiogenesis and development of the intestinal epithelium and have been shown to be essential for the normal development and function of the immune system.[29] Although miniscule inoculations of particular pathogenic strains can cause disease, little is known about whether there are core microbiome profiles that we all share in health and disease.[30–35] Although more studies on unrelated healthy adults have shown substantial diversity in their gut communities, the sampling sizes are often moderate, and how this diversity is affected by the host genetics or relates to function remains obscure.

Distinctive membership and composition of the gut microbiota have been shown to play a significant role in CD pathogenesis.[32,36,37] One recent study of 231 patients with IBD and healthy control individuals[38] showed that microbiome profiles are different between patients with CD and healthy control individuals. Particularly, compared with the healthy controls, the abundance of *Roseburia*, *Phascolarctobacterium*, Ruminococcaceae, and *Faecalibacterium* were reduced and *Clostridium* and *Escherichia/Shigella* were enriched in patients with CD. Some differences were observed only in tissue biopsies but not fecal samples. Another recent study of 447 pediatric patients with CD and 221 control individuals[39] showed that enrichment in Enterobacteriaceae, Pasteurellacaea, Veillonellaceae, and Fusobacteriaceae, and depletion in Erysipelotrichales, Bacteroidales, and Clostridiales, correlates strongly with disease status. This microbiome study also suggested that antibiotic exposure might amplify the microbial dysbiosis associated with CD.

EFFECT OF CROHN DISEASE–ASSOCIATED HOST GENETICS ON GUT MICROBIOME

Because many CD-associated host genes are related to microbial recognition, response, and clearance, it is expected that the variation on those genes may substantially affect the composition or structure of the gut microbiome. Many studies using host candidate gene deletions in animal models have observed associated substantial changes in microbiota. Although few human studies have elucidated the role of host genotype in reshaping the microbiota composition, a recent study of pediatric patients with CD[40] reported the covariations between the host ileal gene expression and the ileal microbiome communities, suggesting a global link between the host genetics and microbiome. Several major CD susceptibility genes have been reported to modulate the gut microbiome. Those genes are involved in 3 host immune pathways.

Recognition of Microbial-Associated Molecular Patterns

NOD2/CARD15 gene is one of the major susceptibility genes for CD.[14,16] Its gene product detects bacterial peptidoglycan found in both gram-positive and gram-negative bacteria and stimulates the host innate immune response. Several animal studies[41–43] reported that the deficiency of *NOD2* in mice resulted in substantially altered gut microbiome composition. At phylum level, the abundance of both ileal-associated and fecal-associated Bacteroidaceae was significantly increased in *NOD2*-deficient mice compared with wild-type mice.[41,42,44] In addition, the overall bacterial loads in the feces and terminal ileum of *NOD2*-deficient mice were significantly increased.[42] This finding might be partly explained because *NOD2* regulate the expression of antimicrobial peptide β-defensin-2.[45] In addition, the *NOD2* gene expression is inducible by the presence of commensal bacteria,[41] suggesting a possible feedback loop in regulating *NOD2* expression.

Consistent with the animal studies, human studies showed that the CD-associated frame-shift *NOD2* variant L1007fsinsC is associated with enhanced mucosal colonization by *Bacteroidetes* and *Firmicutes*[42] compared with the healthy controls. Another 2 human studies combined the 3 major CD risk alleles of *NOD2* (R702W, G908R, and L1007fsinsC) and confirmed that genotype and disease phenotype are associated with shifts in their intestinal microbial compositions.[46–48]

However, 2 recent studies[49,50] reported that only minimal differences were found in gut microbial composition between cohoused, littermate-controlled *NOD2*-deficient and wild-type mice, suggesting that the shifts in bacterial communities were not dependent on genotype but correlated with housing conditions. Although those findings might be partly explained by the restoration of disturbed microbiota because of animal cohousing, more studies are required to fully understand the role of *NOD2* in host-microbe interactions.

Similar to *NOD2/CARD15*, *NOD1/CARD4* also recognizes peptidoglycan found predominantly in gram-negative bacteria. In contrast to *NOD2*, CD susceptibility related to variants of the *NOD1* gene has been suggested but remains controversial.[51–53] One animal study showed that recognition of peptidoglycan from the microbiota by *NOD1*, not *NOD2*, primes systemic innate immunity by enhancing the cytotoxicity of bone-marrow derived neutrophils in response to systemic infection with the bacterial pathogens *Streptococcus pneumoniae* and *Staphylococcus aureus*.[54] However, the interplay between *NOD1* and gut microbiome has not been confirmed in human studies.

Autophagy

One of the major CD susceptibility genes, *ATG16L1* encodes a key component of the autophagy machinery to degrade damaged or obsolete organelles and proteins. Functional studies have shown that *ATG16L1* knockdown in intestinal epithelial cell lines impairs the clearance of *Salmonella typhimurium* infection.[55] In *ATG16L1* expression suppressed mice, studies have shown that microbial compositions were substantially shifted compared with the wild-type controls.[56] In humans, 2 case-control studies[47,48] on carriers with CD-associated *ATG16L1* risk allele T300A confirmed the significant association between host *ATG16L1* gene and the shift of gut microbiome profile.

Maintenance of Epithelial Barrier Integrity

Fucosyltransferase 2 (*FUT2*) is an enzyme that is responsible for the synthesis of the H antigen. The H antigen is an oligosaccharide moiety on the intestinal mucosa that acts as both an attachment site and carbon source for intestinal bacteria. The secretor status determines the expression of the ABH and Lewis histoblood group antigens in the intestinal mucosa. Nonsecretors, who are homozygous for the loss of function nonsense mutation of the *FUT2* gene, have shown increased susceptibility to CD.[57] Several human studies found that the host secretor status, encoded by *FUT2*, altered the intestinal microbiota composition.[7,58,59] Bifidobacterial diversity and abundance were significantly reduced in fecal samples from nonsecretors compared with those from the secretors.[59] The distinct clustering of the overall intestinal microbiota and significant differences in relative abundances of several dominant taxa, including *Clostridium* and *Blautia*, were observed between the nonsecretors and the secretors as well as between the *FUT2* genotypes.[58] In addition, the nonsecretors had lower species richness than the secretors.

Overall, the candidate gene approaches, in which the selected gene is deleted, suppressed, or overexpressed in an animal model or cell line, have shown the host genetic effect on modulating the structure and diversity of the gut microbiota. In addition, even with moderate sample size, emerging evidence from human studies has confirmed the interaction between host genetics and the gut microbiome, supporting the results from animal studies.

FUTURE PERSPECTIVES

CD is a complex disease resulting from both genetic predispositions and environmental factors, including the gut microbiota. Although distinctive membership and composition of the gut microbiota have been shown to play a significant role in CD pathogenesis, because of the sample size, human studies were limited to studying the effect of only 1 or 2 candidate genes on the gut microbiome of patients with CD and unaffected individuals based on the carriage status. Therefore, a large cohort is required to compare the bacterial distribution and abundance in the intestine of the patients with regard to disease status (CD vs no CD) and global genetic networks containing multiple CD risk loci. The gut microbiota profiles generated from this large cohort can be used to develop a predictive model combining both genetic and microbiome signatures to assess the overall risk of CD among individuals. With a better understanding of the microbiome-host gene interplay associated with CD pathogenesis, comprehensive diagnostic tools can be developed to identify individuals at risk for developing CD, as well as to develop novel personalized treatments.

REFERENCES

1. Abraham C, Cho JH. Inflammatory bowel disease. N Engl J Med 2009;361(21): 2066–78.
2. Scaldaferri F, Fiocchi C. Inflammatory bowel disease: progress and current concepts of etiopathogenesis. J Dig Dis 2007;8(4):171–8.
3. Yang H, Li Y, Wu W, et al. The incidence of inflammatory bowel disease in northern China: a prospective population-based study. PLoS One 2014;9(7):e101296.
4. Lakatos PL. Recent trends in the epidemiology of inflammatory bowel diseases: up or down? World J Gastroenterol 2006;12(38):6102–8.
5. Benchimol EI, Fortinsky KJ, Gozdyra P, et al. Epidemiology of pediatric inflammatory bowel disease: a systematic review of international trends. Inflamm Bowel Dis 2011;17(1):423–39.
6. Loftus EV Jr. Clinical epidemiology of inflammatory bowel disease: incidence, prevalence, and environmental influences. Gastroenterology 2004;126(6):1504–17.
7. Rausch P, Rehman A, Kunzel S, et al. Colonic mucosa-associated microbiota is influenced by an interaction of Crohn disease and FUT2 (secretor) genotype. Proc Natl Acad Sci U S A 2011;108(47):19030–5.
8. Jostins L, Ripke S, Weersma RK, et al. Host-microbe interactions have shaped the genetic architecture of inflammatory bowel disease. Nature 2012;491(7422): 119–24.
9. Vasseur F, Sendid B, Jouault T, et al. Variants of NOD1 and NOD2 genes display opposite associations with familial risk of Crohn's disease and anti–Saccharomyces cerevisiae antibody levels. Inflamm Bowel Dis 2012;18(3):430–8.
10. Billmann-Born S, Till A, Arlt A, et al. Genome-wide expression profiling identifies an impairment of negative feedback signals in the Crohn's disease-associated NOD2 variant L1007fsinsC. J Immunol 2011;186(7):4027–38.
11. Cadwell K. Crohn's disease susceptibility gene interactions, a NOD to the newcomer ATG16L1. Gastroenterology 2010;139(5):1448–50.
12. Cooney R, Baker J, Brain O, et al. NOD2 stimulation induces autophagy in dendritic cells influencing bacterial handling and antigen presentation. Nat Med 2010;16(1):90–7.
13. Homer CR, Richmond AL, Rebert NA, et al. ATG16L1 and NOD2 interact in an autophagy-dependent antibacterial pathway implicated in Crohn's disease pathogenesis. Gastroenterology 2010;139(5):1630–41, 1641.e1–2.
14. Hugot JP, Chamaillard M, Zouali H, et al. Association of NOD2 leucine-rich repeat variants with susceptibility to Crohn's disease. Nature 2001;411(6837): 599–603.

15. Kosovac K, Brenmoehl J, Holler E, et al. Association of the NOD2 genotype with bacterial translocation via altered cell-cell contacts in Crohn's disease patients. Inflamm Bowel Dis 2010;16(8):1311–21.

16. Ogura Y, Bonen DK, Inohara N, et al. A frameshift mutation in NOD2 associated with susceptibility to Crohn's disease. Nature 2001;411(6837):603–6.

17. Travassos LH, Carneiro LA, Ramjeet M, et al. Nod1 and Nod2 direct autophagy by recruiting ATG16L1 to the plasma membrane at the site of bacterial entry. Nat Immunol 2010;11(1):55–62.

18. Brest P, Lapaquette P, Mograbi B, et al. Risk predisposition for Crohn disease: a "menage a trois" combining IRGM allele, miRNA and xenophagy. Autophagy 2011;7(7):786–7.

19. Brest P, Lapaquette P, Souidi M, et al. A synonymous variant in IRGM alters a binding site for miR-196 and causes deregulation of IRGM-dependent xenophagy in Crohn's disease. Nat Genet 2011;43(3):242–5.

20. Parkes M, Barrett JC, Prescott NJ, et al. Sequence variants in the autophagy gene IRGM and multiple other replicating loci contribute to Crohn's disease susceptibility. Nat Genet 2007;39(7):830–2.

21. Hampe J, Franke A, Rosenstiel P, et al. A genome-wide association scan of nonsynonymous SNPs identifies a susceptibility variant for Crohn disease in ATG16L1. Nat Genet 2007;39(2):207–11.

22. Gomez-Suaga P, Luzon-Toro B, Churamani D, et al. Leucine-rich repeat kinase 2 regulates autophagy through a calcium-dependent pathway involving NAADP. Hum Mol Genet 2012;21(3):511–25.

23. Friedrichs F, Stoll M. Role of discs large homolog 5. World J Gastroenterol 2006; 12(23):3651–6.

24. Tong M, McHardy I, Ruegger P, et al. Reprograming of gut microbiome energy metabolism by the FUT2 Crohn's disease risk polymorphism. ISME J 2014. [Epub ahead of print].

25. Somerville KW, Logan RF, Edmond M, et al. Smoking and Crohn's disease. BMJ 1984;289(6450):954–6.

26. Jakobsson HE, Jernberg C, Andersson AF, et al. Short-term antibiotic treatment has differing long-term impacts on the human throat and gut microbiome. PLoS One 2010;5(3):e9836.

27. Koren O, Spor A, Felin J, et al. Human oral, gut, and plaque microbiota in patients with atherosclerosis. Proc Natl Acad Sci U S A 2011;108(Suppl 1): 4592–8.

28. Savage DC. Microbial ecology of the gastrointestinal tract. Annu Rev Microbiol 1977;31:107–33.

29. Artis D. Epithelial-cell recognition of commensal bacteria and maintenance of immune homeostasis in the gut. Nat Rev Immunol 2008;8(6):411–20.

30. Gao Z, Tseng CH, Pei Z, et al. Molecular analysis of human forearm superficial skin bacterial biota. Proc Natl Acad Sci U S A 2007;104(8):2927–32.

31. Grice EA, Kong HH, Renaud G, et al. A diversity profile of the human skin microbiota. Genome Res 2008;18(7):1043–50.

32. Qin J, Li R, Raes J, et al. A human gut microbial gene catalogue established by metagenomic sequencing. Nature 2010;464(7285):59–65.

33. Turnbaugh PJ, Hamady M, Yatsunenko T, et al. A core gut microbiome in obese and lean twins. Nature 2009;457(7228):480–4.

34. Turnbaugh PJ, Ley RE, Hamady M, et al. The human microbiome project. Nature 2007;449(7164):804–10.

35. Turnbaugh PJ, Quince C, Faith JJ, et al. Organismal, genetic, and transcriptional variation in the deeply sequenced gut microbiomes of identical twins. Proc Natl Acad Sci U S A 2010;107(16):7503–8.

36. Hartman AL, Lough DM, Barupal DK, et al. Human gut microbiome adopts an alternative state following small bowel transplantation. Proc Natl Acad Sci U S A 2009;106(40):17187–92.

37. Manichanh C, Rigottier-Gois L, Bonnaud E, et al. Reduced diversity of faecal microbiota in Crohn's disease revealed by a metagenomic approach. Gut 2006;55(2):205–11.

38. Morgan XC, Tickle TL, Sokol H, et al. Dysfunction of the intestinal microbiome in inflammatory bowel disease and treatment. Genome Biol 2012;13(9):R79.

39. Gevers D, Kugathasan S, Denson LA, et al. The treatment-naive microbiome in new-onset Crohn's disease. Cell Host Microbe 2014;15(3):382–92.

40. Haberman Y, Tickle TL, Dexheimer PJ, et al. Pediatric Crohn disease patients exhibit specific ileal transcriptome and microbiome signature. J Clin Invest 2014;124(8):3617–33.

41. Petnicki-Ocwieja T, Hrncir T, Liu YJ, et al. Nod2 is required for the regulation of commensal microbiota in the intestine. Proc Natl Acad Sci U S A 2009;106(37): 15813–8.

42. Rehman A, Sina C, Gavrilova O, et al. Nod2 is essential for temporal development of intestinal microbial communities. Gut 2011;60(10):1354–62.

43. Couturler-Maillard A, Secher T, Rehman A, et al. NOD2-mediated dysbiosis predisposes mice to transmissible colitis and colorectal cancer. J Clin Invest 2013;123(2):700–11.

44. Smith P, Siddharth J, Pearson R, et al. Host genetics and environmental factors regulate ecological succession of the mouse colon tissue-associated microbiota. PLoS One 2012;7(1):e30273.

45. Voss E, Wehkamp J, Wehkamp K, et al. NOD2/CARD15 mediates induction of the antimicrobial peptide human beta-defensin-2. J Biol Chem 2006;281(4): 2005–11.

46. Frank DN, Robertson CE, Hamm CM, et al. Disease phenotype and genotype are associated with shifts in intestinal-associated microbiota in inflammatory bowel diseases. Inflamm Bowel Dis 2011;17(1):179–84.

47. Li E, Hamm CM, Gulati AS, et al. Inflammatory bowel diseases phenotype, C. difficile and NOD2 genotype are associated with shifts in human ileum associated microbial composition. PLoS One 2012;7(6):e26284.

48. Zhang T, DeSimone RA, Jiao X, et al. Host genes related to Paneth cells and xenobiotic metabolism are associated with shifts in human ileum-associated microbial composition. PLoS One 2012;7(6):e30044.

49. Shanahan MT, Carroll IM, Grossniklaus E, et al. Mouse Paneth cell antimicrobial function is independent of Nod2. Gut 2014;63(6):903–10.

50. Robertson SJ, Zhou JY, Geddes K, et al. Nod1 and Nod2 signaling does not alter the composition of intestinal bacterial communities at homeostasis. Gut Microbes 2013;4(3):222–31.

51. McGovern DP, Hysi P, Ahmad T, et al. Association between a complex insertion/ deletion polymorphism in NOD1 (CARD4) and susceptibility to inflammatory bowel disease. Hum Mol Genet 2005;14(10):1245–50.

52. Van Limbergen J, Russell RK, Nimmo ER, et al. Contribution of the NOD1/ CARD4 insertion/deletion polymorphism +32656 to inflammatory bowel disease in Northern Europe. Inflamm Bowel Dis 2007;13(7):882–9.

53. Zouali H, Lesage S, Merlin F, et al. CARD4/NOD1 is not involved in inflammatory bowel disease. Gut 2003;52(1):71–4.
54. Clarke TB, Davis KM, Lysenko ES, et al. Recognition of peptidoglycan from the microbiota by Nod1 enhances systemic innate immunity. Nat Med 2010;16(2): 228–31.
55. Rioux JD, Xavier RJ, Taylor KD, et al. Genome-wide association study identifies new susceptibility loci for Crohn disease and implicates autophagy in disease pathogenesis. Nat Genet 2007;39(5):596–604.
56. Simmons A. Crohn's disease: genes, viruses and microbes. Nature 2010; 466(7307):699–700.
57. McGovern DP, Jones MR, Taylor KD, et al. Fucosyltransferase 2 (FUT2) non-secretor status is associated with Crohn's disease. Hum Mol Genet 2010; 19(17):3468–76.
58. Wacklin P, Tuimala J, Nikkila J, et al. Faecal microbiota composition in adults is associated with the FUT2 gene determining the secretor status. PLoS One 2014; 9(4):e94863.
59. Wacklin P, Makivuokko H, Alakulppi N, et al. Secretor genotype (FUT2 gene) is strongly associated with the composition of *Bifidobacteria* in the human intestine. PLoS One 2011;6(5):e20113.

Microscopic Colitis

Darrell S. Pardi, MD, MS

KEYWORDS

- Microscopic colitis • Collagenous colitis • Lymphocytic colitis

KEY POINTS

- Microscopic colitis is a relatively common cause of chronic diarrhea, particularly in older adults.
- After a period of increasing incidence in the United States and Europe, it seems to be stabilizing.
- Colon biopsies are required for diagnosis and should be performed in any patient undergoing colonoscopy to evaluate chronic watery diarrhea.
- The 2 subtypes of microscopic colitis, collagenous and lymphocytic colitis, are similar histologically and clinically and seem to respond similarly to various medical therapies.
- Although there are few controlled trials of therapies for microscopic colitis, the treatment approach presented here often leads to satisfactory control of symptoms, although maintenance therapy is often required.

INTRODUCTION

Microscopic colitis is a relatively common cause of diarrhea, especially in the elderly. Overall, approximately 10% to 15% of patients investigated for chronic watery diarrhea are found to have this diagnosis, although this proportion is much higher in older patients. The diarrhea is often accompanied by other symptoms such as abdominal pain, and therefore, it is difficult to distinguish microscopic colitis from the more common irritable bowel syndrome (IBS) without colonic biopsies. The pathophysiology of microscopic colitis is not well established. Several treatment options are available, although few have been subjected to well-done clinical trials. This article reviews details of these issues.

CLINICAL FINDINGS

Microscopic colitis is characterized by chronic or intermittent watery diarrhea.[1] The severity of diarrhea can range from mild to severe with dehydration and electrolyte abnormalities. Other symptoms are often present, including abdominal pain, weight loss,

This article originally appeared in Clinics in Geriatric Medicine, Volume 30, Issue 1, February 2014.
Disclosures: Consulting: Santarus.
Division of Gastroenterology and Hepatology, Inflammatory Bowel Disease Clinic, Mayo Clinic College of Medicine, 200 First Street SW, Rochester, MN 55905, USA
E-mail address: Pardi.darrell@mayo.edu

and arthralgias, each present in approximately 50% of patients. The weight loss is typically mild but can be significant in some cases. Quality of life is affected in proportion to the degree of diarrhea, abdominal pain, urgency, and incontinence.[2]

It is important to recognize that the symptoms of microscopic colitis are nonspecific. In fact, many patients with microscopic colitis meet the diagnostic criteria for IBS, such as the Manning or Rome criteria.[3] Therefore, these criteria are not specific, and histologic analysis of colon biopsies is required to distinguish microscopic colitis from the much more common IBS.

Microscopic colitis is an umbrella term that encompasses 2 main subtypes: collagenous colitis and lymphocytic colitis. These subtypes have very similar clinical and epidemiologic features, and the main distinction is histologic, as discussed below in the Diagnosis section. Given the significant clinical and histologic overlap between the 2 reports of patients transitioning from one type to the other over time or even having evidence for both types on biopsies from a single colonoscopy, and the similar response to treatments as discussed below in the Treatment section, it is not clear whether lymphocytic and collagenous colitis are 2 separate entities or part of a single disorder.[4] The current approach to these diagnoses is to consider them variants of the same condition.

The colonic mucosa generally appears endoscopically normal, although occasionally mild findings, such as edema or erythema, may be seen. Gross ulcerations suggest an alternate diagnosis, although these can be seen in patients with microscopic colitis who are taking nonsteroidal anti-inflammatory drugs (NSAIDs). Arthralgias are commonly present, and some patients also have increased erythrocyte sedimentation rates or positive results in tests for antinuclear antibodies or other markers of autoimmunity,[5] although these markers are insensitive and nonspecific for microscopic colitis.

Concomitant autoimmune conditions, such as diabetes mellitus, thyroid dysfunction, connective tissue disorders, and psoriasis, occur commonly in patients with microscopic colitis.[5,6] In particular, the association between microscopic colitis and celiac disease is clinically important. As many as 33% of patients with celiac disease have colonic histologic changes that are consistent with microscopic colitis.[7] In a large cohort study of patients with celiac disease, 4.3% were diagnosed with microscopic colitis, 72-fold greater than for patients without celiac disease.[8] Microscopic colitis is therefore more common among patients with celiac disease, and it should be considered in patients who have continued or recurrent diarrhea despite a strict gluten-free diet.[9]

On the other hand, the prevalence of celiac-like changes in the small bowel of patients with microscopic colitis ranges from 2% to 9% in the largest studies reporting this association.[5,6,10] However, in patients with microscopic colitis, celiac serologies are often negative, with anti-endomysial antibodies and anti-tissue transglutaminase antibodies being reported in 0% to 4%.[11,12] Therefore, serologies do not appear to be good diagnostic tools for celiac disease in patients with microscopic colitis. Finally, HLA types of patients with microscopic colitis were similar to those of patients with celiac disease in one study,[12] but not in others.

These data indicate that celiac disease is relatively uncommon in patients with microscopic colitis, and it is probably not necessary to evaluate these patients routinely for celiac disease. However, celiac disease should be considered in patients with features of malabsorption, such as significant weight loss, steatorrhea, and unexplained iron deficiency anemia, as well as those who do not respond to usual therapies, as discussed below in the Treatment section.

There have been a few reports of patients with microscopic colitis later developing inflammatory bowel disease (IBD) and of patients with IBD developing collagenous colitis. However, given the small number of cases, these reports could represent random chance associations. It also is important to recognize that histologic features of IBD, such as Paneth cells metaplasia and distortion of the crypt architecture, may occur in patients with microscopic colitis who otherwise have no evidence of IBD.[13]

The reported natural history of microscopic colitis varies considerably. The rate of symptomatic remission ranges from 59% to 93% in patients with lymphocytic colitis and 2% to 92% in those with collagenous colitis.[1] One study reported spontaneous remission in 15% of patients with collagenous colitis and treatment-induced remission in another 48%.[14] Only 22% required prolonged therapy. In contrast, clinical trials have reported that only 12% to 40% of patients respond to placebo after 6 to 8 weeks,[15–18] and an open-label study of steroid therapy reported that 90% of patients required maintenance therapy.[19]

EPIDEMIOLOGY

Microscopic colitis can develop in patients of any age, including children, but most commonly presents in older adults and the elderly. It is a relatively common finding among patients who undergo colonoscopy with biopsy for evaluation of chronic watery diarrhea, present in 10% to 15% of such patients.[10,20,21] In the elderly, this proportion is even higher.[10] Thus, microscopic colitis should be considered in all patients being evaluated for chronic diarrhea, especially in older patients.

Population-based studies in Europe and North America have reported the incidence of microscopic colitis to be between 1 and 12 per 100,000 person-years.[10,21–25] The reported incidence of collagenous colitis varies from 1.1 to 5.2 per 100,000 person-years and the incidence of lymphocytic colitis from 3.1 to 5.5 per 100,000 person-years.[10,21–25] Several studies reported the overall incidence of microscopic colitis and its subtypes to have increased substantially over time. For example, in a North American study, the incidence of microscopic colitis increased almost 20-fold, from 1.1 per 100,000 person-years to 19.6 per 100,000 person-years, from 1985 to 2001.[24] By the end of the study period, on December 31, 2001, the prevalence of microscopic colitis was 103.0 per 100,000 persons (39.3 for collagenous colitis and 63.7 for lymphocytic colitis).[24] Similarly, a European study reported that the incidence of microscopic colitis increased from 6.8 per 100,000 to 11.8 per 100,000 over a 6-year period.[10] The reasons for these increases in incidence are not clear, but increased awareness, with increasing use of colonoscopy with biopsies to evaluate patients with diarrhea, likely contributed. Indeed, the study from North America showed increasing use of colonoscopy in parallel with the increased incidence of microscopic colitis.

However, more recent data have shown a stabilization in the incidence rates. For example, follow-up data from Swedish and North American populations have shown a stabilization of incidence rates over the last 10 to 15 years.[26,27]

Although microscopic colitis can be diagnosed in patients of any age, it is more common among older individuals. The average age of patients at diagnosis ranges from 53 to 69 years.[6,10,21–23] A Canadian study found that patients older than 65 years were 5.6 times more likely to be diagnosed with microscopic colitis than younger persons.[25] On the other hand, pediatric cases have been reported, and in one study, 25% of patients were younger than 45 years of age.[6,28]

In most reports, microscopic colitis is more common in women than in men, with a female-to-male ratio in collagenous colitis ranging up to 9:1.[21,22,25] The gender ratio in lymphocytic colitis appears to be lower, and some studies reported no significant difference in rates between men and women.[21,24,25,29]

As opposed to other forms of chronic colitis, such as ulcerative colitis, there is no evidence that microscopic colitis is associated with an increased risk of colon cancer.[24,30] Cases of lung cancer have been reported in patients with collagenous colitis,[6,21,30,31] possibly reflecting an association with cigarette smoking, which may be more common in patients with collagenous colitis.[30–32] For example, one study reported that 25% of patients with collagenous colitis smoked cigarettes, compared with only 14% of patients with lymphocytic colitis.[31]

DIAGNOSIS

Grossly, the colon usually appears normal or has mild, nonspecific changes, such as erythema or edema. Colon ulcerations may occasionally be seen, typically reflecting NSAID use.[33] Fecal leukocytes can be present,[5] but are neither sensitive nor specific. Thus, the diagnosis of microscopic colitis relies on colonic histology.

The classic histologic finding in lymphocytic colitis is intraepithelial lymphocytosis (IEL),[31] defined arbitrarily as greater than 20 IEL per 100 epithelial cells. The IEL density is usually more prominent in the surface than the crypt epithelium. In addition, biopsies show a mixed infiltrate of acute and chronic inflammatory cells in the lamina propria. Collagenous colitis has similar inflammatory findings on colonic biopsies, although the IEL infiltrate tends to be less prominent. Therefore, the main distinguishing feature of collagenous colitis is a thickened subepithelial collagen layer. The collagen band thickness in patients with collagenous colitis varies substantially, from 7 to 100 μm, compared with a normal band of approximately 5 μm. In addition, biopsies often show surface epithelium damage including detachment of the epithelium in some cases. It is important to recognize that biopsies can contain neutrophils, with active cryptitis being reported in a third of patients,[13] although acute inflammation should not dominate the inflammatory infiltrate.

PATHOPHYSIOLOGY

The pathophysiology of microscopic colitis is not well understood. Existing mechanistic studies are typically small and often give conflicting results. Several hypotheses have been raised, with proposed mechanisms ranging from autoimmunity/immune dysregulation to a reaction to a luminal antigen such as various medications or infectious agents. It may be that the histologic finding that is currently labeled as "microscopic colitis" is the result of multiple different mechanisms with similar clinical and histologic features. Some of the proposed pathophysiologic mechanisms are discussed.

Genetic Predisposition

Several studies have investigated HLA associations and have found conflicting results. One study reported an HLA pattern similar to that seen in celiac sprue,[12] while another found no HLA association.[34] Abnormal HLA expression on colonocytes also has been described, suggesting that MHC-restricted immune activation could be involved.[35] However, given the conflicting results of these various studies, it is difficult to draw conclusions about the role of HLA haplotypes in microscopic colitis. Familial cases of microscopic colitis have been reported,[32] but the infrequency of this observation suggests that genetic predisposition is not a major factor in this disease.

Reaction to Luminal Antigen

This mechanism is suggested by studies of dietary factors, medications (see below in the Medication Side Effect section), or unspecified agents. For example, microscopic colitis is more common in patients with celiac sprue, and lymphocytic colitis-like changes can be induced in patients with sprue by a gluten enema.[36] Furthermore, symptoms and histologic changes of microscopic colitis may resolve with diversion of the fecal stream.[37] Finally, a lymphocytic colitis-like disorder in dogs resolves with a hypo-allergenic diet.[38] If microscopic colitis is due to an abnormal reaction to a luminal antigen, the immune reaction may have an autoimmune component, given the association with various autoimmune conditions and serologic markers.[11,34,39,40]

Abnormalities in Fluid Homeostasis

Several studies have reported abnormal fluid and electrolyte absorption or secretion in microscopic colitis,[41–43] although another reported normal absorption.[44] Abnormalities of the nitric oxide system[45] and prostaglandin levels[43] have been have been reported, suggesting possible mediators of abnormal secretion. The down-regulation of epithelial tight junction proteins may impair mucosal barrier function, contributing to passive fluid and electrolyte loss.[41]

Bile Acid Malabsorption

Several investigators have studied the role of bile acid malabsorption (BAM) in microscopic colitis, because patients with BAM (eg, after ileal resection) have diarrhea, and colonic infusion of bile acids in animals causes a colitis similar to lymphocytic colitis.[46] Villous atrophy, inflammation, and collagen deposition in the ileum have been reported in patients with microscopic colitis, suggesting a potential mechanism for BAM.[47] However, results of tests for BAM[42,44,47] have been conflicting, and many patients with normal results respond to a bile acid binder,[47] casting doubt on the validity of these tests or the importance of demonstrating BAM for directing therapy.

Infection

Several lines of evidence suggest the possibility of an infectious cause for microscopic colitis. Many patients with microscopic colitis have acute inflammation on biopsy and/or an acute onset of symptoms similar to a gastroenteritis,[4,44] and patients have been reported to respond to antibiotic therapy.[6] Furthermore, microscopic colitis has many features in common with "Brainerd diarrhea," a chronic diarrhea thought to be of infectious origin, which has mucosal lymphocytosis on colon biopsies.[48] Finally, a transgenic mouse model develops a lymphocytic colitis-like phenotype, but only if exposed to colonic bacteria.[49] However, no putative organism has been identified for microscopic colitis.

Medication Side Effect

An association between microscopic colitis and the use of NSAIDs has been reported in some studies but not in others, and some patients with microscopic colitis improve with discontinuation of NSAIDs.[14,50] Several other drugs also have been implicated as possible causes of microscopic colitis, including histamine-2 receptor blockers, carbamazepine, simvastatin, ticlopidine, flutamide, and others. One study assessed the strength of evidence that individual medications or classes of medications cause microscopic colitis and concluded that several drugs had strong evidence.[51] However, there are very few cases of positive drug rechallenge, and the number of cases for any specific drug is small, such that a chance association cannot be excluded. Furthermore, another study showed that some of the drug thought to cause microscopic colitis may simply worsen diarrhea, bringing subclinical cases to diagnosis, but do not actually cause the colitis.[52] Regardless, if a potential case of drug-induced microscopic colitis is identified, discontinuation of the offending medication may lead to symptom resolution.

Hormonal Influence

Microscopic colitis is more common in women, and there is a report of disease resolution during pregnancy,[6] raising the possibility of a hormonal influence, although this mechanism has not been well studied.

Abnormal Collagen Metabolism

Collagen typing studies have identified multiple potential abnormalities in patients with collagenous colitis.[53,54] Some studies suggest that the abnormal collagen layer is part of a reparative process in response to chronic inflammation, whereas others suggest a primary abnormality of collagen synthesis. Pericryptal fibroblasts regulate the production and deposition of basement membrane collagen.[55] In collagenous colitis, they appear to be activated with increased synthetic activity leading to excessive collagen production.[55] However, another study found no evidence for increased collagen synthesis as measured by messenger RNA levels[53] and others have not found elevated levels of fibroblast growth factor.

Transforming growth factor β may play a role in collagen deposition. This growth factor mediates collagen accumulation and, in one study, patients with collagenous colitis had increased expression of transforming growth factor β mRNA.[56] Vascular endothelial growth factor, another important mediator of fibrosis, appears to be upregulated in patients with collagenous colitis.[57] Furthermore, treatment with budesonide reduces vascular endothelial growth factor levels, at least in the lamina propria.[57]

It is likely that any abnormality of the fibroblast sheath is a secondary phenomenon, because it would not explain the inflammatory infiltrate. Furthermore, the severity of diarrhea in collagenous colitis is more strongly associated with the degree of inflammation and not with the thickness of the collagen band.[58]

In summary, various potential pathophysiologic mechanisms have been proposed in microscopic colitis. However, given the small number of patients studied in many of these reports, as well as the often contradictory findings, it is difficult to draw firm conclusions regarding the underlying pathophysiology of lymphocytic or collagenous colitis.

TREATMENT
Pharmacologic Treatment Options

The first step in managing patients with microscopic colitis is to search for exacerbating factors, including a careful dietary history searching for foods that might contribute to diarrhea, such as dairy products in a patient with lactose intolerance or excessive consumption of diet products that contain artificial sweeteners that can lead to diarrhea. It is also important to review the patient's medication list, including over-the-counter products and health food supplements, to search for drugs or other substances that might cause microscopic colitis or exacerbate diarrhea. In some patients, identification and elimination of such a factor may lead to improvement or even resolution of the diarrhea. However, most patients with microscopic colitis will require treatment.

Nonspecific antidiarrheal medications such as loperamide or diphenoxylate can be effective in patients with microscopic colitis[5,6,10] and are often used empirically in patients with mild diarrhea. If these medications are unsuccessful, or for patients with moderate symptoms, bismuth subsalicylate at a dose of 3 tablets (262 mg each) 3 times per day can be successful,[5,59] although one study found that most patients treated with this medication only experience partial response.[5] However, some patients who respond to this therapy achieve a long-lasting remission without maintenance therapy.[59]

For patients with diarrhea that does not respond to bismuth or those with severe symptoms, corticosteroids are typically used. In the largest, uncontrolled observational series, steroids have been the most effective therapies reported. Budesonide is the best-studied treatment for microscopic colitis, with 3 randomized, placebo-controlled induction studies in collagenous colitis[15–17] and 2 in lymphocytic colitis.[18,60] In all of these studies, budesonide was superior to placebo for inducing response, with response rates typically in the 80% to 90% range. Budesonide has fewer side effects than prednisone, and in one uncontrolled study it seemed to be more effective.[19] Therefore, unless cost is a significant concern, budesonide is generally used when corticosteroid therapy is necessary.

Despite the demonstrated efficacy of budesonide for induction, relapse is common (~70%) when it is discontinued.[10,19,61] Therefore, many patients become steroid dependent, and thus, before starting a patient on budesonide, the diagnosis should be reviewed and alternative diagnoses, such as concomitant celiac sprue, should be excluded if not done so already.

Immune suppressing medications such as azathioprine, 6-mercaptopurine, or methotrexate can be helpful in steroid-dependent or steroid-refractory patients.[5,62,63] However, to avoid the risks of immunosuppression, particularly in older patients, many clinicians are using long-term, low-dose budesonide (3–6 mg/d) for patients with steroid-dependent colitis.[64] This practice has been assessed in 2 randomized, placebo-controlled maintenance trials, which demonstrated that budesonide, 6 mg/d, was superior to placebo for maintaining response, at least through 6 months.[65,66] However, even after that duration of treatment, relapse was still high after budesonide was discontinued.

Therefore, if diarrhea recurs soon after completion of a successful course of budesonide (typically 9 mg/d given for 6–8 weeks), it is given again, often at a dose of 6 mg per day. Once remission is re-established, the dose is reduced to 3 mg per day, if possible and then to 3 mg every other day. After 6 to 12 months of therapy, another attempt is made to discontinue budesonide. If relapse occurs again, budesonide is restarted at the lowest effective dose.

Patients treated with long-term budesonide should be monitored for steroid-related side effects, such as hypertension, hyperglycemia, and metabolic bone disease, among others.[64] These patients should avoid consuming grapefruits and grapefruit juice, and any other cytochrome P450 inhibitors, which interfere with budesonide metabolism and predispose to side effects.

It is unusual for a patient not to respond to budesonide,[19] and in these patients, alternate or concomitant diagnoses and noncompliance should be considered. Treatment with an aminosalicylate is often considered as a treatment for these patients, or perhaps even before budesonide is used. However, several large uncontrolled series[5,6,10] have reported that only a minority of patients responds to aminosalicylates, and a recent placebo-controlled study in patients with collagenous colitis was negative.[67]

For patients that do have steroid-resistant microscopic colitis, treatment options include a bile acid binding agent or an immunomodulator, although there are relatively little data on these treatments. Cholestyramine can be effective,[5,6,10] although many patients do not tolerate it because of its texture. Bile-acid binders in tablet form, such as colesevalam or colestipol, might be better tolerated. There have been a few reports of the use of azathioprine,[62] methotrexate,[63] or anti-tumor necrosis factor therapies such as adalimumab and infliximab[68,69] in patients with steroid-refractory microscopic colitis.

Surgical Treatment Options

Patients rarely require surgery for medically refractory microscopic colitis. Reported operations include an ileostomy, with or without a colectomy,[5,37] or ileal pouch anal anastomosis.[70]

SUMMARY

Microscopic colitis is a relatively common cause of chronic diarrhea, particularly in older adults. After a period of increasing incidence in the United States and Europe, it seems to be stabilizing. Colon biopsies are required for diagnosis and should be performed in any patient undergoing colonoscopy to evaluate chronic watery diarrhea. The 2 subtypes of microscopic colitis, collagenous and lymphocytic colitis, are similar histologically and clinically, and seem to respond similarly to various medical therapies. Although there are few controlled trials of therapies for microscopic colitis, the treatment approach presented here often leads to satisfactory control of symptoms, although maintenance therapy is often required.

REFERENCES

1. Pardi DS, Kelly C. Microscopic colitis. Gastroenterology 2011;140:1155–65.
2. Madisch A, Heymer P, Voss C, et al. Oral budesonide therapy improves quality of life in patients with collagenous colitis. Int J Colorectal Dis 2005;20:312–6.
3. Limsui D, Pardi DS, Camilleri M, et al. Symptomatic overlap between irritable bowel syndrome and microscopic colitis. Inflamm Bowel Dis 2007;13:175–81.
4. Jessurun J, Yardley JH, Lee EL, et al. Microscopic and collagenous colitis: different names for the same condition? Gastroenterology 1986;91(6):1583–4.
5. Pardi DS, Ramnath VR, Loftus EV Jr, et al. Lymphocytic colitis: clinical features, treatment, and outcomes. Am J Gastroenterol 2002;97(11):2829–33.
6. Bohr J, Tysk C, Eriksson S, et al. Collagenous colitis: a retrospective study of clinical presentation and treatment in 163 patients. Gut 1996;39(6):846–51.
7. Wolber R, Owen D, Freeman H. Colonic lymphocytosis in patients with celiac sprue. Hum Pathol 1990;21:1092–6.
8. Green PH, Yang J, Cheng J, et al. An association between microscopic colitis and celiac disease. Clin Gastroenterol Hepatol 2009;7:1210–6.
9. Fine KD, Meyer RL, Lee EL. The prevalence and cause of chronic diarrhea in patients with celiac sprue treated with a gluten-free diet. Gastroenterology 1997;112:1830–8.
10. Olesen M, Eriksson S, Bohr J, et al. Microscopic colitis: a common diarrhoeal disease. An epidemiological study in Orebro, Sweden, 1993-1998. Gut 2004; 53(3):346–50.
11. Bohr J, Tysk C, Yang P, et al. Autoantibodies and immunoglobulins in collagenous colitis. Gut 1996;39(1):73–6.
12. Fine KD, Do K, Schulte K, et al. High prevalence of celiac sprue-like HLA-DQ genes and enteropathy in patients with the microscopic colitis syndrome. Am J Gastroenterol 2000;95:1974–82.
13. Ayata G, Ithamukkala S, Sapp H, et al. Prevalence and significance of inflammatory bowel disease-like morphological features in collagenous and lymphocytic colitis. Am J Surg Pathol 2002;26:1414–23.

14. Goff JS, Barnett JL, Pelke T, et al. Collagenous colitis: histopathology and clinical course. Am J Gastroenterol 1997;92:57–60.
15. Bonderup OK, Hansen JB, Birket-Smith L, et al. Budesonide treatment of collagenous colitis: a randomized, double-blind, placebo controlled trial with morphometric analysis. Gut 2003;52:248–51.
16. Baert F, Schmit A, D'Haens G, et al. Budesonide in collagenous colitis: a double-blind placebo-controlled trial with histologic follow-up. Gastroenterology 2002; 122:20–5.
17. Miehlke S, Heymer P, Bethke B, et al. Budesonide treatment for collagenous colitis: a randomized, double-blind, placebo-controlled, multicenter trial. Gastroenterology 2002;123:978–84.
18. Miehlke S, Madish A, Karimi D, et al. A randomized double-blind, placebo-controlled study showing that budesonide is effective in treating lymphocytic colitis. Gastroenterology 2009;136:2092–100.
19. Gentile N, Abdalla A, Khanna S, et al. Outcomes of patients with microscopic colitis treated with corticosteroids: a population-based study. Am J Gastroenterol 2013;108:256–9.
20. Fine KD, Seidel RH, Do K. The prevalence, anatomic distribution, and diagnosis of colonic causes of chronic diarrhea. Gastrointest Endosc 2000;51(3): 318–26.
21. Fernandez-Banares F, Salas A, Forne M, et al. Incidence of collagenous and lymphocytic colitis: a 5-year population-based study. Am J Gastroenterol 1999;94(2):418–23.
22. Bohr J, Tysk C, Eriksson S, et al. Collagenous colitis in Orebro, Sweden, an epidemiological study 1984-1993. Gut 1995;37(3):394–7.
23. Agnarsdottir M, Gunnlaugsson O, Orvar KB, et al. Collagenous and lymphocytic colitis in Iceland. Dig Dis Sci 2002;47(5):1122–8.
24. Pardi DS, Loftus EV Jr, Smyrk TC, et al. The epidemiology of microscopic colitis: a population based study in Olmsted County, Minnesota. Gut 2007; 56(4):504–8.
25. Williams JJ, Kaplan GG, Makhija S, et al. Microscopic colitis-defining incidence rates and risk factors: a population-based study. Clin Gastroenterol Hepatol 2008;6(1):35–40.
26. Gentile NM, Khanna S, Loftus EV Jr, et al. The epidemiology of microscopic colitis in Olmsted County from 2002 to 2010: a population-based study. Clin Gastroenterol Hepatol 2013. [Epub ahead of print]. http://dx.doi.org/10.1016/j. cgh.2013.09.066.
27. Wickbom A, Bohr J, Eriksson S, et al. Stable incidence of collagenous colitis and lymphocytic colitis in Örebro, Sweden, 1999–2008: a continuous epidemiologic study. Inflamm Bowel Dis 2013;19:2387–93.
28. Gremse DA, Boudreaux CW, Manci EA. Collagenous colitis in children. Gastroenterology 1993;104(3):906–9.
29. Olesen M, Eriksson S, Bohr J, et al. Lymphocytic colitis: a retrospective clinical study of 199 Swedish patients. Gut 2004;53(4):536–41.
30. Chan JL, Tersmette AC, Offerhaus GJ, et al. Cancer risk in collagenous colitis. Inflamm Bowel Dis 1999;5(1):40–3.
31. Baert F, Wouters K, D'Haens G, et al. Lymphocytic colitis: a distinct clinical entity? A clinicopathological confrontation of lymphocytic and collagenous colitis. Gut 1999;45(3):375–81.
32. Jarnerot G, Hertervig E, Granno C, et al. Familial occurrence of microscopic colitis: a report on five families. Scand J Gastroenterol 2001;36(9):959–62.

33. Kakar S, Pardi DS, Burgart LJ. Colonic ulcers accompanying collagenous colitis: implication of NSAIDs. Am J Gastroenterol 2003;98:1834–7.
34. Sylwestrowicz T, Kelly JK, Hwang WS, et al. Collagenous colitis and microscopic colitis: the watery diarrhea-colitis syndrome. Am J Gastroenterol 1989;84:763–8.
35. Beaugerie L, Luboinski J, Brousse N, et al. Drug induced lymphocytic colitis. Gut 1994;35:426–8.
36. Dobbins W, Rubin C. Studies of the rectal mucosa and celiac sprue. Gastroenterology 1964;47:471–9.
37. Jarnerot G, Tysk C, Bohr J, et al. Collagenous colitis and fecal stream diversion. Gastroenterology 1995;109:449–55.
38. Nelson RW, Stookey LJ, Kazacos E. Nutritional management of idiopathic chronic colitis in the dog. J Vet Intern Med 1988;2:133–7.
39. Giardiello FM, Lazenby AJ, Bayless TM, et al. Lymphocytic (microscopic) colitis. Clinicopathologic study of 18 patients and comparison to collagenous colitis. Dig Dis Sci 1989;34(11):1730–8.
40. Freeman HJ. Perinuclear antineutrophil cytoplasmic antibodies in collagenous or lymphocytic colitis with or without celiac disease. Can J Gastroenterol 1997;11:417–20.
41. Burgel N, Bojarski C, Mankertz J, et al. Mechanisms of diarrhea in collagenous colitis. Gastroenterology 2002;123(2):433–43.
42. Giardiello FM, Bayless TM, Jessurun J, et al. Collagenous colitis: physiologic and histopathologic studies in seven patients. Ann Intern Med 1987;106:46–9.
43. Rask-Madsen J, Grove O, Hansen MG, et al. Colonic transport of water and electrolytes in a patient with secretory diarrhea due to collagenous colitis. Dig Dis Sci 1983;28:1141–6.
44. Kingham JG, Levison DA, Ball JA, et al. Microscopic colitis—a cause of chronic watery diarrhea. Br Med J 1992;285:1601–4.
45. Lundberg JO, Herulf M, Olesen M, et al. Increased nitric oxide production in collagenous and lymphocytic colitis. Eur J Clin Invest 1997;27:869–71.
46. Chadwick VS, Gaginella TS, Carlson GL, et al. Effect of molecular structure on bile acid induced alterations in absorptive function, permeability and morphology in the perfused rabbit colon. J Lab Clin Med 1979;94:661–74.
47. Einarsson K, Eusufzai S, Johansson U, et al. Villous atrophy of distal ileum and lymphocytic colitis in a woman with bile acid malabsorption. Eur J Gastroenterol Hepatol 1992;4:585–90.
48. Osterholm MT, MacDonald KL, White KE, et al. An outbreak of a newly recognized chronic diarrhea syndrome associated with raw milk consumption. JAMA 1986;256:484–90.
49. Rath HC, Herfarth HH, Ikeda JS, et al. Normal luminal bacteria, especially Bacteroides species, mediate chronic colitis, gastritis, and arthritis in HLA B27/human beta 2 microglobulin transgenic rats. J Clin Invest 1996;98: 945–53.
50. Riddell RH, Tanaka M, Mazzoleni G. Non-steroidal anti-inflammatory drugs as a possible cause of collagenous colitis: a case-control study. Gut 1992;33:683–6.
51. Beaugerie L, Pardi DS. Review article: drug-induced microscopic colitis—proposal for a scoring system and review of the literature. Aliment Pharmacol Ther 2005;22(4):277–84.
52. Fernandez Banarez F, Esteve M, Espinos JC, et al. Drug consumption and the risk of microscopic colitis. Am J Gastroenterol 2007;102:324–30.
53. Aigner T, Neureiter D, Muller S, et al. Extracellular matrix composition and gene expression in collagenous colitis. Gastroenterology 1997;113:136–43.

54. Gunther U, Schuppan D, Bauer M, et al. Fibrogenesis and fibrolysis in collagenous colitis. Am J Pathol 1999;155:493–503.

55. Hwang WS, Kelly JK. Collagenous colitis: a disease of pericryptal fibroblast sheath? J Pathol 1986;149:33–40.

56. Stahle-Backdahl M, Maim J, Veress B, et al. Increased presence of eosinophilic granulocytes expressing transforming growth factor-beta1 in collagenous colitis. Scand J Gastroenterol 2000;35(7):742–6.

57. Griga T, Tromm A, Schmiegel W, et al. Collagenous colitis: implications for the role of vascular endothelial growth factor in repair mechanisms. Eur J Gastroenterol Hepatol 2004;16(4):397–402.

58. Lee E, Schiller LR, Vendrell D, et al. Subepithelial collagen table thickness in colon specimens from patients with microscopic colitis and collagenous colitis. Gastroenterology 1992;103:1790–6.

59. Fine KD, Lee EL. Efficacy of open-label bismuth subsalicylate for the treatment of microscopic colitis. Gastroenterology 1998;114(1):29–36.

60. Pardi DS, Loftus EV, Tremaine WJ, et al. A randomized, double-blind, placebo-controlled trial of budesonide for the treatment of active lymphocytic colitis. Gastroenterology 2009;136:A519.

61. Miehlke S, Madisch A, Voss C, et al. Long-term follow-up of collagenous colitis after induction of clinical remission with budesonide. Aliment Pharmacol Ther 2005;22:1115–9.

62. Pardi DS, Loftus EV, Tremaine WJ, et al. Treatment of refractory microscopic colitis with azathioprine and 6-mercaptopurine. Gastroenterology 2001;120:1483–4.

63. Riddell J, Hillman L, Chiragakis L, et al. Collagenous colitis: oral low-dose methotrexate for patients with difficult symptoms: long-term outcomes. J Gastroenterol Hepatol 2007;22:1589–93.

64. Pardi DS. After budesonide, what next for collagenous colitis? Gut 2009;58:3–4.

65. Bonderup OK, Hansen JB, Teglbjoerg PS, et al. Long-term budesonide treatment of collagenous colitis: a randomised, double-blind, placebo-controlled trial. Gut 2009;58:68–72.

66. Miehlke S, Madish A, Bethke B, et al. Oral budesonide for maintenance treatment of collagenous colitis: a randomized, double-blind, placebo controlled trial. Gastroenterology 2008;135:1510–6.

67. Miehlke S, Madisch A, Kupcinskas L, et al. Double-blind, double-dummy, randomized, placebo-controlled, multicenter trial of Budesonide and mesalamine in collagenous colitis. Gastroenterology 2012;142(Suppl 1):S211.

68. Munch A, Ignatova S, Strom M. Adalimumab in budesonide and methotrexate refractory collagenous colitis. Scand J Gastroenterol 2012;47:59–63.

69. Esteve M, Mahadavan U, Sainz E, et al. Efficacy of anti-TNF therapies in refractory severe microscopic colitis. J Crohns Colitis 2011;5:612–8.

70. Varghese L, Galandiuk S, Tremaine WJ, et al. Lymphocytic colitis treated with proctocolectomy and ileal J-pouch anal anastomosis. Dis Colon Rectum 2002;45:123–6.

Update on Anti-Tumor Necrosis Factor Agents in Crohn Disease

Siddharth Singh, MD, Darrell S. Pardi, MD, MS*

KEYWORDS

- Anti-tumor necrosis factor • Infliximab • Adalimumab • Certolizumab pegol
- Crohn disease

KEY POINTS

- Anti-TNF therapy is effective in induction and maintenance of remission as well as mucosal healing in adults and children with Crohn disease.
- Anti-TNF therapy also decreases the risk of hospitalization and surgery in patients with Crohn disease, improves quality of life, and decreases postoperative recurrence after surgical remission.
- Approximately one-third of patients do not respond to induction therapy with anti-TNF therapy (primary nonresponders).
- Approximately 13% to 20% of initial responders may lose response to anti-TNF therapy annually; these patients may be managed with dose escalation or switching within or outside the anti-TNF class of medications.

INTRODUCTION

Tumor necrosis factor-α (TNF) is a key pro-inflammatory cytokine in Crohn disease (CD).[1] Produced mainly by activated macrophages and T lymphocytes, TNF induces many other pro-inflammatory cytokines, including interleukin-1 and interleukin-6, enhances leukocyte migration by inducing expression of adhesion molecules by endothelial cells and leukocytes, activates leukocytes, induces acute phase reactants and metalloproteinases, and inhibits apoptosis of inflammatory cells. Anti-TNF agents, by binding to membrane-bound and soluble TNF, induce destruction of immune cells by antibody-dependent cellular toxicity, induce T-cell apoptosis by binding to membrane-bound TNF, and neutralize the effects of soluble TNF.[2] Currently,

This article originally appeared in Gastroenterology Clinics, Volume 43, Issue 3, September 2014.

Inflammatory Bowel Disease Clinic, Division of Gastroenterology and Hepatology, Department of Internal Medicine, Mayo Clinic, 200 First Street South West, Rochester, MN 55905, USA
* Corresponding author.
E-mail address: Pardi.Darrell@mayo.edu

anti-TNF agents are the mainstay of treatment for the induction and maintenance of remission in patients with moderate to severe CD.

Three anti-TNF agents have been approved by the US Food and Drug Administration for the management of CD: infliximab (IFX), adalimumab (ADA), and certolizumab pegol (CZP).[2] IFX is a chimeric monoclonal immunoglobulin G1 (IgG1) antibody against TNF composed of 75% human and 25% murine sequences. It is administered intravenously, over 1 to 3 hours, with standard weight-based dosing of 5 mg/kg body weight at weeks 0, 2, and 6 for induction, followed by 5 mg/kg every 8 weeks for maintenance of remission. ADA is a fully human, monoclonal IgG1 antibody against TNF. It is administered subcutaneously with standard dosing of 160 mg and 80 mg at weeks 0 and 2 for induction, followed by 40 mg every 2 weeks for maintenance of remission. CZP contains the Fab fragment of a humanized anti-TNF monoclonal antibody, and to increase plasma half-life, the Fab fragment is covalently attached to a polyethylene glycol moiety, far removed from the antigen-binding site, to prevent interference. Like ADA, it is administered subcutaneously, with standard dosing of 400 mg at weeks 0, 2, and 4 for induction, followed by 400 mg every 4 weeks for maintenance of remission. In this review, the efficacy, predictors of response, primary and secondary nonresponse to anti-TNF therapy, as well as the use of anti-TNF therapy in special situations are discussed. Evidence on optimal use of anti-TNF therapy (step-up vs top-down therapy; withdrawal of anti-TNF therapy), combination immunosuppressive therapy, and therapeutic drug monitoring is discussed elsewhere in this issue.

EFFICACY OF ANTI-TNF THERAPY

The goals of therapy in CD are to induce and maintain corticosteroid-free remission, achieve mucosal healing, improve quality of life, reduce the need for surgery and hospitalization, as well as reduce long-term risk of small intestinal and colorectal adenocarcinoma.[3] Anti-TNF therapy is effective in achieving these goals in moderate to severe luminal CD, especially in steroid-dependent patients, patients intolerant to or with progressive disease despite immunomodulator therapy, and for penetrating CD.[3] It also appears to be an effective maintenance therapy in patients at high risk of CD recurrence after surgically induced remission. Currently, a minority of patients are treated with anti-TNF agents based on nationwide administrative database studies,[4,5] although, with increasing understanding of disease behavior and the potential for disease modification by anti-TNFs, their use is likely to increase.

Clinical Remission

Tables 1 and 2 summarize the key randomized controlled trials (RCTs) of induction and maintenance of remission with anti-TNF therapy in luminal CD. Overall, in RCTs of patients with moderate to severe luminal CD, clinical remission rates at weeks 4 to 12 were 33% to 72% for IFX,[6–8] 21% to 43% for ADA (36%–43% in anti-TNF-naïve patients, 21%–26% in anti-TNF-exposed patients),[9–11] and 22% to 32% for CZP (32%–40% in anti-TNF-naïve patients, 24% in anti-TNF-exposed patients).[12–14] On meta-analysis, remission of CD was achieved in 456/1598 anti-TNF-treated patients (28.5%) at 4 to 12 weeks, compared with 223/1158 placebo-treated patients (19.3%); rates of clinical response were higher.[15] These rates correspond to a 13% lower risk of failure to achieve remission (95% confidence interval [CI], 6%–20%) and 8 patients would need to be treated with IFX to achieve clinical remission in one more patient after induction therapy compared with placebo (number needed

Table 1
Key RCT on the efficacy of anti-TNF therapy for induction of remission in luminal CD

Study, Year of Publication	Location, Time Period	Participants	Intervention (and Comparator)	Outcomes of Interest	Key Results
INFLIXIMAB					
Targan et al,[8] 1997	North America and Europe, 18 sites; 1995–1996	Luminal, moderate-severe CD (CDAI 220–450); 16% Ileal, 54% ileocolonic, 30% colonic; 108 patients	IFX 5 mg/kg, 10 mg/kg, or 20 mg/kg at week 0; placebo	Remission: CDAI <150, week 4 and 12 Response: 70-point decrease in CDAI, week 4 and 12	1. Remission: IFX (all doses) vs placebo: 33% vs 4% (week 4), 24% vs 8% (week 12) 2. Response: IFX (all doses) vs placebo: 65% vs 16% (week 4), 41% vs 12% (week 12)
Lemann et al,[7] 2006	France, 22 sites; 2000–2002	Luminal moderate-severe CD, all patients with steroid-dependent CD; 20% ileal, 51% ileocolonic, 29% colonic; 115 patients	IFX 5 mg/kg or 10 mg/kg at weeks 0, 2, and 6; placebo (all patients received azathioprine or 6-mercaptopurine)	Remission: CDAI <150 (steroid-free), week 12 and 24	1. Steroid-free remission: IFX (all doses) vs placebo: 72% vs 36% (week 12), 53% vs 26% (week 24)
Colombel et al (SONIC),[6] 2010	Multinational, 92 sites; 2005–2008	Luminal, moderate-severe CD (CDAI 220–450), all patients were immunomodulator-naive; 36% ileal, 42% ileocolonic, 22% colonic; 508 patients	IFX 5 mg/kg at weeks 0, 2, and 6, and then every 8 wk; azathioprine 2.5 mg/kg/d; IFX + azathioprine (combination)	Remission: CDAI <150 (steroid-free), week 10 Response: 100-point decrease in CDAI, week 10 Mucosal healing: absence of mucosal ulceration at week 26 in patients who had confirmed mucosal ulceration at baseline	1. Steroid-free remission: IFX vs AZA (vs combination): 37% vs 24% (vs 47%) 2. Response: IFX vs AZA (vs combination): 56% vs 39% (vs 69%) 3. Mucosal healing: IFX vs AZA (vs combination): 30% vs 16% (vs 44%)

(continued on next page)

Table 1
(continued)

Study, Year of Publication	Location, Time Period	Participants	Intervention (and Comparator)	Outcomes of Interest	Key Results
ADALIMUMAB					
Hanauer et al (CLASSIC-I),[9] 2006	Multinational, 55 sites; 2002–2003	Luminal, moderate-severe CD (CDAI 220–450): 62% ileal, 9% ileocolonic, 25% colonic; 299 patients	ADA 40/20 mg, 80/40 mg, or 160/80 mg at weeks 0 and 2; placebo (excluded patients with previous anti-TNF therapy)	Remission: CDAI <150, week 4 Response: 100-point decrease in CDAI, week 4	1. Remission: ADA 160/80 vs placebo: 36% vs 12% 2. Response: ADA 160/80 vs placebo: 50% vs 25%
Sandborn et al (GAIN),[10] 2007	North America and Europe, 52 sites; 2005–2006	Luminal, moderate-severe CD (CDAI 220–450), with prior intolerance to IFX or loss of response; 325 patients	ADA 160/80 mg at weeks 0 and 2; placebo	Remission: CDAI <150, week 4 Response: 100-point decrease in CDAI, week 4	1. Remission: ADA vs placebo: 21% vs 7% 2. Response: ADA vs placebo: 38% vs 25%
Watanabe et al,[11] 2012	Japan, 2007	Luminal, moderate-severe CD (CDAI 220–450): 113 patients	ADA 80/40 mg, or 160/80 mg at weeks 0 and 2; placebo	Remission: CDAI <150, week 4 Response: 100-point decrease in CDAI, week 4; analysis stratified by previous anti-TNF exposure	In anti-TNF exposed patients: 1. Remission: ADA 160/80 vs placebo: 26% vs 8% 2. Response: ADA 160/80 vs placebo: 42% vs 15% In anti-TNF naïve patients: 3. Remission: ADA 160/80 vs placebo: 43% vs 20% 4. Response: ADA 160/80 vs placebo: 50% vs 20%

CERTOLIZUMAB PEGOL

Study	Setting	Population	Treatment	Outcome	Results
Schreiber et al,[14] 2005	Multinational, 58 centers; 2001–2002	Luminal, moderate-severe CD (CDAI 220–450); 291 patients	CZP 100 mg, 200 mg, or 400 mg at weeks 0, 4, and 8; placebo	Remission: CDAI <150, week 12; Response: 100-point decrease in CDAI, week 12	1. Remission: CZP (all doses) vs placebo: 24% vs 23% 2. Response: CZP (all doses) vs placebo: 39% vs 36%
Sandborn et al (PRECISE 1),[13] 2007	Multinational, 171 centers; 2003–2005	Luminal, moderate-severe CD (CDAI 220–450); 28% ileal, 48% ileocolonic, 24% colonic; 659 patients	Certolizumab 400 mg at weeks 0, 2, and 4; placebo	Remission: CDAI <150, week 6; Response: 100-point decrease in CDAI, week 6; analysis stratified by previous anti-TNF exposure	1. Remission: CZP vs placebo: 22% vs 17% 2. Response: CZP vs placebo: 35% vs 27% In anti-TNF exposed patients: 3. Response: CZP vs placebo: 24% vs 20% In anti-TNF naïve patients: 4. Response: CZP vs placebo: 40% vs 29%
Sandborn et al,[84] 2011	Multinational, 120 sites; 2008–2009	Luminal, moderate-severe CD (CDAI 220–450): 27% ileal, 41% ileocolonic, 29% colonic; 421 patients	Certolizumab 400 mg at weeks 0, 2, and 4; placebo (excluded patients with previous anti-TNF therapy)	Remission: CDAI <150, week 6; Response: 100-point decrease in CDAI, week 6	1. Remission: CZP vs placebo: 32% vs 25% 2. Response: CZP vs placebo: 40% vs 34%

Abbreviation: CDAI, Crohn disease activity index.
Data from Refs.[6–14,84]

Table 2
Key RCT on the efficacy of anti-TNF therapy for maintenance of remission in patients with luminal CD

Study, Year of Publication	Location, Time Period	Participants	Intervention (and Comparator)	Outcomes of Interest	Key Results
INFLIXIMAB					
Rutgeerts et al,[31] 2004	North America and Europe, 17 sites;	Luminal, moderate-severe CD (CDAI 220–450); 14% ileal, 55% ileocolonic, 31% colonic; 73 patients	Initial response to placebo or single-dose IFX (5, 10, or 20 mg/kg) (CR-70) (nonresponders given IFX 10 mg/kg at week 12), then responders randomized to IFX 10 mg/kg at 8-weekly intervals thereafter; placebo	Relapse: CDAI ≥150, or need for surgery, or escalation of medical therapy, week 44 Maintenance of remission: CDAI <150, week 44	1. Relapse: IFX vs placebo: 51% vs 81% 2. Remission: IFX vs placebo: 49% vs 19%
Hanauer et al (ACCENT-I),[16] 2002	Multinational, 55 sites	Luminal, moderate-severe CD (CDAI 220–400); 22% ileal, 55% ileocolonic, 22% colonic; 335 patients	Initial response to open-label single-dose IFX (5 mg/kg), then responders (CR-70), randomized to IFX 5 mg/kg at week 2 and 6, then 5 mg/kg or 10 mg/kg at 8-weekly intervals thereafter; placebo	Relapse: CDAI ≥150, or need for surgery, or escalation of medical therapy, week 30 Maintenance of remission: CDAI <150, week 30	1. Relapse: IFX vs placebo: 58% vs 79% 2. Remission: IFX vs placebo: 42% vs 21%
ADALIMUMAB					
Colombel et al (CHARM),[18] 2007	Multinational, 92 sites; 2003–2005	Luminal and penetrating, moderate-severe CD (CDAI 220–450); 499 patients	Initial open-label ADA 80/40, then randomized (stratified by responder status) at week 4 to ADA 40 mg weekly or 40 mg every other week thereafter; placebo	Relapse: CDAI ≥150, week 56 Maintenance of remission in week 4-responders: CDAI <150, week 56 in patients with 70-point decrease in CDAI at week 4	1. Relapse: ADA vs placebo: 62% vs 88% 2. Remission, in week 4 responders: ADA vs placebo: 38% vs 12%

Sandborn et al (CLASSIC-II),[19] 2007	North America and Europe, 53 sites; 2002–2005	Luminal, moderate-severe CD (CDAI 220–450), enrolled in CLASSIC-I trial: included only patients in remission 4 and 8 wk after 2 induction doses of ADA; 55 patients	Initial ADA or placebo as part of CLASSIC-I, then patients with remission (CDAI <150 at week 4 and after 40 mg open-label at week 8) randomized to ADA 40 mg weekly or 40 mg every other week, thereafter; placebo	Relapse: CDAI $\geq$150, week 56 Maintenance of remission: CDAI <150, week 56	1. Relapse: ADA vs placebo: 19% vs 56% 2. Remission: ADA vs placebo: 81% vs 44%
CERTOLIZUMAB PEGOL					
Schreiber et al (PRECISE 2),[20] 2007	Multinational, 147; 2004–2005	Luminal and penetrating, moderate-severe CD (CDAI 220–450); 428 patients	Initial open-label CZP 400 mg at weeks 0, 2, 4, then patients with response (CR100) at week 6, randomized to CZP 400 mg every 4 wk; placebo	Relapse: CDAI $\geq$150, week 26 Maintenance of remission: CDAI <150, week 26	1. Relapse: CZP vs placebo: 52% vs 72% 2. Remission: CZP vs placebo: 29% vs 48%

Abbreviation: CDAI, Crohn disease activity index.
Data from Refs.[16,18–20,31]

to treat [NNT], 8; 95% CI, 6–17). At 10 to 12 weeks, induction therapy with IFX achieved remission in 45.3% of patients (compared with 25.3% of patients treated with placebo); this corresponds to a 32% lower risk of failure to achieve remission (95% CI, 10%–48%) and NNT of 4 (95% CI, 3–7). Likewise, induction therapy with ADA achieved remission in 24.2% of patients (compared with 9.1% of patients treated with placebo); this corresponds to a 15% lower risk of failure to achieve remission (95% CI, 9%–21%) and an NNT of 7 (95% CI, 5–12.5). On the other hand, on meta-analysis of 4 RCTs of CZP induction therapy, remission was achieved in 24.7% of CZP-treated patients and 21% of placebo-treated patients. Induction therapy with CZP was not superior to placebo in achieving remission (relative risk [RR], 0.95; 95% CI, 0.90–1.01). However, it should be noted that there were differences in trial design, especially for CZP, which may account for some of the differences in the observed efficacy of these agents.

In RCTs evaluating maintenance of remission after open-label induction, clinical remission rates at weeks 30 to 56 were 42% to 49% for IFX,[16,17] 38% to 81% for ADA,[11,18,19] and 48% for CZP in luminal CD.[20] On pooling data from 5 RCTs of maintenance therapy with anti-TNF, 44.1% of initial responders to induction therapy, who continued on anti-TNF therapy, were able to maintain remission 26 to 60 weeks later; in contrast, only 21.6% of patients treated with placebo were able to maintain remission.[15] The RR of relapse with anti-TNF compared with placebo was 0.71 (95% CI, 0.65–0.76), with the corresponding NNT to prevent one CD patient from relapsing of 4 (95% CI, 3–5). For IFX, ADA, and CZP, the RR of relapse after achieving remission, compared with placebo was 0.72 (95% CI, 0.63–0.83), 0.54 (95% CI, 0.27–1.07), and 0.73 (0.63–0.85), respectively. Steroid-free remission was reported in 12% to 16% of patients at weeks 48 to 52 for IFX and 23% to 29% for ADA.[21]

Similar results have been observed for clinical response (defined as decrease in Crohn Disease Activity Index score by 70 points) to anti-TNF therapy.[22] Patients treated with anti-TNF agents were 64% more likely to achieve clinical response at week 4 after induction therapy than placebo (RR, 1.64; 95% CI, 1.37–1.95); likewise, among patients with initial response to induction therapy, maintenance therapy with anti-TNF agents was twice as likely to maintain clinical response than placebo (RR, 2.06; 95% CI, 1.32–3.23).

Table 3 summarizes the RCTs of fistula healing with anti-TNF therapy. Of note, only IFX has been specifically studied with fistula healing as the primary endpoint in an RCT in patients with penetrating CD[23,24]; RCTs of other agents have reported fistula healing as a secondary endpoint in a subset of patients with penetrating disease. In these RCTs, complete fistula closure rates at weeks 18 to 56 were 36% to 46% for IFX,[23,24] 33% for ADA,[18] and 30% to 54% for CZP[13,20]; fistula closure was observed in only 8% to 12% of ADA-treated patients in short-term 4-week induction trials.[9,10] On meta-analysis, the RR of failing to achieve fistula healing with anti-TNF therapy was 0.80 (95% CI, 0.65–0.98) when short-term trials were excluded.[15] Partial fistula healing rates (at least 50% reduction in the number of draining fistulae) are expectedly higher, with 62% of IFX-treated patients achieving partial response, as compared with 26% of placebo-treated patients.[23]

Long-term follow-up of patients enrolled in these RCTs demonstrate continued benefit with extended use of anti-TNF agents. In a follow-up of the CHARM and ADHERE trials, of the 329 patients with an initial 4-week response to ADA, more than 30% maintained clinical remission extending to 4 years.[25] In a subset of patients who were in remission at week 54, more than half maintained remission at the end of 4 years of follow-up. In a prospective cohort study of 469 patients with CD treated with IFX, 61% of those with response to induction therapy had sustained benefit at end of 4.5 years of follow-up; the estimated 5-year sustained benefit was 56%.[26]

Mucosal Healing

Mucosal healing has been associated with clinical response, durable steroid-free remission, reduced need for surgery and hospitalization, and reduced risk of colitis-associated colorectal cancer.[27,28] In a Norwegian population-based cohort study of patients with CD, mucosal healing 1 year after diagnosis was associated with decreased need for corticosteroids and a trend toward lower risk of intestinal resection over the next 7 years, as compared with patients with continued endoscopic disease activity.[29] In the endoscopic substudy of the "top-down/step-up" study of newly diagnosed, treatment-naïve patients with CD, patients with complete mucosal healing 2 years after treatment initiation were 4.3 times more likely to maintain steroid-free remission 3 and 4 years after treatment initiation.[30]

Anti-TNF agents are currently the most effective agents in achieving mucosal healing. In the ACCENT I trial, scheduled IFX induction at weeks 0, 2, and 6 led to mucosal healing in 29% of patients, as compared with 3% patients given only a single dose of IFX at week 10; subsequent scheduled IFX maintenance every 8 weeks led to mucosal healing in 44% of patients at week 54, as compared with 18% patients who received episodic IFX.[16,31] In the SONIC trial, IFX monotherapy achieved mucosal healing in 30% of patients, as compared with only 16% of azathioprine-treated patients at week 26; combination therapy with IFX and azathioprine was superior to either of these strategies with 44% of patients achieving mucosal healing.[6] In the EXTEND trial, patients who received scheduled ADA were more likely than placebo-treated patients to achieve mucosal healing at both weeks 12 (27% vs 13%) and 52 (24% vs 0%), respectively.[32] Similar results were observed with CZP: rates of complete endoscopic remission and mucosal healing at week 10 and 54 compared with placebo were 10% and 4%, and 14% and 8%, respectively.[33] Differences in the definition of endoscopic remission and mucosal healing partly account for the differences observed in rates of mucosal healing for different anti-TNF agents.

Although retrospective studies and post-hoc analysis of RCTs have demonstrated better outcomes associated with achievement of mucosal healing, prospective data on the ability of mucosal healing to modify natural history of CD are lacking. Moreover, the definition of mucosal healing has been variable across studies, and it is not clarified in the literature how mucosal healing should ideally be defined in CD (ie, whether it should be based on biochemical, endoscopic, radiographic, or histologic parameters, or a combination of these). Although the understanding of mucosal healing continues to evolve, it is premature to recommend universal treatment to achieve mucosal healing.

Quality of Life in CD

Multiple RCTs have demonstrated improvement in health-related quality of life in patients who respond to anti-TNF therapy. In the CHARM trial of maintenance therapy with ADA in patients with moderate to severe CD, patients who continued ADA for maintenance reported significantly less depression, fewer fatigue symptoms, greater improvements in the inflammatory bowel disease (IBD) questionnaire, greater Short Form Health Survey-36 physical component summary scores, and less abdominal pain from weeks 12 to 56, compared with patients who were assigned to placebo after ADA induction therapy.[34] In the open-label, multicenter CARE trial of ADA in patients with moderate to severe CD, 60% of IFX-naïve patients

Table 3
Key RCT on the efficacy of anti-TNF therapy for treatment of enterocutaneous and perianal fistulae in patients with penetrating CD

Study, Year of Publication	Location, Time Period	Participants	Intervention (and Comparator)	Outcomes of Interest	Key Results
INFLIXIMAB					
Present et al,[23] 1999	US and Europe, 12 sites; 1996	Penetrating CD, single or multiple draining enterocutaneous or perianal fistulae; 94 patients	IFX 5 mg/kg or 10 mg/kg at weeks 0, 2, and 6; placebo	Fistula remission: absence of any draining fistula at 2 consecutive visits, week 18. Fistula improvement: reduction of number of draining fistulae by ≥50% (fistula response) at 2 consecutive visits, week 18	1. Fistula remission: IFX (all doses) vs placebo: 46% vs 13% 2. Fistula improvement: IFX (all doses) vs placebo: 62% vs 26%
Sands et al (ACCENT-II),[24] 2004	Multinational, 45 sites; 2000–2001	Penetrating CD, single or multiple draining enterocutaneous or perianal fistulae	Initial response to open-label IFX (5 mg/kg, at weeks 0, 2, and 6), then responders (fistula improvement) randomized at week 14 to IFX 40 mg every 8 wk thereafter; placebo	Fistula remission: absence of any draining fistulae, week 54	1. Fistula remission: IFX vs placebo: 36% vs 19%
ADALIMUMAB					
Hanauer et al (CLASSIC-I),[9] 2006	Multinational, 55 sites; 2002–2003	Enterocutaneous or perianal fistulae at baseline; 32 patients	ADA 40/20 mg, 80/40 mg, or 160/80 mg at weeks 0 and 2; placebo (excluded patients with previous anti-TNF therapy)	Fistula remission: absence of any draining fistula at 2 consecutive visits, week 4. Fistula improvement: reduction of number of draining fistulae by ≥50% (fistula response) at 2 consecutive visits, week 4	1. Fistula remission: ADA (all doses) vs placebo: 12% vs 17% 2. Fistula improvement: ADA (all doses) vs placebo: 23% vs 33%

Study	Location, sites; years	Patient population	Treatment	Definition	Results
Sandborn et al (GAIN),[10] 2007	North America and Europe, 52 sites; 2005–2006	Luminal and penetrating, moderate-severe CD, with enterocutaneous or perianal fistulae at baseline in CD patients with prior intolerance to IFX or loss of response (excluded primary nonresponders to IFX); 45 patients	ADA 160/80 mg at weeks 0 and 2; placebo	Fistula remission: absence of any draining fistula at 2 consecutive visits, week 4. Fistula improvement: reduction of number of draining fistulae by ≥50% (fistula response) at 2 consecutive visits, week 4	1. Fistula remission: ADA vs placebo: 8% vs 5%. 2. Fistula improvement: ADA vs placebo: 20% vs 15%
Colombel et al (CHARM),[18] 2007	Multinational, 92 sites; 2003–2005	Luminal and penetrating, moderate-severe CD, with enterocutaneous or perianal fistulae at baseline; 117 patients	Initial response to open-label ADA 80/40, then randomized at week 4 to ADA 40 mg weekly or 40 mg every other week thereafter; placebo	Fistula remission: absence of any draining fistula at 2 consecutive visits, weeks 26 and 56	1. Fistula remission: ADA (all doses) vs placebo: 30% vs 13% (week 26), 33% vs 13% (week 56)

CERTOLIZUMAB PEGOL

Study	Location, sites; years	Patient population	Treatment	Definition	Results
Sandborn et al (PRECISE 1),[13] 2007	Multinational, 171 centers; 2003–2005	Luminal and penetrating, moderate-severe CD, with enterocutaneous or perianal fistulae at baseline; 107 patients	Certolizumab 400 mg at weeks 0, 2, and 4, then 400 mg at 4-weekly intervals thereafter; placebo	Fistula remission: absence of any draining fistula at 2 consecutive visits, week 26	1. Fistula remission: CZP vs placebo: 30% vs 31%
Schreiber et al (PRECISE 2),[20] 2007	Multinational, 147 centers; 2004–2005	Luminal and penetrating, moderate-severe CD, with enterocutaneous or perianal fistulae at baseline; 58 patients	Initial response to open-label certolizumab (400 mg at weeks 0, 2, 4), then responders (CR-100) randomized to certolizumab 400 mg at week 8; then 400 mg at 4-weekly intervals thereafter; placebo	Fistula remission: absence of any draining fistulae on gentle compression at any 2 consecutive visits after baseline, week 26	1. Fistula remission: CZP vs placebo: 54% vs 43%

Abbreviation: CDAI, Crohn disease activity index.
Data from Refs.[9,10,13,18,20,23,24]

achieved clinically important improvements on the short IBD questionnaire, and 51% had improved work productivity.[35] Overall, at week 20, 64% of IFX-naïve patients achieved clinically important improvement in total activity impairment with ADA therapy. Based on these findings, the investigators concluded that ADA therapy resulted in a per-patient indirect cost savings of €2577, owing to reductions in CD-related work loss and productivity impairment, with work productivity improving as early as 4 weeks after initiation. Similar improvements in work productivity, daily activities, and health-related quality of life were observed in patients with active CD treated with CZP.[36]

Hospitalization and Surgery in CD

Anti-TNF therapy has been associated with decreased risk of hospitalization and surgery in patients with CD, in both RCTs and observational studies. In the ACCENT I trial in patients with moderate to severe CD, patients treated with scheduled IFX were significantly less likely to require hospitalization or surgery, as compared with patients treated with episodic IFX.[31] Likewise, in the ACCENT II study of patients with fistulizing CD, those who initially responded to IFX therapy and then received IFX maintenance had significantly fewer mean hospitalization days (0.5 vs 2.5 days, $P<.05$), mean number (per 100 patients) of hospitalizations (11 vs 31, $P<.05$), all surgeries and procedures (65 vs 126, $P<.05$), inpatient surgeries and procedures (7 vs 41, $P<.01$), and major surgeries (2 vs 11, $P<.05$), compared with those who received placebo maintenance.[37] In a meta-analysis of 3 RCTs, IFX use was associated with a 52% lower risk of hospitalization (odds ratio [OR], 0.48; 95% CI, 0.34–0.67) and 69% lower risk of surgery at 1 year (OR, 0.31 95% CI, 0.15–0.64), as compared with placebo[38]; likewise, on meta-analysis of 9 observational studies, patients treated with IFX had a 72% lower risk of hospitalization (OR, 0.28; 95% CI, 0.18–0.46), and 68% lower risk of surgery (OR, 0.32; 95% CI, 0.21–0.49), as compared with patients not on IFX. In a single-center, retrospective cohort study, initiation of IFX was associated with decreased risk of surgery (11% vs 24%, $P<.001$) and hospitalization (55% vs 31%, $P<.001$), and a shorter duration of hospital stay (6.3 d/y vs 11.3 d/y, $P<.001$) compared with the pre-IFX period.[39]

Similar benefits have also been observed with ADA. In the CHARM trial in responders to initial open-label ADA, patients who received maintenance ADA were less likely to have all-cause or CD-related hospitalization, as compared with patients randomized to placebo.[40] The rate of all-cause hospitalization at 12 months in ADA-treated and placebo-treated patients was 12.6% and 25.2%, respectively. Long-term efficacy data on the risk of hospitalization and surgery are not available for CZP currently, but are expected to be similar.

COMPARATIVE EFFECTIVENESS OF ANTI-TNF AGENTS

Despite multiple trials demonstrating the superiority of anti-TNF agents over placebo, there are no comparative-effectiveness clinical trials comparing one agent to another. Clinical trials have suggested that a 4-week induction of remission rates may be slightly lower with ADA and CZP, as compared with IFX, although it is not valid to directly compare results across clinical trials. In an open-label, single-center SWITCH trial of patients with CD with sustained clinical response on maintenance IFX, elective switching from IFX to ADA was associated with intolerance or loss of efficacy in 47% of patients switched to ADA, compared with 16% of patients continued on IFX.[41] In an observational comparative-effectiveness cohort study comparing outcomes in first-time users of anti-TNF agents among Medicare beneficiaries, Osterman and colleagues[42] found no significant difference among IFX-treated or ADA-treated patients with CD, although numerically the risk of surgery was lower in IFX-treated patients (5.5 vs 6.9 surgeries per 100 person-years; adjusted hazard ratio [HR], 0.79; 95% CI, 0.60–1.05). Given the Medicare population, most patients in this study were older than 65 years of age, and hence, were not representative of the average patient with CD; interestingly, in a subset of patients younger than 65 years, it appeared that IFX use was associated with lower risk of surgery as compared with ADA (adjusted OR, 0.66; 95% CI, 0.47–0.93).

In a Bayesian network meta-analysis of 17 RCTs on the efficacy of anti-TNF therapy in first-time users with moderate to severe CD, induction therapy with IFX was 4.2 times more likely to achieve clinical remission than CZP (OR, 4.2; 95% CI, 1.4–14.3) but was comparable to ADA (OR, 2.0; 95% CI, 0.5–9.1) (Singh S, personal observation, 2014). IFX, ADA and CZP were comparable to each other in maintaining remission among responders to induction therapy. As noted above, there were differences in trial design, especially for CZP, which may account for some of the differences in the observed efficacy of these agents. Hence, in the absence of any direct comparison, the quality of evidence is low and warrants further evaluation through prospective studies.

PREDICTORS OF RESPONSE TO ANTI-TNF THERAPY

Several clinical and biologic factors have been identified that may predict response to anti-TNF therapy in CD.[43–45] The most consistent and predictive factor is a shorter duration of disease. In the CHARM trial with ADA, remission rates approached 60% in patients who had CD for less than 2 years compared with 40% ($P<.05$) in those with a longer duration of disease.[18] Presence of an inflammatory and not fibrostenotic CD phenotype, isolated colonic disease, less severe disease, nonsmoking status, and young age may also be associated with better response to anti-TNF therapy.[43,45–49] In patients with penetrating CD, the presence of a rectovaginal fistula may be associated with poor response to IFX.[50]

Among biologic factors, an elevated CRP, and a return to normal after initiation of therapy, predicts a good response to anti-TNF therapy. In a Belgian cohort of IFX-treated patients, baseline CRP greater than 5 mg/L before the start of IFX was associated with higher response (76%) compared with patients with normal CRP (46%; OR of nonresponse to anti-TNF in patients with high CRP, compared with patients with normal CRP, 0.26; 95% CI, 0.11–0.63)[51]; similar results have also been observed with ADA,[13,14] but not with CZP.[52] Serologic markers may also predict response to anti-TNF therapy: increased perinuclear anti-neutrophil cytoplasmic antibodies (pANCA) levels may be associated with decreased response to IFX in patients with CD, particularly in the absence of associated ASCA antibodies, although these findings are not consistent.[53,54] Pharmacogenomic studies have suggested genetic markers that may be potential predictors of response to anti-TNF therapies. Genetic variants in the TNF and TNF receptor pathways or NOD2 mutations have not shown a consistent relationship with IFX response.[44] Consistent with the observation that IFX acts through induction of apoptosis of activated T cells, a Belgian cohort of 287 patients found that the presence of 3 single nucleotide polymorphisms in apoptosis-related genes influenced short-term response to IFX in luminal and penetrating CD and developed an "apoptotic pharmacogenetic index," which correlates with IFX response and remission.[55,56]

Composite models based on genotype, phenotype, and serologic biomarkers have been proposed that may identify patients who would be anti-TNF responsive, with good discriminatory value.[57] However, these findings are preliminary and warrant further validation in a prospective cohort of patients.

Primary Nonresponse to Anti-TNF Therapy

Primary nonresponse refers to lack of clinical improvement with induction therapy with anti-TNF, typically assessed 8 to 12 weeks after initiation of therapy. Approximately one-third of patients are classified as primary nonresponders.[45] Lack of response may be due to an alternative pro-inflammatory pathway beyond TNF-mediated inflammation, a differential role of TNF in certain stages of disease, individual differences in bioavailability and pharmacokinetics, inadequate concentrations of a biologic secondary to immunogenicity (innate neutralizing or nonneutralizing antibodies, or unmeasured or unknown antibody), or other factors that increase drug clearance, including high consumption in severe disease. Other, as yet unidentified, factors may play a role, such as genetic or serologic backgrounds of individual patients or absence of inflammation accounting for clinical symptoms.[43,45]

The best treatment strategy for patients with primary nonresponse to anti-TNF agents is unclear. Clinical trials of ADA and CZP typically excluded patients who were primary nonresponders to IFX or another anti-TNF agent. Only a few uncontrolled studies have evaluated the efficacy of secondary anti-TNF therapy in primary nonresponders with CD, with suboptimal results. In a cohort of 118 patients treated with ADA at Mayo Clinic, 9 patients were primary nonresponders to IFX. Of these 9 patients, only 1 patient had complete clinical response (11.1%), compared with 47.8% of patients with loss of response to IFX who achieved complete clinical response on switching to ADA therapy.[58] In the open-label, multicenter CHOICE trial of 673 patients with penetrating CD with previous failure of IFX (17% primary nonresponders), ADA achieved complete fistula healing in 30.8% of primary nonresponders and 40.0% of patients with loss of response to IFX.[59] In contrast, in another open-label, multicenter European trial of ADA therapy in patients with luminal CD (the CARE study), similar rates of response were observed in IFX primary nonresponders and those who discontinued IFX because of secondary loss of response or adverse events; clinical remission was achieved in 29% of IFX primary nonresponders by week 4, and 37% by week 20, and 38% and 43% by weeks 4 and 20, respectively, in patients who discontinued IFX because of other reasons.[60]

The availability of alternative biologic agents, such as an IL-12/23 antagonist (ustekinumab) and leukocyte trafficking blockers (natalizumab, vedolizumab), has increased options available to physicians and patients in the management of patients with primary nonresponse to anti-TNF.[61–63] Surgical resection may be an option for patients with limited disease extent.

Loss of Response to Anti-TNF Therapy

Loss of response, or secondary failure, refers to recurrence of disease activity during maintenance therapy after achieving an appropriate induction response. Multiple factors contribute to loss of response: subtherapeutic drug levels, either secondary to immunogenicity or other factors that increase drug clearance (such as high consumption in severe disease), shift in the dominant mechanism of inflammation to a non-TNF-mediated pathway (loss of the pharmacodynamic effect), or development of symptoms unrelated to active inflammation (for example, concomitant bacterial overgrowth, bile salt-induced diarrhea, irritable bowel syndrome, gastrointestinal infections such as *Clostridium difficile*, or the development of fibrostenotic disease).[43,45]

In a systematic review of 16 studies of IFX on 2236 patients with CD followed for 6284 person-years, the annual risk for loss of IFX response was estimated to be

13%.[64] The mean time to loss of response or need for dose intensification varied from 9.5 months to 18 months. Likewise, on systematic review of 11 studies of ADA, the annual risk of loss of response was 20%, and a significant proportion of patients required ADA dose intensification annually.[65] It is important to note that the incidence of loss of response is not linear: two-thirds of patients who lose response to anti-TNF do so within the first 12 months of therapy, and the remaining third do so at a much slower rate. Typically, the rate of loss of response within 12 months of anti-TNF therapy in CD patients ranges between 23% and 46% for both IFX and ADA.[66]

Predictors of loss of response to anti-TNF therapy include a combination of demographic (male gender, current/former smoker status, family history of IBD), disease-specific (isolated colonic disease, presence of extra-intestinal manifestations, longer disease duration, greater baseline disease activity), previous therapy-related (previous primary nonresponse to anti-TNF agent and anti-TNF-exposed status), and other drug-related characteristics (concomitant corticosteroid use, no deep remission, use of suboptimal doses, and low trough anti-TNF level).[65,66]

Strategies for management of loss of response are discussed in detail elsewhere in this issue. Dose intensification may be an effective strategy for management of loss of response, especially in patients with subtherapeutic drug levels. In the ACCENT I trial, 88% of patients who had initially responded to IFX but lost response during maintenance therapy regained response by increasing the dose to 10 mg/kg.[17] In a pooled analysis of 9 studies, ADA dose escalation led to regain of response in 71%, with remission in 40% of patients.[65] Switching to another anti-TNF is another effective strategy. The efficacy of a second anti-TNF agent in patients with loss of response to the first anti-TNF agent has been specifically studied in 2 RCTs. In the GAIN trial, 325 patients with moderate to severe CD with loss of response or intolerance to IFX were randomized to receive induction ADA therapy or placebo.[19] At week 4, 21% of ADA-treated patients achieved remission as compared with only 7% of placebo-treated patients. Similarly, in the WELCOME trial, 539 CD patients with loss of response or intolerance to IFX received open-label CZP and subsequently responders were randomized to maintenance CZP every 2 or 4 weeks. Overall, 62% of the participants achieved clinical response, with 39% achieving remission at week 6.[12] At week 26, 30% of patients remained in remission with maintenance CZP.

In patients who have lost response to 2 anti-TNF agents, treatment with a third anti-TNF can also be considered. In a single-center retrospective cohort study of 63 patients with IBD (57 with CD) with loss of response to 2 anti-TNF agents, the probability of remaining on the third anti-TNF, 1 and 2 years after commencement, was 55% and 37%, respectively.[67] Primary nonresponse to the first anti-TNF agent (HR, 6.4; 95% CI, 2.5–16.1) and persistent disease activity 3 months after initiation of the third anti-TNF agent (HR, 3.2; 95% CI, 1.3–7.8) were predictive of poor response to the third anti-TNF agent.

ANTI-TNF USE IN SPECIAL SITUATIONS
Postoperative Prophylaxis

In a small, single-center, placebo-controlled RCT, Regueiro and colleagues[68] observed that patients randomized to IFX within 4 weeks after surgery were significantly less likely to develop endoscopic recurrence 12 months after therapy (9.1%), as compared with placebo (84.6%); none of the patients who received IFX developed clinical recurrence. In a subsequent 5-year, open-label prospective follow-up of this cohort, patients who continued on IFX had a 13.5 times lower risk of endoscopic recurrence than patients who chose not to use IFX.[69] This initial study on efficacy of

IFX for postoperative prophylaxis is being followed up with a large, multicenter RCT. In a comparative-efficacy RCT, Savarino and colleagues[70] observed that patients randomized to ADA after surgical remission of CD were significantly less likely to develop endoscopic (6.3%) and clinical (12.5%) recurrence than patients who received azathioprine (64.7%, 64.7%) or 5-aminosalicylates (83.3%, 50.0%) 2 years after randomization. Hence, for patients at highest risk of recurrence after surgical resection of CD (young adults, with a history of penetrating CD, prior intestinal resection, perianal disease, and active smoking), anti-TNF therapy started within 4 weeks of surgery may be the preferred strategy. Follow-up endoscopic evaluation 9 to 12 months after initiation of postoperative prophylaxis is useful to ensure appropriate response.

Pediatric CD

The safety and efficacy of anti-TNF therapy in patients who had failed conventional therapy with corticosteroids and immunomodulators have also been established in pediatric CD, although there are no placebo-controlled RCTs. In the multicenter, open-label REACH study of 112 children, mean age 13.3 years, Hyams and colleagues[71] observed that 10-week clinical remission and response rate after induction therapy with IFX were 58.9% and 88.4%, respectively. Among patients who responded to induction IFX therapy, 55.8% and 63.5% were in clinical remission and response at week 54. In addition, IFX therapy was associated with improvement in quality of life, decreased corticosteroid requirement as well as increase in height. Likewise, in another multicenter, open-label, IMAgINE 1 trial, Hyams and colleagues[72] observed that of 188 patients who received open-label induction therapy with ADA, 82.4% had a clinical response at week 4% and 27.7% achieved clinical remission. Of the patients who had an initial response, 33.5% were in clinical remission at week 26. The superiority of anti-TNF therapy over immunomodulators in early, inflammatory CD was observed in a prospective cohort study. In analyzing data from the RISK study, Walters and colleagues[73] observed that early treatment with anti-TNF (within 3 months of CD diagnosis) was superior to immunomodulator monotherapy in achieving remission (85.3% vs 60.4%) and improved overall clinical and growth outcomes at 1 year. In a retrospective, multicenter RESEAT cohort of 100 pediatric CD patients who had previously been treated with IFX, Rosh and colleagues[74] observed clinical response rates with ADA of 70% and 71% at 6 and 12 months, respectively, and 33% and 42% steroid-free clinical remission rates, respectively. Hence, anti-TNF agents are effective in inducing and maintaining clinical remission, mucosal healing, improving quality of life, and growth in pediatric CD; they also appear to be safe.[75] However, it is unclear whether top-down therapy with early use of aggressive anti-TNF with or without concomitant immunomodulators is superior to step-up therapy in children with CD.

CD in the Elderly

There is an increasing incidence of CD in the elderly, who generally have a milder course with predominant colonic involvement. Anti-TNF medications are used in only 2% to 9% of elderly patients with IBD.[76] In a population-based cohort of elderly patients, the cumulative probability of receiving anti-TNF agents at 5 and 10 years was 5% and 9%, respectively.[77] In a study of 54 elderly patients with CD, the rate of complete and partial response to anti-TNF therapy was 61%, as compared with 83% with younger patients; 70% of elderly patients had discontinued anti-TNF therapy after a mean follow-up of 2 years.[78] There is a higher rate of adverse events with use of biologic therapy in the elderly than in younger patients. In the authors' experience of 58 elderly IBD patients treated with anti-TNF, 22% developed a serious infection, as compared with 8% of younger patients, even after adjusting for disease extent, severity, and comorbidities.[79] In an Italian cohort of 95 elderly patients with IBD (58 with CD) treated with anti-TNF agents, 11% developed serious infection and 10% died; the corresponding proportions in elderly IBD patients not treated with anti-TNF agents were 2.6% and 1%, respectively.[80] Hence, although anti-TNF agents are effective for treatment of CD in elderly patients, there is a higher incidence of adverse events, particularly of infections, which requires careful monitoring.

Extra-intestinal Manifestations

Anti-TNF agents are effective in the management of ankylosing spondylitis, regardless of the presence of coexistent IBD.[81] In a controlled study of 24 patients with active or quiescent CD and spondyloarthropathy, patients treated with scheduled IFX had rapid and significant improvement in gastrointestinal as well as articular and periarticular manifestations of spondyloarthropathy and peripheral arthritis.[82] IFX is also effective for the treatment of pyoderma gangrenosum. In a multicenter, placebo-controlled trial of 30 patients with pyoderma gangrenosum (19 with associated IBD), a single dose of IFX 5 mg/kg was associated with a reduction in size, depth, and degree of undermining of skin lesions in 46% of patients, as compared with only 6% of placebo-treated patients. Following open-label IFX infusions, by week 6, 69% of patients had clinical improvement. Likewise, the safety and efficacy of anti-TNF therapy have been demonstrated in patients with IBD-associated immune-mediated ocular diseases such as uveitis.[83]

SUMMARY

Anti-TNF therapy is the cornerstone of management of moderate to severe luminal and penetrating CD, effective in inducing and maintaining clinical remission, inducing mucosal healing, improving quality of life, and decreasing risk of surgery and hospitalization. Future research in comparative effectiveness of the different anti-TNF agents is warranted. In addition, a better understanding of predictors of clinical response, primary nonresponse, and secondary failure is required to enable greater optimization of anti-TNF therapy.

REFERENCES

1. Abraham C, Cho JH. Inflammatory bowel disease. N Engl J Med 2009;361(21): 2066–78.
2. Nielsen OH, Ainsworth MA. Tumor necrosis factor inhibitors for inflammatory bowel disease. N Engl J Med 2013;369(8):754–62.
3. Lichtenstein GR, Hanauer SB, Sandborn WJ, et al. Management of Crohn's disease in adults. Am J Gastroenterol 2009;104(2):465–83.
4. Herrinton LJ, Liu L, Fireman B, et al. Time trends in therapies and outcomes for adult inflammatory bowel disease, Northern California, 1998-2005. Gastroenterology 2009;137(2):502–11.
5. Long MD, Martin C, Sandler RS, et al. Increased risk of pneumonia among patients with inflammatory bowel disease. Am J Gastroenterol 2013;108(2): 240–8.
6. Colombel JF, Sandborn WJ, Reinisch W, et al. Infliximab, azathioprine, or combination therapy for Crohn's disease. N Engl J Med 2010;362(15):1383–95.
7. Lemann M, Mary JY, Duclos B, et al. Infliximab plus azathioprine for steroid-dependent Crohn's disease patients: a randomized placebo-controlled trial. Gastroenterology 2006;130(4):1054–61.

8. Targan SR, Hanauer SB, van Deventer SJ, et al. A short-term study of chimeric monoclonal antibody cA2 to tumor necrosis factor alpha for Crohn's disease. Crohn's Disease cA2 Study Group. N Engl J Med 1997;337(15):1029–35.

9. Hanauer SB, Sandborn WJ, Rutgeerts P, et al. Human anti-tumor necrosis factor monoclonal antibody (adalimumab) in Crohn's disease: the CLASSIC-I trial. Gastroenterology 2006;130(2):323–33.

10. Sandborn WJ, Rutgeerts P, Enns R, et al. Adalimumab induction therapy for Crohn disease previously treated with infliximab: a randomized trial. Ann Intern Med 2007;146(12):829–38.

11. Watanabe M, Hibi T, Lomax KG, et al. Adalimumab for the induction and maintenance of clinical remission in Japanese patients with Crohn's disease. J Crohns Colitis 2012;6(2):160–73.

12. Sandborn WJ, Abreu MT, D'Haens G, et al. Certolizumab pegol in patients with moderate to severe Crohn's disease and secondary failure to infliximab. Clin Gastroenterol Hepatol 2010;8(8):688–95.

13. Sandborn WJ, Feagan BG, Stoinov S, et al. Certolizumab pegol for the treatment of Crohn's disease. N Engl J Med 2007;357(3):228–38.

14. Schreiber S, Rutgeerts P, Fedorak RN, et al. A randomized, placebo-controlled trial of certolizumab pegol (CDP870) for treatment of Crohn's disease. Gastroenterology 2005;129(3):807–18.

15. Ford AC, Sandborn WJ, Khan KJ, et al. Efficacy of biological therapies in inflammatory bowel disease: systematic review and meta-analysis. Am J Gastroenterol 2011;106(4):644–59.

16. Hanauer SB, Feagan BG, Lichtenstein GR, et al. Maintenance infliximab for Crohn's disease: the ACCENT I randomised trial. Lancet 2002;359(9317):1541–9.

17. Rutgeerts P, D'Haens G, Targan S, et al. Efficacy and safety of retreatment with anti-tumor necrosis factor antibody (infliximab) to maintain remission in Crohn's disease. Gastroenterology 1999;117(4):761–9.

18. Colombel JF, Sandborn WJ, Rutgeerts P, et al. Adalimumab for maintenance of clinical response and remission in patients with Crohn's disease: the CHARM trial. Gastroenterology 2007;132(1):52–65.

19. Sandborn WJ, Hanauer SB, Rutgeerts P, et al. Adalimumab for maintenance treatment of Crohn's disease: results of the CLASSIC II trial. Gut 2007;56(9):1232–9.

20. Schreiber S, Khaliq-Kareemi M, Lawrance IC, et al. Maintenance therapy with certolizumab pegol for Crohn's disease. N Engl J Med 2007;357(3):239–50 [Erratum appears in N Engl J Med 2007;357(13):1357].

21. Peyrin-Biroulet L, Deltenre P, Suray N, et al. Efficacy and safety of tumor necrosis factor antagonists in Crohn's disease: meta-analysis of placebo-controlled trials. Clin Gastroenterol Hepatol 2008;6(6):644–53.

22. Kawalec P, Mikrut A, Wisniewska N, et al. Tumor necrosis factor-alpha antibodies (infliximab, adalimumab and certolizumab) in Crohn's disease: systematic review and meta-analysis. Arch Med Sci 2013;9(5):765–79.

23. Present DH, Rutgeerts P, Targan S, et al. Infliximab for the treatment of fistulas in patients with Crohn's disease. N Engl J Med 1999;340(18):1398–405.

24. Sands BE, Anderson FH, Bernstein CN, et al. Infliximab maintenance therapy for penetrating Crohn's disease. N Engl J Med 2004;350(9):876–85.

25. Panaccione R, Colombel JF, Sandborn WJ, et al. Adalimumab maintains remission of Crohn's disease after up to 4 years of treatment: data from CHARM and ADHERE. Aliment Pharmacol Ther 2013;38(10):1236–47.

26. Eshuis EJ, Peters CP, van Bodegraven AA, et al. Ten years of infliximab for Crohn's disease: outcome in 469 patients from 2 tertiary referral centers. Inflamm Bowel Dis 2013;19(8):1622–30.

27. Neurath MF, Travis SP. Mucosal healing in inflammatory bowel diseases: a systematic review. Gut 2012;61(11):1619–35.

28. Peyrin-Biroulet L, Ferrante M, Magro F, et al. Results from the 2nd Scientific Workshop of the ECCO. I: impact of mucosal healing on the course of inflammatory bowel disease. J Crohns Colitis 2011;5(5):477–83.

29. Froslie KF, Jahnsen J, Moum BA, et al. Mucosal healing in inflammatory bowel disease: results from a Norwegian population-based cohort. Gastroenterology 2007;133(2):412–22.

30. Baert F, Caprilli R, Angelucci E. Medical therapy for Crohn's disease: top-down or step-up? Dig Dis 2007;25(3):260–6.

31. Rutgeerts P, Feagan BG, Lichtenstein GR, et al. Comparison of scheduled and episodic treatment strategies of infliximab in Crohn's disease. Gastroenterology 2004;126(2):402–13.

32. Rutgeerts P, Van Assche G, Sandborn WJ, et al. Adalimumab induces and maintains mucosal healing in patients with Crohn's disease: data from the EXTEND trial. Gastroenterology 2012;142(5):1102–11.

33. Hebuterne X, Lemann M, Bouhnik Y, et al. Endoscopic improvement of mucosal lesions in patients with moderate to severe ileocolonic Crohn's disease following treatment with certolizumab pegol. Gut 2013;62(2):201–8.

34. Loftus EV, Feagan BG, Colombel JF, et al. Effects of adalimumab maintenance therapy on health-related quality of life of patients with Crohn's disease: patient-reported outcomes of the CHARM trial. Am J Gastroenterol 2008;103(12):3132–41.

35. Louis E, Lofberg R, Reinisch W, et al. Adalimumab improves patient-reported outcomes and reduces indirect costs in patients with moderate to severe Crohn's disease: results from the CARE trial. J Crohns Colitis 2013;7(1):34–43.

36. Feagan BG, Sandborn WJ, Wolf DC, et al. Randomised clinical trial: improvement in health outcomes with certolizumab pegol in patients with active Crohn's disease with prior loss of response to infliximab. Aliment Pharmacol Ther 2011;33(5):541–50.

37. Lichtenstein GR, Yan S, Bala M, et al. Infliximab maintenance treatment reduces hospitalizations, surgeries, and procedures in penetrating Crohn's disease. Gastroenterology 2005;128(4):862–9.

38. Costa J, Magro F, Caldeira D, et al. Infliximab reduces hospitalizations and surgery interventions in patients with inflammatory bowel disease: a systematic review and meta-analysis. Inflamm Bowel Dis 2013;19(10):2098–110.

39. Taxonera C, Rodrigo L, Casellas F, et al. Infliximab maintenance therapy is associated with decreases in direct resource use in patients with luminal or penetrating Crohn's disease. J Clin Gastroenterol 2009;43(10):950–6.

40. Feagan BG, Panaccione R, Sandborn WJ, et al. Effects of adalimumab therapy on incidence of hospitalization and surgery in Crohn's disease: results from the CHARM study. Gastroenterology 2008;135(5):1493–9.

41. Van Assche G, Vermeire S, Ballet V, et al. Switch to adalimumab in patients with Crohn's disease controlled by maintenance infliximab: prospective randomised SWITCH trial. Gut 2012;61(2):229–34.

42. Osterman MT, Haynes K, Delzell E, et al. Comparative effectiveness of infliximab and adalimumab for Crohn's disease. Clin Gastroenterol Hepatol 2013. http://dx.doi.org/10.1016/j.cgh.2013.06.010.

43. D'Haens GR, Panaccione R, Higgins PD, et al. The London Position Statement of the World Congress of Gastroenterology on Biological Therapy for IBD with the European Crohn's and Colitis Organization: when to start, when to stop, which drug to choose, and how to predict response? Am J Gastroenterol 2011; 106(2):199–212.

44. Gerich ME, McGovern DP. Towards personalized care in IBD. Nat Rev Gastroenterol Hepatol 2013. http://dx.doi.org/10.1038/nrgastro.2013.242.

45. Yanai H, Hanauer SB. Assessing response and loss of response to biological therapies in IBD. Am J Gastroenterol 2011;106(4):685–98.

46. Arnott ID, McNeill G, Satsangi J. An analysis of factors influencing short-term and sustained response to infliximab treatment for Crohn's disease. Aliment Pharmacol Ther 2003;17(12):1451–7.

47. Lichtenstein GR, Olson A, Travers S, et al. Factors associated with the development of intestinal strictures or obstructions in patients with Crohn's disease. Am J Gastroenterol 2006;101(5):1030–8.

48. Parsi MA, Achkar JP, Richardson S, et al. Predictors of response to infliximab in patients with Crohn's disease. Gastroenterology 2002;123(3):707–13.

49. Vermeire S, Louis E, Carbonez A, et al. Demographic and clinical parameters influencing the short-term outcome of anti-tumor necrosis factor (infliximab) treatment in Crohn's disease. Am J Gastroenterol 2002;97(9):2357–63.

50. Topstad DR, Panaccione R, Heine JA, et al. Combined seton placement, infliximab infusion, and maintenance immunosuppressives improve healing rate in penetrating anorectal Crohn's disease: a single center experience. Dis Colon Rectum 2003;46(5):577–83.

51. Louis E, Vermeire S, Rutgeerts P, et al. A positive response to infliximab in Crohn disease: association with a higher systemic inflammation before treatment but not with -308 TNF gene polymorphism. Scand J Gastroenterol 2002;37(7): 818–24.

52. Shao LM, Chen MY, Cai JT. Meta-analysis: the efficacy and safety of certolizumab pegol in Crohn's disease. Aliment Pharmacol Ther 2009;29(6): 605–14.

53. Esters N, Vermeire S, Joossens S, et al. Serological markers for prediction of response to anti-tumor necrosis factor treatment in Crohn's disease. Am J Gastroenterol 2002;97(6):1458–62.

54. Taylor KD, Plevy SE, Yang H, et al. ANCA pattern and LTA haplotype relationship to clinical responses to anti-TNF antibody treatment in Crohn's disease. Gastroenterology 2001;120(6):1347–55.

55. Hlavaty T, Ferrante M, Henckaerts L, et al. Predictive model for the outcome of infliximab therapy in Crohn's disease based on apoptotic pharmacogenetic index and clinical predictors. Inflamm Bowel Dis 2007;13(4):372–9.

56. Hlavaty T, Pierik M, Henckaerts L, et al. Polymorphisms in apoptosis genes predict response to infliximab therapy in luminal and penetrating Crohn's disease. Aliment Pharmacol Ther 2005;22(7):613–26.

57. Dubinsky MC, Mei L, Friedman M, et al. Genome wide association (GWA) predictors of anti-TNFalpha therapeutic responsiveness in pediatric inflammatory bowel disease. Inflamm Bowel Dis 2010;16(8):1357–66.

58. Swoger JM, Loftus EV, Tremaine WJ, et al. Adalimumab for Crohn's disease in clinical practice at Mayo Clinic: the first 118 patients. Inflamm Bowel Dis 2010;16(11):1912–21.

59. Lichtiger S, Binion DG, Wolf DC, et al. The CHOICE trial: adalimumab demonstrates safety, fistula healing, improved quality of life and increased work

productivity in patients with Crohn's disease who failed prior infliximab therapy. Aliment Pharmacol Ther 2010;32(10):1228–39.

60. Lofberg R, Louis EV, Reinisch W, et al. Adalimumab produces clinical remission and reduces extraintestinal manifestations In Crohn's disease: results from CARE. Inflamm Bowel Dis 2012;18(1):1–9.

61. Sandborn WJ, Colombel JF, Enns R, et al. Natalizumab induction and maintenance therapy for Crohn's disease. N Engl J Med 2005;353(18):1912–25.

62. Sandborn WJ, Feagan BG, Rutgeerts P, et al. Vedolizumab as induction and maintenance therapy for Crohn's disease. N Engl J Med 2013;369(8):711–21.

63. Sandborn WJ, Gasink C, Gao LL, et al. Ustekinumab induction and maintenance therapy in refractory Crohn's disease. N Engl J Med 2012;367(16):1519–28.

64. Gisbert JP, Panes J. Loss of response and requirement of infliximab dose intensification in Crohn's disease: a review. Am J Gastroenterol 2009;104(3):760–7.

65. Billioud V, Sandborn WJ, Peyrin-Biroulet L. Loss of response and need for adalimumab dose intensification in Crohn's disease: a systematic review. Am J Gastroenterol 2011;106(4):674–84.

66. Ben-Horin S, Chowers Y. Review article: loss of response to anti-TNF treatments in Crohn's disease. Aliment Pharmacol Ther 2011;33(9):987–95.

67. de Silva PS, Nguyen DD, Sauk J, et al. Long-term outcome of a third anti-TNF monoclonal antibody after the failure of two prior anti-TNFs in inflammatory bowel disease. Aliment Pharmacol Ther 2012;36(5):459–66.

68. Regueiro M, Schraut W, Baidoo L, et al. Infliximab prevents Crohn's disease recurrence after ileal resection. Gastroenterology 2009;136(2):441–50.

69. Regueiro M, Kip KE, Baidoo L, et al. Postoperative therapy with infliximab prevents long-term Crohn's disease recurrence. Clin Gastroenterol Hepatol 2014. http://dx.doi.org/10.1016/j.cgh.2013.12.035.

70. Savarino E, Bodini G, Dulbecco P, et al. Adalimumab is more effective than azathioprine and mesalamine at preventing postoperative recurrence of Crohn's disease: a randomized controlled trial. Am J Gastroenterol 2013;108(11): 1731–42.

71. Hyams J, Crandall W, Kugathasan S, et al. Induction and maintenance infliximab therapy for the treatment of moderate-to-severe Crohn's disease in children. Gastroenterology 2007;132(3):863–73.

72. Hyams JS, Griffiths A, Markowitz J, et al. Safety and efficacy of adalimumab for moderate to severe Crohn's disease in children. Gastroenterology 2012;143(2): 365–74.

73. Walters TD, Kim MO, Denson LA, et al. Increased effectiveness of early therapy with anti-tumor necrosis factor-alpha vs an immunomodulator in children with Crohn's disease. Gastroenterology 2014;146(2):383–91.

74. Rosh JR, Lerer T, Markowitz J, et al. Retrospective evaluation of the safety and effect of adalimumab therapy (RESEAT) in pediatric Crohn's disease. Am J Gastroenterol 2009;104(12):3042–9.

75. Dulai PS, Thompson KD, Blunt HB, et al. Risks of serious infection or lymphoma with anti-tumor necrosis factor therapy for pediatric inflammatory bowel disease: a systematic review. Clin Gastroenterol Hepatol 2014. http://dx.doi.org/10.1016/j.cgh.2014.01.021.

76. Katz S, Surawicz C, Pardi DS. Management of the elderly patients with inflammatory bowel disease: practical considerations. Inflamm Bowel Dis 2013; 19(10):2257–72.

77. Charpentier C, Salleron J, Savoye G, et al. Natural history of elderly-onset inflammatory bowel disease: a population-based cohort study. Gut 2014;63(3):423–32.

78. Desai A, Zator ZA, de Silva P, et al. Older age is associated with higher rate of discontinuation of anti-TNF therapy in patients with inflammatory bowel disease. Inflamm Bowel Dis 2013;19(2):309–15.

79. Bhushan A, Pardi DS, Loftus EV, et al. Association of age with adverse events from biologic therapy in patients with inflammatory bowel disease. Gastroenterology 2010;138:S413.

80. Cottone M, Kohn A, Daperno M, et al. Advanced age is an independent risk factor for severe infections and mortality in patients given anti-tumor necrosis factor therapy for inflammatory bowel disease. Clin Gastroenterol Hepatol 2011;9(1): 30–5.

81. Spadaro A, Lubrano E, Marchesoni A, et al. Remission in ankylosing spondylitis treated with anti-TNF-alpha drugs: a national multicentre study. Rheumatology (Oxford) 2013;52(10):1914–9.

82. Generini S, Giacomelli R, Fedi R, et al. Infliximab in spondyloarthropathy associated with Crohn's disease: an open study on the efficacy of inducing and maintaining remission of musculoskeletal and gut manifestations. Ann Rheum Dis 2004;63(12):1664–9.

83. Barrie A, Regueiro M. Biologic therapy in the management of extraintestinal manifestations of inflammatory bowel disease. Inflamm Bowel Dis 2007; 13(11):1424–9.

84. Sandborn WJ, Schreiber S, Feagan BG, et al. Certolizumab pegol for active Crohn's disease: a placebo-controlled, randomized trial. Clin Gastroenterol Hepatol 2011;9(8):670–8.

An Update on Anti-TNF Agents in Ulcerative Colitis

Mark A. Samaan, MBBS[a], Preet Bagi, MD[b], Niels Vande Casteele, PharmD, PhD[b], Geert R. D'Haens, MD, PhD[a], Barrett G. Levesque, MS, MD[b],*

KEYWORDS

- Ulcerative colitis • UC • Anti-TNF • Infliximab • Adalimumab • Golimumab

KEY POINTS

- Large randomized controlled trials have demonstrated the efficacy of multiple anti- tumor necrosis factor (TNF) agents in delivering mucosal healing, reducing clinical disease activity, and improving long-term outcomes in patients with moderate-to-severe ulcerative colitis.
- A head-to-head trial has shown that infliximab may be as effective as cyclosporin when used as rescue therapy in severe colitis.
- Combining infliximab with an Immunomodulator is more effective than infliximab alone in inducing a response in moderate-to-severe ulcerative colitis.
- Therapeutic drug monitoring and dose optimization of anti-TNF agents can maximize their efficacy.

INTRODUCTION

The advent of biologic therapies has led to significant changes in treatment strategies for ulcerative colitis (UC). Before biologic therapies, options for treatment primarily consisted of the stepwise use of mesalamine, corticosteroids, and immunomodulators for disease of increasing severity. Mesalamine was used to achieve and maintain remission in mild-to-moderate cases with the addition of corticosteroids for those failing to respond or with severe disease.[1,2] Patients with colitis refractory to intravenous (IV) corticosteroids received cyclosporin[3] or underwent colectomy. Over the past decade, multiple clinical trials have shown the efficacy of anti-tumor necrosis factor-α (anti-TNF) therapies for these patients with moderate-to-severe UC.[4–6] Therefore, anti-TNF agents are key tools in current treatment algorithms for both chronically active and acute severe UC.[7]

This article originally appeared in Gastroenterology Clinics, Volume 43, Issue 3, September 2014.

[a] Department of Gastroenterology, Academic Medical Centre, Meibergdreef 9, Amsterdam 1105 AZ, The Netherlands; [b] Division of Gastroenterology, University of California, San Diego, 9500 Gilman Drive, La Jolla, CA 92093-0956, 92103, USA
* Corresponding author.
E-mail address: bglevesque@ucsd.edu

Clinics Collections 7 (2015) 501–516
http://dx.doi.org/10.1016/j.ccol.2015.06.034

The effectiveness of biologic agents has also changed treatment goals in UC, which is evident in the evolution of endpoints used for clinical trials and targets used in clinical practice.[8] Conventional and established goals of treatment focused predominantly on achieving symptomatic remission. The cessation of corticosteroid use and achieving mucosal healing (MH) were secondary goals.[9] However, in the era of anti-TNF agents with the ability to heal colonic mucosa when other drugs have failed, MH and steroid-free clinical remission have gained prominence as therapeutic targets.

In this update, data are reviewed from randomized controlled trials (RCTs) and comparative effectiveness research and the impact of anti-TNF agents on long-term disease outcomes and their safety data is assessed. In addition, ongoing research is discussed on the pharmacokinetics and pharmacodynamics of TNF-antagonists in UC. Also considered is what may lie ahead as it is aimed to maximize the benefit this group of drugs can deliver.

INFLIXIMAB

Infliximab (Remicade) is a chimeric IgG_1 monoclonal antibody that binds with high affinity and specificity to soluble TNF-α. This process prevents the proinflammatory cytokine binding to cell receptors and propagating the inflammatory cascade.[10] Infliximab also mediates inflammatory processes by binding to membrane-bound TNF-α on inflammatory cells, thereby inducing apoptosis.[11] Infliximab is administered as an IV infusion with weight-based dosing and a regimen that includes an induction phase followed by maintenance treatment.

The first randomized, placebo-controlled study of infliximab for UC was published in 2001. Described as a pilot study, it included just 11 patients with severely active, steroid-refractory UC (defined as a Truelove and Witts[12] score >10 and Blackstone[13] endoscopic grade of 3 or 4). Although the trial was not sufficient to draw meaningful conclusions, it provided an initial signal of the drug's efficacy with response seen in 4 of the 8 patients treated, compared with none in the placebo group.[14] This study was followed by several uncontrolled trials[15,16] before a larger randomized, double-blind, placebo-controlled trial using only a single dose of 4 to 5 mg/kg of infliximab was carried out in Sweden.[17] That study included 45 patients with moderate, severe, or fulminant colitis (based on the Seo[18] or fulminant colitis index[19]) who were refractory to conventional therapies. Their results demonstrated the value of infliximab as a rescue therapy with 7 of 24 (29%) treated patients requiring colectomy at 3 months compared with 14 of 21 (67%) given placebo ($P = .017$). The first RCT to implement an induction regimen of 5 mg/kg at 0, 2, and 6 weeks demonstrated the superiority of infliximab when compared with IV methylprednisolone.[20]

Clinical Efficacy: Moderate-to-Severe Disease and Maintenance Therapy

Infliximab has also been evaluated for use in patients with ongoing moderate to severely active UC, despite conventional therapy. In 2005, infliximab became the first anti-TNF agent approved by the US Food and Drug Administration (FDA) for use in moderate-to-severe UC. A year later, this approval was extended to include maintenance, as well as induction therapy, and European approval was also granted. This evidence was generated in 2 large, randomized, placebo-controlled, double-blind trials[4]: Active Ulcerative Colitis Trials 1 and 2 (ACT 1 and ACT 2). The 2 trials ran concurrently for 3 years at multiple sites over 4 continents. Each trial included 364 patients and studied the effect of infliximab given at doses of 5 or 10 mg/kg at weeks 0, 2, and 6 followed by maintenance treatment scheduled at 8 weekly intervals. Both studies included patients with moderate-to-severe disease activity (defined as a Mayo[21] score >6, with an endoscopic subscore of ≥2) and their inclusion criteria regarding concomitant medications differed only slightly. Both included patients taking corticosteroids and/or thiopurines as well as those who were no longer taking them but had previously failed or had contraindications (or intolerance) to these medications in the past. In addition to these groups, ACT 2 also included 5-aminosalicylate drugs using the same criteria. Therefore, patients did not necessarily need to be receiving corticosteroids at baseline (61% and 51% were in ACT 1 and 2, respectively). Although the 2 studies had identical induction regimens, the duration of treatment and follow-up period differed. Patients were given maintenance treatment until week 46 in ACT 1 and followed until 56 weeks. In ACT 2, the corresponding time points were week 22 and 30. Clinical response at week 8 was the primary endpoint of the ACT trials. The authors defined this as a decrease from baseline in the total Mayo score of at least 3 points and at least 30%, with an accompanying decrease in the subscore for rectal bleeding of at least 1 point or an absolute subscore for rectal bleeding of 0 or 1. Both trials showed that patients treated with infliximab (at either dose) were significantly more likely to have a clinical response at week 8 and 30. The 2 dosing regimens delivered similar efficacy, and response rates at these time points in treated patients were greater than 60% at week 8 and greater than 47% at week 30. Placebo response rates were less than 38% and 30% at the corresponding time points. With its extended follow-up period, ACT 1 showed this response to be durable at week 54 with 45.5% and 44.3% of treated patients (5 mg/kg and 10 mg/kg, respectively) responding compared with 19.8% on placebo. Clinical remission rates followed a similar pattern to clinical response and the effect of infliximab was again significant. In ACT 1, remission rates at 54 weeks were 34.7%, 34.4%, and 16.5% of patients treated with infliximab 5 mg/kg, 10 mg/kg, or placebo, respectively ($P = .01$).

Corticosteroid-Free Remission

Remission In the absence of corticosteroid treatment has become an important endpoint for clinical trials in UC. Of the 61% of patients in ACT 1 on steroids at baseline, the proportion in clinical remission following corticosteroid cessation at week 30 was significantly higher with infliximab 5 mg/kg than with placebo (24.3% vs 10.1%, respectively; $P = .03$). The durability of this effect was evident at week 54 when the corresponding corticosteroid-free remission rates were 25.7% versus 8.9%, respectively ($P = .006$). Furthermore, at baseline, the median dose was 20 mg/d in all groups. By week 54, this had fallen to 5 mg/d in the group given infliximab 5 mg/kg, whereas it remained at 20 mg/d in the placebo group.

Mucosal Healing

MH is an outcome measure with important implications for remission rates, future steroid use, and risk of colectomy in UC. Evidence is growing that complete mucosal reconstitution or significant improvement of endoscopic appearance can have multiple clinical benefits.[22,23] MH was defined in the trials as a Mayo endoscopic subscore of 0 or 1 following treatment. Analysis of data from ACT 1 using this definition showed that at all time points, 5 mg/kg infliximab was significantly superior to placebo in this regard. At week 8, 62% achieved MH on this dose compared with 33.9% on placebo. This difference was maintained at weeks 30 (50.4% vs 24.8%, respectively) and 54 (45.5% vs 18.2%, respectively) with all comparisons reaching statistical significance ($P<.001$).

As debate is on-going[23] regarding whether Mayo grade 1 (abnormal vascular pattern and some friability but no erosions, ulcerations, or active bleeding) should be included in the group achieving MH, subgroup analysis including only those with grade 0 (completely normal mucosa) has subsequently been carried out.[24] Using this more stringent definition, MH was achieved in 22.3% of infliximab patients and 12.4% of placebo patients at week 8, and 32.2% and 15.7%, respectively, at week 54.

Hospitalizations, Colectomy, and Long-Term Efficacy

Hospitalization and colectomy rates from the ACT trials were studied in a post-hoc analysis, which included 630 (87%) of the original 728 patients.[25] When assessed at week 54, the cumulative incidence of colectomy was 10% in the infliximab-treated group compared with 17% in the placebo group ($P = .02$). Infliximab therefore delivers an absolute risk reduction of 7% for colectomy in patients with moderate-to-severe UC. In their post-hoc analysis, the authors also showed that infliximab halved the rate of hospital admissions compared with placebo. Through week 54, there were 40 hospitalizations per 100 patient-years (PY) in the placebo group and 20 per 100 PY with infliximab ($P = .003$).

To assess the long-term efficacy, effect on quality of life (QoL), and safety of infliximab, a 3-year open-label extension to the ACT trials was carried out.[26] Any patient participating in the original trials who could benefit from ongoing treatment, as deemed by the investigator (without specific criteria), was eligible for inclusion. Ongoing infliximab, given at 8 weekly intervals, was shown to deliver maintained clinical benefit and health-related QoL while reducing corticosteroid use.

Combination Therapy Versus Monotherapy

Panaccione and colleagues[27] conducted the UC SUCCESS trial to compare the efficacy of infliximab monotherapy with the combination of infliximab and azathioprine. To compare these 2 approaches, they recruited 239 biologic-naïve patients with moderate-to-severe UC (Mayo score $\geq$6). Ninety percent were azathioprine-naïve and 10% had stopped azathioprine more than 3 months before trial entry. The original trial design had planned the enrollment of 600 patients to the first phase (described here) to allow 200 to subsequently enter a longer-term observational study in the second phase. However, enrollment was terminated prematurely by the sponsor, because of higher than expected serious infusion reactions with an intermittent infliximab regimen in an unrelated study of patients with psoriasis.[28] Patients were randomized to 1 of 3 treatment arms: azathioprine and placebo; infliximab and placebo; infliximab and azathioprine. A standard induction regimen of 5 mg/kg infliximab and/or 2.5 mg/kg azathioprine was administered to the relevant groups and endpoints were judged at week 16. The primary endpoint investigated was steroid-free remission (defined as total Mayo score $\leq$2 with no subscore >1). In this regard, combination therapy performed significantly better than either infliximab (40% vs 22%, $P = .017$) or azathioprine (40% vs 24%, $P = .032$) alone. Patients on combination therapy were significantly more likely to achieve MH (endoscopic Mayo of 0 or 1) than those on azathioprine monotherapy. MH rates were 63% with combination therapy compared with 55% with infliximab monotherapy ($P = .295$) and 37% with azathioprine monotherapy ($P = .001$).

Safety

The TREAT (Crohn Therapy, Resource, Evaluation, and Assessment Tool) registry was designed specifically to investigate the long-term safety of anti-TNF therapy in patients with Crohn disease (CD).[29] More than 5 years of data from this ongoing, prospective, observational study was published in 2012 and, although the study only includes patients with CD, results are certainly relevant to anti-TNF-treated patients with UC. Based on analysis of more than 6000 patients, the authors demonstrated no increase in mortality or neoplasia between patients receiving infliximab and those receiving other treatments only. Analysis of this data also confirmed the increased risk of serious infections that had been previously seen (hazard ratio 1.98; 95% confidence interval [CI] 1.11, 1.84; P = .006). It should be noted, however, that increased risk was not relative to cumulative infliximab dose because neither the number of infusions nor the dose escalation to 10 mg/kg significantly impacted it.

Of significant concern in the treatment of fulminant colitis with infliximab is its possible effect on postoperative complication rates among nonresponder who require colectomy. This group of patients are often already at increased risk of infectious complications owing to the use of immunomodulators and corticosteroids. A literature review[30] and meta-analysis[31] of trials have been conducted to examine this issue. Although the studies included[17,32–36] are all retrospective, use different endpoints, and report mixed results, limited conclusions can be drawn. It seems that if the use of preoperative infliximab increases the risk of postoperative complications (infectious or otherwise) at all, the effect is minimal.

Clinical Efficacy: Rescue Therapy

Before infliximab, therapeutic options for patients with severe or fulminant colitis unresponsive to IV corticosteroids were only cyclosporin or colectomy. Given the risks for toxicity with cyclosporin,[37] the benefit of infliximab in clinical trials of moderate-to-severe UC suggested a potential alternative for patients hospitalized with severe UC. However, until recently the 2 agents had not been compared in a head-to-head trial to assess their relative efficacy. This comparison was recently carried out in a study involving 27 centers in France and Belgium as part of a parallel, open-label, RCT.[38] Patients experiencing a severe flare (defined as a Lichtiger[39] score >10) with an insufficient response to IV corticosteroids received either cyclosporin (2 mg/kg/d for 1 week, followed by oral drug until day 98) or infliximab (5 mg/kg at 0, 2, and 6 weeks). All 115 patients included were naïve to the trial agents and those with a satisfactory response to either drug commenced azathioprine at day 7. The primary outcome was "treatment failure," and the authors defined this as the absence of a clinical response at day 7, a relapse between day 7 and day 98, absence of steroid-free remission at day 98, a severe adverse event leading to treatment interruption, colectomy, or death. Failure of therapy was seen in 60% (35) of those receiving cyclosporin and 54% (31) given infliximab (absolute risk difference 6%, 95% CI −7 to 19; odds ratio 1.3, 95% CI 0.6–2.7). Roughly 85% of patients in both groups had a clinical response at day 7 measured by the Lichtiger score (a secondary endpoint). The proportion of severe adverse events was also similar among the 2 arms with 9 (16%) and 14 (25%) suffering these in the cyclosporin and infliximab groups, respectively. No deaths and few serious infections were reported. Overall, the authors concluded that treatment choice should be guided by physician and center experience. When considered in the context of the monitoring cyclosporin blood levels, the significant potential toxicity of cyclosporin, and the emerging evidence regarding the pharmacodynamics of infliximab, infliximab may soon become the rescue therapy of choice for many practitioners.[40] The overriding practical issue in relation to cyclosporin is that its use is restricted to centers that can regularly monitor concentrations and have sufficient clinical experience in the use of drugs not routinely used in outpatient practices. Evidence has also emerged demonstrating that patients with severe, steroid-refractory colitis may fail to respond to infliximab because of accelerated clearance of the drug.[41] Dose optimization with higher or more frequent doses may therefore improve response rates, an aspect that was not studied in the head-to-head comparison. This theory is supported by post-hoc analysis from the ACT 1 and 2 demonstrating that higher infliximab trough concentrations were associated with greater likelihood of response, remission, and MH than were low or absent trough concentrations.[42]

It is also important to consider the patient who has a severe flair despite thiopurine maintenance therapy in whom there is no subsequent maintenance option if rescue cyclosporin is chosen and succeeds. Infliximab, therefore, has a significant advantage in this group. Further data regarding the efficacy and cost-effectiveness of each agent will be available when the UK-wide CONSTRUCT trial (COmparison of iNfliximab and cyclosporin in STeroid Resistant Ulcerative Colitis: a Trial) is completed in August 2014.

ADALIMUMAB

After FDA approval of infliximab for induction and maintenance of UC, the next anti-TNF agent to achieve FDA approval for the treatment of UC was adalimumab (Humira). Adalimumab is a TNF-α targeted fully human monoclonal antibody. It is administered via the subcutaneous route and is FDA approved as therapy for moderate-to-severe CD as well. In addition, adalimumab is currently in use for the therapy for psoriasis, psoriatic arthritis, rheumatoid arthritis, and ankylosing spondylitis. Initially, case reports and many small open-label studies showed efficacy in UC.[43–46] Recently, a multicenter RCT, ULTRA1, was conducted to examine the efficacy of adalimumab in induction of clinical remission in moderate-to-severe UC.[5] This phase III, randomized, double-blind, placebo-controlled study was conducted across 94 European and North American centers. Enrolled subjects were required to have a full Mayo score ranging from 6 to 12, with an endoscopic subscore of 2 to 3. Subjects were required to be anti-TNF naïve. Prior failure of oral corticosteroid and/or immunomodulator therapy with azathioprine or 6-mercaptopurine was required for study enrollment. Subjects were randomized to either placebo or induction with subcutaneous adalimumab 160/80 mg or 80/40 mg. This dosing selection was based on adalimumab dosing in the CHARM and CLASSIC-I CD trials and regulatory agency guidance.[47,48] The 160/80 mg group received subcutaneous adalimumab 160 mg at week 0, 80 mg at week 2, followed by 40 mg at weeks 4 and 6. The 80/40 mg group received 80 mg at week 0 followed by 40 mg at weeks 2, 4, and 6.

The study's primary endpoint was the proportion of subjects in clinical remission by week 8, defined as a composite Mayo score less than or equal to 2 with no individual subscore of 1 or more. At the study's end, the adalimumab 160/80 mg group achieved clinical remission in 18.5% of subjects, which was double the placebo rate of 9.2% ($P = .031$). The adalimumab 80/40 mg group reached a clinical remission rate that was similar to placebo at 10% ($P = .833$). Furthermore, secondary endpoints revealed that the adalimumab 160/80 mg group did achieve greater rates of MH, clinical response, and improvement to less than or equal to 1 in all components of the Mayo score in comparison to placebo. Subanalyses revealed that subjects with a greater composite Mayo score on study entry, CRP more than or equal to 10 mg/L at baseline, and higher study entry weight achieved lower rates of remission than those with a lower Mayo score. The safety profile of adalimumab appeared to be comparable to that of placebo. Overall, the results of ULTRA1 conclude that adalimumab 160/80 mg is effective for induction of remission in moderate-to-severe UC subjects who are failing corticosteroids and/or thiopurines. The optimal dose regimen in UC may, however, not have been reached because the dose-response curve suggests that efficacy may be improved with doses more than the current standard dosing regimen.

Following ULTRA1, the ULTRA2 study was conducted as a phase III, randomized, double-blind, placebo-controlled trial to examine the efficacy of adalimumab in long-term maintenance of remission in moderate-to-severe UC.[49] Before enrollment, subjects were required to have 3 months of active moderate-to-severe UC defined as a composite Mayo score of 6 to 12 and an endoscopic subscore of 2 or more. Subjects had moderate-to-severe UC despite corticosteroid or azathioprine/6-meroaptopurine. Concomitant 5-ASA therapy was allowed but not a requirement, and prior use of infliximab was permitted after a more than or equal to 8-week washout period. In total, 40% of subjects had prior anti-TNF exposure. Randomization to placebo or subcutaneous adalimumab 160 mg at week 0, 80 mg at week 2, and then 40 mg every other week was done in a 1:1 fashion. After week 12, subjects who showed poor response were able to enter the open-label phase using adalimumab 40 mg every other week. In addition, subjects were permitted to dose escalate to adalimumab 40 mg every week in the case of inadequate response to every other week dosing.

The study followed subjects for a total of 52 weeks with assessments of primary and secondary endpoints at weeks 8, 32, and 52. The primary endpoint of clinical remission was defined as a composite Mayo score less than or equal to 2 with no individual subscore greater than 1. By week 8, 16.5% of subjects who received adalimumab were in clinical remission, whereas the placebo remission rate was 9.3% ($P = .019$). By week 52, remission rates were 17.3% and 8.5% in the adalimumab and placebo group, respectively ($P = .004$). Secondary endpoints included clinical response and MH. Clinical response was defined as a decrease in Mayo score of more than or equal to 3 from baseline and a decrease in Mayo score more than or equal to 30% from baseline and decrease in rectal bleeding subscore more than or equal to 1 or an absolute score of 0 or 1. By week 8, the adalimumab group achieved clinical response in 50.4% of subjects compared with 34.6% in the placebo group ($P<.001$). By week 52, the adalimumab group revealed response in 30.2% compared with 18.3% placebo response ($P = .002$). MH was achieved by reaching an endoscopic subscore of 0 or 1. At week 8, 41.1% of subjects achieved MH compared with 31.7% on placebo ($P = .032$). In comparison, by week 52, the adalimumab group achieved MH in 25% compared with 15.4% in the placebo group ($P = .009$). Further subanalyses revealed that subjects who were anti-TNF naïve had a greater chance of achieving clinical remission at weeks 8 and 52 compared with the anti-TNF exposed group. Safety results were also comparable between the treatment and placebo groups.

An additional study analyzing the safety of adalimumab using a benefit-to-risk balance assessed the likelihood of achieving efficacy without serious adverse events in the intention-to-treat group.[50] This analysis showed a favorable adverse event profile and overall positive benefit/risk balance when remission or response was achieved at weeks 8 and 52 in adalimumab-treated subjects. One notable difference between the ULTRA2 trial and the infliximab trials (ACT 1 and 2) is that the infliximab studies did not allow for rescue therapy. Another variation is that a significant portion of the ULTRA2 subjects had been exposed to anti-TNF, whereas all the infliximab study subjects were anti-TNF naïve at enrollment. These variations may explain in part the lower remission rates seen with adalimumab versus infliximab.

In summary, the ULTRA2 study results confirm findings from ULTRA1. Combined, these studies show that adalimumab 160 mg at week 0, 80 mg at week 2, followed by 40 mg every other week is effective in induction and maintenance of remission in moderate-to-severe UC.

To study the long-term safety of adalimumab, the PYRAMID registry was initiated in 2007.[51] In common with the TREAT registry for infliximab, only patients with CD are included, but once again the results are also certainly of relevance to those on long-term adalimumab treatment of UC. Although not due for completion until 2015 with a planned 6-year study duration for each patient, an interim safety analysis was carried out at year 3. This study demonstrated very low rates of opportunistic infection (0.1 per 100 PY) as well as malignancy (0.6 per 100 PY) and lymphoma (<0.1 per 100 PY) with no new safety signals. At that point, more than 8000 PY had been studied with a median exposure to adalimumab of 19 months, suggesting that long-term treatment can be considered safe.

GOLIMUMAB

In 2013, the FDA expanded the armamentarium for treatment of moderate-to-severe UC with the approval of golimumab (Simponi), a fully human monoclonal antibody to TNF-α administered subcutaneously. Golimumab is also approved for the treatment of rheumatoid arthritis, psoriatic arthritis, and ankylosing spondylitis. PURSUIT-SC was a randomized, double-blind, placebo-controlled integrated phase 2 and 3 study to assess the safety as well as efficacy of golimumab in inducing remission in moderate-to-severe UC subjects.[6] Subjects were required to have had failed or inadequately responded to standard therapy including oral 5-aminosalyciates, thiopurines, or oral corticosteroids. Prior anti-TNF therapy was an exclusion criterion. A composite Mayo score of 6 to 12 with an endoscopic subscore of 2 or more was required for study entry. The initial phase 2 portion of the study was conducted to determine the dose-response relationship of subcutaneous golimumab, and this information was applied to the phase 3 efficacy portion. Enrolled subjects were randomized to either placebo or 1 of 3 induction regimens 2 weeks apart (100/50 mg, 200/100 mg, or 400/200 mg). After safety, pharamacokinetic, and efficacy analyses, the 200/100 mg and 400/200 mg doses were selected for continuation in the phase 3 study portion. For the phase 3 portion, subjects were assessed at week 6 for primary and secondary endpoints. The study's primary endpoint was week 6 clinical response measured by a decline in the baseline composite Mayo score by 30% or more and 3 points or more (with a bleeding subscore of 0 or 1 or decrease ≥1). Clinical remission was a secondary endpoint and was defined by the authors as a composite Mayo score less than or equal to 2 and no subscore greater than 1. In addition, week 6, MH was also assessed and defined as an endoscopy subscore of 0 or 1. QoL assessment was made as well using the Inflammatory Bowel Disease Questionnaire (IBDQ). By the end of phase 3, the study demonstrated favorable findings for primary and all secondary endpoints. A larger proportion of subjects in the 400/200 mg golimumab group had achieved clinical response, clinical remission, or MH or had greater IBDQ scores when compared with placebo. Clinical response was greatest in the 400/200 mg (54.9%) and 200/100 mg (51%) groups compared with placebo (30.3%), indicating that the study was able to meet its primary endpoint. Improvement in MH was noted at week 2 and was greater by week 6 in the 400/200 mg and 200/100 mg groups compared with placebo. Furthermore, mean C-reactive protein concentrations declined to a greater extent in the 400/200 mg and 200/100 mg groups compared with placebo. Adverse events were similar in the treatment and placebo groups with the most notable being headache and nasopharyngitis. There was no noted dose-dependent accumulation of adverse events. In summary, induction with 400/200 mg and 200/100 mg of golimumab at weeks 0 and 2 resulted in statistically significant induction of remission by week 6 in subjects suffering from moderate-to-severe UC.

Additional analysis of serum golimumab concentration using a validated assay revealed that serum concentrations were dose-proportional and those with higher serum concentrations had greater rates of clinical response and remission and greater improvement in median composite Mayo scores.

All subjects from the PURSUIT-SC study were eligible for enrollment in the PURSUIT-Maintenance study in which subjects received 54 weeks of golimumab

50 mg or 100 mg every 4 weeks as maintenance.[52] This study's primary endpoint of maintenance of clinical response by week 54 was achieved at rates of 49.7% and 47% in the 100 mg and 50 mg groups, respectively, compared with 31.2% placebo response. Secondary endpoints of clinical remission, MH, and corticosteroid-free remission by week 54 were greater in the 100 mg and 50 mg golimumab groups compared with placebo.

It is too early for any safety registry data for golimumab in inflammatory bowel disease (IBD) to mirror the results from infliximab (TREAT[29]) and adalimumab (PYRAMID[51]) registries. However, safety analyses were made as part of the PURSUIT trials. Overall, the safety signals were reassuring and consistent with experience gained from use in rheumatoid arthritis but should prompt a note of caution.[53] Four cases of tuberculosis were seen, all in golimumab-treated patients (who were also receiving corticosteroids) living in endemic regions, with one resulting death. This finding should serve to underscore the importance of robust pretreatment screening for tuberculosis in clinical practice.

ALTERING PRACTICE? TREATING TO TARGET, MUCOSAL, AND HISTOLOGIC HEALING

Progress related to the advent of anti-TNF agents has seen MH become an established endpoint for clinical trials. In conjunction with this, interest in alternative, nonclinical endpoints has also grown. Histologic healing is one such alternative and offers significant promise. As is the case with ongoing endoscopic activity, studies have shown that clinical remission in the presence of ongoing histologic inflammation is less durable than if histologic healing is achieved.[54,55] Also, mirroring the situation in MH, a validated definition for histologic healing remains elusive. Nonetheless, it is likely to feature to some degree as an endpoint in future clinical trials,[56] possibly alongside MH as a part of a composite endpoint.

To investigate the feasibility of using these endpoints as targets in a predefined treatment algorithm for UC, Bouguen and colleagues[8] performed a retrospective cohort study of 60 patients undergoing serial endoscopies. Multivariate analysis demonstrated that anti-TNF use at baseline (along with disease duration <2 years and family history of IBD) predicted MH (hazard ratio 4.47; 95% CI 1.58–11.96). Although anti-TNF treatment during the course of the study (median follow-up 76 weeks) was not associated with higher rates of MH, use of the treatment algorithm approach was. This approach was based on adapting therapy to the target of MH, meaning optimizing biologic therapy by increasing the dose, adjusting to target serum infliximab concentrations, switching biologics, and adding immunosuppressive agents as needed to reach MH. Using this approach allowed 60% of those with endoscopic disease at baseline to achieve MH (with a stringent definition of Mayo 0) at week 76. A similar pattern was seen on a microscopic level, whereby adjustments in medical therapy in response to ongoing histologic activity resulted in higher rates of histologic healing. Preliminary experience regarding treat-to-target algorithms has also been gained from those used in the management of rheumatoid arthritis. The structure of a corresponding proposal for specific recommendations in IBD can be made based on these (Fig. 1).[57] However, long-term studies with similar algorithms are necessary, and it appears that this type of target-driven approach could optimize the benefit gained from anti-TNF agents.

THERAPEUTIC DRUG MONITORING

In the setting of anti-TNF treatment optimization as suggested in the algorithm by Bouguen and colleagues,[57] therapeutic drug monitoring (TDM) could be an objective

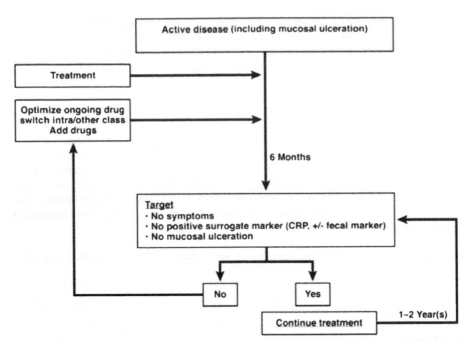

Fig. 1. Schematic representation for a treat-to-target based strategy for UC. On the basis of preliminary experience from RA, proposal algorithm for UC includes careful selection of patients to active treatment, use of MH as the optimal target, and a time frame to assess treatment efficacy.

tool to guide treatment decisions. Prospective studies using TDM are currently, however, lacking.

Concentration-Effect Relationship

The correlation between anti-TNF trough concentrations, anti-drug antibodies, and clinical outcomes, such as clinical response, remission, and MH, has been investigated. In a retrospective study including 115 UC patients treated with 3-dose induction followed by scheduled maintenance infliximab, the authors found that detectable as opposed to undetectable infliximab trough concentrations were associated with clinical remission (69% vs 15%; P<.001), endoscopic improvement (76% vs 28%; P<.001), and endoscopic remission (27% vs 8%; P = .021).[58] Moreover, an undetectable infliximab trough concentration predicted an increased risk for colectomy (odds ratio 9.3; 95% CI 2.9 to 29.9; P<.001). This dichotomous cutoff of presence or absence of detectable infliximab trough concentration was later refined in a follow-up study including 134 patients with steroid refractory active UC treated with 3-dose induction followed by scheduled maintenance therapy.[59] An infliximab trough concentration greater than 2 μg/mL, without or with Antibodies Toward Infliximab, was associated with a higher rate of clinical steroid-free remission (69% vs 16%; P<.001) that was sustained over the follow-up period of a median of 19.9 months. These results were recently corroborated in a post-hoc analysis of the ACT 1 and 2 trials whereby the proportion of patients achieving clinical response, remission, and MH at week 8, 30, and 54 increased with increasing quartiles of infliximab concentration.[42] Interestingly, the same concentration-effect relationship (although it was dose-proportional) was observed in the PURSUIT trial as the change from baseline Mayo score and rates of clinical response and clinical remission at week 6 increased with increasing quartiles of serum golimumab concentration.[6] In the subsequent maintenance trial with golimumab, a combined analysis of patients randomized to golimumab 50-mg and 100-mg groups showed that greater proportions of patients in the higher serum golimumab concentration quartiles achieved clinical response through week 54 or clinical remission at both weeks 30 and 54 when compared with those in the lower serum concentration quartiles.[52] MH has emerged as an important target and it is therefore of interest to investigate the correlation between MH and anti-TNF trough concentrations. In a cross-sectional study in 40 IBD patients treated with adalimumab therapy, the outcome of endoscopic evaluation was correlated to the adalimumab trough concentration.[60] The authors found that an absence of MH was associated with an adalimumab trough concentration less than 4.9 mg/mL (likelihood ratio, 4.3; sensitivity, 66%; specificity, 85%). Although the authors did not find these results to vary with type of IBD, the number of CD and UC patients did become small in subgroup analysis (22 and 18 patients, respectively). Nevertheless, these concentration-effect relationships indicate that when the predefined target is not met, a TDM approach with measurement of serum anti-TNF drug concentrations could be used to optimize anti-TNF treatment further.

TDM-guided Treatment

In a simulated model, Velayos and colleagues[61] showed that a testing-based strategy is more cost-effective than the empiric dose-escalation strategy to address secondary loss of response. In a recent Scandinavian RCT of 69 CD patients with secondary loss of response, the TDM strategy was shown to reduce treatment costs with up to 34% at similar efficacy rates (a response rate of 58% vs 53% for the testing-based and empiric approach, respectively).[62] A similar approach can be applied to further optimize treatment in patients who have insufficient response to the drug (**Table 1**). When response to the current anti-TNF is inadequate and the patient has adequate anti-TNF trough concentrations, switching to an out-of-class drug may be the preferred strategy. In this case, patients might not respond to the drug because of pharmacodynamic problems (a non-TNF-driven disease). In the case of a low anti-TNF trough concentration, dose optimization should be considered if antidrug antibodies are absent. If antidrug antibodies are sustained, the preferred strategy is to switch to another anti-TNF drug. These therapeutic monitoring strategies must be confirmed in UC in prospective clinical trials.

Table 1
TDM algorithm used to optimize anti-TNF therapy in patients failing to improve with standard dosing

		Serum Anti-TNF Trough Concentration	
		Low	Adequate
Antidrug antibodies (ADA)	Undetectable Low titers	Dose optimize Switch within class or Consider dose optimization or Consider addition of immunomodulator (transient ADA)	Switch out of class
	High titers	Switch within class	

SUMMARY

This update has served to illustrate the significant progress made in the treatment of UC during the anti-TNF era. Considered together, this group of trials has demonstrated the value of an effective class of UC therapy. The results have brought about an increasingly widespread use of anti-TNF agents for UC and may yet see these agents being used earlier in the disease course.[9] The evidence gained from them, along with growing clinical experience, has opened up multiple new avenues of investigation. The predominant thrust of more recent research has concerned maximizing the benefit of these agents and has centered on treat-to-target strategies and the use of TDM. However, there is a lack of prospective trials comparing the efficacy of anti-TNF agents in clinical trials. Meta-analysis techniques may be attempted to compare therapies across trials; however, these are limited by not only the difference in inclusion criteria in the placebo arms but also the different pharmacokinetic properties of each anti-TNF agent, which may require unique dosing for their optimal efficacy in UC. Cluster randomization trials in UC will provide large-scale tests of the effectiveness of anti-TNF agent treatment strategies and their effect on outcomes such as costs, hospitalizations, and surgeries. Along with these well-established long-term outcomes, it may now be time also to consider additional outcomes, such as improvement in function or disability scores.[9,63]

The focus of anti-TNF research should now broaden to include comparative effectiveness trials.[64] The potential benefits of trials designed to compare these medications directly include the identification of optimal treatments, a better understanding of their relative economic impacts, and greater applicability to everyday practice.[65] The fact these issues remain unresolved demonstrates that, although anti-TNF agents have delivered on their early promise, there remains significant progress still to be made.

CONFLICTS OF INTEREST PAST 12 MONTHS

M.A. Samaan, P. Bagi: none.

N. Vande Casteele is a Postdoctoral Fellow of the Research Foundation-Flanders (FWO), Belgium. He has served as a consultant for MSD and Janssen Biologics. He has received payment for development of educational presentations, including service on speakers bureaus from AbbVie.

G. D'Haens has received consulting fees from Abbott/Abbvie, ActoGeniX NV, Amgen, AM-Pharma BV, Boehringer Ingelheim, ChemoCentryx, Centocor/Jansen Biologics, Cosmo Technologies, Elan/Biogen, EnGene Inc, Ferring Pharmaceuticals, Gilead Sciences, Given Imaging, GSK, Merck Research Laboratories, Merck Serono, Millenium Pharmaceuticals, Novo Nordisk, NPS Pharmaceuticals, PDL Biopharma, Pfizer, Receptos, Salix Pharmaceuticals, Schering Plough, Shire Pharmaceuticals, Sigmoid Pharma Ltd, Teva Pharmaceuticals, Tillotts Pharma AG, UCB Pharma; research grants from Abbvie, GSK, Falk, Janssen, Merck, Given Imaging; payments for lectures/speakers bureaus from Abbvie, Jansen, Merck, Takeda, UCB, Shire.

B.G. Levesque has received consulting fees from Prometheus Laboratories, Santarus Inc.

REFERENCES

1. Schroeder KW. Role of mesalazine in acute and long-term treatment of ulcerative colitis and its complications. Scand J Gastroenterol Suppl 2002;(236): 42–7.

2. Sninsky CA, Cort DH, Shanahan F, et al. Oral mesalamine (Asacol) for mildly to moderately active ulcerative colitis. A multicenter study. Ann Intern Med 1991; 115(5):350–5.

3. Rogler G. Medical management of ulcerative colitis. Dig Dis 2009;27(4):542–9.

4. Rutgeerts P, Sandborn WJ, Feagan BG, et al. Infliximab for induction and maintenance therapy for ulcerative colitis. N Engl J Med 2005;353(23):2462–76.

5. Reinisch W, Sandborn WJ, Hommes DW, et al. Adalimumab for induction of clinical remission in moderately to severely active ulcerative colitis: results of a randomised controlled trial. Gut 2011;60(6):780–7.

6. Sandborn WJ, Feagan BG, Marano C, et al. Subcutaneous golimumab induces clinical response and remission in patients with moderate-to-severe ulcerative colitis. Gastroenterology 2014;146(1):85–95.

7. Panaccione R, Rutgeerts P, Sandborn WJ, et al. Review article: treatment algorithms to maximize remission and minimize corticosteroid dependence in patients with inflammatory bowel disease. Aliment Pharmacol Ther 2008;28(6):674–88.

8. Bouguen G, Levesque BG, Pola S, et al. Feasibility of endoscopic assessment and treating to target to achieve mucosal healing in ulcerative colitis. Inflamm Bowel Dis 2014;20:231–9.

9. Danese S, Colombel JF, Peyrin-Biroulet L, et al. Review article: the role of anti-TNF in the management of ulcerative colitis – past, present and future. Aliment Pharmacol Ther 2013;37(9):855–66.

10. Rutgeerts P, Van Assche G, Vermeire S. Optimizing anti-TNF treatment in inflammatory bowel disease. Gastroenterology 2004;126(6):1593–610.

11. Wilhelm SM, McKenney KA, Rivait KN, et al. A review of infliximab use in ulcerative colitis. Clin Ther 2008;30(2):223–30.

12. Truelove SC, Witts LJ. Cortisone in ulcerative colitis; final report on a therapeutic trial. Br Med J 1955;2(4947):1041–8.

13. Blackstone MO. Endoscoppic interpretation. New York: Raven Press; 1984.

14. Sands BE, Tremaine WJ, Sandborn WJ, et al. Infliximab in the treatment of severe, steroid-refractory ulcerative colitis: a pilot study. Inflamm Bowel Dis 2001;7(2):83–8.

15. Chey WY, Hussain A, Ryan C, et al. Infliximab for refractory ulcerative colitis. Am J Gastroenterol 2001;96(8):2373–81.

16. Kohu A, Prantera C, Pera A, et al. Anti-tumor necrosis factor alpha (infliximab) in the treatment of severe ulcerative colitis: result of an open study on 13 patients. Dig Liver Dis 2002;34:626–30.

17. Jarnerot G, Hertervig E, Friis-Liby I, et al. Infliximab as rescue therapy in severe to moderately severe ulcerative colitis: a randomized, placebo-controlled study. Gastroenterology 2005;128(7):1805–11.

18. Seo M, Okada M, Yao T, et al. An index of disease activity in patients with ulcerative colitis. Am J Gastroenterol 1992;87(8):971–6.

19. Lindgren SC, Flood LM, Kilander AF, et al. Early predictors of glucocorticosteroid treatment failure in severe and moderately severe attacks of ulcerative colitis. Eur J Gastroenterol Hepatol 1998;10(10):831–5.

20. Armuzzi A, De Pascalis B, Lupascu A, et al. Infliximab in the treatment of steroid-dependent ulcerative colitis. Eur Rev Med Pharmacol Sci 2004;8(5):231–3.

21. Schroeder KW, Tremaine WJ, Ilstrup DM. Coated oral 5-aminosalicylic acid therapy for mildly to moderately active ulcerative colitis. A randomized study. N Engl J Med 1987;317(26):1625–9.

22. Pineton de Chambrun G, Peyrin-Biroulet L, Lemann M, et al. Clinical implications of mucosal healing for the management of IBD. Nat Rev Gastroenterol Hepatol 2010;7(1):15–29.

23. Neurath MF, Travis SP. Mucosal healing in inflammatory bowel diseases: a systematic review. Gut 2012;61(11):1619–35.
24. Rutgeerts P. Landmark data in early IBD patients: time to change your practice? BMJ Satellite Symposium. 2009:3–5.
25. Sandborn WJ, Rutgeerts P, Feagan BG, et al. Colectomy rate comparison after treatment of ulcerative colitis with placebo or infliximab. Gastroenterology 2009; 137(4):1250–60 [quiz: 1520].
26. Reinisch W, Sandborn WJ, Rutgeerts P, et al. Long-term infliximab maintenance therapy for ulcerative colitis: the ACT-1 and -2 extension studies. Inflamm Bowel Dis 2012;18(2):201–11.
27. Panaccione R, Ghosh S, Middleton S, et al. Combination therapy with infliximab and azathioprine is superior to monotherapy with either agent in ulcerative colitis. Gastroenterology 2014;146(2):392–400.e3.
28. Reich K, Wozel G, Zheng H, et al. Efficacy and safety of infliximab as continuous or intermittent therapy in patients with moderate-to-severe plaque psoriasis: results of a randomized, long-term extension trial (RESTORE2). Br J Dermatol 2013;168(6):1325–34.
29. Lichtenstein GR, Feagan BG, Cohen RD, et al. Serious infection and mortality in patients with Crohn's disease: more than 5 years of follow-up in the TREAT registry. Am J Gastroenterol 2012;107(9):1409–22.
30. Ali T, Yun L, Rubin DT. Risk of post-operative complications associated with anti-TNF therapy in inflammatory bowel disease. World J Gastroenterol 2012;18(3): 197–204.
31. Yang Z, Wu Q, Wu K, et al. Meta-analysis: pre-operative infliximab treatment and short-term post-operative complications in patients with ulcerative colitis. Aliment Pharmacol Ther 2010;31(4):486–92.
32. Selvasekar CR, Cima RR, Larson DW, et al. Effect of infliximab on short-term complications in patients undergoing operation for chronic ulcerative colitis. J Am Coll Surg 2007;204(5):956–62 [discussion: 962–3].
33. Schluender SJ, Ippoliti A, Dubinsky M, et al. Does infliximab influence surgical morbidity of ileal pouch-anal anastomosis in patients with ulcerative colitis? Dis Colon Rectum 2007;50(11):1747–53.
34. Mor IJ, Vogel JD, da Luz Moreira A, et al. Infliximab in ulcerative colitis is associated with an increased risk of postoperative complications after restorative proctocolectomy. Dis Colon Rectum 2008;51(8):1202–7 [discussion: 1207–10].
35. Kunitake H, Hodin R, Shellito PC, et al. Perioperative treatment with infliximab in patients with Crohn's disease and ulcerative colitis is not associated with an increased rate of postoperative complications. J Gastrointest Surg 2008; 12(10):1730–6 [discussion: 1736–7].
36. Ferrante M, Vermeire S, Fidder H, et al. Long-term outcome after infliximab for refractory ulcerative colitis. J Crohns Colitis 2008;2(3):219–25.
37. Arts J, D'Haens G, Zeegers M, et al. Long-term outcome of treatment with intravenous cyclosporin in patients with severe ulcerative colitis. Inflamm Bowel Dis 2004;10(2):73–8.
38. Laharie D, Bourreille A, Branche J, et al. Ciclosporin versus infliximab in patients with severe ulcerative colitis refractory to intravenous steroids: a parallel, open-label randomised controlled trial. Lancet 2012;380(9857):1909–15.
39. Lichtiger S. Cyclosporine therapy in inflammatory bowel disease: open-label experience. Mt Sinai J Med 1990;57(5):315–9.
40. Levesque BG, Sandborn WJ. Infliximab versus ciclosporin in severe ulcerative colitis. Lancet 2012;380(9857):1887–8.

41. Kevans D, Murthy S, Iacono A, et al. Accelerated clearance of infliximab during induction therapy for acute ulcerative colitis is associated with treatment failure. Gastroenterology 2012;142(5 Suppl 1):S384–5.

42. Reinisch W, Feagan BG, Rutgeerts PJ, et al. Infliximab concentration and clinical outcome in patients with ulcerative colitis. Gastroenterology 2012;142(5 Suppl 1): S114.

43. Afif W, Leighton JA, Hanauer SB, et al. Open-label study of adalimumab in patients with ulcerative colitis including those with prior loss of response or intolerance to infliximab. Inflamm Bowel Dis 2009;15(9):1302–7.

44. Barreiro-de Acosta M, Lorenzo A, Dominguez-Munoz JE. Adalimumab in ulcerative colitis: two cases of mucosal healing and clinical response at two years. World J Gastroenterol 2009;15(30):3814–6.

45. Peyrin-Biroulet L, Laclotte C, Roblin X, et al. Adalimumab induction therapy for ulcerative colitis with intolerance or lost response to infliximab: an open-label study. World J Gastroenterol 2007;13(16):2328–32.

46. Taxonera C, Estelles J, Fernandez-Blanco I, et al. Adalimumab induction and maintenance therapy for patients with ulcerative colitis previously treated with infliximab. Aliment Pharmacol Ther 2011;33(3):340–8.

47. Hanauer SB, Sandborn WJ, Rutgeerts P, et al. Human anti-tumor necrosis factor monoclonal antibody (adalimumab) in Crohn's disease: the CLASSIC-I trial. Gastroenterology 2006;130(2):323–33 [quiz: 591].

48. Colombel JF, Sandborn WJ, Rutgeerts P, et al. Adalimumab for maintenance of clinical response and remission in patients with Crohn's disease: the CHARM trial. Gastroenterology 2007;132(1):52–65.

49. Sandborn WJ, van Assche G, Reinisch W, et al. Adalimumab induces and maintains clinical remission in patients with moderate-to-severe ulcerative colitis. Gastroenterology 2012;142(2):257–65.e1–3.

50. Sandborn WJ, Colombel JF, D'Haens G, et al. One-year maintenance outcomes among patients with moderately-to-severely active ulcerative colitis who responded to induction therapy with adalimumab: subgroup analyses from ULTRA 2. Aliment Pharmacol Ther 2013;37(2):204–13.

51. D'Haens G, Reinisch W, Satsangi J, et al. PYRAMID registry: an observational study of adalimumab in Crohn's disease: results at year 3. Inflamm Bowel Dis 2011;17:S21.

52. Sandborn WJ, Feagan BG, Marano C, et al. Subcutaneous golimumab maintains clinical response in patients with moderate-to-severe ulcerative colitis. Gastroenterology 2014;146(1):96–109.e1.

53. Hanauer SB. Still in pursuit. Gastroenterology 2014;146(1):13–5.

54. Bitton A, Peppercorn MA, Antonioli DA, et al. Clinical, biological, and histologic parameters as predictors of relapse in ulcerative colitis. Gastroenterology 2001; 120(1):13–20.

55. Riley SA, Mani V, Goodman MJ, et al. Microscopic activity in ulcerative colitis: what does it mean? Gut 1991;32(2):174–8.

56. Peyrin-Biroulet L, Bressenot A, Kampman W. Histologic remission: the ultimate therapeutic goal in ulcerative colitis? Clin Gastroenterol Hepatol 2014;12:929–34.e2.

57. Bouguen G, Levesque BG, Feagan BG, et al. Treat to target: a proposed new paradigm for the management of crohn's disease. Clin Gastroenterol Hepatol 2013. [Epub ahead of print].

58. Seow CH, Newman A, Irwin SP, et al. Trough serum infliximab: a predictive factor of clinical outcome for infliximab treatment in acute ulcerative colitis. Gut 2010; 59(1):49–54.

59. Murthy S, Kevans D, Seow CH, et al. Association of serum infliximab and antibodies to infliximab to long-term clinical outcome in acute ulcerative colitis. Gastroenterology 2012;142(5 Suppl 1):S-388.
60. Roblin X, Marotte H, Rinaudo M, et al. Association between pharmacokinetics of adalimumab and mucosal healing in patients with inflammatory bowel diseases. Clin Gastroenterol Hepatol 2014;12(1):80–4.e2.
61. Velayos FS, Kahn JG, Sandborn WJ, et al. A test-based strategy is more cost effective than empiric dose escalation for patients with Crohn's disease who lose responsiveness to infliximab. Clin Gastroenterol Hepatol 2013;11(6): 654–66.
62. Steenholdt C, Brynskov J, Thomsen OO, et al. Individualised therapy is more cost-effective than dose intensification in patients with Crohn's disease who lose response to anti-TNF treatment: a randomised, controlled trial. Gut 2014; 63:919–27.
63. Peyrin-Biroulet L, Cieza A, Sandborn WJ, et al. Development of the first disability index for inflammatory bowel disease based on the international classification of functioning, disability and health. Gut 2012;61(2):241–7.
64. Cheifetz AS, Melmed GY, Spiegel B, et al. Setting priorities for comparative effectiveness research in inflammatory bowel disease: results of an international provider survey, expert RAND panel, and patient focus groups. Inflamm Bowel Dis 2012;18(12):2294–300.
65. Roland M, Torgerson DJ. What are pragmatic trials? BMJ 1998;316(7127):285.

Acute Gastroenteritis

Nancy S. Graves, MD

KEYWORDS

- Gastroenteritis • Infectious • Vomiting • Diarrhea • Abdominal pain

KEY POINTS

- Acute gastroenteritis is a common infectious disease syndrome, causing a combination of nausea, vomiting, diarrhea, and abdominal pain. The Centers for Disease Control and Prevention (CDC) estimate there are more than 350 million cases of acute gastroenteritis in the United States annually, and 48 million of these cases are caused by foodborne bacteria.
- Traveler's diarrhea affects more than half of people traveling from developed countries to developing countries. Prevention can be summarized by the caution, "boil it, cook it, peel it, or forget it."
- Except in cases of fever, bloody diarrhea, immunocompromised patients, or patients with significant comorbidities, identifying a specific pathogen is rarely indicated in acute bacterial gastroenteritis because illness is usually self-limited.
- In both adult and pediatric patients, the prevalence of *Clostridium difficile* is increasing in the United States. Contact precautions, public health education, and prudent use of antibiotics are still necessary goals. Complicating these efforts are that there is increasing antibiotic resistance to *C difficile* and a new strain, NAP1/027/III, has been emerging since the early 2000s. This new strain has a high association with community onset and has been linked to increasing frequency and severity of illness. There is research into the possibility that the community onset may be related to animals and to retail meat, where the new strain has been detected.
- Preventing dehydration or providing appropriate rehydration is the primary supportive treatment of acute gastroenteritis.

INTRODUCTION
Definition

Gastroenteritis is inflammation of the stomach, small intestine, or large intestine, leading to a combination of abdominal pain, cramping, nausea, vomiting, and diarrhea. Acute gastroenteritis usually lasts fewer than 14 days. This is in contrast to persistent gastroenteritis, which lasts between 14 and 30 days, and chronic gastroenteritis, which lasts more than 30 days.[1]

This article originally appeared in Primary Care: Clinics in Office Practice, Volume 40, Issue 3, September 2013.
Department of Family and Community Medicine, Milton S. Hershey Medical Center, Penn State Hershey, 500 University Drive, Hershey, PA 17033, USA
E-mail address: ngraves@hmc.psu.edu

Clinics Collections 7 (2015) 517–531
http://dx.doi.org/10.1016/j.ccol.2015.06.035
2352-7986/15/$ – see front matter

Epidemiology

In the United States, acute gastroenteritis is often viewed as a nuisance rather than the life-threatening illness it can be in developing countries. Although significant morbidity and mortality have been attributed to acute diarrheal illnesses in the United States, epidemiologic studies in this country have not been as comprehensive as those conducted in developing nations. The CDC, however, estimate that there are more than 350 million cases of acute diarrheal illnesses in the United States annually. Acute gastroenteritis compares with upper respiratory illnesses as the most common infectious disease syndrome.[2,3]

Using data from the National Center for Health Statistics, the CDC recently reported that deaths from all-cause gastroenteritis increased from approximately 7000 to more than 17,000 per year from 1999 to 2007. Adults over 65 years old made up 83% of these deaths and C difficile accounted for two-thirds of these deaths, reflecting that the most significant morbidity and mortality are experienced by the extremes of age.[4]

Etiology

Etiology of acute gastroenteritis

Acute gastroenteritis is caused by many infectious agents as listed in **Table 1**.

Assessing the precise incidence and cause of acute infectious gastroenteritis is made difficult because not everyone reports their symptoms or seeks medical care. In addition, stool cultures, which are used to identify bacterial causes of gastroenteritis, are only positive in 1.5% to 5.6% of cases.[5]

Viral causes of acute gastroenteritis are dominated by rotavirus and norovirus. In the United States, it is estimated that 15 to 25 million episodes of viral gastroenteritis occur each year, leading to 3 to 5 million office visits and 200,000 hospitalizations.[6,7]

Rotavirus causes a particularly severe dehydrating gastroenteritis that affects young children. The severity of the infection is made worse by malnourishment, making rotavirus a significant cause of mortality in children worldwide, responsible for approximately 500,000 deaths annually.[8,9] The introduction of the rotavirus vaccine in the United States and Europe has been effective at reducing rotavirus gastroenteritis. There has been a 67% decrease in positive laboratory diagnosis attributed to vaccination.[10]

Norovirus, however, causes the most outbreaks of nonbacterial acute gastroenteritis in all age groups. It often occurs in epidemic outbreaks in schools, nursing homes, cruise ships, prisons, and other group settings. Symptoms of severe vomiting are usually self-limited, lasting 12 to 60 hours. Transmission of this stable virus is through the fecal-oral route, with viral shredding lasting on average 10 to 14 days after onset of symptoms.[11]

Table 1
Infectious causes of acute gastroenteritis

Viral: 50%–70%	Bacterial: 15%–20%	Parasitic: 10%–15%
Norovirus	Shigella	Giardia
Rotavirus	Salmonella	Amebiasis
Enteric adenovirus types 40 and 41	Campylobacter	Cryptosporidium
Astrovirus	E coli	Isospora
Coronavirus	Vibrio	Cyclospora
Some picornaviruses	Yersinia	Microsporidium
	C difficile	

Rotavirus and enteric adenovirus can be detected by rapid assays for the viral antigen in stool. Norovirus is best detected by reverse transcriptase–polymerase chain reaction.

Medications and toxic ingestions that cause acute diarrhea or gastroenteritis include those listed in **Table 2**.

Etiology of chronic gastroenteritis

Causes of persistent or chronic gastroenteritis include parasitic infections, medications, inflammatory bowel disease (ulcerative colitis, Crohn disease, collagenous colitis, and microscopic colitis), irritable bowel syndrome, eosinophilic gastroenteritis, celiac disease, lactose intolerance, colorectal cancer, bowel obstruction, malabsorption, and ischemic bowel.

Immunocompromised hosts are most vulnerable to chronic gastroenteritis infections. *Crytosporidium* has been a cause of chronic diarrhea in persons with AIDS. It is also responsible for large outbreaks in day care centers and public swimming pools and has contaminated public water supplies. One of the reasons for these outbreaks is that the oocytes are resistant to bleach or other disinfectants, making them easily transmittable by contact with contaminated surfaces or by person-to-person contact. *Giardia* is another common cause of chronic gastroenteritis. It is found in contaminated streams but is also common in day care centers and swimming pools. *Giardia* causes bloating, flatulence, and explosive, pale, foul-smelling diarrhea.

TYPES OF ACUTE GASTROENTERITIS

The remainder of this article focuses on acute bacterial gastroenteritis, reviewing the common pathogens that cause traveler's gastroenteritis, foodborne gastroenteritis, and antibiotic-associated gastroenteritis. Each section addresses transmission, pathophysiology, the incubation period, symptoms, symptom duration, management, and prevention.

Traveler's Diarrhea

Travelers to developing countries often present to their primary care providers with concerns about traveler's diarrhea and how to avoid or treat this problem should it occur; 40% to 60% of travelers to developing countries acquire this problem. It should also be considered if diarrhea develops within 10 days of their return home.

For epidemiologic reasons, traveler's diarrhea is divided into classic, moderate, and mild forms.

Table 2
Medications and toxic ingestions that cause acute diarrhea or gastroenteritis

Medications	Toxic Ingestions
Antibiotics	Organophosphates
Laxative abuse	Poisonous mushrooms
Sorbitol	Arsenic
Colchicine	Ciguatera or scombroid
Cardiac antidysrhythmics	
Nonsteroidal anti-inflammatory drugs[12]	
Chemotherapeutics	
Antacids	

- Classic: 3 of more unformed bowel movements per 24 hours plus 1 of the following: nausea, vomiting, fever, abdominal pain, and blood in the stool
- Moderate: 1 to 2 unformed bowel movements per 24 hours plus 1 of the above symptoms OR more than 2 unformed bowel movements
- Mild: 1 to 2 unformed bowel movements

Transmission
Traveler's diarrhea is usually transmitted by contaminated food or water. It can be caused by bacteria, viruses, or parasites. Bacteria cause the majority of cases of traveler's diarrhea. The most common are enterotoxigenic *E coli* (ETEC), followed by *Salmonella*, *Campylobacter jejuni*, and *Shigella*. In 1 study of 322 patients, ETEC caused 12% of bacterial traveler's diarrhea, *Salmonella* 8%, *Campylobacter jejuni* 6%, and *Shigella* less than 1%. In another study of 636 travelers, ETEC caused 30% and enteroaggregative *E coli* caused 26% of cases.[13,14]

Coinfection with an additional pathogen was found in 20% of travelers.[14]

Areas of the world with the highest risk are countries in Asia, outside of Singapore, on the African continent, outside of South Africa, and in Central and South America.

Pathogenesis
Pathogenesis is discussed in detail for each bacterial cause.

Incubation
Incubation is 4 to 14 days after arrival in a developing nation.

Symptoms
Common symptoms include malaise, anorexia, abdominal pain and cramping, watery diarrhea, nausea and vomiting, and low-grade fever. If caused by *Campylobacter jejuni* or *Shigella*, symptoms may progress to colitis, bloody diarrhea, and tenesmus.

Duration
Duration is 1 to 5 days and generally self-limited, but, in 8% to 15% of cases, symptoms last longer than 1 week.[15] If bloating, nausea, or other gastrointestinal symptoms persist for more than 14 days, consider alternative diagnoses, such as parasitic infection.

Diagnosis
The diagnosis is often clinical and confirmation is usually not pursued because traveler's diarrhea is self-limited. Stool cultures may be useful in patients with severe symptoms, prolonged illness, bloody diarrhea, and fever. Stool cultures, however, do not differentiate between nonpathogenic *E coli* and ETEC or enteroaggregative *E coli*.

Treatment

- Fluid replacement is the mainstay of symptomatic treatment, plus or minus diet restrictions. There is limited information about whether a clear liquid diet versus an unrestricted diet significantly changes the duration or severity of symptoms because traveler's diarrhea is usually self-limited, lasting 3 to 5 days. Oral rehydration is ideal, but intravenous hydration may be necessary in the setting of dehydration.
- Antibiotics may shorten the course by 1 to 2 days. Travelers often request a prescription for antibiotics that may be taken at the onset of symptoms. Ciprofloxacin (500 mg as a single dose or twice a day for 1–2 days) is commonly sufficient, although resistance to quinolones is increasing, especially for *Campylobacter jejuni*. Quinolones are not Food and Drug Administration approved for pregnancy

or for treating traveler's diarrhea in children. Azithromycin is appropriate in these groups. In adults, a single 1-g dose is effective. In children, recommended dosing is 10 mg/kg as a single dose, not to exceed 1 g. Rifaximin (200 mg 3 times a day) has been shown effective and, with increasing quinolone resistance, it is increasingly used.[16]

- Antimotility agents, such as loperamide or diphenoxylate, can decrease stool frequency but do not alter the course of the infection. Their use should be avoided in cases of fever or rectal bleeding.
- *Lactobacillus GG*, a specific probiotic, has been shown to decrease diarrhea caused by the pathogens that typically cause traveler's gastroenteritis. Other *Lactobacillus* preparations, however, using nonviable probiotics, have not.[17,18]

Prevention

In 2001, the Infectious Diseases Society of America (IDSA) published guidelines to assist travelers in decreasing their chances of contracting traveler's diarrhea:

- Water must be boiled for 3 minutes to kill pathogens. Two drops of bleach or 5 drops of iodine kill pathogens in water within 30 minutes.
- Freezing does not kill pathogens. Avoid ice, request bottled beverages, and use a straw versus a glass.
- Fruit that must be peeled is safe. Fruit that is not peeled or raw vegetables should be avoided.
- Steam table buffets pose a high risk of contracting traveler's gastroenteritis.
- Communal condiments are frequently contaminated and should be avoided.

Medications, such as H_2 blockers and proton pump inhibitors, can increase susceptibility to traveler's diarrhea. These medications lower gastric acidity and can increase the chance of contracting traveler's diarrhea by allowing more pathogens to survive transit to the small bowel. Similarly, conditions or medications that slow gastric motility allow the number of pathogens to accumulate.

Foodborne Acute Gastroenteritis

The CDC estimate that 48 million cases of foodborne bacterial gastroenteritis occur annually in the United States, leading to 125,000 hospitalizations, 3000 deaths, and costs greater than $150 billion.[2] The Foodborne Disease Active Surveillance Network (or Food-Net program) was established in 1996 by the CDC to track foodborne gastrointestinal illnesses in the United States. Data from this 10-site study that covers 46 million cases suggests that 1 in 5 episodes of gastroenteritis are caused by foodborne pathogens. Data from 2010 show little significant overall change in the known foodborne causes of acute gastroenteritis over the past 4 years. The data did, however, show a decline in Shiga toxin–producing *E coli* O157:H7 and *Shigella*. *Vibrio* gastroenteritis increased over this time period and Salmonella incidence was unchanged, despite increasing awareness and efforts to decrease these infections. In general, treatment of foodborne gastroenteritis can range in cost from $78 in Montana to $162 in New Jersey. The total cost per case, including productivity losses, can be as high as $1506, as noted in Connecticut.[3] There is also research suggesting, however, a significant presence of unspecified agents causing 38.4 million cases of foodborne acute gastroenteritis.[19] Reasons for this include a limited amount of data because not all cases of foodborne gastroenteritis are reported nor is a specific etiology identified; other microbes or chemicals in food could cause or contribute to illness; and, finally, new causes being discovered and known causes, such as *C difficile*, not thought to be transmitted by food, have been detected in retail meat products,[19] suggesting a new route of transmission.

Pathogenesis

The pathogenesis of foodborne gastroenteritis can be broken down into 3 mechanisms:

1. Pathogens that make a toxin in the food before it is consumed (preformed toxin)
2. Pathogens that make a toxin in the gastrointestinal tract, after the food is ingested
3. Pathogens that invade the bowel wall and directly break down the epithelial lining, releasing factors that cause an inflammatory diarrhea.

1. Preformed toxins: *Staphylococcus aureus* and *Bacillus cereus* produce heat-stable enterotoxins in the food before it is consumed.

> Transmission: These pathogens are usually transmitted by a food handler and often found in summer picnic foods.
> *S aureus*: grows well in dairy, meat, eggs, and salads
> *Bacillus cereus*: grows in starchy foods, such as rice, but is also found in beef, pork, and vegetables
> Incubation: 1–6 hours. Ingestion of preformed toxins leads to rapid onset of symptoms.
> Pathophysiology: These bacteria usually affect the small intestine, causing nausea, profuse vomiting, and abdominal pain/cramping. The emetic enterotoxin can be found in vomitus and the food. Testing is rarely conducted, however, because illnesses are self-limited. In cases of preformed toxins, there is no risk of person-to-person spread.
> Symptoms: Sudden onset of nausea and vomiting after eating suggests ingestion of a preformed toxin.
> Diagnosis: Stool studies are not contributory. Diagnosis is usually made based on history and food diary.
> Treatment: No antibiotics needed because it is a preformed enterotoxin.
> Supportive care and parenteral antiemetics help control vomiting.
> Prognosis: Rapid spontaneous recovery in 1 day is typical.

2. Pathogens that transmit illness by making a toxin after consumption
a. *C perfringens*
> Transmission: ingestion of spores that have germinated in food products, such as beef, pork, home canned foods, and poultry[1]
> Pathophysiology: Once spores reach the small intestine, they produce an enterotoxin, leading to watery diarrhea.
> Incubation: 6–48 hours
> Symptoms: frequent watery stools and abdominal cramping; rarely, fever, nausea, and vomiting
> Duration: usually less than 24 hours
> Treatment: Rarely does a patient need intravenous fluids. Antibiotics are of no use given the short duration of symptoms.
> Diagnosis: Usually unnecessary given the short lived nature of this illness, but fecal leukocytes are present because this is an inflammatory gastroenteritis.
> Prognosis: Self-limited, rarely lasting more than 24 hours. Ingestion of type C strain of these bacteria, however, can lead to a serious illness, enteritis necroticans (pigbel). Symptoms include severe abdominal pain, vomiting, diarrhea, and possible shock and can be rapidly fatal.
> Prevention: Do not keep foods that have already been cooked warm for long periods of time.
b. ETEC
> Transmission: ingestion of food or water contaminated by infected fecal matter

Pathophysiology: Bacteria attach to the wall of the small bowel and enterotoxins are released, drawing fluid and electrolytes from the mucosa into the lumen, causing profuse watery diarrhea.

Incubation: 24–72 hours after ingestion

Symptoms: wide-ranging, from mild to severe diarrhea

Duration: 48–72 hours

Treatment: hydration plus ciprofloxacin (500 mg twice daily × 3 days) or Bactrim DS (twice daily × 3 days)

Prevention: safe preparation of food and the avoidance of keeping foods that have already been cooked warm for long periods of time

3. Pathogens that directly invade the bowel wall causing inflammatory diarrhea

a. Enterohemorrhagic *E coli* (EHEC) (Shiga toxin producing)

E coli O157:H7 is 1 of at least 30 serotypes of *E coli* that make shiga-like toxin. It was discovered in 1982, after 2 outbreaks traced to undercooked beef. In May 2011, another serotype, O104:H4, was discovered in Germany.[20] The CDC estimate 110,000 cases and 2100 hospitalizations annually in the United States.[1]

Transmission: These bacteria are present in the intestines of cows and transferred initially through processing and then ingested through undercooked animal food products. Transmission can also occur through contaminated water, raw milk, unpasteurized apple cider, petting zoos, and day care centers.[1]

Pathophysiology: Bacteria attack epithelial cells of the cecum and the large bowel. The shiga-like toxins, called verotoxins, destroy the cells, leading to hemorrhagic colitis.

Incubation: 1–9 days, with 3–4 days typical

Symptoms: Watery diarrhea develops that quickly becomes bloody. Elevated white cell count, abdominal pain, cramping, and vomiting are also commonly seen. The absence of fever (or only a low-grade fever) helps differentiate EHEC from other bacterial causes of bloody acute gastroenteritis.

Duration: 1 week for uncomplicated EHEC infection

Diagnosis: The CDC recommend all stool cultures be screened for *E coli* O157:H and certainly all bloody stool samples. Fecal leukocytes are present in 50% of cases. *E coli* O157:H7 can be screened for using a sorbitol MacConkey agar. Both stool cultures and toxin assays are recommended.

Complications: Hemolytic uremic syndrome (HUS) is associated with Shiga toxin 2 and is a complication seen in 6% to 9% of EHEC causes of acute gastroenteritis.[21] The CDC estimate that greater than 90% of HUS is associated with *E coli* O157:H7. HUS is often seen in children younger than 4 years old and the elderly. There is some concern that empiric antibiotic use may increase the risk of developing HUS.[22] Long-term sequelae caused by this complication include, hypertension, proteinuria, decreased glomerular filtration rate, and, less commonly, seizure, coma, or motor deficits.[23]

Thrombotic thrombocytopenia purpura, which shares many similar features with HUS, presents with prominent neurologic findings rather than renal failure. Rarely, pseudomembranous colitis is associated with *E coli* O157:H7.

Treatment: Treatment is largely supportive. Antibiotics do not shorten the duration of illness and should be avoided. There is some thought that empiric antibiotics or antiperistaltics may increase the chance of developing complications.[24]

Prognosis: Uncomplicated cases resolve spontaneously in 7 to 10 days. A carrier state may last an additional 1 to 2 weeks. Hospitalization is required for 23% to 47% of patients, median length of stay 6 to 14 days. Mortality rate is 1% to 2% and is highest in the elderly population.[1]

Prevention: The best prevention is practicing good hand hygiene and fully cooking meat. In addition, the Department of Agriculture has been improving and continues to improve the slaughter process.

b. Salmonella

Transmission: Salmonella is transmitted through the consumption of contaminated raw or undercooked eggs, meats, raw milk, ice cream, peanuts, fruits, and vegetables. Transmission also occurs through contact with infected animals, such as turtles and pet ducklings.[11]

Pathophysiology: bacteria that survive the acidity of the stomach, colonize the intestine, and move across the intestinal epithelium, either by direct invasion of enterocytes or through dendritic cells inserted into epithelial cells. Once present, the inflammatory process begins releasing cytokines, neutrophils, macrophages, and T cells and B cells. This inflammatory response decreases normal intestinal flora and allows the pathogen to proliferate. The nontyphoid Salmonella produce a more localized response and the typhi serotype (the cause of typhoid fever) tends to be more invasive and more often results in bacteremia.[25]

Incubation: 6–48 hours[11]

Duration: 1–7 days

Symptoms: nausea, vomiting, fever, cramping abdominal pain, possibly bloody diarrhea

Treatment: not usually recommended. Exceptions include severe illness, extremes of age, valvular heart disease, uremia, or malignancy. In the case of these exceptions, a third-generation cephalosporin or fluoroquinolone for 5 to 7 days is indicated.

Complications: Antibiotic use can increase carrier state. Additional complications include transient reactive arthritis, which can be seen in up to 30% of adult patients, and Reiter syndrome, which occurs in 2% of patients.

Prognosis: Most patients recover in 2 to 5 days. Sustained or intermittent bacteremia may occur in immunocompromised patients.

c. *Campylobacter jejuni*

Population: usually under 5 years of age

Transmission: handling or eating raw or undercooked poultry or raw milk or cheeses, by contaminated drinking water, or by handling infected animals[1]

Pathophysiology: direct invasion of epithelial cells of the colon inducing inflammation

Incubation: 1 to 10 days

Duration: 5 to 14 days

Symptoms: Usually rapid onset with fever, chills, headache, and malaise followed by abdominal pain, nausea, vomiting, and diarrhea. Diarrhea may be grossly bloody or melanotic in 60% to 90% of patients.

Treatment: Empiric antibiotics are not recommended in healthy patients. Stool culture is appropriate. Antibiotics shorten the illness by 1 to 1.5 days. Erythromycin or azithromycin × 5 days (resistance to fluoroquinolones).

Complications: *Campylobacter jejuni* gastroenteritis is associated with postinfectious Guillain-Barré syndrome, incidence 1 per 1000. In cases of more severe symptoms, this can be less reversible.[26]

Prognosis: Most patients recover within 1 week. Relapses are common but tend to be milder than the original infection. Fatalities are rare.

d. *Vibrio parahaemolyticus*

It is not common in the United States, but worldwide this pathogen is the most common cause of bacterial gastroenteritis.[1]

Transmission: eating contaminated seafood, crabs, oysters, or clams or by exposure of an open wound to contaminated seawater (Gulf of Mexico). It has been transmitted through airline food.

Pathophysiology: production of a heat-stable enterotoxin, inducing a secretory diarrhea and hemolysis

Incubation: 6 hours to 4 days

Duration: self-limited up to 3 days, commonly 24 to 48 hours

Symptoms: abrupt onset of severe watery diarrhea, abdominal cramping, nausea, and vomiting are common symptoms. Fever occurs less commonly.

Diagnosis: can be cultured on thiosulfate citrate–bile salts sucrose if ingestion of contaminated seafood within 3 days before testing[1]

Treatment: tetracycline × 3 days, ciprofloxacin × 1 dose, or chloramphenicol

e. Shigella

Population: usually has an impact on children less than 5 years of age. It is rare in the United States.

Transmission: consumption of contaminated food or water or by person-to-person or fecal-oral route

Pathophysiology: invades colonic epithelia cells; Shiga toxin causes inflammation and results in hemorrhagic colitis.[1]

Incubation: 1 to 6 days

Duration: self-limiting, lasting 2 to 5 days

Symptoms: Fever, cramping abdominal pain, and diarrhea that is often bloody. Infants may not have bloody diarrhea.

Treatment: ciprofloxacin (500 mg twice a day × 3–5 days), trimethoprim/sulfamethoxazole (160 mg twice a day × 3–5 days), or azithromycin (500 mg once daily for 3 days).

Prognosis: Most patients recover in 1 week. Untreated patients shed bacteria in stool for 2 weeks. Relapse occurs in 10% of patients if not treated with antibiotics.

Antibiotic-Associated Diarrhea

Antibiotic-associated diarrhea is also called *C difficile* colitis. This infection often occurs in hospitalized patients, with increasing risk correlating with length of hospital stay. The use of multiple antibiotics and duration of antibiotic are associated with an increased risk of *C difficile* infection. Patients older than 65 years of age and those who are immunocompromised are at an increased risk of developing *C difficile* colitis, likely related to comorbid conditions.[27] The prevalence of *C difficile* associated colitis is increasing in the United States, both in pediatric and adult admissions. From 2001 to 2006, pediatric *C difficile* admissions increased from 2.6 to 4 cases per 1000.[28] The National Hospital Discharge Survey found the rate for *C difficile* colitis increased from 31 per 100,000 in 1996 to 61 per 100,000 in 2003.[29]

Antibiotics most often associated with *C difficile* infection are flouroquinolones, clindamycin, cephalosporins, and penicillins. Those least associated with *C difficile* infection include doxycycline, aminoglycosides, vancomycin, and metronidazole. Proton pump inhibitors have also been associated with increased susceptibility to *C difficile* infection. Studies found that the use proton pump inhibitors increased the risk 1.4 to 2.75 times compared with those without proton pump inhibitor use.[30]

Transmission
Transmission occurs by fecal-oral route and colonization occurs because antibiotic use has disturbed the normal flora of the intestinal tract.

Pathophysiology
C difficile is an anaerobic bacterium that forms spores capable of producing exotoxins. The spores are heat resistant, acid resistant, and antibiotic resistant. They are also resistant to alcohol-based hand sanitizer, so caregivers must wash their hands in soap and water. Once in the colon, the bacteria become functional and produce toxin A (enterotoxin) and toxin B (cytotoxin). Both toxins lead to inflammation, mucosal injury, and secretory diarrhea.[31] Although toxin B is more virulent than toxin A, they both inactivate regulatory pathways, causing cell apoptosis, mucosal ulceration, and neutrophil chemotaxis to produce the pseudomembranes, common in this infection.[32] Pseudomenbranes are composed of neutrophils, fibrin, epithelial debris, and mucin. Pseudomembranes are not found in all patients, for example, those with ulcerative colitis or who are on immunosuppressive agents, such as steroids or cyclosporine.[33] The hypothesized reason for this is that pseudomembranes develop because of the host immunoreactions.[33]

A new strain of C difficile, hypervirulent North American pulsed-field type 1 (NAP1/027/III), has been suspected in epidemic outbreaks since the early 2000s. It produces a binary toxin in addition to larger quantities of toxin A and toxin B and is associated with increasing incidence and severity of illness. It is resistant to fluoroquinolones.[1] It is associated with community onset and there is concern for transmission via animals and retail meat.[34]

Incubation and duration
Symptom onset may start during use of antibiotics or up to 3 to 4 weeks after antibiotic completion. Symptoms can resolve after stopping the offending antibiotic or follow a complicated and prolonged course.

Symptoms
Patients can present with abdominal pain and mild to moderate watery diarrhea. C difficile can also present with fever, nausea, severe abdominal pain, profuse diarrhea, and, possibly, bloody diarrhea.

Diagnosis
C difficile toxin assay is widely used and available. It must be done on liquid or unformed stool. Stool cultures are sensitive but not clinically useful because results are not rapid. Also, C difficile is present in stool of healthy people and infants. Fecal leukocyte testing is not diagnostic. Sigmoidoscopy and colonoscopy is occasionally used but the risk of perforation is possible. A complete blood cell count to identify leukocytosis and thrombocytosis, albumin level, and lactate may also be useful.

Treatment
Discontinuation of the offending antibiotic is one of the first steps in treatment. According to IDSA treatment guidelines, mild to moderate disease should be treated with metronidazole (500 mg 3 times daily × 10–14 days) and severe disease should be treated with vancomycin (125 mg 4 times daily for 10–14 days). For a first recurrence, treat the same as the initial episode. For a second recurrence, however, use of vancomycin in a tapered or pulsed dose is recommended.

A Cochrane review from 2008 concluded that there is inconclusive evidence supporting the benefit of probiotics in the treatment of *C difficile*. Stool transplantation in patients with recurrent or refractory *C difficile* colitis may be useful.[35] Antiperistaltic medications should be avoided, because they increase the risk for toxic megacolon.

Complications
Complications include toxic megacolon.

Prevention
Use contact precautions—isolate patients in private rooms and gown and glove all visitors and health care workers. Mandate that everyone wash hands with soap and water (**Table 3**).

EVALUATION OF PATIENTS PRESENTING WITH SIGNS AND SYMPTOMS OF ACUTE GASTROENTERITIS, ETIOLOGY UNKNOWN
History

Important questions to consider when exploring the history of acute gastroenteritis are listed in (**Box 1**).

Physical Examination Findings

1. Abnormal vital signs: fever and/or orthostatic blood pressure, and/or tachycardia, and/or pain
2. Clinical signs of dehydration include the following: dry mucus membranes, decreased skin turgor, absent jugular vein pulsations, mental status changes

These and other physical examination findings, such as abdominal pain, have poor predictive value but contribute to the diagnosis and help with appropriate management of the illness.

Diagnostics

Test if symptoms are prolonged or severe or if the patient was recently hospitalized or has fever, bloody stool, systemic illness, recent antibiotic use, or day care center attendance. Assess serum electrolytes, serum urea nitrogen, creatinine to evaluate hydration, and acid-base status. A complete blood cell count is nonspecific but, if eosinophils are elevated, a parasitic infection should be considered.

Table 3
Onset, duration, and symptoms as caused by specific bacteria

Bacteria	Onset	Duration	Signs
Salmonella	6–48 h	1–7 d	N, V, F, P, ± blood
Campylobacter	1–10 d	5–14 d	F, H, P, N, V ± blood
Vibrio	6 h–4 d	SL (up to 3 d)	N, V, D
Shigella	1–6 d	SL (2–3 d)	F, P, D, ± blood
ETEC	1–3 d	2–3 d	D
C perfringens	8–16 h	Less than 24 h	P, D
EHEC	1–9 d	1 wk	N, P, D + blood
C difficile	4–5 d	Variable	F, N, P, D ± blood

Abbreviations: D, diarrhea; F, fever; H, headache; N, nausea; P, abdominal pain; SL, self-limiting; V, vomiting.

> **Box 1**
> **Questions to consider in the evaluation of patient with signs and symptoms of acute gastroenteritis**
>
> 1. Abrupt or gradual onset of symptoms. In cases of foodborne illness, how many hours after eating before symptoms onset?
> 2. Duration of symptoms
> 3. Characteristics of stool: watery, bloody, mucus, and color
> 4. Frequency and quantity of bowel movements.
> 5. Presence of fever, tenesmus, nausea, vomiting, headache, abdominal pain, malaise
> 6. Recent hospitalization, recent antibiotic use
> 7. Recent travel, pets, occupational exposures
> 8. Food history, specifically consumption of raw milk, cheese, undercooked beef, pork, poultry
> 9. Immunocompromised
> 10. Family members, coworkers, or other close contacts with similar symptoms
> 11. Evidence of dehydration: thirst, tachycardia, decreased urine output, lethargy, orthostasis

1. Fecal leukocytes and occult blood: The presence of these suggests a bacterial cause of the acute gastroenteritis. The sensitivity of fecal leukocyte testing varies tremendously. A meta-analysis reported that at 70% sensitivity, fecal leukocytes were only 50% specific for an inflammatory process.[36]
2. Fecal lactoferrin: Use when an inflammatory process is considered or when there is fever, tenesmus, or bloody stool. It is a more sensitive test for fecal leukocytes, because lactoferrin is a marker for fecal leukocytes, with sensitivity and specificity between 90% and 100%. Test is not readily available.[5]
3. Stool cultures: The IDSA published guidelines for diagnosis and management of infectious gastroenteritis in 2001, but controversy remains as to when stool cultures are most useful. This controversy is not helped by the low rate of positive stool cultures.[1]
   - According to IDSA recommendations, stool cultures are appropriate if symptoms do not quickly resolve, if fever or bloody stool are present, if patients' comorbidities put them at risk for complications, or if patients are immunocompromised. Culture for Salmonella, shigella, campylobacter, E coli O157:H7 (also do Shiga toxin assay if blood in stool).
   - Food handlers may require negative cultures to return to work.
4. *C difficile* assay: if hospitalized or if recent antibiotics or chemotherapy
5. Stool ova and parasites: Generally, testing stool for ova and parasites is low yield and not cost effective. It is appropriate if symptoms and exposure history support a parasitic or protozoal etiology, bloody diarrhea without fecal leukocytes, or persistent diarrhea in day care centers or aer associated with a community waterborne outbreak. In these cases, 3 samples, taken on 3 consecutive days, should be sent to catch parasite excretion.

Treatment

General recommendations
Guidelines emphasize hydration or rehydration plus diet changes and bowel rest. Oral rehydration is best, if possible, and is often underutilized in the United States. In

---

Box 2
WHO rehydration recommendations

Manufactured 1-L solutions contain

- 3.5 g Sodium chloride

- 2.5 g Sodium bicarbonate

- 1.5 g Potassium chloride

- 20 g Glucose

Home 1-L solutions contain[37]

- ½ Teaspoon salt

- ½ Teaspoon baking soda

- 4 Teaspoons sugar

---

diarrheal illnesses that involve the small intestine, oral rehydration is effective because the small bowel can still absorb water but requires sodium-glucose cotransport. To provide the glucose and electrolytes, the World Health Organization recommends rehydration with water containing salt, sodium bicarbonate, and glucose. Gatorade and other sports drinks do not contain sufficient salt (**Box 2**).

Antibiotics

Empiric antibiotics should be used with caution. IDSA treatment guidelines from 2001 suggest empiric treatment of moderate to severe traveler's gastroenteritis; those with more than 8 stools per day, dehydration, symptoms more than a week; or immuno-compromised patients. Empiric treatment can also be considered with the presence of fever and bloody stools. Empiric treatments include ciprofloxacin (500 mg twice a day for 3 to 5 days), norfloxacin (400 mg twice a day for 3–5 days), or levofloxacin (500 mg daily for 3–5 days). In areas where fluoroquinolone resistance is a problem, azithromycin (500 mg daily for 3 days) is recommended. Specific treatments of other pathogens are discussed previously. These treatment guidelines, however, are for immunocompetent patients. For immunocompromised hosts, antibiotic treatment should be extended for 7 to 10 days and may be considered when not recommended for immunocompetent patients and there is a lower threshold for hospitalization.

Dietary modifications

A short period of clear liquids with adequate electrolyte replacement is generally ideal. In patients with watery diarrhea, boiled rice, potato, noodles or oats with salt, soup, crackers, or bananas are recommended. This is often referred to as the BRAT diet—bananas, rice, applesauce, and toast. Avoid high-fat foods until normal bowel function returns. Secondary lactose malabsorption or intolerance occurs after infectious gastroenteritis and may last for several weeks, so avoiding lactose-containing foods during this time is appropriate.[38]

REFERENCES

1. Craig S, Zich DK. Gastroenteritis. In: Marx JA, editor. Rosen's emergency medicine. 7th edition. 2009; p. 1200.
2. Mead PS, Slutsker L, Dietz V, et al. Food-related illness and death in the United States. Emerg Infect Dis 1999;5:607.

3. Scharff RL. Health-related costs from foodborne illness and death in the United States. The Produce Safety Project at Georgetown University. Available at: www.producesafetyproject.org. Accessed March, 2013.
4. CDC Division of News and Electronic Media. Deaths from gastroenteritis double. Available at: www.cdc.gov. Accessed March 14, 2012.
5. Guerrant RL, Van Gilder T, Steiner TS, et al. Practice guidelines for the management of infectious diarrhea. Clin Infect Dis 2001;32:337–8.
6. Matson DO, Estes MK. Impact of rotavirus infection at a large pediatric hospital. J Infect Dis 1990;162:598.
7. Tucker AW, Haddix AC, Bresee JS, et al. Cost-effectiveness analysis of a rotavirus immunization program for the United States. JAMA 1998;279:1371.
8. Grimwood K, Buttery JP. Clinical update: rotavirus gastroenteritis and its prevention. Lancet 2007;370:302.
9. Parashar UD, Burton A, Lanata C, et al. Global mortality associated with rotavirus disease among children 2004. J Infect Dis 2009;200(Suppl 1):S9.
10. Parashar UD, Glass RI. Rotavirus vaccines—early success, remaining questions. N Engl J Med 2009;360:1063.
11. Getto L, Zeserson E, Breyer M. Vomitting, diarrhea, constipation and gastroenteritis. Emerg Med Clin North Am 2011;29:224.
12. Etienney I, Beaugerie L, Viboud C, et al. Non-steroidal anti-inflammatory drugs as a risk factor for acute diarrhea: case crossover study. Gut 2003;52(2):260–3.
13. Steffen R, Collard F, Tornieporth N, et al. Epidemiology, etiology and impact of travelers' diarrhea in Jamaica. JAMA 1999;281:811.
14. Adachi JA, Jiang ZD, Mathewson JJ, et al. Enteroaggregative Escherichia coli as a major etiologic agent in traveler's diarrhea in 3 regions of the world. Clin Infect Dis 2001;32:1706.
15. Rendi-Wagner P, Kollaritsch H. Drug prophylaxis for travelers' diarrhea. Clin Infect Dis 2002;34:628.
16. Steffen R, Sack DA, Riopel L, et al. Therapy of travelers' diarrhea with rifaximin on various continents. Am J Gastroenterol 2003;98:1073.
17. Hilton E, Kolakowski P, Singer C, et al. Efficacy of Latobacillis GG as a diarrheal prevention in travelers. J Travel Med 1997;4:41.
18. Briand V, Buffet P, Genty S, et al. Absence of efficacy of nonviable Lactobacillus acidophilus for thr prevention of treavelers' diarrhea: a randomized, double-blind, controlled study. Clin Infect Dis 2006;43:1170.
19. Scallan E, Griffin PM, Angulo F, et al. Foodborne illness acquired in the United States-unspecified agents. Emerg Infect Dis 2011;17(1). Available at: www.cdc.gov/eid. Accessed March 2013.
20. Frank C, Weber D, Cramer JP, et al. Eipdemic profile of Shiga-toxin-producing Escherichia coli O104:H4 outbreak in Germany. N Engl J Med 2011;365:1771.
21. Tarr PI, Gordon CA, Chandler WL. Shiga-toxin-producing Escherichia coli and haemolytic uraemic syndrome. Lancet 2005;365:1073.
22. Wong CS, Jelacic S, Habeeb RL, et al. The risk of the hemolytic-uremic syndrome after antibiotic treatment of Escherichia coli O157:H7 infections. N Engl J Med 2000;342:1930.
23. Rosales A, Hofer J, Zimmerhackl LB, et al. Need for long-term follow-up in enterhemorrhagic Escherchia coli-associated hemolytic uremic syndrome due to late-emerging sequelae. Clin Infect Dis 2012;54:1413.
24. Nelson JM, Griffin PM, Jones TF, et al. Antimicrobial and antimotility agent use in persons with shiga toxin-producing Escherichia coli O157:H7 infection in FoodNet Sites. Clin Infect Dis 2011;52:1130.

25. Giannella RA. Salmonella. In: Baron S, editor. Medical microbiology. 4th edition. Galveston (TX). Chapter 21. Available at: www.ncbi.nlm.nih.gov/books/NBK8435. Accessed March 2013.

26. Nachamkin I, Allos BM, Ho T, Campylobacter species and Guillain-Barre syndrome. Clin Microbiol Rev 1998;11:555.

27. Campbell RR, Beere D, Wilcock GK, et al. Clostridium difficile in acute and long-stay elderly patients. Age Ageing 1988;17:333.

28. Kim J, Smathers SA, Prasad P, et al. Epidemiological features of Clostridium difficile-associated disease among inpatients at children's hospitals in the United States, 2001-2006. Pediatrics 2008;122(6):1266–70.

29. MacDonald CL, Owings M, Jernigan DB. Clostridium difficile infection in patients discharged from US short-stay hospitals, 1996-2003. Emerg Infect Dis 2006; 12(3):409–14.

30. Dial S, Delaney JA, BArkun AN, et al. Use of gastric acid-suppressive agents and the risk of community-acquired Clostridium difficile-associated disease. JAMA 2005;294:2989.

31. Sears CL, Kaper JB. Enteric bacterial toxins: mechanisms of action and likage to intestinal secretion. Microbiol Rev 1996;60:167.

32. Kuehne SA, Cartman ST, Heap JT, et al. The role of toxin A and toxin B in Clostridium difficile infection. Nature 2010;467:711.

33. Nomura K, Fujimotos Y, Yamashta M, et al. Absence of pseudomembranes in Clostridium difficile-associated diarrhea in patients using immunosuppression agents. Scand J Gastroenterol 2009;44:74–8.

34. Mulvey MR, Boyd DA, Gravel D, et al. Hypervirulent Clostridium difficile strains in hospitalized patients, Canada. Emerg Infect Dis 2010;16(4):678–81 (sited May 13, 2013). Available at: http://wwwnc.cdc.gov/eid/article/16/4/09-1152.htm. Accessed March 2013.

35. van Nood E, Vrieze A, Nieuwdorp M, et al. Duodenal infusion of donor feces for recurrent Clostridium difficile. N Engl J Med 2013;368(5):407.

36. Huicho L, Sanchez D, Contreras M, et al. Occult blood and fecal leukocytes as screening tests in childhood infectious diarrhea:an old problem revisited. Pediatr Infect Dis J 1993;12:474.

37. de Zoysa I, Kirkwood B, Feachem R, et al. Preparation of sugar-salt solutions. Trans R Soc Trop Med Hyg 1984;78:260.

38. DuPont HL. Guidelines on acute infectious diarrhea in adults. The Practice Parameters Committee of the American College of Gastroenterology. Am J Gastroenterol 1997;92:1962.

Treating Foodborne Illness

Theodore Steiner, MD

KEYWORDS

- Antiemetics • Antidiarrheals • Diarrhea • Antibiotics

KEY POINTS

- Most foodborne illnesses are self-limited without treatment, but may have important long-term consequences in immune-compromised hosts and children.
- Oral rehydration therapy and other supportive measures have a significant impact on morbidity and mortality caused by enteric infections.
- Randomized, controlled trials have shown that antibiotic treatment improves outcomes in selected foodborne infections and specific hosts, although in general the benefits are relatively mild.

INTRODUCTION

Foodborne illnesses are among the most frequent diseases experienced worldwide. Most cases in developed countries are mild and self-limited, but severe and life-threatening complications do occur, even in previously healthy people. However, the greatest burden of disease is in developing areas, where gastrointestinal infections are a leading cause of mortality in early childhood and in patients with human immunodeficiency virus (HIV)/AIDS. Although many of these infections are capable of being spread through person-to-person contact, contaminated food and particularly water remain important transmission vehicles.

In addition to infectious agents, food and water can be the vehicle for transmission of illness caused by toxins, including those that originate from microbes (eg, *Staphylococcus aureus* enterotoxins, botulinum toxin) and environmental sources (eg, heavy metals, pesticides, mushrooms). This review focuses on those foodborne illnesses of microbial origin, but treating physicians need to remain aware of the possibility of environmental toxin ingestion, because the therapeutic and epidemiologic implications can be different.

PATIENT EVALUATION OVERVIEW

As a general rule, it is difficult if not impossible to definitively identify the specific cause of a foodborne illness from the clinical presentation alone. However, a thorough history

This article originally appeared in Infectious Disease Clinics, Volume 27, Issue 3, September 2013.
Infectious Disease, University of British Columbia, Rm. D452 HP East, VGH, Vancouver, British Columbia V5Z 3J5, Canada
E-mail address: tsteiner@mail.ubc.ca

Clinics Collections 7 (2015) 533–554
http://dx.doi.org/10.1016/j.ccol.2015.06.036

(including symptoms, exposure, and timing) can almost always allow the treating clinician to identify the presenting syndrome, which guides the appropriate diagnostic and therapeutic algorithms. There are a few syndromes that are so characteristic that they can be diagnosed with high accuracy from the history alone (for example, ciguatera after consumption of barracuda, or norovirus infection during an institutional outbreak).

The major clinical syndromes of foodborne illness and some of the leading causes include:

- Acute bacterial toxin ingestion. The patient who ingests food that was improperly handled or stored, allowing for growth of toxigenic organisms, generally becomes ill 1 to 8 hours later with the abrupt onset of severe nausea and vomiting, sometimes followed by abdominal pain/cramps and watery diarrhea. Fever is usually absent and symptoms should resolve within 24 hours.[1] In some cases (such as with nonemetic *Bacillus cereus*), cramping and diarrhea are the predominant symptoms.[2] Many patients who present with this syndrome are already better by the time they are seen by a care provider. Often, there is a clear food exposure (such as a picnic or other informal gathering) and others attending the same event have a similar illness at the same time. The major causes are *Staphylococcus aureus*, *Bacillus cereus*, and *Clostridium perfringens*, and commonly implicated foods include prepared salads that are not kept cold enough during storage.
- Viral gastroenteritis. This category contains similar illnesses caused by a growing number of recognized viruses. Although most exposure is through direct contact, food can also be a source when it is handled by any person shedding virus.
  - Norovirus and related viruses. A patient exposed to norovirus generally presents after an incubation period of 12 to 48 hours with abrupt onset of nausea and vomiting followed by watery diarrhea.[3] Norovirus infections can easily be confused with acute bacterial toxin ingestion, but rather than resolving within a few hours, symptoms generally last for 1 to 3 days, and can be more prolonged in young children and the elderly. Many patients have an obvious exposure to a sick family member or coworker, but during annual winter outbreaks, there may be no clear source of the infection. Several more recently described enteric viruses can produce a similar syndrome.
  - Rotavirus syndrome. Rotavirus is most common and most dangerous in children, in whom it typically presents with diarrhea and fever, which can lead to fatal dehydration if not treated appropriately. Symptoms may be prolonged,[4] although the mean is about 6 days.[5] Immunity is not lifelong and rotavirus infection can present in healthy adults. An extended duration of symptoms and relative lack of vomiting can sometimes help to distinguish rotavirus from norovirus.[6]
- Microbial neurotoxin exposure. This term refers to ingestion of stable, preformed toxins produced by bacteria or protozoa that concentrate in foods and disseminate in the individual after ingestion. In a few of these cases, there is an acute gastrointestinal syndrome of nausea, vomiting, intestinal pain, or diarrhea immediately after ingestion, but generally the predominant symptoms occur after the toxin reaches its target cells. Some important examples include:
  - Botulism. *Clostridium botulinum* is a common environmental contaminant, and forms spores that are resistant to boiling. When canned products are not sterilized properly, the organism can germinate and produce the highly lethal botulinum toxins, which impair neurotransmitter function in motor neurons, leading to paralysis. The disease usually presents with descending paralysis,

beginning with the cranial nerves, and if not appropriately recognized and treated with antitoxin, can lead to diffuse paralysis, requiring respiratory support for a period of weeks.[7] The major item in the differential diagnosis is Guillain-Barré syndrome.

o Ciguatera. Ciguatoxins are a family of neurotoxins produced by ocean dinoflagellates that become concentrated as they move up the food chain, concentrating in tissues of large predator fish (particularly barracuda, red snapper, and other tropical and subtropical species). After an acute nonspecific gastrointestinal syndrome, ciguatera progresses to neurologic symptoms, which may include neuropathic pain, cold allodynia, headache, ataxia, and confusion.[8] Symptoms generally last for days to weeks (or occasionally years), and clinical relapses can occur after periods of well-being.

o Scombroid. Histidine in improperly stored fish can be converted to bioactive histamine, which is relatively heat stable. Patients who ingest large quantities of histamine can present with acute onset of headache, flushing, tachycardia, and occasionally diarrhea and nausea. These symptoms are self-limited to a few hours to days.

- Small intestinal infection. Infectious agents that colonize the small intestine can produce symptoms through toxin production or local tissue invasion.

o Nontoxigenic organisms (eg, *Giardia, Cryptosporidium, Cyclospora*) frequently lead to an inflammatory response that causes villous blunting, fluid hypersecretion, and impaired absorption. This response produces a syndrome of abdominal cramping, bloating, flatulence, and watery or loose stools, occasionally with a greasy appearance caused by fat malabsorption. Nausea may be present, but vomiting is generally less prominent. Symptoms may persist for days or weeks, depending on the organism. A history of consumption of untreated water (eg, from lakes or streams) or travel to a developing area is often present in these cases.

o Toxin-producing bacteria (such as *Vibrio cholerae* and enterotoxigenic *Escherichia coli*) also produce mild mucosal inflammation, but most symptoms are caused by effects of the toxins on the epithelium, leading to fluid hypersecretion. Patients typically present with acute onset of nausea, occasionally vomiting, and high-volume, watery diarrhea. Fever, if present, is low-grade. If untreated, the illness is short-lived (typically <3 days), but can be fatal if appropriate rehydration is not provided.

- Inflammatory diarrhea. Invasive infections can present with a nonspecific diffuse gastroenteritis or a more characteristic dysentery syndrome. The symptoms are not specific enough to provide a diagnosis without microbiological investigation.

o Inflammatory enterocolitis typically presents as diarrhea, significant abdominal pain, and fever. Nausea and vomiting may be present but are typically not the major symptoms. Patients may pass frequent, low-volume stools with blood or pus, or may have larger watery stools. The presence of a high fever and duration for more than 48 hours can usually help to distinguish this syndrome from viral gastroenteritis. Although foodborne bacteria such as *Salmonella* and *Campylobacter* are common causes, *Clostridium difficile* can present in an identical fashion and must be considered in any patient with recent hospitalization, antibiotic use, or gastrointestinal surgery.

o Dysentery refers to colonic infection presenting with tenesmus and bloody or mucusy, small-volume stools, typically with fever and considerable discomfort. Although this infection is classically associated with *Shigella* or *Entamoeba histolytica* infection, it is neither sensitive nor specific for these organisms, but clearly warrants evaluation and appropriate treatment. The differential diagnosis includes ulcerative colitis and sexually transmitted proctitis.

- Hemorrhagic colitis. This syndrome classically consists of acute onset of watery diarrhea and abdominal cramps and tenderness, progressing to frankly bloody diarrhea and severe abdominal pain, but with a conspicuous absence of fever in most cases.[9,10] Although intestinal symptoms are self-limited, the disease can progress to hemolytic-uremic syndrome (HUS) with potentially fatal consequences. There is no clear evidence for benefit, and some evidence for harm, with the use of antibiotics in this syndrome, which makes it important to recognize (discussed in detail later).
- Enteric fever. *Salmonella enterica* serovar Typhi and related strains can be transmitted through food and water after contamination by infected individuals. After ingestion, the bacteria invade the intestinal epithelium and take up residence in macrophages, which disseminate the organism. The typical presentation involves fever, abdominal discomfort, headache, and other nonspecific symptoms.[11] These symptoms often progress in a stepwise fashion, becoming more severe until either resolution or fatal complications result. Because the symptoms are so nonspecific, enteric fever should be considered in the differential diagnosis of fever in endemic areas or travelers to these areas, in whom it can be confused with malaria or dengue fever, particularly early in its course.
- Other pathogen-specific conditions. There are certain pathogens that are foodborne but do not fit easily into the other categories. Some examples are:
  - *Listeria monocytogenes.* This gram-positive bacillus grows well at refrigerator temperatures and is classically associated with ingestion of unpasteurized cheese or contaminated cold cuts. It frequently causes a nonspecific diarrheal illness, but this can be followed by bacteremia with meningitis or endocarditis, particularly in immune-compromised hosts, and fetal loss in pregnant women.
  - *Yersinia enterocolitica.* This organism can present as a nonspecific inflammatory enterocolitis, but has a propensity to cause mesenteric adenitis that can mimic acute appendicitis or ileal Crohn disease.
  - Helminthic infections. Various cestodes (tapeworms), trematodes (flukes), and nematodes (roundworms) are transmitted primarily through contaminated food or water. They are described in **Table 1**.
  - *Toxoplasma gondii.* This apicomplexan protozoon causes systemic infection after ingestion of infectious cysts. This infection can occur through 2 means. Food or water can be directly contaminated with oocysts excreted by cats, which are the definitive host for the organism. In addition, other animals that have ingested toxoplasma oocysts can develop infectious muscle cysts, allowing for transmission through contaminated meat. Although toxoplasmosis is benign in most people, immunocompromised hosts are at particular risk of serious consequences, and primary infection during pregnancy can lead to severe fetal anomalies.

NONPHARMACOLOGIC TREATMENT OPTIONS

Most foodborne illnesses are self-limited and require only symptomatic treatment, but there are certain diseases in which specific therapy is indicated by either randomized, controlled trial (RCT) data or expert opinion based on case series in the setting of severe illness. In the case of diarrheal foodborne infections, even in the absence of effective specific therapy, it is important to provide supportive treatment whenever possible to prevent potentially fatal complications, which include:

Table 1
Treatment of foodborne helminthic pathogens

Pathogen	Presentation of Infection	Complications if Untreated	Recommended Treatment
Nematodes			
Trichinella spp	Muscle cysts: intense pain, orbital edema	Rare cardiac or neurological involvement	Supportive care; albendazole ± corticosteroids
Ascaris lumbricoides	Usually asymptomatic	Obstruction with heavy worm burden, biliary sepsis	Single-dose pyrantel, levamisole, mebendazole, albendazole
Trichuris trichiura	Usually asymptomatic	Heavy infestation can lead to rectal prolapse	Mebendazole
Anisakis	Acute nausea, vomiting, abdominal pain	Self-limited	Worm may self-expel as a result of vomiting; can be extracted endoscopically
Cestodes			
Taenia solium	Adult phase: asymptomatic; cyst phase: seizures	Parenchymal brain calcifications leading to seizure foci	Adult worm: praziquantel Cysts: early phase: albendazole or praziquantel, often with steroids Late phase: treatment benefit unclear
Taenia saginata, Hymenolepis nana, Diphyllobothrium latum, and others	Generally asymptomatic	Rarely, vitamin deficiencies; growth impairment in children	Praziquantel or niclosamide
Echinococcus spp	Gradually expanding cyst	Compression of surrounding viscera; anaphylaxis caused by cyst rupture	Surgical removal, PAIR (percutaneous aspiration, injection, reaspiration). Treatment with albendazole or praziquantel alone occasionally successful
Trematodes			
Paragonimus westermani	Cough, dyspnea	Can mimic tuberculosis	Praziquantel
Fasciola hepatica	Typically asymptomatic	Biliary scarring, obstruction	Triclabendazole
Liver flukes	Acute phase nonspecific; chronic phase asymptomatic	Carcinoma of biliary tract	Praziquantel

- Volume depletion
- Electrolyte disturbances
- Nutritional deficiencies (particularly in children)
- Sepsis
- HUS

Oral Rehydration Therapy

The best studied of these nonpharmacologic treatments is oral rehydration therapy (ORT). ORT has been shown in numerous RCTs to improve outcomes in severe diarrheal illnesses, particularly cholera. Choleratoxin and related bacterial enterotoxins act by inducing hypersecretion of salts and water by intestinal crypt cells. The villi and their ability to absorb fluid are relatively preserved. Villous epithelial cells express several transport proteins that facilitate nutrient and salt absorption; one of the most highly expressed is SGLT-1, which cotransports 1 glucose molecule and 2 Na^+ ions, bringing more than 200 water molecules from the lumen into the enterocyte, leading to considerable water absorption.[12] Related cotransporters for other carbohydrates and amino acids are also active. As a result, administration of an ORT containing glucose and Na^+ in the appropriate concentrations (close to a 1:1 Molar ratio) leads to water absorption that can effectively balance out the hypersecretion, improving diarrhea and maintaining the patient's health until an appropriate immune response (or antibiotic treatment) clears the infecting organism. Standard ORT solutions also contain bicarbonate or citrate to correct acidosis and potassium to replace intestinal losses.

Progressive refinements in ORT have been made since its initial discovery. Current recommendations are found in **Table 2**. In particular, a reduction in the osmolarity has been recommended since 2004 based on several strong studies showing better control of diarrheal volume, albeit with occasional asymptomatic hyponatremia.[13,14] In addition, glucose polymers (eg, rice or wheat starch) have been shown in several large RCTs (and confirmed by a meta-analysis) to be superior to glucose in terms of duration of symptoms and need for rescue intravenous fluids.[15] However, some of these studies compared starch-based oral rehydration solution (ORS) with high-osmolarity glucose-based ORS. In addition, the differences between solutions are generally more pronounced in cholera than in other dehydrating diarrheal illnesses.

If the World Health Organization (WHO) ORS salts are not available, a simple home recipe is found in **Table 2**. The solution should taste similar to tears. Plain water or water with a bit of salt added are preferable to hyperosmolar home remedies like ginger ale or apple juice, which contain a high carbohydrate/sodium ratio, and can lead to greater intestinal fluid losses. Use of hypo-osmolar solutions can lead to asymptomatic hyponatremia, but this is preferable to potentially life-threatening dehydration.

Other Nonpharmacologic Treatments for Foodborne Illness

- Micronutrients.
  - Zinc deficiency is common in poor, developing areas with limited dietary diversity. Although young infants are relatively replete from maternal sources, older infants and children can suffer considerable gastrointestinal losses because of recurrent diarrheal episodes, leading to frank deficiency and resulting hypersusceptibility to infectious diarrhea. A recent meta-analysis of zinc supplementation trials[16] found that overall there was a small but statistically significant improvement in the duration of diarrhea with zinc administration compared with placebo. This effect was most pronounced in children older than 6 months

Table 2
**Recommended oral rehydration solutions http://www.who.int/maternal_child_adolescent/
documents/fch_cah_06_1/en/**

Source	Carbohydrate	Sodium Chloride	Other Salts	Indication
Recommended				
World Health Organization reduced-osmolarity ORS	Glucose 13.5 g/L (75 mM)	2.6 g/L (75 mM Na+, 65 mM Cl−)	KCl 1.5 g/L (20 mM K+); trisodium citrate 2.9 g/L (10 mM citrate)	Recommended for all diarrheal illness
Acceptable range	≥Na+ concentration but <111 mM	60–90 mM Na+; 50–80 mM Cl−	15–25 mM K+; 8–12 mM citrate	If World Health Organization solution not available
Starch-based ORS	50–80 g/L cooked rice powder	2.6 g/L (75 mM Na+, 65 mM Cl−)	KCl 1.5 g/L (20 mM K+); trisodium citrate 2.9 g/L (10 mM citrate)	More effective than standard ORS in cholera
Home-made ORS	2 level tablespoonsful sugar (30 g)	Half a level teaspoonful salt (2.5 g)	Add 0.5 c. (125 mL) orange juice or mashed banana	Per liter of clean water
Not Recommended				
Sugared carbonated soft drink	700 mM	2 mM	Low in K+	Osmolarity too high: can exacerbate dehydration
Apple juice	690 mM	3 mM	32 mM	Same
Gatorade	255 mM	20 mM	3 mM	Hyperosmolar
Tea	As desired	0	0	Inadequate electrolyte replacement

and in studies in Asia, where zinc-deficient diets are more common. No overall effect on mortality was identified, and zinc administration was associated with increased vomiting in children. There remains insufficient evidence to know whether zinc supplementation is beneficial in developed areas.[17]

○ Vitamin A is another micronutrient frequently low in developing areas, and deficiency is associated with xerophthalmia and blindness as well as childhood mortality. Several RCTs have examined the benefits of vitamin A supplementation to improve childhood mortality, and a meta-analysis found a significant improvement in overall mortality and specifically mortality caused by diarrhea.[18] However, use of vitamin A in the treatment of acute diarrheal episodes is not beneficial.[19]

• Feeding. Adults and older children with enteric infection often suffer from anorexia during their illness, and may experience transient weight loss, but generally recover quickly. The same is not true for young children, in whom repeated episodes of diarrheal illness, particularly persistent episodes (those lasting >14 days), can lead to permanent deficits in growth and even cognitive development.[20,21] Specific feeding approaches to prevent this situation have not yet been identified. Infants are at even greater risk, because they cannot control their own food and fluid intake. Cultural practices such as withholding breastfeeding during diarrheal illness can lead to fatal consequences, and parents should be encouraged to continue feeding infants normally as tolerated.[22]

- Infection control and public health considerations. Many foodborne infections are highly transmissible, and efforts should be made to limit spread, particularly in health care settings. The Society for Healthcare Epidemiology of America recommends that all hospitalized patients who develop diarrhea be placed on contact isolation (gown and gloves) and in a private room where possible, to reduce the spread of *Clostridium difficile*.[23] Often, more intensive measures such as closure of wards and banning of visitation are required during norovirus outbreaks.[3] In addition, many enteric infections must be reported to public health authorities. This strategy is instrumental for outbreak identification and also to advise people at risk of transmission (such as food service workers) when it is safe for them to resume work.

- Probiotics. There has been considerable interest in the use of nonpathogenic bacteria and yeast supplementation to prevent or treat infectious diarrhea. It is hypothesized that these organisms would colonize the intestine heavily to reduce the environmental niche for the offending pathogen, and many clinical studies have been performed. There is no solid evidence for a clear benefit of any specific probiotic preparation in the treatment of foodborne illness, although some have been proved to improve diarrheal symptoms in specific situations (such as irritable bowel syndrome[24] and antibiotic-associated diarrhea in children[25]). There is some trial evidence that addition of *Lactobacillus* GG to ORS can improve pediatric infectious diarrhea,[26] but not enough to warrant a universal recommendation.[22]

PHARMACOLOGIC TREATMENT OPTIONS

Pharmacologic treatments for foodborne infections include drugs used for symptomatic benefit, such as antiemetics, antispasmodics, and antimotility agents, and drugs used specifically to treat infection. Most of the latter are antimicrobials, although there are some agents that are not antibiotics per se, but either facilitate the activity of antibiotics (such as proton pump inhibitors in the treatment of *Helicobacter pylori* infection) or target microbial toxins (such as cholestyramine used in the treatment of *Clostridium difficile* infection). Antimicrobials are discussed later for each specific infectious syndrome.

Drugs used specifically to treat the symptoms of foodborne illness include:

- Antimotility agents. One of the most troubling symptoms of foodborne illness is diarrhea, particularly when prolonged. There are several available agents that act to reduce stool frequency, volume, and urgency, which can allow patients to carry out their daily activities more comfortably. These drugs are effective, particularly in relatively mild illness. For example, in combination with antibiotics, they significantly shorten the duration of illness in travelers' diarrhea.[27] However, they are not effective in high-volume secretory diarrhea (eg, cholera) or in inflammatory colitis. They are relatively contraindicated during inflammatory diarrheal illness because of a risk of potentially fatal complications such as toxic megacolon.[28] For example, rare fatal cases of *Campylobacter* infection were reported in association with antimotility drug use.[29] Moreover, use of antimotility drugs has been associated with worse outcomes (including HUS) in hemorrhagic colitis.[30] However, a retrospective review of patients with *Clostridium difficile* infection found no harmful effect of antimotility agents when coadministered with metronidazole or vancomycin.[31] The most recent Infectious Diseases Society of

America guidelines (2001) recommend avoiding these agents during bloody diarrhea or proven infection with enterohemorrhagic *E coli*.

Specific antimotility agents include:

- o Loperamide. This opioid agonist acts largely on μ-opioid receptors in the intestinal myenteric plexus, reducing intestinal motility and increasing transit time. This situation can reduce cramping and allows greater contact time with the colonic mucosa, reducing diarrheal volume.[32] It is available over the counter as a generic medication in many countries (including the United States and Canada) for treatment of adults and children older than 2 years. Side effects include constipation and bloating; in addition, coadministration with *P*-glycoprotein inhibitors (such as quinidine) can lead to accumulation in the central nervous system, with central opioid activity as a result, leading to sedation and analgesia.

- o Diphenoxylate/atropine. This combination drug, marketed for years as Lomotil, combines an opioid agonist (diphenoxylate) with the anticholinergic agent atropine. It is generally reserved for more chronic intestinal disorders rather than foodborne illness, because of its increased side effects, which include dry mouth, blurry vision, and sedation from the anticholinergic action.

- o Opiates. All opiate agonist drugs have the potential to decrease motility and reduce diarrhea as a result of their effects on intestinal neurons. Generally, their sedating qualities and potential for dependence preclude their routine use for foodborne illness in modern times, although preparations such as paregoric and tincture of opium were used through much of the twentieth century and are still available in some countries.

- Antispasmodics. These drugs are muscarinic cholinergic antagonists that act to reduce the intensity of smooth muscle contractions in the intestinal wall. These drugs can provide relief from pain caused by abdominal cramping, but are also associated with anticholinergic side effects, and the potential to induce toxic megacolon, although there are no reports of this occurring in infectious diarrhea. Currently used drugs in this class include butylscopolamine (Buscopan), hyoscyamine, dicycloverine, and the older drugs scopolamine and atropine.

- Bismuth salts. Bismuth subsalicylate is marketed worldwide as an agent to treat diarrhea, nausea, and dyspepsia. Its precise mechanism of action is unknown, but it does have antisecretory, antiinflammatory, and antibacterial properties. It is more effective than placebo in the prevention of travelers' diarrhea,[33,34] although antimicrobials are preferred for treatment based on clinical trial evidence.[35] It is a weak antacid but can reduce gastric discomfort, possibly because of the antiinflammatory activity of the salicylate moiety. Because it contains a salicylate, it should not be used in children with fever, because of risk of Reye syndrome. It also causes black discoloration of stool.

- Other antidiarrheals. Clay minerals have been used for years to treat diarrhea, and a combination of kaolin and pectin (Kaopectate) was marketed in the United States. This antidiarrheal was later (around 1990) changed to a different mineral, attapulgite. However, a review by the US Food and Drug Administration in 2003 found insufficient evidence of efficacy of attapulgite in earlier studies and withdrew approval for the drug as an antidiarrheal. The manufacturer changed the formulation in the United States to contain bismuth subsalicylate instead of attapulgite, although the latter is still available in Canada. Racecadotril is an enkephalinase inhibitor marketed in Europe but not North America; there is evidence of benefit in childhood diarrhea.[36,37]

- Antiemetics. Nausea and vomiting can be the most unpleasant symptoms of foodborne illness. They can also impair the ability to use oral rehydration, leading to hospital admissions for intravenous therapy, particularly in children. There are many different classes of antiemetics for various indications, although surprisingly few have been studied in acute gastroenteritis.
  - 5-HT_3 receptor antagonists. These drugs inhibit serotonin signaling in the brain chemoreceptor trigger zone, impairing the central nausea/vomiting response. They also inhibit serotonin signaling in the enteric nervous system. They were initially marketed for the prevention and treatment of chemotherapy-induced emesis, but because of their safety and efficacy, their use has expanded to other indications. The only member of this class studied in foodborne illness is ondansetron, which has been shown in several RCTs to effectively improve nausea and vomiting in children with gastroenteritis.[38] Recent meta-analyses have confirmed that this drug is safe and effective in reducing vomiting, need for intravenous hydration, and immediate hospitalization in children with acute gastroenteritis.[39,40] It can be administered orally or intravenously. Some studies have shown an increase in diarrhea, but this has been inconsistent.
  - Dopamine antagonists. Before the introduction of 5-HT_3 antagonists, these antagonists were the mainstay of antiemetic therapy, although they have fallen out of favor because of increased side effects, which include sedation and rare extrapyramidal neurologic symptoms (akathisia, muscle stiffness). Drugs in this class specifically used as antiemetics include prochlorperazine, domperidone, and metoclopramide. Metoclopramide also has prokinetic activity. Metoclopramide was shown to be equivalent to ondansetron in 1 RCT in children,[41] although the study was underpowered to show a significant difference. One RCT in adults found prochlorperazine to be slightly better than ondansetron in nausea scores but equivalent in terms of reducing vomiting.[42]
  - Antihistamines. Histaminergic neurons are found in the emesis pathway from the chemoreceptor trigger zone to the vomiting center in the brainstem, and numerous over-the-counter and prescription agents that block histamine 1 receptors are marketed as antiemetics. Their primary benefit is in motion sickness rather than acute gastroenteritis. Dimenhydrinate (Gravol, Dramamine) is specifically marketed for nausea, although the only RCT in acute gastroenteritis[43] found a reduction in vomiting but not need for intravenous fluids or hospitalization. These drugs are generally very sedating.
  - Ginger. Ginger root preparations have been used as a folk remedy for nausea and vomiting for years, and recent clinical trials have begun to study the activity of ginger in a rigorous fashion, but not in acute gastroenteritis. A recent meta-analysis found insufficient evidence of activity in chemotherapy-induced nausea and vomiting.[44]
  - Acupuncture/acupressure. Acupuncture by a trained practitioner or self-stimulation of the ventral surface of the wrist have been studied as treatments for anesthesia-induced and chemotherapy-induced nausea and vomiting. One small, noncontrolled study found good success in the treatment of vomiting in acute gastroenteritis in children.[45]
- Treatments for noninfectious/toxin-mediated food poisoning. The major benefit in this category is the treatment of botulism with antitoxin antibodies, which, when administered promptly, can stop symptoms from progressing but cannot reverse the effect on neurons that have already bound the toxin.[46] Equine trivalent, pentavalent, and heptavalent preparations have been used but can cause

serum sickness reactions; a human immunoglobulin Ig-based product is available for infants. Scombroid poisoning responds to antihistamine drugs, although it is self-limited regardless. There are no antitoxin agents for ciguatera and related illnesses, and supportive/symptomatic treatment is recommended. Intravenous mannitol was suggested in case reports[47] to be beneficial, but a more recent clinical trial found no efficacy, and as a result this is no longer recommended.[48]

ANTIMICROBIAL THERAPIES FOR FOODBORNE ILLNESS

Antimicrobials are of no use in toxin-mediated foodborne illness, including those caused by ingestion of bacterial, preformed toxins. In addition, there are no agents to treat viral gastroenteritis. Bacterial and protozoal agents, on the other hand, are almost always susceptible to 1 or more commercially available antibiotics. Before instituting treatment of one of these infections, is it important to consider the following:

- Does this infection need to be treated? Most causes of foodborne illness are self-limited and specific antibiotic treatment in general provides only modest benefit. Nevertheless, certain infections (*Shigella*, typhoid fever) have clear RCT evidence of a benefit of treatment. However, many other infections lack evidence of a benefit of antibiotic treatment, even when the isolate and drug susceptibilities are known (eg, *Yersinia enterocolitica*). In addition, there are some infections (nontyphoidal *Salmonella*) in which treatment can benefit some patients but lead to unwanted outcomes in others. There is competing evidence of both harm and benefit of antibiotics in the treatment of hemorrhagic colitis caused by enterohemorrhagic and related strains of E coli, and as a result, treatment is not generally recommended.
- Should the syndrome be treated before the cause is known? In some cases, the clinical features are enough to warrant specific antibiotic treatment even without a clear cause. The best example of this is travelers' diarrhea, in which empiric antibiotic treatment has been shown in many RCTs to shorten the severity and duration of illness (reviewed in Ref.[49]). There is also evidence that empiric treatment of severe diarrhea that persists beyond 72 hours is beneficial, although the choice of agent depends on the index of suspicion and the local susceptibility patterns (see later discussion).[50] However, treatment should generally be avoided in the syndrome of hemorrhagic colitis (frankly bloody diarrhea without fever), for reasons discussed later.
- Which antibiotic should be used? The broad variety of infectious agents that can, in many cases, produce indistinguishable clinical syndromes makes treatment challenging. Moreover, many of the drugs studied in well-designed RCTs can no longer be recommended because of increasing resistance, which can vary according to geographic area. Whenever possible, treatment should be tailored based on culture and susceptibility reports; when this is not feasible, an updated knowledge of local susceptibility patterns should guide therapy as much as possible.

A list of major bacterial and protozoal pathogens and the recommended antibiotic treatment is shown in **Tables 3** and **4**. Specific cases meriting mention are the following:

- *Salmonella.* *Salmonella* gastroenteritis is a self-limited illness, and treatment with antibiotics can prolong the duration of shedding and lead to some clinical

Table 3
Treatment of foodborne protozoal pathogens

Pathogen	Presentation of Infection	Complications if Untreated	Recommended Treatment
Giardia lamblia	Small bowel syndrome	Self-limited but often prolonged	Tinidazole, albendazole, metronidazole
Cryptosporidium	Small bowel syndrome; fulminant chronic diarrhea in AIDS	In AIDS, fatal wasting syndrome and dehydration; cholangiopathy	Nitazoxanide in immune competent; antiretroviral therapy in AIDS
Cyclospora cayetanensis	Small bowel syndrome; fatigue	Self-limited but often prolonged	TMP-SMX; ciprofloxacin if allergic
Microsporidia (*Enterocytozoon bieneusi, Encephalitozoon intestinalis*)	Chronic diarrhea in AIDS; rarely in transplant recipients	Wasting syndrome; cholangiopathy	Antiretrovirals or reduce immune suppression; albendazole for *Encephalitozoon intestinalis*
Entamoeba histolytica	Asymptomatic colonization to severe dysenteric colitis	Ameboma, liver abscess, other parenchymal abscess	Invasive disease: tinidazole or metronidazole, followed by paromomycin or iodoquinol Asymptomatic cyst passer: paromomycin or iodoquinol
Blastocystis hominis	Generally asymptomatic; some patients experience diarrhea, bloating, flatulence, and so forth	None	Treatment controversial; metronidazole, TMP-SMX, iodoquinol may be effective
Toxoplasma gondii	Acute: localized or disseminated lymphadenopathy, sometimes with fever; rarely chorioretinitis, encephalitis	Reactivation in immune compromise to encephalitis or chorioretinitis; fetal anomalies if acquired during pregnancy	Acute: treatment not clearly indicated[86] Reactivation: TMP-SMX or pyrimethamine/sulfadiazine or pyrimethamine/clindamycin
Trypanosoma cruzi	Rarely acquired through ingestion of crushed trematode bugs in food (eg, sugar cane juice)	Chronic sequelae of Chagas disease: organomegaly; chagoma in immune compromise	Acute or early chronic disease: benznidazole Late chronic disease with organomegaly: treatment benefit remains uncertain Chagoma: benznidazole

Abbreviation: TMP-SMX, trimethoprim-sulfamethoxazole.

relapses.[51] A recent meta-analysis[52] found no overall benefit of antibiotic treatment of *Salmonella* gastroenteritis in healthy adults, and confirmed increased likelihood of shedding the organism at 30 days. Most of the studies were considered to have low-quality evidence. Nevertheless, it is recommended not to use antibiotics in uncomplicated cases. Some experts do recommend treatment of severe cases (requiring hospitalization, high fever, multiple daily stools) based on efficacy in 1 RCT. In addition, treatment of children younger than 2 years and elderly patients is recommended by many experts.

One important consideration is that *Salmonella* can cause prolonged, metastatic, or lethal infection in immune-compromised hosts. These hosts include patients with AIDS, solid organ transplants, asplenia, or corticosteroid treatment. Although there are no RCT data in these cases, it is recommended that they be treated, given the relatively high risk of prolonged or recurrent bacteremia (reviewed in Ref.[53]).

- *Shigella.* Shigellosis can produce a particularly severe colitis, and is an independent risk factor for mortality in children hospitalized with diarrhea.[54] Although the illness is self-limited in most patients, antibiotics have been shown in several studies to shorten the duration of both illness and bacterial shedding, and because *Shigella* spreads readily from person to person, it is generally recommended that all cases be treated.[55] Antibiotic resistance has been increasing in different parts of the world.[56] In North America, most isolates remain susceptible to ciprofloxacin and third-generation cephalosporins.

- *Campylobacter.* Fatalities caused by *Campylobacter jejuni* gastroenteritis are rare, although bacteremias do occur, largely in immunocompromised hosts, with a mortality in those cases of 15% in 1 series.[57] A recent meta-analysis found that antibiotic treatment in uncomplicated cases does shorten the duration of illness, particularly when administered early, but the effect is modest.[58] Many patients are already better, or beyond the window of antibiotic usefulness, by the time the culture result is received. However, many experts do recommend treating severe cases and cases in immune-compromised hosts. As with most other bacterial diarrheal pathogens, *Campylobacter* is becoming increasingly resistant to first-line agents in some parts of the world, although macrolides (eg, azithromycin) remain active against most US isolates.[59]

- Enterohemorrhagic *E coli* (EHEC). The gastrointestinal symptoms of EHEC infection are self-limited, but the major complication, HUS, can be fatal or lead to permanent neurologic or renal sequelae. The predominant pathogen in this class, *E coli* O157:H7, remains antibiotic sensitive.[60] However, there is strong evidence from in vitro and animal models that antibiotics can induce increased toxin release from EHEC, leading to worse outcomes. For *E coli* O157:H7, the best evidence against the use of antibiotics was a prospective study of infected children in the United States,[61] in which antibiotic use was an independent risk factor for HUS in multivariate analysis, controlling for disease severity. However, the data were derived from only 10 HUS cases, and the antibiotics used were trimethoprim-sulfamethoxazole and β-lactam drugs. In contrast, retrospective data from the large Japanese outbreak in the late 1990s suggested that fosfomycin (the most commonly used antibiotic in that outbreak) was protective against HUS when used in the first 2 days of illness.[62] However, given the absence of RCT data and, more importantly, no good evidence of benefit, most authorities recommend against antibiotic treatment of *E coli* O157:H7 infection. In patients who do develop HUS, the C5 complement inhibitor eculizumab has been reported to be beneficial in a

Table 4
Treatment of bacterial foodborne and waterborne pathogens

Pathogen	Syndrome	Benefits of Treatment	Risks of Treatment	Recommendation	Recommended Drugs
Nontyphoidal *Salmonella*	Inflammatory diarrhea	Shortens duration of illness; prevents bacteremic seeding	Prolonged shedding; risk of clinical relapse	Treat only specific hosts (extremes of age, immune compromised, asplenic, and so forth)	TMP-SMX, FQ, Ceph3, amoxicillin
Typhoid fever	Enteric fever	Improves survival, eliminates shedding in most	Some patients may remain colonized and infectious	Treat	Ceph3; FQ, TMP-SMX if from area of low resistance
Shigella spp	Inflammatory diarrhea or dysentery	Reduced duration of illness, reduced shedding	Minimal	Treat	FQ, Ceph3, azithromycin; TMP-SMX if susceptible
Campylobacter spp	Inflammatory diarrhea	Reduced duration of illness if started early	Minimal	Consider treatment in severe or persistent cases	Azithromycin, FQ if from susceptible area
Enterohemorrhagic *E coli*	Hemorrhagic colitis	Reduces shedding; may or may not reduce risk of HUS	Increased toxin release and potential predisposition to HUS	Do not treat (from current evidence)	
Enteropathogenic *E coli*	Infantile diarrhea	ORS life saving; no evidence antibiotics are helpful	Unknown	Antibiotics not indicated for infantile diarrhea	
Enterotoxigenic *E coli*	Travelers' diarrhea	Significantly shortens duration of illness	Minimal	Empirical treatment indicated for travelers' diarrhea	Azithromycin, FQ, TMP-SMX, rifaximin

Enteroaggregative E coli	Endemic diarrhea, travelers' diarrhea, prolonged diarrhea in AIDS	Improves symptoms in AIDS; treatment of travelers' diarrhea beneficial as for ETEC	Unknown	Empirical treatment indicated for travelers' diarrhea; treat if found in persistent diarrhea	FQ, TMP-SMX, Ceph3, azithromycin
Yersinia spp	Inflammatory diarrhea or pseudoappendicitis	Reduces shedding but does not improve clinical outcomes	Unknown	No clear recommendation	Usually resistant to ampilillin and Ceph1
Listeria monocytogenes	Nonspecific gastroenteritis; bacteremia; meningitis; endocarditis	Treatment of invasive disease improves mortality	Minimal	Treat invasive disease or disease in pregnant women	Ampicillin or penicillin; TMP-SMX if allergic
Vibrio cholerae	Fulminant watery diarrhea	Self-limited without antibiotics but antibiotics shorten illness	Minimal	ORS as mainstay; antibiotics if feasible	Doxycycline, FQ, TMP-SMX
Noncholera Vibrio	Inflammatory or nonspecific diarrhea	No evidence for benefit	Minimal	Consider treating severe cases	Doxycycline, FQ
Aeromonas hydrophila	Inflammatory or nonspecific diarrhea	Most cases self-limited; case series of benefit in prolonged illness[87]	Minimal	Treat severe or prolonged cases (>7–10 d)	TMP-SMX, doxycycline, FQ

Abbreviations: Ceph1/3, first-generation/third-generation cephalosporin; FQ, fluoroquinolone; TMP-SMX, cotrimoxazole.

small case series,[63] although prospective, randomized data are lacking. Plasma exchange is frequently used, although it also lacks supporting randomized data.

- Enteroaggregative Shiga toxin–producing *E coli* O104:H4. This strain caused a large European foodborne outbreak of hemorrhagic colitis in 2011, in which the HUS rates in adults were a frightening 22%.[64] This isolate carried an extended-spectrum β-lactamase, rendering it resistant to cephalosporins, but it remained susceptible to fluoroquinolones, rifaximin, and azithromycin. There are conflicting reports as to whether antibiotics induce toxin production and release from this strain.[65,66] No randomized data are available on antibiotic use and the risk of HUS with this infection, but many patients in the outbreak received treatment with antibiotics, and no association with worse outcome was found. Treatment with ciprofloxacin was associated with reduced HUS risk in 1 case series.[67] Another case series[68] found reduced duration of shedding in patients who received azithromycin, with no apparent effect on HUS onset or outcomes, which could have implications for reducing secondary spread. There is insufficient evidence that antibiotics are either harmful or beneficial in O104:H4 infection, but the outbreak data are still being analyzed. In 1 prospective case series,[9] eculizumab was not found to be beneficial in 7 patients with severe HUS with neurologic symptoms. Plasma exchange was also not found to be beneficial in 1 case-control study.[69]

- *Giardia.* Metronidazole for 7 days has long been the recommended treatment of giardiasis, and although generally effective, it is poorly tolerated by many patients. Newer drugs active against *Giardia* have advantages of shorter treatment duration or better side-effect profile, although the studies comparing them have not been of high quality. A recent meta-analysis[70] found that tinidazole, nitazoxanide, and albendazole are likely to be as effective as metronidazole, and with generally fewer side effects. Relapses are not uncommon after metronidazole treatment, and resistance can develop. The optimal treatment in these cases remains uncertain.

- *Cryptosporidium.* This protozoan is a common cause of self-limited infections in immune-competent children and adults, although symptoms can be prolonged in some cases. In contrast, patients with advanced HIV/AIDS or other severe immune defects can develop devastating, fatal diarrheal illness. The only drug approved for this infection, nitazoxanide, provides modest symptomatic benefit in immune-competent hosts, with significantly better symptom resolution and decreased shedding at 4 days.[71] However, results in patients with HIV infection have been less encouraging, particularly in those with CD4 counts less than $50/\mu L$[72] and in children in developing areas,[73] as confirmed in 1 meta-analysis.[74] The mainstay of treatment of cryptosporidiosis in HIV/AIDS is antiretroviral therapy, which leads to lasting remission, although relapse of infection can occur if therapy is stopped.[75]

- *Entamoeba histolytica.* Metronidazole has been the mainstay of therapy for invasive amebiasis for years, although a recent meta-analysis of 8 RCTs[76] found that tinidazole is equally effective but with a shorter treatment duration and better side-effect profile. Nevertheless, metronidazole remains a first-line agent for invasive disease. It is recommended to use a luminal agent such as paromomycin to clear cysts after treatment of invasive disease, because nitroimidazoles do not reliably eradicate the cyst form. *Entamoeba histolytica* can be mistaken under microscopy for the nonpathogenic *Entamoeba dispar*, which does not require treatment.

TREATMENT RESISTANCE/COMPLICATIONS

Antibiotic resistance among enteric pathogens is continuously evolving, but large geographic differences remain. For example, fluoroquinolone resistance rates among *Campylobacter* isolates are more than 95% in Thailand,[77] but less than 20% in North America.[78] The driving forces behind evolving resistance include widespread human prescription as well as animal feed supplementation. It is important for treating practitioners to review the most recent available data on local resistance patterns when selecting empirical antibiotics to treat an enteric infection, and to follow the antibiotic sensitivity report on an isolate when available.

In general, treatment courses for foodborne infections are short and well tolerated. As with any antibiotic, allergic reactions and secondary *Clostridium difficile* infection are ever-present concerns. Among nonantibiotic agents, the greatest concern is with inappropriate use of antimotility agents during inflammatory or hemorrhagic colitis, because of a potential to increase the risk of toxic megacolon or HUS, respectively.

EVALUATION OF OUTCOME AND LONG-TERM RECOMMENDATIONS

In general, patients recover quickly from foodborne infections and permanent sequelae are relatively rare. Stool analysis for test of cure is not generally recommended for individual patients, although screening of certain individuals (such as food preparation workers) may be indicated for public health reasons.[79] Although most patients can expect to recover fully from a foodborne illness, population-based studies from large-scale outbreaks such as the *E coli* O157:H7 and *Campylobacter* outbreak in Walkerton, ON in 2000, have shown an increased risk of postinfectious irritable bowel syndrome[80,81]; moreover, the rates of chronic kidney disease and hypertension are increased in those who recover from HUS.[82] *Campylobacter* is a well-recognized trigger for Guillain-Barré syndrome.[83] Moreover, population studies suggest that an acute episode of infectious gastroenteritis is associated with about a 2-fold increased risk of developing Inflammatory bowel disease.[84] Any enteric infection can precipitate reactive arthritis, which can be self-limited to a few weeks or months, or evolve into a chronic spondyloarthropathy. It is not known whether antibiotic treatment of these infections affects these long-term risks; it does not seem to improve outcomes in established reactive arthritis.[85]

SUMMARY/DISCUSSION

Foodborne illnesses come from a wide variety of infectious and noninfectious sources, and can produce several relatively distinct clinical syndromes. Recognition of these syndromes, along with a careful exposure history, can usually provide enough information to guide rational use of diagnostic testing, empiric supportive therapy, and occasionally specific antimicrobial therapy. With appropriate treatment of dehydration (ideally with ORS), the risk of mortality or long-term morbidity is generally low. Key recent advances in the management of foodborne illness include the introduction of reduced-osmolarity ORS, the benefit of zinc supplements in children in developing areas, and the usefulness of ondansetron in pediatric gastroenteritis. Antimicrobial therapy still plays a small role in enteric foodborne infections. The most worrisome foodborne illness in otherwise healthy people in developed countries is hemorrhagic colitis, with its attendant risks of HUS. Moreover, patients with immune compromise are at risk for potentially devastating consequences of enteric infection. Most of the world's children, who live in impoverished areas without appropriate sanitation, remain vulnerable to repeated bouts of foodborne illness, which are frequently fatal and in survivors produce long-term consequences that are only now beginning to be appreciated.

REFERENCES

1. Le Loir Y, Baron F, Gautier M. *Staphylococcus aureus* and food poisoning. Genet Mol Res 2003;2(1):63–76.
2. Stenfors Arnesen LP, Fagerlund A, Granum PE. From soil to gut: *Bacillus cereus* and its food poisoning toxins. FEMS Microbiol Rev 2008;32(4):579–606.
3. Division of Viral Diseases, National Center for Immunization and Respiratory Diseases, Centers for Disease Control and Prevention. Updated norovirus outbreak management and disease prevention guidelines. MMWR Recomm Rep 2011; 60(RR-3):1–18.
4. Carr ME, McKendrick GD, Spyridakis T. The clinical features of infantile gastroenteritis due to rotavirus. Scand J Infect Dis 1976;8(4):241–3.
5. Uhnoo I, Olding-Stenkvist E, Kreuger A. Clinical features of acute gastroenteritis associated with rotavirus, enteric adenoviruses, and bacteria. Arch Dis Child 1986;61(8):732–8.
6. Bresee JS, Marcus R, Venezia RA, et al. The etiology of severe acute gastroenteritis among adults visiting emergency departments in the United States. J Infect Dis 2012;205(9):1374–81.
7. Centers for Disease Control and Prevention (CDC). Recognition of illness associated with the intentional release of a biologic agent. MMWR Morb Mortal Wkly Rep 2001;50(41):893–7.
8. Wong CK, Hung P, Lee KL, et al. Features of ciguatera fish poisoning cases in Hong Kong 2004-2007. Biomed Environ Sci 2008;21(6):521–7.
9. Ullrich S, Bremer P, Neumann-Grutzeck C, et al. Symptoms and clinical course of EHEC O104 infection in hospitalized patients: a prospective single center study. PLoS One 2013;8(2):e55278.
10. Griffin PM, Ostroff SM, Tauxe RV, et al. Illnesses associated with *Escherichia coli* O157:H7 infections. A broad clinical spectrum. Ann Intern Med 1988;109(9): 705–12.
11. Thriemer K, Ley BB, Ame SS, et al. Clinical and epidemiological features of typhoid fever in Pemba, Zanzibar: assessment of the performance of the WHO case definitions. PLoS One 2012;7(12):e51823.
12. Gagnon MP, Bissonnette P, Deslandes LM, et al. Glucose accumulation can account for the initial water flux triggered by Na+/glucose cotransport. Biophys J 2004;86(1 Pt 1):125–33.
13. Multicentre evaluation of reduced-osmolarity oral rehydration salts solution. International Study Group on Reduced-osmolarity ORS solutions. Lancet 1995; 345(8945):282–5.
14. Santosham M, Fayad I, Abu Zikri M, et al. A double-blind clinical trial comparing World Health Organization oral rehydration solution with a reduced osmolarity solution containing equal amounts of sodium and glucose. J Pediatr 1996;128(1):45–51.
15. Gregorio GV, Gonzales ML, Dans LF, et al. Polymer-based oral rehydration solution for treating acute watery diarrhoea. Cochrane Database Syst Rev 2009;(2):CD006519.
16. Lazzerini M, Ronfani L. Oral zinc for treating diarrhoea in children. Cochrane Database Syst Rev 2013;(1):CD005436.
17. Salvatore S, Hauser B, Devreker T, et al. Probiotics and zinc in acute infectious gastroenteritis in children: are they effective? Nutrition 2007;23(6):498–506.

18. Mayo-Wilson E, Imdad A, Herzer K, et al. Vitamin A supplements for preventing mortality, illness, and blindness in children aged under 5: systematic review and meta-analysis. BMJ 2011;343:d5094.

19. Fischer Walker CL, Black RE. Micronutrients and diarrheal disease. Clin Infect Dis 2007;45(Suppl 1):S73-7.

20. Moore SR, Lima NL, Soares AM, et al. Prolonged episodes of acute diarrhea reduce growth and increase risk of persistent diarrhea in children. Gastroenterology 2010;139(4):1156–64.

21. Oria RB, Patrick PD, Zhang H, et al. APOE4 protects the cognitive development in children with heavy diarrhea burdens in Northeast Brazil. Pediatr Res 2005; 57(2):310–6.

22. Guarino A, Albano F, Ashkenazi S, et al. European Society for Paediatric Gastroenterology, Hepatology, and Nutrition/European Society for Paediatric Infectious Diseases evidence-based guidelines for the management of acute gastroenteritis in children in Europe. J Pediatr Gastroenterol Nutr 2008;46(Suppl 2):S81–122.

23. Cohen SH, Gerding DN, Johnson S, et al. Clinical practice guidelines for *Clostridium difficile* infection in adults: 2010 update by the Society for Healthcare Epidemiology of America (SHEA) and the Infectious Diseases Society of America (IDSA). Infect Control Hosp Epidemiol 2010;31(5):431–55.

24. Whelan K. Probiotics and prebiotics in the management of irritable bowel syndrome: a review of recent clinical trials and systematic reviews. Curr Opin Clin Nutr Metab Care 2011;14(6):581–7.

25. Johnston BC, Goldenberg JZ, Vandvik PO, et al. Probiotics for the prevention of pediatric antibiotic-associated diarrhea. Cochrane Database Syst Rev 2011;(11):CD004827.

26. Szajewska H, Mrukowicz JZ. Probiotics in the treatment and prevention of acute infectious diarrhea in infants and children: a systematic review of published randomized, double-blind, placebo-controlled trials. J Pediatr Gastroenterol Nutr 2001;33(Suppl 2):S17–25.

27. Riddle MS, Arnold S, Tribble DR. Effect of adjunctive loperamide in combination with antibiotics on treatment outcomes in traveler's diarrhea: a systematic review and meta-analysis. Clin Infect Dis 2008;47(8):1007–14.

28. Butler T. Loperamide for the treatment of traveler's diarrhea: broad or narrow usefulness? Clin Infect Dis 2008;47(8):1015–6.

29. Smith GS, Blaser MJ. Fatalities associated with *Campylobacter jejuni* infections. JAMA 1985;253(19):2873–5.

30. Bell BP, Griffin PM, Lozano P, et al. Predictors of hemolytic uremic syndrome in children during a large outbreak of *Escherichia coli* O157:H7 infections. Pediatrics 1997;100(1):E12.

31. Koo HL, Koo DC, Musher DM, et al. Antimotility agents for the treatment of *Clostridium difficile* diarrhea and colitis. Clin Infect Dis 2009;48(5):598–605.

32. Baker DE. Loperamide: a pharmacological review. Rev Gastroenterol Disord 2007;7(Suppl 3):S11–8.

33. Steffen R. Worldwide efficacy of bismuth subsalicylate in the treatment of travelers' diarrhea. Rev Infect Dis 1990;12(Suppl 1):S80–6.

34. DuPont HL, Ericsson CD, Farthing MJ, et al. Expert review of the evidence base for prevention of travelers' diarrhea. J Travel Med 2009;16(3):149–60.

35. Shlim DR. Update in traveler's diarrhea. Infect Dis Clin North Am 2005;19(1): 137–49.

36. Lehert P, Cheron G, Calatayud GA, et al. Racecadotril for childhood gastroenteritis: an individual patient data meta-analysis. Dig Liver Dis 2011;43(9):707–13.

37. Szajewska H, Ruszczynski M, Chmielewska A, et al. Systematic review: racecadotril in the treatment of acute diarrhoea in children. Aliment Pharmacol Ther 2007;26(6):807–13.
38. Freedman SB, Adler M, Seshadri R, et al. Oral ondansetron for gastroenteritis in a pediatric emergency department. N Engl J Med 2006;354(16):1698–705.
39. Carter B, Fedorowicz Z. Antiemetic treatment for acute gastroenteritis in children: an updated Cochrane systematic review with meta-analysis and mixed treatment comparison in a Bayesian framework. BMJ Open 2012;2(4). http://dx.doi.org/10.1136/bmjopen, 2011-000622.
40. Fedorowicz Z, Jagannath VA, Carter B. Antiemetics for reducing vomiting related to acute gastroenteritis in children and adolescents. Cochrane Database Syst Rev 2011;(9):CD005506.
41. Al-Ansari K, Alomary S, Abdulateef H, et al. Metoclopramide versus ondansetron for the treatment of vomiting in children with acute gastroenteritis. J Pediatr Gastroenterol Nutr 2011;53(2):156–60.
42. Patka J, Wu DT, Abraham P, et al. Randomized controlled trial of ondansetron vs. prochlorperazine in adults in the emergency department. West J Emerg Med 2011;12(1):1–5.
43. Uhlig U, Pfeil N, Gelbrich G, et al. Dimenhydrinate in children with infectious gastroenteritis: a prospective, RCT. Pediatrics 2009;124(4):e622–32.
44. Lee J, Oh H. Ginger as an antiemetic modality for chemotherapy-induced nausea and vomiting: a systematic review and meta-analysis. Oncol Nurs Forum 2013;40(2):163–70.
45. Anders EF, Findeisen A, Lode HN, et al. Acupuncture for treatment of acute vomiting in children with gastroenteritis and pneumonia. Klin Padiatr 2012; 224(2):72–5.
46. Tacket CO, Shandera WX, Mann JM, et al. Equine antitoxin use and other factors that predict outcome in type A foodborne botulism. Am J Med 1984;76(5): 794–8.
47. Palafox NA, Jain LG, Pinano AZ, et al. Successful treatment of ciguatera fish poisoning with intravenous mannitol. JAMA 1988;259(18):2740–2.
48. Schnorf H, Taurarii M, Cundy T. Ciguatera fish poisoning: a double-blind randomized trial of mannitol therapy. Neurology 2002;58(6):873–80.
49. Kollaritsch H, Paulke-Korinek M, Wiedermann U. Traveler's diarrhea. Infect Dis Clin North Am 2012;26(3):691–706.
50. Dryden MS, Gabb RJ, Wright SK. Empirical treatment of severe acute community-acquired gastroenteritis with ciprofloxacin. Clin Infect Dis 1996; 22(6):1019–25.
51. Neill MA, Opal SM, Heelan J, et al. Failure of ciprofloxacin to eradicate convalescent fecal excretion after acute salmonellosis: experience during an outbreak in health care workers. Ann Intern Med 1991;114(3):195–9.
52. Onwuezobe IA, Oshun PO, Odigwe CC. Antimicrobials for treating symptomatic non-typhoidal Salmonella infection. Cochrane Database Syst Rev 2012;(11):CD001167.
53. Gordon MA. Salmonella infections in immunocompromised adults. J Infect 2008; 56(6):413–22.
54. Uysal G, Sokmen A, Vidinlisan S. Clinical risk factors for fatal diarrhea in hospitalized children. Indian J Pediatr 2000;67(5):329–33.
55. Metzler AE, Burri HR. The etiology of "malignant catarrhal fever" originating in sheep: serological findings in cattle and sheep with ruminant gamma herpesviruses. Tierarztl Prax 1991;19(2):135–40.

56. Rahman M, Shoma S, Rashid H, et al. Increasing spectrum in antimicrobial resistance of *Shigella* isolates in Bangladesh: resistance to azithromycin and ceftriaxone and decreased susceptibility to ciprofloxacin. J Health Popul Nutr 2007;25(2):158–67.

57. Fernandez-Cruz A, Munoz P, Mohedano R, et al. *Campylobacter* bacteremia: clinical characteristics, incidence, and outcome over 23 years. Medicine (Baltimore) 2010;89(5):319–30.

58. Ternhag A, Asikainen T, Giesecke J, et al. A meta-analysis on the effects of antibiotic treatment on duration of symptoms caused by infection with *Campylobacter* species. Clin Infect Dis 2007;44(5):696–700.

59. Wang X, Zhao S, Harbottle H, et al. Antimicrobial resistance and molecular subtyping of *Campylobacter jejuni* and *Campylobacter coli* from retail meats. J Food Prot 2011;74(4):616–21.

60. Beier RC, Poole TL, Brichta-Harhay DM, et al. Disinfectant and antibiotic susceptibility profiles of *Escherichia coli* O157:H7 strains from cattle carcasses, feces, and hides and ground beef from the United States. J Food Prot 2013; 76(1):6–17.

61. Wong CS, Jelacic S, Habeeb RL, et al. The risk of the hemolytic-uremic syndrome after antibiotic treatment of *Escherichia coli* O157:H7 infections. N Engl J Med 2000;342(26):1930–6.

62. Ikeda K, Ida O, Kimoto K, et al. Effect of early fosfomycin treatment on prevention of hemolytic uremic syndrome accompanying *Escherichia coli* O157:H7 infection. Clin Nephrol 1999;52(6):357–62.

63. Lapeyraque AL, Malina M, Fremeaux-Bacchi V, et al. Eculizumab in severe Shiga-toxin-associated HUS. N Engl J Med 2011;364(26):2561–3.

64. Frank C, Werber D, Cramer JP, et al. Epidemic profile of Shiga-toxin-producing *Escherichia coli* O104:H4 outbreak in Germany. N Engl J Med 2011;365(19): 1771–80.

65. Corogeanu D, Willmes R, Wolke M, et al. Therapeutic concentrations of antibiotics inhibit Shiga toxin release from enterohemorrhagic *E. coli* O104:H4 from the 2011 German outbreak. BMC Microbiol 2012;12:160.

66. Bielaszewska M, Idelevich EA, Zhang W, et al. Effects of antibiotics on Shiga toxin 2 production and bacteriophage induction by epidemic *Escherichia coli* O104:H4 strain. Antimicrob Agents Chemother 2012;56(6):3277–82.

67. Geerdes-Fenge HF, Lobermann M, Nurnberg M, et al. Ciprofloxacin reduces the risk of hemolytic uremic syndrome in patients with *Escherichia coli* O104:H4-associated diarrhea. Infection 2013;41(3):669.

68. Nitschke M, Sayk F, Hartel C, et al. Association between azithromycin therapy and duration of bacterial shedding among patients with Shiga toxin-producing enteroaggregative *Escherichia coli* O104:H4. JAMA 2012;307(10):1046–52.

69. Menne J, Nitschke M, Stingele R, et al. Validation of treatment strategies for enterohaemorrhagic *Escherichia coli* O104:H4 induced haemolytic uraemic syndrome: case-control study. BMJ 2012;345:e4565.

70. Granados CE, Reveiz L, Uribe LG, et al. Drugs for treating giardiasis. Cochrane Database Syst Rev 2012;(12):CD007787.

71. Rossignol JF, Kabil SM, el-Gohary Y, et al. Effect of nitazoxanide in diarrhea and enteritis caused by *Cryptosporidium* species. Clin Gastroenterol Hepatol 2006; 4(3):320–4.

72. Rossignol JF, Hidalgo H, Feregrino M, et al. A double-'blind' placebo-controlled study of nitazoxanide in the treatment of cryptosporidial diarrhoea in AIDS patients in Mexico. Trans R Soc Trop Med Hyg 1998;92(6):663–6.

73. Amadi B, Mwiya M, Sianongo S, et al. High dose prolonged treatment with nitazoxanide is not effective for cryptosporidiosis in HIV positive Zambian children: a randomised controlled trial. BMC Infect Dis 2009;9:195.

74. Abubakar I, Aliyu SH, Arumugam C, et al. Prevention and treatment of cryptosporidiosis in immunocompromised patients. Cochrane Database Syst Rev 2007;(1):CD004932.

75. Carr A, Marriott D, Field A, et al. Treatment of HIV-1-associated microsporidiosis and cryptosporidiosis with combination antiretroviral therapy. Lancet 1998; 351(9098):256–61.

76. Gonzales ML, Dans LF, Martinez EG. Antiamoebic drugs for treating amoebic colitis. Cochrane Database Syst Rev 2009;(2):CD006085.

77. Boonmar S, Morita Y, Fujita M, et al. Serotypes, antimicrobial susceptibility, and gyr A gene mutation of *Campylobacter jejuni* isolates from humans and chickens in Thailand. Microbiol Immunol 2007;51(5):531–7.

78. Thakur S, Zhao S, McDermott PF, et al. Antimicrobial resistance, virulence, and genotypic profile comparison of *Campylobacter jejuni* and *Campylobacter coli* isolated from humans and retail meats. Foodborne Pathog Dis 2010;7(7): 835–44.

79. Guerrant RL, Van Gilder T, Steiner TS, et al. Practice guidelines for the management of infectious diarrhea. Clin Infect Dis 2001;32(3):331–51.

80. Thabane M, Simunovic M, Akhtar-Danesh N, et al. An outbreak of acute bacterial gastroenteritis is associated with an increased incidence of irritable bowel syndrome in children. Am J Gastroenterol 2010;105(4):933–9.

81. Zanini B, Ricci C, Bandera F, et al. Incidence of post-infectious irritable bowel syndrome and functional intestinal disorders following a water-borne viral gastroenteritis outbreak. Am J Gastroenterol 2012;107(6):891–9.

82. Clark WF, Sontrop JM, Macnab JJ, et al. Long term risk for hypertension, renal impairment, and cardiovascular disease after gastroenteritis from drinking water contaminated with *Escherichia coli* O157:H7: a prospective cohort study. BMJ 2010;341:c6020.

83. Kalra V, Chaudhry R, Dua T, et al. Association of *Campylobacter jejuni* infection with childhood Guillain-Barre syndrome: a case-control study. J Child Neurol 2009;24(6):664–8.

84. Garcia Rodriguez LA, Ruigomez A, Panes J. Acute gastroenteritis is followed by an increased risk of inflammatory bowel disease. Gastroenterology 2006;130(6): 1588–94.

85. Fryden A, Bengtsson A, Foberg U, et al. Early antibiotic treatment of reactive arthritis associated with enteric infections: clinical and serological study. BMJ 1990;301(6764):1299–302.

86. Gilbert RE, See SE, Jones LV, et al. Antibiotics versus control for toxoplasma retinochoroiditis. Cochrane Database Syst Rev 2002;(1):CD002218.

87. Vila J, Ruiz J, Gallardo F, et al. *Aeromonas* spp. and traveler's diarrhea: clinical features and antimicrobial resistance. Emerg Infect Dis 2003;9(5):552–5.

Infections in Travelers

Mayan Bomsztyk, MD*, Richard W. Arnold, MD

KEYWORDS

- Travel medicine • Traveler's diarrhea • Malaria • Dengue • Leishmaniasis
- Immunosuppressed traveler

KEY POINTS

- The pretravel clinic visit is an integral part of disease prevention for travel.
- Traveler's diarrhea is common and generally occurs between 4 and 14 days after arrival.
- Fever in a returning travel is malaria until proved otherwise and can present months after return from endemic area.
- Most rashes and upper respiratory symptoms in travelers are not specifically related to a travel-related cause.
- The US Centers for Disease Control and the World Health Organization maintain helpful Web sites for both patient and physician.

INTRODUCTION

Every year more than 50 million people from developed nations visit the developing world.[1] Many of these travelers experience some sort of health issue and seek medical attention. In a 2000 study of 784 American travelers,[2] 64% reported some form of illness, and 12% of these travelers sought medical attention. Travelers seek medical attention for many different reasons, but the causes of their concerns can be broadly categorized as trauma-related, routine, or travel-associated illness. This article primarily focuses on the prevention and treatment of travel-associated illnesses.

The pretravel clinic visit is critical in the prevention of travel-related illness. It has 4 aims: baseline health assessment, review of itinerary, administration of appropriate vaccines, and counseling.[2] Although it is impossible to completely eliminate all risks associated with travel, a pretravel clinic visit can help prepare the patient to minimize risk and self-manage many diseases that may develop.

Once home, the 4 most common complaints of the returning traveler are diarrhea, rash, fever, and upper respiratory infection (URI).

This article originally appeared in Medical Clinics, Volume 97, Issue 4, July 2013.
Department of Medicine, University of Washington, 4245 Roosevelt Way Northeast, Seattle, WA 98105, USA
* Corresponding author.
E-mail address: mayanb@uw.edu

Clinics Collections 7 (2015) 555–578
http://dx.doi.org/10.1016/j.ccol.2015.06.037

PRETRAVEL VISIT

A thorough preclinic visit should include the following elements: (1) review of the itinerary; (2) review of past medication history and chronic medications; (3) administration of appropriate immunizations; (4) advice on prevention and self-treatment of common travel-related infections and assembling a medical kit; (5) provision of prescriptions and medical records when relevant.

Itinerary review should include dates of travel, specific sites of travel (eg, cities and regions), including layovers. During the itinerary review, the lodging arrangements and the style of trip should also be assessed. For instance, there are different risk factors for travelers staying at large hotel franchises and spas, travelers staying in youth hostels, and trekkers who are camping. In addition, the risk for travelers who reside in areas for substantial periods is increased over short-stay travelers.

The health assessment should include a review of past medical history, focusing on conditions that might be affected by travel, for instance, pulmonary diseases and air travel or coagulopathies and long periods of sitting. Current prescriptions should be reviewed and refilled to ensure that the patient has an adequate supply of appropriate medications during travel. Patients on antiretroviral medications or immunosuppression for organ transplant should take a supply equal to twice the anticipated quantity of pills needed for the duration of their travel. Other specific considerations for immunosuppressed patients are covered in a separate section.

Insurance coverage for travel visits varies by insurance carrier, as does appropriate bill coding. Some insurance plans allow billing of new (99201-99205) and established (99241-99245) patient evaluation/management (E/M) service for travel medicine visits. If the patient has been referred by a primary care physician, some plans allow billing outpatient consultation E/M service codes (99241-99245). Patients need to contact their insurer before their visit to see what services are covered.

Immunizations

Immunizations are an integral part of the pretravel visit. Multiple factors should be taken into consideration, including travel destination and climate, travel duration, severity of potential disease versus the risk of adverse effect from vaccination, activities planned, whether the trip is urban, rural, or remote from medical care, time remaining before departure, vaccine availability, cost, and the number of doses needed, history of allergy to vaccines or their components, pregnancy, and immunosuppression (**Box 1**). Multiple inactive vaccines can be conveniently and effectively administered at a single clinic visit.[3] Administration of multiple live vaccines sequentially can impair the immune response; therefore, they should be given either simultaneously or separated by at least 4 weeks. Interruption in a vaccine series does not require restarting the series; generally the series can resume from the last

---

Box 1
Considerations for administering vaccines

History of allergy

Pregnancy or immunosuppression

Destination and travel duration

Severity of disease versus risk of adverse effect from vaccination

Urban, rural, or remote from medical care

Vaccine availability, cost, and number of doses needed

administered dose. For instance, if a patient is receiving the hepatitis B series and receives the first and second injection at the appropriate interval (0 and 1 month) but misses the 6-month shot, the patient can receive it as soon as convenient without restarting the series de novo.

The US Centers for Disease Control (CDC) divides immunizations into routine, required, and recommended. Routine vaccines are necessary for protection from diseases that are potential risks in many parts of the world, for instance influenza or tetanus. Some patients may need boosters, especially for tetanus, pertussis, and diphtheria.

The only required vaccination by International Health Regulations, an international legal entity subscribed to by all member states of the World Health Organization (WHO), is yellow fever for travel to specific countries in sub-Saharan Africa and tropical South America. The Saudi Arabian government requires meningococcal vaccine for annual travel during the Hajj,[4] a ritual pilgrimage to Mecca made by more than 3 million Muslims annually.

Recommended vaccines may protect travelers from disease present in other parts of the world and prevent importation of nonendemic infectious diseases when the traveler returns home. Recommendations change frequently and up-to-date information can be found on the CDC Web site (http://www.cdc.gov/vaccines/). Examples of recommended vaccines (depending on travel destination) include hepatitis A, typhoid fever, meningococcus, and Japanese encephalitis (**Table 1**).

COUNSELING
Traveler's Diarrhea

Because it is impossible to tell which foods and water are safe, travelers should be educated in prevention and self-treatment of traveler's diarrhea. There are passive and active precautions. Passive actions include avoiding tap water and ice, salads, unpasteurized dairy products, thin-skinned fruits, and raw seafood. Active measures include drinking only boiled water or carbonated beverages or using a portable water filter. Iodine and chlorine alone are inadequate, because they do not eliminate all enteric pathogens. Taking bismuth prophylactically has been shown to provide up to 65% protection from diarrhea, although 2 tabs must be used 4 times a day to achieve the anticipated efficacy. Less frequent and lower doses still provide some protection, but efficacy may be reduced to between 30% and 40%.[5] Studies on

Table 1 Vaccines and abbreviated recommendations	
Vaccine	Notes
Hepatitis A	Travelers to Central or South America, parts of Asia and Africa
Japanese encephalitis	Travelers who plan to spend >1 mo in endemic areas (most of Asia and parts of Western Pacific) during Japanese encephalitis virus transmission season (varies depending on destination)
Meningococcal	Travelers visiting sub-Saharan Africa during dry season (December–June)
Typhoid	Travelers to Asia, Africa, the Caribbean, and Central or South America, especially those who will have prolonged exposure to potentially contaminated food or drink
Yellow fever	Travelers to endemic areas in South America and sub-Saharan Africa

Data from Centers for Disease Control and Prevention. CDC Health Information for International Travel 2012. New York: Oxford University Press; 2012; and Hill DR, Ericsson CD, Pearson RD, et al. The practice of travel medicine: guidelines by the Infectious Diseases Society of America. Clin Infect Dis 2006;43:1499–539.

probiotics for prophylaxis of traveler's diarrhea have been variable and inconclusive.[6] Antibiotic prophylaxis of traveler's diarrhea is generally inappropriate in a healthy host.

Counseling on how to self-manage traveler's diarrhea is invaluable. Mild cases, defined as 1 to 2 unformed stools in 24 hours, may require no treatment other than oral fluids to maintain hydration. More severe cases benefit from antibiotic treatment. Self-treatment with antibiotics generally improves symptoms within 36 hours. A 2000 Cochrane meta-analysis[7] found that antibiotics reduced both the duration and the severity of traveler's diarrhea. Choice of antibiotic and duration of treatment depend on location of travel.

For otherwise healthy travelers, it is reasonable to provide a 3-day course of cipro-floxacin 500 mg twice a day with instructions to take if unformed stool count exceeds more than 3 per day and is associated with other gastrointestinal symptoms or fever.[8] A shorter course of ciprofloxacin has also proved effective,[9] and patients should be counseled that symptoms need to be reassessed after the first 24 hours, and if resolved, the course can be shortened. Otherwise, completion of the 3-day course is advised. For patients traveling to Southeast Asian countries, where quinolone-resistant *Campylobacter* is prevalent (check the CDC Web site for up-to-date resistance patterns), azithromycin is the preferred antimicrobial agent.[10] For these patients, azithromycin 1000 mg by mouth once should be provided.[11] Rifaxamin is an alternative for otherwise uncomplicated traveler's diarrhea in a healthy host; however, it is not first-line therapy, because of concern for decreased efficacy in more severe cases.[8]

Insect-Borne Diseases

In areas where insect-borne diseases are a significant risk, travelers should wear protective clothing, use bed netting and N,N-diethylmetatoluamide (DEET). Other types of insect repellant have been found inferior. The length of effectiveness is directly related to concentration of DEET. For example, 23.8% DEET is effective for approximately 5 hours, whereas 4.75% is effective for only 88 minutes.[12] Permethrin-based insecticide should be sprayed on clothing and bed nets to decrease risk of mosquitos and tick bites.[11,13]

Malaria deserves special mention, because it infects approximately 30,000 European and North American travelers per year.[14] The Infectious Disease Society of America (IDSA) recommends the ABCD approach to malaria. A stands for risk-awareness. The risk of contracting malaria varies with the destination, season, climate, altitude, and number of mosquito bites; up-to-date information is available on the CDC Web site. B is for bite-avoidance (see earlier discussion on avoiding insect bites in general). C is for chemoprophylaxis compliance. Prophylaxis is recommended for all travelers to endemic areas. Prophylaxis medications suppress malaria by killing asexual blood stages of the parasite before they can cause disease. Therefore, protective levels must be present when parasites emerge from the liver. Effective prophylaxis must start before first possible exposure and continue for a period after the last potential mosquito bite. The timing of starting and stopping prophylaxis varies by regimen, with some regimens needing to be started several weeks before departure, whereas others must be continued after the traveler returns home.[11] There are many options for malaria prophylaxis, although in practice the decision is often made easier by the combination of timing of departure, willingness to take a daily medication, and tolerance of potential side effects. One recommended approach is depicted in **Table 2**.

Table 2
Malaria prophylaxis options by destination

Destination	Suspected Organism	Medication	Special Considerations
Central America (west of the Panama Canal), Mexico, Haiti, Dominican Republic, most of the Middle East, states of former Soviet Union, northern Africa, Argentina, Paraguay and parts of China	Chloroquine-sensitive *P falciparum*	Chloroquine	**Chloroquine** Needs to be taken 1–2 wk before departure and 4 wk after return Once weekly
South America, including Panama (east of Panama Canal) but excluding Argentina and Paraguay, Asia, Southeast Asia, sub-Saharan Africa and Oceania	Chloroquine-resistant *P falciparum*	Atovaquone-proguanil Doxycycline Mefloquine	**Atovaquone-proguanil** Needs to be taken daily More expensive **Doxycycline** Needs to be taken daily and for 4 wk after return Can cause sun sensitivity **Mefloquine:** Avoid in patients with seizures, psychiatric or cardiac conduction issues Needs to be started 2 wk before and continued 4 wk after
Rural, forested areas of the Thailand-Burma and Thailand-Cambodia borders, western provinces of Cambodia	Multidrug-resistant *P falciparum*	Atovaquone-proguanil Doxycycline	**Atovaquone-proguanil** Needs to be taken daily More expensive **Doxycycline** Needs to be taken daily and for 4 wk after return Can cause sun sensitivity

Data from Centers for Disease Control and Prevention. CDC Health Information for International Travel 2012. New York: Oxford University Press; 2012; and Hill DR, Ericsson CD, Pearson RD, et al. The practice of travel medicine: guidelines by the Infectious Diseases Society of America. Clin Infect Dis 2006;43:1499–539.

Sexual Activity

Studies suggest that travelers may engage in more high-risk sexual behavior than they would otherwise, including sex with new partners and unprotected sex. The percentage of travelers who are sexually active with a new partner abroad depends on the population surveyed. A UK study surveying travelers 18 to 35 years old who traveled without a partner found a sexual activity rate of 10%, and of these only 75% used condoms consistently.[15] A Norwegian study that surveyed clients of a sexually transmitted infection clinic found a sexual activity rate of 41%.[16] High-risk sexual activity increases the risk of human immunodeficiency virus (HIV), hepatitis B, and other sexually transmitted diseases. Travelers who may have sex with new partners abroad should bring latex condoms, because some studies have shown those manufactured abroad may be more prone to breakage.[11,17,18] Populations found to be more likely to engage in sexual activity with new partners abroad or to have unprotected sex include younger travelers (<25 years age), men who have sex with men,[19] expatriates,[19] military personnel,[20] and sex tourists[18] (defined as those who travel with explicit intention of engaging in sexual activity). In these populations, discussion about how to obtain pre-exposure or postexposure prophylaxis for sexually transmitted infections is appropriate. Symptoms and signs of sexually transmitted infections, such as dysuria, purulent drainage, pruritus, and genital lesions, should be discussed with all patients.

Animal Exposure

In many parts of the world, rabies is present in the dog population. Travelers from countries with universal rabies vaccination of dogs are rarely aware of rabies risk. Rabies transmission from dog bites is a major problem in Africa, parts of Asia, and Central and South America. Travelers should be advised to avoid dogs when traveling and assume that there are no friendly dogs. If travelers are bitten by dogs while traveling in a high-risk area, they need postexposure prophylaxis as soon as possible.

Reptile and amphibian exposure is more likely in travelers. Turtles, iguanas, geckos, snakes, frogs, and toads are all prevalent in many warm climates, and may be featured in petting zoos and for hire photographic opportunities. All these creatures frequently spread *Salmonella*. It is best to advise to avoid them to decrease *Salmonella* transmission. If there is any exposure, good hand washing and use of antibacterial hand gel is a must. Antibacterial hand gel is a crucial part of the travel medical kit.

SYMPTOMS IN THE RETURNING TRAVELER
Traveler's Diarrhea

Background
Traveler's diarrhea affects 20% to 60% of travelers to resource-poor destinations[21] and is defined by 3 or more loose stools in 24 hours with or without cramps, nausea, fever, or vomiting. The destinations with highest risk are South Asia, Africa, and Latin America. Travel to other developed countries carries some risk but is lower (<10%).[22] The median time of onset of symptoms is approximately 1 week after arrival to destination. The illness tends to be self-limited, lasting several days, although it can occasionally last more than 2 weeks in 5% to 10% of cases. Although rarely life threatening, traveler's diarrhea can significantly affect the planned activities of a traveler.

Epidemiology
Most cases of traveler's diarrhea do not have an identifiable cause. In a 1999 study of 322 travelers returning from Jamaica,[23] only 32% had an identifiable cause. Of those with an identifiable cause, the most common pathogens were bacterial, but viruses and parasites were also common. The most common bacterial cause was enterotoxic *Escherichia coli*, followed by *Salmonella* species, *Campylobacter jejuni,* and *Shigella* species. The most common viral causes were rotavirus and enteric adenovirus. Parasitic causes included *Giardia lamblia, Cryptosporidium, Cyclospora* and *Entamoeba histolytica.*

Diagnosis
For patients with mild to moderate traveler's diarrhea and no fever, hematochezia or tenesmus, the diagnosis of traveler's diarrhea may be made on clinical grounds. One recommended approach is outlined in **Fig. 1**. Routine stool culture should not be reflexively ordered because it cannot distinguish between pathogenic and nonpathogenic strains of *Escherichia coli*, and the results of the stool culture might not affect management. However, if the patient reports fever, bloody, stool or tenesmus, a culture is warranted. Any patient who has recently taken antibiotics should have stool sent for testing for *Clostridium difficile*. Because parasitic infections are less common, an examination of stool for ova and parasites is often not initially indicated. If diarrhea persists more than 1 week despite appropriate antibiotic

Clinical Diagnosis	Species , geographic distribution	Recommended Drug	Additional Comments
Uncomplicated Malaria	*P. ovale, P. malariae, P knowlesi* malaria OR *P. Falciparum* from Central America (West of the Panama Canal), Haiti, the Dominican Republic and most of the Middle East Or *P. vivax* from all regions except Papau New Guinea or Indonesia	Chloroquine	For *P. vivax* and *P. ovale,* add primaquine
	Chloroquine-resistant *P. falciparum* from all other malarious regions not specified elsewhere OR *P. vivax* from Papau New Guinea or Indonesia	Atovaquone-proguanil OR Artemether-lumefantrine OR Quinine+ doxycycline, tetracycline or clindamycin OR Mefloquine	For *P. vivax*, add primaquine
	Multidrug-resistant *P. falciparum* from Southeast Asia	Atovaquone-proguanil OR Artemether-lumefantrine OR Quinine+ doxycycline, tetracycline or clindamycin	
Complicated Malaria	*P. falciparum*	Quinidine gluconate+ doxycycline, tetracycline or clindamycin OR Artesunate	Considered exchange transfusion in patients with parasitemia >10%, altered mental status, pulmonary edema or renal complications

Fig. 1. Approach to workup of traveler's diarrhea by patient history.

treatment, then parasitic infections should be considered. In this setting, stool should be examined for ova and parasites to assess for *Cryptosporidium* and *Cyclospora*, antigen testing for *Entamoeba histolytica* and immunoassay for *Giardia*.

Treatment

Treatment has 3 main components: volume repletion, symptom management, and treatment of the underlying infection. The most common serious complication of traveler's diarrhea is volume depletion. In mild to moderate cases, broth, juice, or similar liquids suffice. In the case of severe diarrhea, oral rehydration solution should be used. Commercial products are available, or the solution can be made inexpensively by mixing one-half tablespoon of table salt, one-half tablespoon of baking soda, and 4 tablespoons of sugar into 1 L of water.

The second component of treatment is aimed at helping symptoms. Bismuth is helpful in controlling nausea, and loperamide can help with decreasing number of loose stools. Several studies have shown that combination of an antibiotic and loperamide is safe and provides more rapid symptom relief than either agent alone.[24]

The infection must be addressed. Antibiotic regimens do not vary from self-treatment recommendations.

SKIN LESIONS IN THE TRAVELER
Background

The differential for skin lesions in a returning traveler can be overwhelming; this section focuses on the most common and the most serious infections with cutaneous manifestations. Approximately 10% of returning travelers experience some form of a skin disorder,[2] and skin disorders account for 18% of posttravel clinic visits.[25] Despite travel to exotic locales, many travel-related skin lesions have pedestrian causes. Travelers frequently experience sexually transmitted infections, sunburns, allergic reactions, scabies, staphylococcal, and streptococcal infections. Chronic skin conditions like acne or allergic dermatitis can flare in tropical locations.

Epidemiology

The GeoSentinel network, a collaboration between the International Society for Tropical Medicine and the CDC, found the most common skin-related diagnoses in returning travelers were cutaneous larva migrans (CLM) and insect bite-related disease, including superinfected bites, skin abscess, and allergic reaction (**Table 3**).

Leishmaniasis and dengue accounted for approximately 3% of cases in the Geo-Sentinel study and should be included in the differential diagnosis, given their potential severity. The largest study before the GeoSentinel study was a 1995 French study[26] that found similar results, but myiasis (9%) and tungiasis (6%) were also common. In the French study, there was a disproportionate travel to Africa, which likely explains the higher frequency of these generally uncommon diseases. The distinctive characteristics of CLM, leishmaniasis, myiasis, and tungiasis are described in this section, but discussion of dengue infections is deferred to the section on fever and the returning traveler.

CLM

CLM is caused by animal hook worms that can be found worldwide, but infection is more frequent in Southeast Asia, Africa, South America, Caribbean, and the southeastern part of the United States.[27] Humans are infected with CLM after contact with ground contaminated with feces from infected animals, generally dogs and cats. The larvae penetrate human skin and migrate through the subcutaneous tissue. The migration causes the characteristic serpiginous pattern of CLM (**Fig. 2**). The rash

Table 3
Most frequent diagnosis in returning travelers with dermatologic diagnoses

Diagnosis (N)	% of all Dermatologic Diagnoses
All (4742)	100
CLM (465)[a]	9.8
Insect bite (388)	8.2
Skin abscess (366)	7.7
Superinfected skin bite (324)	6.8
Allergic rash (263)	5.5
Rash, unknown cause (262)	5.5
Dog bite (203)	4.3
Superficial fungal infection (190)	4
Dengue (159)[a]	3.4
Leishmaniasis (158)[a]	3.3
Myiasis (126)[a]	2.7
Spotted fever group rickettsiae (72)[a]	1.5
Scabies (71)	1.5
Cellulitis (70)	1.5

[a] Travel-related illness.
Data from Lederman ER, Weld LH, Elyazar IR, et al. Dermatologic conditions of the ill returned traveler: an analysis from the GeoSentinel Surveillance Network. Int J Infect Dis 2008;12:593.

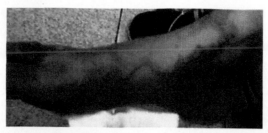

Fig. 2. A cutaneous serpentinelike track characteristic of CLM. (*From* Hamat RA, Rahman AA, Osman M, et al. Cutaneous larva migrans: a neglected disease and possible association with the use of long socks. Trans R Soc Trop Med Hyg 2010;104:171; with permission.)

is usually seen within days of exposure. Lesions may be papular or vesiculobullous and are prone to bacterial superinfection. Common locations are buttocks, thighs, and feet. Lesions may be associated with pruritus or pain. Diagnosis is made from clinical history and appearance. Eosinophilia is rarely present. Although cutaneous disease is self-limited, treatment shortens duration and reduces risk of superinfection. The preferred agent is ivermectin, although albendazole may be used as an alternative.[28] Hematogenous spread to the lungs is a rare complication, commonly presenting as respiratory symptoms approximately 1 week after the cutaneous eruption. No specific diagnostic test is available, and the treatment is the same as for the cutaneous infection.

Leishmaniasis

Leishmaniasis is present in more than 80 countries throughout Africa, Asia, southern Europe, and Latin America. Cutaneous leishmaniasis has 4 superficial manifestations: localized, recidivans, diffuse, and mucosal. The localized cutaneous form occurs on any exposed area of skin, starting as a red papule that enlarges to form a painless ulcer with heaped up margins and granulomatous tissue at the base (**Fig. 3**). These lesions are self-limited and the rate of resolution is determined by the particular infective species. A hypopigmented scar after ulcer resolution is common. Leishmaniasis recidivans is uncommon, and is caused by *Leishmania tropica* infections in the Middle East. After resolution of the primary lesion, a few remaining pathogens cause new papules to occur around the margins of the scar. These papules can appear, ulcerate, and heal repeatedly over decades. In patients with an impaired cell-mediated immune response, diffuse cutaneous leishmaniasis can occur. Instead of a primary lesion that ulcerates, the organism disseminates to macrophages in other areas of the skin. Diffuse cutaneous leishmaniasis characteristically has a relapsing or chronically progressive course that may cause significant deformity. Mucosal leishmaniasis occurs as a late-stage complication of less than 5% of cases of *L braziliensis* infection, which is endemic to Latin America. Months to years after primary lesion has resolved, recurrence at a distant mucosal site may occur.

Leishmaniasis traditionally has been diagnosed by microscopic visualization of the organism in a tissue sample. The burden of disease is determined by duration of infection (more chronic lesions have a lower burden[29]), and therefore lack of organism does not necessarily exclude diagnosis. Depending on the clinical facility, 4 processes are recommended: direct microscopy, culture, histology, and polymerase chain reaction (PCR).[30] PCR can be used for speciation when the location of travel has more than 1 endemic species. Speciation can be important because different species are associated with different clinical entities and prognosis. Tissue samples

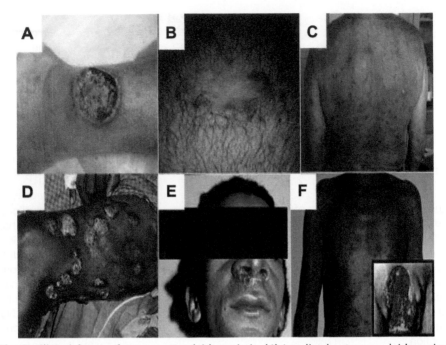

Fig. 3. Clinical forms of tegumentary leishmaniasis. (*A*) Localized cutaneous leishmaniasis presenting as a single ulcer on the leg. (*B*) Leishmaniasis recidiva cutis presenting as papules and vesicles around the healed lesion of cutaneous leishmaniasis on the leg. (*C*) Disseminated cutaneous leishmaniasis presenting as numerous small ulcers on the back. (*D*) Disseminated cutaneous leishmaniasis presenting as tumoral lesions and nodules associated with crusts and several scars from previous injuries on the left thigh. (*E*) Mucocutaneous leishmaniasis lesion in the nose and infiltration in the nasal mucosa. (*F*) Atypical cutaneous leishmaniasis in a patient infected with HIV presenting with multiple macules on the chest and abdomen. (*Insert* in *F*) Extensive ulcer on the penis of a patient with AIDS. (*Courtesy of* [*A*] Luiza K. Oyafuso, Instituto de Infectologia Emilio Ribas, São Paulo, Brazil; [*B*] Maria Edileuza Brito, Centro de Pesquisas Aggeu Magalhães, Fundação Oswaldo Cruz, Brazil; [*C*] Edgar M. Carvalho, Universidade Federal da Bahia, Brazil; and [*D*] Jackson M.L. Costa, Centro de Pesquisas Gonçalo Muniz, Fundação Oswaldo Cruz, Brazil.)

can be obtained by skin scraping, aspirate, or biopsy, which is preferred. If biopsy is possible, the lesion should be biopsied at the active edge, which is likely to have a higher parasite burden.

The treatment goals for leishmaniasis include resolution of active infection, reducing scarring, and decreasing recurrence. Choice and duration of therapy depend on its manifestation (cutaneous versus mucosal) and warrants involvement of a specialist. Traditionally, courses of intravenous (IV) pentavalent antimonials were used for 20 to 28 days. Single-dose IV liposomal amphotericin is becoming more commonly used.[30]

Myiasis

Myiasis is found in tropical and subtropical areas. The most common presentation of myiasis in a returning traveler is furuncular myiasis, caused by the botfly or the tumbu fly. In each instance, larvae penetrate skin and develop in subdermal tissue. There is typically 1 larva per lesion, although multiple lesions may be present. Patients may describe an enlarging insect bite of up to 3 cm in diameter and a crawling sensation or episodic pain near the lesion. There may be serosanguineous discharge from a central punctum or a small, white structure protruding from the lesion. Diagnosis is made by clinical history and physical examination. Removal of the intact larvae is curative. Different approaches for removal can be used. One option is to occlude with petroleum jelly the skin aperture through which the larva breathes and extract the larva when it moves closer to the surfaces to get air (**Fig. 4**). Larvae that die during occlusion are difficult to remove and often trigger an intense inflammatory reaction. Removal via manual expression and extraction through a small incision are preferable when possible.

Tungiasis

Like myiasis, tungiasis is found in subtropical and tropical destinations. Tungiasis is caused by the female sand flea, which can penetrate the human skin, usually on the feet or hands. Tungiasis causes skin inflammation, severe pain, itching, and a lesion at the site of infection that is characterized by a black dot at the center of a swollen red papule, surrounded by what looks like a white halo. The flea produces eggs that are expelled through the host's skin. Diagnosis is made by the clinical history and physical examination. Confirmation is made by identification of the organism after removal. Treatment is achieved by removal of the flea.

THE RETURNING TRAVELER AND FEVER
Background

Fever in a returning traveler can herald significant illness. In the GeoSentinel study, fever was the chief complaint for 28% of patients seeking posttravel care. In this study, 26% of patients with fever required hospitalization.[31] Globally, on return from the developing world, approximately 3% of travelers experience fever.[2] More than 17% of travelers with fever have a vaccine-preventable infection or *falciparum* malaria, which is preventable with chemoprophylaxis, underscoring the importance of the pre-travel visit.

Epidemiology of Fever in Returning Travelers

In the GeoSentinel study, the most common causes of fever in returning travelers were malaria, dengue, rickettsial infections, typhoid, or paratyphoid fever (otherwise known

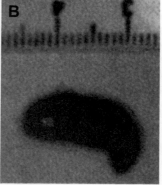

Fig. 4. (*A*) Boillike lesion on the trunk discharging serosanguineous fluid secondary to botfly myiasis infestation. (*B*) Botfly larva after removal from the boillike lesion. (*Data from* Morris-Jones R, Morris-Jones S. Travel-associated skin disease. Infect Dis Clin North Am 2012;26(3):680.)

as enteric fever).[31] Depending on travel destinations, leptospirosis, Chikungunya fever, and hepatitis A should also be considered as the cause of febrile systemic illness in returning travelers.

Diagnostic Algorithm of Fever in Returning Travelers

If a returning traveler presents with fever, the diagnosis of malaria must first be considered. If malaria is possible, based on timing and location of travel, obtain thin and thick smears. Repeat serial blood smears every 6 to 8 hours for 48 hours. If the malaria evaluation is negative or is unlikely based on other factors, evaluate based on localizing symptoms and signs as you would in any febrile patient. If there are no localizing symptoms or signs, consider dengue, rickettsiosis, enteric fever, and other causes of fever based on location of travel.

MALARIA
Background

Any patient who has visited a malaria endemic area in the last 4 years and reports fever should be evaluated for malaria, even if afebrile at presentation. In the GeoSentinel study, 20% of travelers who sought medical attention for fever eventually were diagnosed with malaria.[31] Thirty-three percent of patients with febrile illness who eventually died had malaria.

Malaria is caused by 1 of 5 protozoan species of the genus *Plasmodium: falciparum, vivax, ovale, malariae,* or *knowlesi. Anopheles* mosquito is the vector for malaria. After introduction of the organism through mosquito bite, the incubation period depends on the malaria species, but it is generally between 10 and 35 days, although *P vivax* and *ovale* can present up to 4 years after exposure, because of latent forms hiding in the liver. Fever is caused when the intracellular pathogen bursts from the erythrocyte.

Classification

Uncomplicated malaria is characterized by absence of end-organ dysfunction, although it can be associated with anemia and jaundice. Additional criteria for uncomplicated malaria include a parasite burden (defined as percent of infected erythrocytes) of less than 5% and the ability to take medications orally.[14] Complicated malaria is usually caused by *P falciparum*, although increasingly *P vivax* and *P knowlesi* are recognized to cause complicated malaria.

Cerebral malaria is defined by altered mental status, seizure, or coma. Risk factors include extremes of age, immunocompromised status (including HIV and asplenia), and pregnancy. Without treatment, cerebral malaria is uniformly fatal. Thus, prompt recognition and initiation of therapy are critical. Even with therapy, mortality remains 15% and 20%, and some patients may have permanent cognitive sequelae from infection.[32]

Clinical Presentation

Initially, patients with malaria may experience high fevers at irregular intervals throughout the day. As the infection progresses, rupture of infected red cells tends to synchronize, leading to characteristic day-to-day fever patterns. The pattern of fever depends on the particular species of malaria. *P falciparum, vivax* and *ovale* have a roughly 48-hour cycle, and *P malaria,* 72 hours.

There is no symptom or sign that is pathognomonic for malaria. Clinical features that may suggest malaria include fever without localizing symptoms, enlarged spleen, thrombocytopenia, and hyperbilirubinemia.[33]

The pathophysiology of malaria is related to the cytoadherence of red blood cells. This factor can lead to small infarcts, capillary leakage, and organ dysfunction. Clinical manifestations may include altered mental status, seizure, acute respiratory distress syndrome, metabolic acidosis, renal failure, hemoglobinuria (blackwater fever), hepatic failure, coagulopathy with or without disseminated intravascular coagulation, severe anemia or massive intravascular hemolysis, and hypoglycemia.

Diagnosis

The classic diagnostic test for malaria is examination of Giemsa-stained blood smears by light microscopy (**Fig. 5**). Two different smear preparations are ordered when there is concern for malaria. Thin smear allows for speciation and staging of the parasite in its life cycle. Thick smear allows more sensitivity, because more red blood cells are lysed and therefore more parasites released in the same area compared with the thin smear. The first test is positive in 95% of infected patients, but given the nature of cyclic parasitemia, exclusion of malaria requires smear evaluation every 6 to 12 hours for 48 hours.

Light microscopy has several disadvantages: it is labor intensive, requires considerable training, and is time consuming. Rapid diagnostic tests detect malaria antigen in a small amount of blood by immunochromatographic assay, with monoclonal antibodies directed against parasite antigen impregnated on a test strip. Commercial tests are manufactured with different combinations of target antigens to suit the local malaria epidemiology.[34] In 2007, the US Food and Drug Administration approved the first rapid detection test for use in the United States. Any positive rapid detection test result must be confirmed by microscopy; microscopy is also important for speciation and determination of parasite burden. PCR is available, but it is not used in the initial evaluation. PCR is used in some settings to determine the species of parasite after the diagnosis of malaria has been established.[14]

Treatment

Treatment of malaria is influenced by patient-specific factors (age, background of immunity, pregnancy, ability to take oral medications), species-specific factors, and local

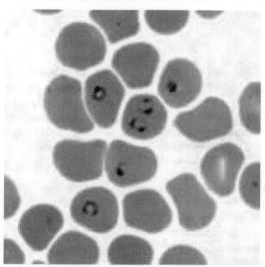

Fig. 5. *P falciparum* trophozyte seen on thin smear with Giemsa stain. (*Courtesy of* CDC.)

factors (drug resistance patterns, government treatment guidelines, tolerability, and drug availability) (**Table 4**). The same medication should not be used for treatment that the patient used for prophylaxis, in case a drug-resistant strain has been selected.

Non-*falciparum* malaria, (*vivax, malariae,* and *ovale*) should generally be treated with chloroquine, but chloroquine-resistant *vivax* has been reported recently in Papua New Guinea and Indonesia and chloroquine-resistant *malariae* has been reported in Sumatra.[35,36] In addition, primaquine is required in *P vivax* and *ovale* infections to eradicate the parasites that survive in the liver. Combination therapy generally prevents relapse in most *P vivax* and *ovale* infections, but primaquine-tolerant strains of *P vivax* have emerged in Oceania and East Africa, and longer and higher doses of primaquine are required in these areas for radical cure.

P falciparum treatment depends on sensitivity patterns in the particular area where the infection was acquired. *P falciparum* originating from Central America west of the Panama Canal, Haiti, the Dominican Republic, and much of the Middle East can be treated with chloroquine. However, there is developing resistance to this regimen. *P falciparum* acquired elsewhere should be treated with atovaquone-proguanil; artemether-lumefantrine; quinine plus doxycycline, tetracycline, or clindamycin; or mefloquine.[14,35] Mefloquine should not be used in patients who return from Cambodia and Thailand, because cases of mefloquine resistance have been reported.

Complicated disease, pregnancy, or severe nausea and vomiting necessitates admission to hospital and involvement of a specialist. Standard treatment of severe disease includes quinidine gluconate plus doxycycline, tetracycline, or clindamycin. Use of artesunate is becoming more common, and requires involvement of the CDC. Randomized controlled trials in endemic regions have shown a 30% reduction in mortality with artesunate-based regimens compared with quinine-based regimens.[37] Exchange transfusion should be considered in patients with parasite burden greater than 10%, altered mental status, pulmonary edema, or renal complications. The CDC Web site (http://www.cdc.gov/malaria/diagnosis_treatment/treatment.html) provides up-to-date information regarding the frequently changing epidemiology and resistance patterns and describes how to obtain artesunate in the United States. This Web site should be reviewed before initiation of malaria treatment.

DENGUE FEVER
Background

Dengue is endemic in Puerto Rico, Latin American, Africa, and Southeast Asia. There are periodic outbreaks in Samoa and Guam.[38] The dengue virus is a single-stranded RNA virus with 4 serotypes. Clinically, this description means that infection with 1 serotype provides immunity only for that particular serotype. The virus is carried by the *Aedes* mosquito, a silent daytime feeder with bites that frequently go unnoticed. The incubation period ranges from 2 to 14 days, and therefore it is effectively excluded as a cause of febrile illness in a traveler whose symptoms started more than 14 days after return.

Both viral and host characteristics influence the clinical presentation of dengue. There are several theories as to which combination of factors results in a more severe presentation.[39] Most evidence suggests that most severe dengue fever occurs in individuals who have been infected with dengue more than 1 time. Other theories include the hypothesis that different dengue viruses have inherently different levels of virulence, or that more severe clinical presentations involve abnormalities in T-cell response or autoimmune phenomena.

Table 4
Malaria treatment

Clinical Diagnosis	Species, Geographic Distribution		Recommended Drug	Additional Comments
Uncomplicated malaria	*P ovale, P malariae, P knowlesi* malaria or *P falciparum* from Central America (west of the Panama Canal), Haiti, the Dominican Republic and most of the Middle East or *P vivax* from all regions except Papa New Guinea or Indonesia	Chloroquine For *P vivax* and *P ovale*, add primaquine	Chloroquine-resistant *P falciparum* from all other malarious regions not specified elsewhere or *P vivax* from Papua New Guinea or Indonesia	Atovaquone-proguanil or artemether-lumefantrine or quinine + doxycycline, tetracycline or clindamycin or mefloquine	For *P vivax*, add primaquine	Multidrug-resistant *P falciparum* from Southeast Asia	Atovaquone-proguanil or artemether-lumefantrine or quinine + doxycycline, tetracycline or clindamycin
Complicated malaria	*P falciparum*		Quinidine gluconate + doxycycline, tetracycline or clindamycin or artesunate	Considered exchange transfusion in patients with parasitemia >10%, altered mental status, pulmonary edema, or renal complications

Data from Centers for Disease Control and Prevention. Treatment of malaria (guidelines for clinicians). Available at: http://www.cdc.gov/malaria/diagnosis_treatment/treatment.html. Accessed April 10, 2013.

Classification and Clinical Presentation

Dengue disease occurs as a spectrum of disease severity. WHO guidelines categorize dengue disease as nonsevere and severe. Nonsevere dengue fever is an acute febrile illness with 2 more of the following manifestations: headache, retro-orbital pain, myalgia, arthralgia (which prompted the name breakbone fever), rash, leucopenia, and mild hemorrhagic symptoms. The triad of skin rash (**Fig. 6**), thrombocytopenia, and leukopenia in a febrile returning traveler is suggestive of dengue infection.[33]

The nonsevere group is further subdivided by the presence of warning signs.[40] Warning signs that usually arise between day 3 and 7 of fever may indicate the development of severe dengue fever. The warning signs include mucosal bleeding, emesis, hematemesis, severe abdominal pain, painful hepatomegaly, breathing discomfort, lethargy, and fatigue. These symptoms often occur as patients defervesce.

Severe dengue is defined by plasma leakage, fluid accumulation, respiratory distress, severe bleeding, and organ impairment. Patients with severe dengue manifest many or all of the warning signs. Severe dengue seems to occur less frequently among travelers than it does in native populations. Native populations might be more susceptible because they are more likely to be infected sequentially by 2 dengue serotypes (secondary infection hypothesis). An alternative explanation is that most exposed travelers are younger adults, who are less likely to develop severe disease compared with the very old or very young.[41]

Diagnosis

Diagnosis is often made based on clinical presentation, but serology and molecular tests are available. The choice of confirmatory diagnostic test depends on timing of the patient's presentation. If the patient presents with at least 3 days of acute febrile illness, measurement of antidengue IgM is recommended. If before 3 days or the antidengue IgM is negative and clinic suspicion remains high, PCR for dengue viral RNA can be performed, although viral RNA clears from the bloodstream early in the course of the infection.

Treatment

Supportive care is the only management available for treatment of dengue.

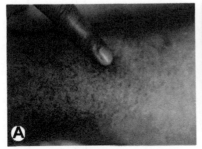 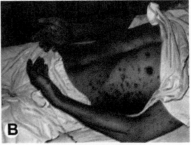

Fig. 6. Cutaneous manifestations of dengue. (*A*) Early maculopapular nonpruritic rash usually seen at the time of defervescence. (*B*) Late hemorrhagic and purpuric skin changes of a patient with severe dengue fever. (*Courtesy of* James H. Maguire, MD, Centers for Disease Control and Prevention, Atlanta, GA.)

RICKETTSIAL INFECTIONS
Background

Rickettsiosis is the term used for a spectrum of diseases caused by the intracellular bacteria *Rickettsia*, which invade endothelial cells and produce a vasculitis. There are multiple ectoparasite vectors for *Rickettsia*, including lice, ticks, fleas, and mites.

Classification

Rickettsiosis is divided into 3 main biogroups: typhus, spotted fever, and scrub typhus. The 4 most common rickettsioses seen in the traveler include murine typhus, Mediterranean spotted fever, African tick bite fever, and scrub typhus.[42] Each disease is caused by a different species, carried by different vector, has a different geographic distribution, and has different clinical presentation and sequelae.

Clinical Presentation

The combination of fever and cutaneous eruptions (**Fig. 7**) suggests rickettsiosis in a traveler returning from an endemic region.[33]

Diagnosis

As with Rocky Mountain spotted fever, rickettsial infections are primarily diagnosed clinically based on epidemiology and the history and physical examination findings. Rickettsiosis can be confirmed by 1 of 4 methods: isolation of the organism, serology, PCR, and immunologic detection in tissue samples.

Treatment

First-line treatment of all rickettsioses is doxycycline. Presumptive treatment is recommended whenever the diagnosis Is suspected, because making the diagnosis during the acute phase can be difficult.

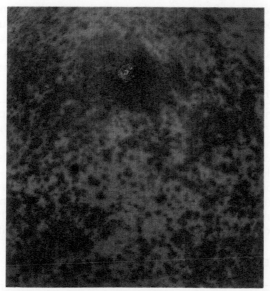

Fig. 7. Rickettsial infection leading to a maculopapular eruption on the back with a central necrotic area where the tick bite occurred. (*Data from* Morris-Jones R, Morris-Jones S. Travel-associated skin disease. Infect Dis Clin North Am 2012;26(3):688.)

ENTERIC FEVER
Background

Enteric fever encompasses both typhoid and paratyphoid fever and is common through most parts of the world except industrialized regions in North America, western Europe, Australia, and Japan.[43] *Salmonella enterica* serotypes *typhi* and *paratyphi* cause clinically indistinguishable entities; however, there are vaccines against serotype *typhi*, but not *paratyphi*. This gram-negative organism is ingested, survives gastric acidity, and invades gut epithelium. From there, it invades lymphatic tissue and can spread hematogenously and lymphatically.

Incubation period depends on amount of pathogen ingested, host age, and immune status, but generally is 7 to 14 days.[44]

Clinical Presentation

The classic clinical triad is abdominal pain, fevers, and chills. The patient may experience incremental increase in fever over the first week, increasing at a rate of 0.5°C to 1.0°C a day. A plateau of fevers ranging from 39 to 41 for 2 weeks follows. Generally, this plateau phase is not seen in the traveler, as opposed to the endemic population in a developing country, because travelers are more apt to seek care at earlier stages. On examination, relative bradycardia may be seen as well as hepatosplenomegaly, although neither of these findings is specific. Rose spots are lightly erythematous, nonblanching plaques 2 to 4 mm in diameter and are seen in 5% to 30% of patients with typhoid. Children and patients with HIV are more likely to present with diarrhea, whereas adults are more likely to complain of constipation. Complications occur in 10% to 15% of patients and are particularly likely in patients who have been ill for more than 2 weeks. Among the numerous complications are gastrointestinal bleeding, intestinal perforation, and typhoid encephalopathy.

Diagnosis

Enteric fever is diagnosed by blood or stool culture, but cultures may be negative if antibiotics have been given before obtaining the sample. Blood cultures have 60% to 80% sensitivity and are the standard diagnostic test. Stool culture has a sensitivity of 35%. If cultures remain negative and diagnosis remains uncertain, bone marrow biopsy is the most useful test, with a sensitivity of 90%. Serologic tests are not useful.[45]

Vaccination and Treatment

First-line treatment of enteric fever is 3 to 5 days quinolone (except for norfloxacin) antibiotic therapy.[46] The first-line agent for quinolone-resistant typhoid has not been determined; azithromycin, third-generation cephalosporins, and long, high-dose courses of quinolones have been proposed. The CDC recommends injectable third-generation cephalosporins.[41]

There are 2 modestly effective vaccines available for typhoid fever. The parental version takes advantage of IgG-mediated cell immunity; the oral form takes advantage of IgA secretory immunity. At best, parental vaccination is only 70% efficacious for preventing typhoid fever; oral vaccination is estimated to be less effective.[47]

RESPIRATORY INFECTION
Background

Respiratory infections occur in up to 20% of travelers.[2] The GeoSentinel study found that the most common diagnosis for URI was nonspecified URI, followed by pharyngitis and tonsillitis. The most common diagnoses for lower respiratory tract infections were bronchitis, pneumonia, and influenza. Thus, most travelers returning with respiratory complaints have diagnoses that are common in the developed world.[48]

Outbreaks are often linked to group settings, such as cruises or tour groups. Several pathogens have been associated with outbreaks including *influenza, Legionella, coronavirus,* and *histoplasma.* The risk for tuberculosis among immunocompetent travelers is low.

Diagnosis

Identification of the specific agent in the outpatient setting causing respiratory symptoms in an immunocompetent host is usually unnecessary.

Treatment

In some patients with influenza, treatment with oseltamivir might be appropriate. There is no effective specific therapy for noninfluenza respiratory viruses in immunocompetent adults. Treatment of bacterial pneumonia should be based on antibiotic sensitivity and local guidelines.

THE IMMUNOSUPPRESSED TRAVELER
Special Considerations in Patients with HIV

Fifty-nine countries have restrictions regarding travelers with HIV visiting their country, including deportation if HIV status is discovered. Four countries bar entry to any patient with HIV: Sudan, Yemen, United Arab Emirates, and Brunei.[49] Up-to-date information is available at http://www.unaids.org and should be reviewed before travel.

Killed or inactivated vaccines are safe in HIV-positive patients. For maximal effectiveness, vaccines should be administered when CD4 counts have peaked on effective antiretroviral therapy.[50]

There is increased incidence, prevalence, and severity of malaria in HIV-infected individuals.[51] Although there is no special precaution for patients with HIV that would not be indicated for immunocompetent patients (ie, nets, DEET, and strict prophylaxis compliance), the increased risk of infection and severe disease underscores their importance. The incidence of clinical episodes of malaria was found to be higher in individual with CD4 cell counts less then 200 cells/μL than in those with CD4 cell counts greater than 500 cells/μL.[52] Patients with CD4 less than 200 should be advised to postpone their travel until their counts rebound. The pharmacy should review any possible interactions between antiretroviral medications and malaria prophylaxis.

Routine antimicrobial prophylaxis for traveler's diarrhea for patients with HIV is not recommended. If severe immunosuppression is present and the trip cannot be postponed, a preventive regimen of daily-dose quinolone or rifaximin is appropriate.[28,53] As is the case in the immunocompetent patient, most HIV-infected travelers who develop traveler's diarrhea can be treated with ciprofloxacin. However, if diarrhea persists, in addition, a stool sample should be submitted for *Giardia* antigen, specific instructions for *Microsporidia* and *Cryptosporidium parvum* staining and ova and parasite (O&P) examination to look for *Cyclospora cayatenensis* and *Isospora belli.*

Special Considerations in Solid Organ Transplant Patients

The greatest risk for infection is during the 6 months after transplantation, when immunosuppression is highest[54,55]; travel should be postponed until this period has lapsed. Patients on antirejection drugs should avoid volume depletion, because many antirejection drugs are nephrotoxic and are more likely to cause acute kidney injury. Therefore, patients on antirejection drugs should be counseled to start volume repletion and should be given antibiotics and loperamide to start promptly for even mild traveler's diarrhea. Malaria prophylaxis may interact with antirejection drugs; thus, levels need to be monitored by a pharmacist before departure.

Special Considerations in Asplenic Patients

Splenectomy (whether functional or surgical) is not a contraindication to any vaccine. In addition, asplenic patients are particularly susceptible to encapsulated organisms and should have already been vaccinated against *Streptococcus pneumoniae* (within 5 years), *Neisseria meningitis* (within 3 years) and *Haemophilus influenza* (once). These vaccinations should be administered at travel visit if the traveler has not previously received them.[56] Although patients with asplenia are not at higher risk of influenza, it may predispose to invasive *Streptococcus pneumoniae*, and thus should also be immunized for flu at their pretravel visit if this has not already been done. Patients with asplenia should be promptly treated with antibiotics at the onset of any febrile illness or after any animal bite. Given that travelers may not have ready access to medical care, asplenic patients should be given a course of amoxicillin/clauvanate, which should be adequate initial treatment of both fever and animal bite prophylaxis. Taking antibiotics in this setting is an adjunct to seeking prompt medical care, not a replacement, and this distinction needs to be explicitly stated. Asplenic patients should also wear an alert bracelet. Asplenic patients with malaria may have delayed clearance of parasites from the bloodstream despite appropriate treatment.[57] They should receive a follow-up blood smear after treatment is complete.

Special Consideration in Patients on Corticosteroids or Tumor Necrosis Factor α

Patients taking greater than the equivalent 20 mg/d prednisone for more than 2 weeks should be considered immunosuppressed.[58] Live vaccines should not be administered, and immune response to inactivated vaccines may be insufficient. Physicians should wait more than 1 month after steroid discontinuation before administering vaccines. There is a paucity of data on administration of live vaccines to patients on tumor necrosis factor α (TNF-α) inhibitors, and they should be avoided in these patients.

The differential diagnosis in patients on corticosteroids and TNF-α inhibitors is necessarily broad, because they may present atypically. In addition, these patients have an increased risk for infections not otherwise commonly seen in other travelers, including tuberculosis and invasive fungal diseases.

Special Consideration in Patients on Oncologic Medications

The CDC considers patients on alkylating agents (cyclophosphamide), antimetabolites (azathioprine), and chemotherapeutic agents (including weekly methotrexate but excluding tamoxifen) to be severely immunosuppressed. Live vaccines should not be administered for at least 3 months after therapy has been discontinued.

SUMMARY

The pretravel clinic visit is an integral part of disease prevention for travel. The intended trip should be reviewed in depth with the patient to assess for risks particular to certain countries and conditions. Appropriate immunizations should be reviewed and administered; up-to-date recommendations are listed by location on the CDC Web site. Patients should be counseled on insect bite and traveler's diarrhea avoidance measures. Safe sex practices should be reinforced. Patients can be given antibiotics to take in case of moderate or severe traveler's diarrhea.

Traveler's diarrhea is common and generally occurs between 4 and 14 days after arrival.[10] Viral causes as well as most bacterial causes are usually self-limited, lasting several days. Mild diarrhea should be treated with volume repletion and symptoms management with loperamide and bismuth. If symptoms last longer than a week or bloody diarrhea is present, stool cultures should be obtained. If diarrhea has been present for more than a week despite antibacterial treatment, parasitic causes should be considered and stool O&P, and examinations for *Cryptosporidium*, *Cyclospora*, and so forth should be sent.

Skin lesions in a returning traveler are often secondary to conditions commonly seen in developed countries. CLM develops its pathognomonic serpiginous appearance 2 to 3 days after the larva has entered the human host. Diagnosis is clinical and can be treated with ivermectin or albendazole. Leishmaniasis has 4 different cutaneous manifestations. The interval from infection to clinical manifestation can range from weeks to years depending on the particular species and host immune status. Leishmaniasis is diagnosed by obtaining a tissue sample and performing microscopy, histology, PCR, or culture. Treatment is lengthy and should involve a specialist. Myiasis and tungiasis are diagnosed clinically and are treated by removal of the parasite.

Fever in a returning traveler is malaria until proved otherwise and can present months after return from endemic area. Evaluation involves thin and thick blood smears, the decision whether to admit, and treatment based on species and resistance patterns. The dengue incubation period is less than a week and can be excluded in any patient who presents with a fever more than 14 days after return. Dengue has a spectrum of severity and treatment is supportive. The incubation period and clinical presentation of rickettsiosis depend on the particular infective species; diagnosis is primarily clinical and treatment is doxycycline. Enteric fever presents as abdominal pain, fever, and chills. Incubation is generally from 1 to 2 weeks and is less likely in patients who present more than 3 weeks after return from endemic countries. Blood cultures are the diagnostic standard and infections are treated with a quinolone.

Patients with underlying immunosuppression need to receive tailored advice at their pretravel clinic visit. Immunosuppressed patients may have contraindications to live vaccines and impaired immune response to inactive vaccines. On return, the differential to a returning immunosuppressed patient must be broader because they may present atypically and are also susceptible to a wider range of pathogens.

Travel medicine continues to grow as international tourism and patient medical complexity increases. This article reflects the state of the discipline, but new recommendations on immunizations, resistance patterns, and treatment modalities constantly change. The CDC and WHO maintain helpful Web sites for both patient and physician. With thoughtful preparation and prevention, risks can be minimized and travel can continue as safely as possible.

REFERENCES

1. Spira A. Preparing the traveler. Lancet 2003;361:1368–81.
2. Hill DR. Health problems in a large cohort of Americans traveling to developing countries. J Travel Med 2000;7:259–66.
3. National Center for Immunization and Respiratory Diseases. General recommendations on immunization: recommendations of the Advisory Committee on Immunization Practices. MMWR Recomm Rep 2011;60(2):1–64.
4. Health information for travelers to Saudi Arabia. On: CDC Travelers Health Website. Available at: http://wwwnc.cdc.gov/travel/destinations/saudi-arabia.htm. Accessed December 12, 2012.

5. Steffen R, DuPont HL, Heusser R, et al. Prevention of traveler's diarrhea by the tablet form of bismuth subsalicylate. Antimicrob Agents Chemother 1986;29:625–7.

6. Ericsson CD. Nonantimicrobial agents in the prevention and treatment of traveler's diarrhea. Clin Infect Dis 2005;41:S557–63.

7. De Bruyn G, Hahn S, Borwick A. Antibiotic treatment for travellers' diarrhea. Cochrane Database Syst Rev 2000;(3):CD002242.

8. Castelli F, Saleri N, Tomasoni LR, et al. Prevention and treatment of traveler's diarrhea: focus on antimicrobial agents. Digestion 2006;73(Suppl 1):109–18.

9. Salam I, Katelaris P, Leigh-Smith S, et al. Randomized trial of single-dose ciprofloxacin for travellers' diarrhoea. Lancet 1994;344:1537–9.

10. Kuschner RA, Trofa AF, Thomas RJ, et al. Use of azithromycin for the treatment of *Campylobacter* enteritis in travelers to Thailand, an area where ciprofloxacin resistance is prevalent. Clin Infect Dis 1995;21:536–41.

11. Hill DR, Ericsson CD, Pearson RD, et al. The practice of travel medicine: guidelines by the Infectious Diseases Society of America. Clin Infect Dis 2006;43: 1499–539.

12. Fradin MS, Day JF. Comparative efficacy of insect repellents against mosquito bites. N Engl J Med 2002;347:13–8.

13. Nevill CG, Some ES, Mung'ala VO, et al. Insecticide-treated bednets reduce mortality and severe morbidity from malaria among children on the Kenyan coast. Trop Med Int Health 1996;1:139–46.

14. Malaria. In: World Health Organization Website. Available at: http://www.who.int/topics/malaria/en/. Accessed December 14, 2012.

15. Bloor M, Thomas M, Hood K, et al. Differences in sexual risk behaviour between young men and women travelling abroad from the UK. Lancet 1998;352:1664–8.

16. Tveit KS, Nilsen A, Nyfors A. Casual sexual experience abroad in patients attending an STD clinic and at high risk for HIV infection. Genitourin Med 1994;70:12–4.

17. Marrazzo JM. Sexual tourism: implications for travelers and the destination culture. Infect Dis Clin North Am 2005;19:103–20.

18. Hamlyn E, Peer A, Easterbrook P. Sexual health and HIV in travellers and expatriates. Occup Med 2007;57:313–21.

19. Hill DR. Occurrence and self-treatment of diarrhea in a large cohort of Americans traveling to developing countries. Am J Trop Med Hyg 2000;62:585–9.

20. Malone JD, Hyams KC, Hawkins RE, et al. Risk factors for sexually transmitted diseases among deployed U.S. military personnel. Sex Transm Dis 1993;20: 294–8.

21. Hill DR, Beeching NJ. Traveler's diarrhea. Curr Opin Infect Dis 2010;23:481–7.

22. Steffen R. Epidemiologic studies of the travelers' diarrhea, severe gastrointestinal infections and cholera. Rev Infect Dis 1986;8(Suppl 2):S122–30.

23. Steffen R, Collard F, Tornieporth N, et al. Epidemiology, etiology, and impact of traveler's diarrhea in Jamaica. JAMA 1999;281:811–7.

24. Riddle MS, Arnold S, Tribble DR. Effect of adjunctive loperamide in combination with antibiotics on treatment outcomes in traveler's diarrhea: a systematic review and meta-analysis. Clin Infect Dis 2008;47:1007–14.

25. Lederman ER, Weld LH, Elyazar IR, et al. Dermatologic conditions of the ill returned traveler: an analysis from the GeoSentinel Surveillance Network. Int J Infect Dis 2008;12:593–602.

26. Caumes E, Carrière J, Guermonprez G, et al. Dermatoses associated with travel to tropical countries: a prospective study of the diagnosis and management of 269 patients presenting to a tropical disease unit. Clin Infect Dis 1995;20:542–8.

27. Hochedez P, Caumes E. Hookworm related cutaneous larva migrans. J Travel Med 2007;14:326–33.
28. Caumes E, Carriere J, Datry A, et al. A randomized trial of ivermectin versus albendazole for the treatment of cutaneous larva migrans. Am J Trop Med Hyg 1993;49:641–4.
29. Andrade-Narvaez FJ, Medina-Peralta S, Vargas-Gonzalez A, et al. The histopathology of cutaneous leishmaniasis due to Leishmania (Leishmania) mexicana in the Yucatan peninsula, Mexico. Rev Inst Med Trop Sao Paulo 2005;47:191–4.
30. Ameen M. Cutaneous leishmaniasis: advances in disease pathogenesis, diagnostics and therapeutics. Clin Exp Dermatol 2010;35:699–705.
31. Wilson ME, Weld LH, Boggild A, et al. Fever in returned travelers: results from the GeoSentinel Surveillance Network. Clin Infect Dis 2007;44:1560–8.
32. Kihara M, Carter JA, Newton CR. The effect of Plasmodium falciparum on cognition: a systematic review. Trop Med Int Health 2006;11:386–97.
33. Bottieau E, Clerinx J, Van den Enden E, et al. Fever after a stay in the tropics: diagnostic predictors of the leading tropical conditions. Medicine 2007;86: 18–25.
34. Wongsrichanalai C, Barcus MJ, Muth S, et al. A review of malaria diagnostic tools. Am J Trop Med Hyg 2007;77:119–27.
35. White NJ. The treatment of malaria. N Engl J Med 1996;335:800–6.
36. Maguire JD, Sumawinata IW, Masbar S, et al. Chloroquine-resistant Plasmodium malariae in south Sumatra, Indonesia. Lancet 2002;360:58–60.
37. Dondorp A, Nosten F, Stepniewska K, et al. Artesunate versus quinine for treatment of severe falciparum malaria: a randomised trial. Lancet 2005;366:717–25.
38. Tomashek KM. Dengue fever and dengue hemorrhagic fever. In: 2012 Yellow Book-Traveler's Health. Available at: http://wwwnc.cdc.gov/travel/yellowbook/2012/chapter-3-infectious-diseases-related-to-travel/dengue-fever-and-dengue-hemorrhagic-fever.htm. Accessed January 3, 2013.
39. Halstead SB. Controversies in dengue pathogenesis. Paediatr Int Child Health 2012;32:5–9.
40. Nathan MB, Dayal-Drager R, Guzman M. Dengue: guidelines for diagnosis, treatment, prevention and control. 2009. Available at: http://whqlibdoc.who.int/publications/2009/9789241547871_eng.pdf. Accessed January 3, 2013.
41. Wilder-Smith A. Dengue infections in travelers. Paediatr Int Child Health 2012; 32:28–32.
42. Jensenius M, Fournier PE, Raoult D. Rickettsioses and the international traveler. Clin Infect Dis 2004;39:1493–9.
43. Bhattarai A, Mintz E. Typhoid and paratyphoid fever. In: 2012 Yellow Book-Traveler's Health. Available at: http://wwwnc.cdc.gov/travel/yellowbook/2012/chapter-3-infectious-diseases-related-to-travel/typhoid-and-paratyphoid-fever.htm. Accessed January 3, 2013.
44. Parry CM, Hien TT, Dougan G, et al. Typhoid fever. N Engl J Med 2002;347: 1770–82.
45. Edelman R, Levine MM. Summary of an international workshop on typhoid fever. Rev Infect Dis 1986;8:329–49.
46. White NJ, Parry CM. The treatment of typhoid fever. Curr Opin Infect Dis 1996;9: 298–302.
47. Typhoid immunization: recommendations of the Advisory Committee on Immunization Practices (ACIP). MMWR Morb Mortal Wkly Rep 1994;43:1–7.
48. Leder K, Sundararajan V, Wald L, et al. Respiratory tract infections in travelers: a review of the GeoSentinel surveillance network. Clin Infect Dis 2003;36:399–406.

49. Mapping of restrictions on the entry, stay and residence of people living with HIV 2009. Available at: http://www.unaids.org/en/media/unaids/contentassets/dataimport/pub/report/2009/jc1727_mapping_en.pdf. Accessed January 3, 2013.

50. McCarthy AE, Mileno MD. Prevention and treatment of travel-related infections in compromised hosts. Curr Opin Infect Dis 2006;19:450–5.

51. Kublin JG, Steketee RW. HIV infection and malaria–understanding the interactions. J Infect Dis 2006;193:1–3.

52. Laufer MK, van Oosterhout JJ, Thesing PC, et al. HIV-associated immunosuppression on malaria infection and disease in Malawi. J Infect Dis 2006;193: 872–8.

53. Franco-Paredes C, Hidron A, Tellez I, et al. HIV infection and travel: pretravel recommendations and health-related risks. Top HIV Med 2009;17:2–11.

54. Kofidis T, Pethig K, Ruther G, et al. Traveling after heart transplantation. Clin Transplant 2002;16:280–4.

55. Boggild AK, Sano M, Humar A, et al. Travel patterns and risk behavior in solid organ transplant recipients. J Travel Med 2004;11:37–43.

56. Watson DA. Pretravel health advice for asplenic individuals. J Travel Med 2003; 10:117–21.

57. Chotivanich K, Udomsangpetch R, McGready R, et al. Central role of the spleen in malaria parasite clearance. J Infect Dis 2002;185:1538–41.

58. Jong EC, Freedman DO. Immunocompromised Traveler. In: 2012 Yellow Book-Traveler's Health. Available at: http://wwwnc.cdc.gov/travel/yellowbook/2012/chapter-8-advising-travelers-with-specific-needs/immunocompromised-travelers.htm. Accessed January 3, 2013.

Clostridium difficile Infection

Christopher L. Knight, MD[a],*, Christina M. Surawicz, MD[b]

KEYWORDS

- *Clostridium difficile* • Metronidazole • Fecal microbiota transplantation

KEY POINTS

- *Clostridium difficile* infection (CDI) is increasing in prevalence and severity.
- Major risk factors include antibiotic use, age, exposure to the organism in health care settings, and (likely) use of proton-pump inhibitors.
- Prevention of transmission is essential in reducing nosocomial outbreaks.
- Oral metronidazole (500 mg 3 times daily for 10 days) is the therapy of choice for mild to moderate disease.
- Oral vancomycin (125 mg 4 times daily for 10 days) is the therapy of choice for severe disease and pregnant/lactating women.
- High-dose oral vancomycin (250–500 mg 4 times daily for 10 days) and intravenous metronidazole are the therapies of choice for complicated disease.
- Rectal vancomycin enemas can be given in patients with ileus, abdominal distention, and anatomic/surgical abnormalities that prevent oral antibiotics from reaching the colon.
- The first recurrence of CDI should be treated the using the same protocol as for initial infection.
- The second recurrence should be treated with oral vancomycin using an extended "pulsed" course.
- The best treatment for third and subsequent recurrences remains unclear, but fecal microbiota transplantation shows considerable promise.

MICROBIOLOGY

In 1935, microbiologists isolated a new species of gram-positive, spore-forming bacteria from human feces. The difficulty of its isolation, requiring an anaerobic environment, gave it its name: *Bacillus difficilis*. In the 1970s, it was recognized that toxins produced by this organism, renamed *Clostridium difficile*, were a major cause of pseudomembranous colitis.[1,2] The 2 primary toxins, toxin A and toxin B, both cause injury

This article originally appeared in Medical Clinics, Volume 97, Issue 4, July 2013.
[a] Division of General Internal Medicine, Department of Medicine, University of Washington School of Medicine, 4245 Roosevelt Way Northeast, Box 354760, Seattle, WA 98109, USA;
[b] Division of Gastroenterology, Department of Medicine, University of Washington School of Medicine, 325 9th Avenue, Box 359773, Seattle, WA 98104, USA
* Corresponding author.
E-mail address: cknight@uw.edu

to intestinal mucosa, but toxin B is much more potent than toxin A, thought to be the reason why some strains of *C difficile* remain pathogenic despite producing only toxin B.[3] The ability of *C difficile* to form spores that resist many common disinfectants and can survive for months on environmental surfaces makes it particularly prone to nosocomial transmission.

In 2002, hospitals in Québec and southern Canada began to report dramatically increased rates of *C difficile* infection (CDI). This and several subsequent outbreaks were eventually attributed to a newly epidemic strain of *C difficile*. The strain has been named based on the microbiologic techniques used to identify it: North American pulsed-field gel electrophoresis type 1, restriction endonuclease analysis type BI, and PCR ribotype 027, or NAP1/BI/027. This strain produces dramatically more toxin A and B in vitro than do conventional strains of pathogenic *C difficile*, causing more severe disease.[4]

EPIDEMIOLOGY AND RISK FACTORS

Both the incidence and the severity of CDI have been rising since 2001. From 2000 to 2005, the rate of hospitalizations reporting CDI doubled from 5.5 per 10,000 to 11.2 per 10,000 population, with a similar increase in age-adjusted case-fatality rate from 1.2% to 2.2%.[5] Much of the increase is seen in older patients with exposure to health care settings such as long-term care facilities and hospitals.[6] However, *C difficile* is also emerging in a pathogen in populations previously thought to be at low risk, such as pregnant women hospitalized for delivery and patients without prior exposure to health care settings.[7–9]

Antibiotic Exposure

Exposure to antibiotics remains the preeminent risk factor for CDI. Any antibiotic can cause CDI, commonly clindamycin, penicillins, cephalosporins, and fluoroquinolones, and especially multiple antibiotics. CDI has also been reported with exposure to metronidazole and vancomycin, which are used for treatment.[10] The effect of antibiotics is presumed to be disruption of the normal gut microbiota, thus allowing proliferation of *C difficile*.[11]

Antibiotics are the most significant risk factor, and their effect can persist for weeks to months after they are stopped. A case-control study done in the Netherlands showed a 7- to 10-fold increased risk for CDI during antibiotic therapy that persisted for the first month after stopping antibiotics. The risk gradually declined over the following 2 months, returning to baseline 3 months after stopping antibiotic therapy. There was a trend toward increased risk with longer overall duration of antibiotics, although differences were not statistically significant.[12]

Exposure to Toxigenic C difficile

The other major risk factor for health care–associated CDI is exposure to settings where the organism is prevalent. Risk for CDI has been shown to correlate with length of hospital stay, but recently discharged patients and patients who live in long-term care facilities or other health care settings are also at increased risk.[13] By definition, community-acquired CDI is not associated with exposure to a health care setting.

Age

Older age is a well-established risk factor for health care–associated CDI. From 2000 to 2005, the majority of United States hospitalizations with CDI occurred in a group between 65 and 84 years of age, and patients older than 85 are at even higher risk.

Data are more limited for community-acquired infection, but some studies suggest that younger people are at risk. The median age of patients with community-associated CDI tends to be lower, and a study of community-associated CDI in North Carolina showed a higher incidence in the 45- to 64-year-old age group than in those older than 65.[13,14]

Gastric Acid Suppression

Despite a large number of studies regarding an association between gastric acid suppression and CDI, the subject remains somewhat controversial. Many studies evaluated hospitalized patients but some also studied outpatients. Most, but not all, show an increased risk of CDI associated with the use of proton-pump inhibitors (PPIs). Some studies have shown a lesser increase in risk with the use of H2-receptor antagonists, suggesting a correlation with degree of acid suppression.[15,16] Multiple recent meta-analyses of PPI use in patients with CDI have found pooled estimates of between 1.7- and 2.1-fold increase in risk, favoring an association.[17–19]

Inflammatory Bowel Disease

The generalized increase in the incidence of CDI in recent years has been accompanied by a parallel increase in rates among patients with inflammatory bowel disease (IBD). Patients with ulcerative colitis appear to be at particularly high risk, with a tripling of incidence between 1998 and 2005 in one study.[20] In addition to higher incidence rates, patients with IBD present a clinical challenge because CDI can mimic the symptoms of an IBD flare. Patients with IBD who also have CDI have higher rates of colectomy and a 4-fold increase in mortality. Patients with IBD may also experience unique complications of CDI, including pouchitis in patients status post colectomy with ileoanal reconstruction.[21]

CLINICAL MANIFESTATIONS AND DIAGNOSIS
Clinical Manifestations and Disease Severity

The cardinal symptom of CDI is watery diarrhea, which can be up to 10 to 15 stools per day. Diarrhea of CDI is rarely bloody, although it can be in severe cases. Some patients may lose significant amounts of serum proteins in stool, causing hypoalbuminemia, edema, and ascites.[22] In addition, fever ($\geq$38.0°C), abdominal distension, and leukocytosis ($\geq$15–20,000 white blood cells/mm^3) are significant indicators of severe disease, likely to cause admission to the intensive care unit, surgery for complications of CDI, or death.[23] Leukocytosis may precede diarrhea. A retrospective review of 60 patients with unexplained leukocytosis reported 35 (58%) with *C difficile* toxin in their stool. Of these patients, 30 (86%) eventually had symptoms consistent with colitis, but for 16 (53%) leukocytosis was noted before any mention of colitis symptoms.[24]

Patients with severe CDI frequently have abdominal pain caused by ileus, colonic dilation, and even toxic megacolon. Marked leukocytosis (sometimes as high as 50,000/μL) and lactic acidosis are worrisome signs and should prompt surgical consultation.

Pseudomembranous Colitis

Patients with CDI frequently have pathognomonic findings on lower endoscopy. *C difficile* colitis can be nonspecific or there may be release of proteins and inflammatory cells, which coalesce to form yellowish pseudomembranes (**Fig. 1**). Although a typical endoscopic appearance is virtually pathognomonic for CDI, endoscopy is rarely needed as a diagnostic test when CDI is suspected, because of the availability of less invasive stool studies and the risk of perforation in patients with severe colitis.

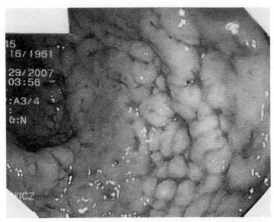

Fig. 1. Confluent pseudomembranes in a patient with *Clostridium difficile* colitis.

Diagnostic Studies

The past gold-standard test for the diagnosis of CDI was the cytotoxin neutralization assay. Culture alone is insufficient because some *C difficile* isolates are nontoxigenic.[25] However, these tests are expensive and time consuming, so they have largely been replaced by more rapid assays.

Enzyme immunoassay (EIA) tests are available for toxins A and B, as well as glutamate dehydrogenase (GDH), an enzyme produced by *Clostridium* species. EIA tests for toxins A and B have a sensitivity of 75% to 95% and a specificity of 83% to 98% in comparison with cytotoxin neutralization assays.[26] GDH may be easier to detect by EIA testing and is sometimes used as an initial screen, but a positive GDH test does not distinguish between toxigenic and nontoxigenic strains. A negative GDH test has good negative predictive value, but a positive GDH test requires additional testing to confirm presence of toxin. GDH testing has been reported to have sensitivities from 75% to more than 90%, with negative predictive values of 95% to 100% in the appropriate clinical setting.[27]

The newest testing methodologies are nucleic acid amplification tests, including polymerase chain reaction (PCR) and loop-mediated isothermal amplification tests. These tests detect genes residing within the pathogenicity locus of the *C difficile* genome such as the toxin A gene (tcdA), toxin B gene (tcdB), and the toxin regulatory gene (tcdC). Overall performance for gene amplification assays shows sensitivities of 90% to 100% with specificities of 94% to 100%.[28] In a head-to-head comparison, gene amplification significantly outperformed EIA-based testing.[29]

Although not needed for diagnosis, computed tomography (CT) imaging of the abdomen can be useful in assessing disease severity. Colon-wall thickening (**Fig. 2**), dilation of the colon, and ascites are all concerning findings. CT can also be helpful in ruling out other pathologic processes, and in determining the presence of perforation.

Surveillance and Repeat Testing

Clinical guidelines issued jointly by the Society for Healthcare Epidemiology of America (SHEA) and the Infectious Disease Society of America (IDSA) recommend evaluating only diarrheal stool from patients thought have symptomatic CDI, unless the patient has ileus, in which case a rectal swab may be used to obtain a specimen for PCR testing.[30] There is no benefit to testing multiple stool specimens. It is not advisable to

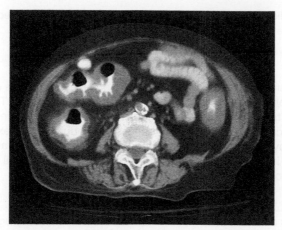

Fig. 2. Colon wall thickening on abdominal computed tomography imaging. Oral contrast fills the lumen of the colon.

retest patients for "clearance" of *C difficile,* because successfully treated patients may continue to have a positive test for CDI for as long as 30 days after starting therapy.[31]

PREVENTION

It is crucial that efforts focus on prevention of initial CDI, especially in health care settings. The cornerstones of these efforts are reduction in the overuse of antimicrobials and efforts to prevent transmission from patient to patient.

Antimicrobial Stewardship

Exposure to antibiotics is the primary risk factor for CDI. Although any antibiotic can cause CDI, the more antibiotics the patient is exposed to and the greater the duration, the higher the risk. There have been multiple studies demonstrating a reduced risk of CDI when institutions initiate programs to limit the use of high-risk antimicrobials.[32–34] In one study an effort to optimize antimicrobial use in response to an epidemic of the NAP1/BI/027 hypervirulent strain reduced nosocomial CDI by 60%.[34] There is also a joint IDSA/SHEA guideline on establishing an institutional program to enhance antimicrobial stewardship.[35]

Reduction of Transmission

C difficile is particularly problematic in health care settings because in its spore form it is resistant to commonly used disinfectants. Alcohol, the active ingredient in many hand gels and cleansers, has been shown to be ineffective against *C difficile* spores.[36] Hand washing with soap and water or chlorhexidine is preferable. Use of gloves when handling body substances was associated with a significant reduction incidence of CDI in one randomized study.[37] Use of surface disinfectants specifically active against *C difficile* has also been shown to be helpful.[38,39]

Probiotics

Probiotics, such as *Lactobacillus* preparations and *Saccharomyces boulardii,* have been shown to reduce overall rates of antibiotic-associated diarrhea. Although most studies focusing specifically on *C difficile* have been small and have not had significant results, a meta-analysis of combining the results of multiple studies showed a statistically significant 66% reduction in CDI. Both *Lactobacillus*-based and *Saccharomyces*-based preparations appeared to be effective.[40]

TREATMENT

Although exposure to antimicrobials is a key part of the pathogenesis of CDI, once the infection is established, antimicrobials are necessary for treatment. Three agents are used for primary treatment of CDI: metronidazole (Flagyl), vancomycin (Vancocin), and fidaxomicin (Dificid). Other drugs have been studied but are not extensively used. Choice of therapy depends on the severity of the patient's illness, and whether one is treating initial infection or recurrent CDI. If possible, antibacterial agents that are not being used to treat CDI should be stopped.

Metronidazole

Metronidazole is a nitroimidazole antibiotic that has broad activity against anaerobic bacteria (including *C difficile*) in vitro. Unlike other agents commonly used to treat CDI, orally administered metronidazole is well absorbed in the proximal gut. However, in patients with colitis, metronidazole and its primary metabolite, hydroxymetronidazole, reach sufficient endoluminal concentrations to have antibacterial activity. In patients without diarrhea, fecal concentrations of metronidazole and metabolites are much lower, suggesting that the infection itself allows metronidazole to reach effective levels in the colon, either by altering the permeability of the colon mucosa or disrupting reabsorption of metronidazole secreted from the biliary tract.[41] Because metronidazole is able to reach the colon via the bloodstream, it can be given intravenously for the treatment of CDI, unlike vancomycin and fidaxomicin.

Metronidazole's primary advantages over other antimicrobials are low cost and lack of concerns about antimicrobial resistance. At the time of writing, a full course of vancomycin costs nearly 100 times as much as a course of metronidazole, and fidaxomicin is even more expensive. Although *C difficile* itself is not typically resistant to vancomycin, other gram-positive organisms are developing vancomycin resistance, providing a compelling reason to avoid its use when other agents might be effective.

Metronidazole's disadvantages relative to other agents relate primarily to adverse effects from systemic absorption, including nausea, a metallic taste in the mouth, and occasionally a disulfiram-like reaction when patients consume alcohol. Metronidazole also readily crosses the placenta and is excreted in breast milk; it has been implicated in facial anomalies when used during the first trimester, making it contraindicated in pregnant and lactating women. Long-term use of metronidazole (2–4 weeks or more) has been associated with a peripheral neuropathy, which is problematic for treating patients with recurrent CDI.[42] There is also limited evidence that metronidazole is less effective than vancomycin in patients with severe CDI (see the section on comparative effectiveness).

Vancomycin

Vancomycin is a glycopeptide antibiotic that is poorly absorbed from the gastrointestinal tract when administered orally. It has broad activity against gram-positive organisms, including *C difficile*. Vancomycin's primary advantage over metronidazole is lack of systemic absorption and the accompanying toxicities. There is also some evidence of greater efficacy in severe CDI (see the section on comparative effectiveness). Its primary disadvantage is cost: the oral form of vancomycin is particularly expensive in the United States. Because of this, some hospitals and compounding pharmacies use the intravenous form administered orally. Anecdotally this appears to be effective, although patients may report a bad taste with this formulation. There is also concern about fostering vancomycin resistance among other organisms, particularly entero-cocci, when using vancomycin to treat CDI. This aspect remains largely theoretical at this point, although one study of 301 patients showed decreased acquisition rates of vancomycin-resistant enterooooooi with fidaxomicin treatment for CDI when com-pared with vancomycin.[43]

Fidaxomicin

Fidaxomicin is a macrocyclic antibiotic with particularly potent activity against *C difficile*. It is active against some other gram-positive organisms, including enterococci, staph-ylococci, and other clostridial species, but less so than vancomycin. It has little activity against other common bowel flora, particularly gram-negative species.[44] Fidaxomicin has been approved by the United States Food and Drug Administration for the treatment of *C difficile* colitis, based primarily on the results of one randomized controlled trial, which enrolled 629 patients and randomized them to fidaxomicin or vancomycin. Equiv-alent cure rates (88% vs 86%) were found, but some patients receiving fidaxomicin had a somewhat lower recurrence rate than those receiving vancomycin, only apparent in patients without the NAP1/BI/027 hypervirulent strain of *C difficile*.[45] This result gives fidaxomicin an apparent clinical edge over vancomycin. However, the duration of follow-up in the study (4 weeks) may not have been long enough to capture recurrence in all patients. Fidaxomicin is significantly more expensive than oral vancomycin, and dramatically more so than metronidazole. There is also a relative lack of both empirical data and clinical experience, as it is a new therapeutic agent.

Comparative Effectiveness of Antimicrobials

Numerous controlled trials have evaluated the relative effectiveness of various antimi-crobials. Several compare metronidazole and vancomycin, and showed no difference in patients with mild to moderate CDI. In patients with severe CDI, two trials showed a benefit of vancomycin over metronidazole, although one is based on a limited analysis of a small subgroup.[46,47]

A systematic review published in 2011 found that metronidazole, vancomycin, and fidaxomicin were all equally effective for initial therapy. The investigators concur that fidaxomicin appears to have a lower risk of recurrence, but find the evidence supporting superiority of vancomycin in severe CDI to be insufficient, and encourage additional studies.[48]

Antiperistaltic Agents

Antiperistaltic agents (such as loperamide) are generally avoided in the treatment of CDI. The 2010 SHEA/IDSA guidelines recommend against their use "as they may obscure symptoms and precipitate toxic megacolon."[30]

Management of Initial Infection

Assessment of disease severity is a cornerstone of determining treatment for initial CDI. Unfortunately there are no universally accepted or validated criteria for severe disease. The 2010 SHEA/IDSA guidelines propose criteria based on expert opinion, which include as markers of severe disease leukocytosis with a white blood cell count of 15,000 cells/mL or higher, or a serum creatinine level greater than or equal to 1.5 times the patient's baseline level. The guidelines refer to CDI with hypotension, shock, ileus, or megacolon as "complicated" CDI.[30] Other criteria used in research studies in-clude fever or hypothermia, hypoalbuminemia, and advanced age.[47,49] Ultimately, assessment of disease severity relies on the clinical judgment of the treating clinician. The authors suggest criteria to assess severity and a treatment algorithm in **Fig. 3**.

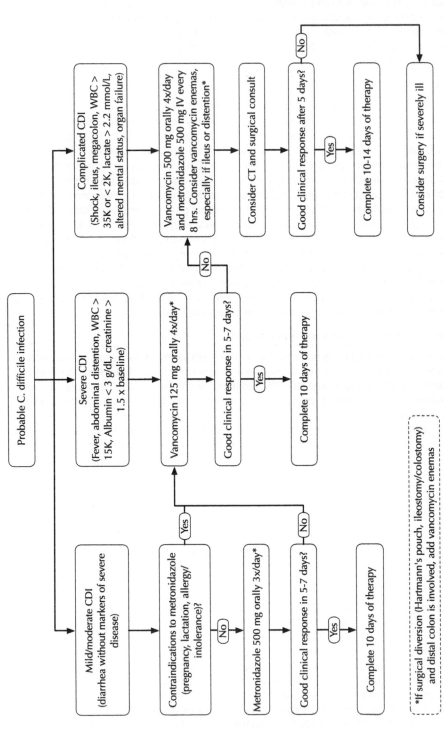

Fig. 3. Algorithm for treatment of initial and first recurrence of *Clostridium difficile* infection. CDI, *C difficile* infection; IV, intravenous; K, thousand; WBC, white blood cells.

Treatment of mild to moderate CDI

Based on evidence showing therapeutic equivalence between metronidazole and van-comycin, the best initial therapy for mild or moderate CDI in patients without contrain-dications (pregnancy, lactation, allergy/intolerance) is metronidazole, 500 mg 3 times daily for 10 days. Patients who have contraindications or are unable to tolerate metro-nidazole should be treated with oral vancomycin, 125 mg 4 times daily for 10 days. Most patients will recover within the first week of therapy.[50] For those who fail to respond after 5 to 7 days, the authors recommend switching to oral vancomycin.

Patients with surgical or anatomic abnormalities in whom oral antibiotics cannot reach the colon (eg, Hartmann pouch, ileostomy, or diverting colostomy) should be given vancomycin enemas (500 mg in 500 mL saline) if the distal colon is involved.[51]

Treatment of severe CDI

Although the data supporting the benefit of vancomycin over metronidazole in severe CDI are limited, it is prudent to start initial treatment with oral vancomycin (125 mg 4 times daily) in patients with fever, leukocytosis, hypoalbuminemia, or worsened renal function (see **Fig. 1**). Patients who fail to respond to low-dose vancomycin after 5 to 7 days may benefit from escalation to high-dose (250–500 mg every 6 hours) oral van-comycin plus intravenous metronidazole, 500 mg 3 times a day.[30,31] Patients who develop ileus, abdominal distention, severe colitis, ascites, or other markers of compli-cated CDI should be treated with oral vancomycin, intravenous metronidazole, and possibly vancomycin enemas.

Treatment of complicated CDI

Patients with complicated CDI (markers include shock, hypotension, ileus, megacolon, severe leukocytosis or leukopenia, elevated serum lactate, altered mental status, and end-organ failure) should be treated with high-dose (500 mg every 6 hours) oral vanco-mycin plus intravenous metronidazole, 500 mg 3 times a day.[30,31] Patients with ileus, abdominal distention, megacolon, or surgical/anatomic abnormalities in whom oral an-tibiotics cannot reach the colon (eg, Hartmann pouch, ileostomy, or diverting colos-tomy) should also be given vancomycin enemas (500 mg in 500 mL saline).[51]

Early surgical consultation is suggested for patients with complicated CDI. Several case series have demonstrated better outcomes with early surgery in patients with fulminant colitis.[52–54] CT of the abdomen may be valuable in assessing disease severity and the need for surgical intervention.

Management of Recurrent Infection

Between 15% and 20% of patients treated for CDI will experience a recurrence of dis-ease within 30 days of initial therapy.[10] Roughly half of recurrent disease is caused by new infection and half by the original organism.[55] Making the distinction clinically is diffi-cult, and does not change management. The most important risk factor for recurrent CDI is intercurrent antibiotic use to treat another infection while completing CDI therapy. Impaired host immune response may be a factor: toxin A is immunogenic, and the pres-ence of antibody to toxin A is associated with a decreased risk of recurrence.[56]

Treatment of first recurrence

Treatment of the first recurrence of CDI follows the same protocol as for initial infec-tion. There is no evidence of increased efficacy of metronidazole or vancomycin, regardless of the drug used for the initial infection.[46] However, patients with severe or complicated recurrent CDI should be treated with vancomycin using the same pa-rameters as for initial infection.

Treatment of second recurrence

Patients with a second recurrence of CDI should be treated with vancomycin rather than metronidazole because of the risk of metronidazole toxicity, especially neurotoxicity, with repeat dosing.[42] Tapering the vancomycin dose or using intermittent "pulsed" dosing may reduce the risk of a subsequent recurrence. One cohort study of patients with recurrent CDI showed that the recurrence rate in the group with pulsed dosing every 2 to 3 days was 14%, compared with 31% with tapered dosing and 40% to 50% with conventional dosing.[57]

Both case series and a randomized trial have shown potential for rifampin and rifaximin to reduce recurrence.[58] However, the randomized study was underpowered to show significant differences, and reports of emerging rifampin resistance suggest that additional study is needed.[59] Rates of recurrence have been shown to be lower with fidaxomicin than with vancomycin when used for initial therapy, but this has never been studied in recurrent CDI.[45]

Treatment of third and subsequent recurrences

Patients with a third or subsequent recurrence of CDI have several therapeutic options, none of which have been definitively studied. Perhaps the most intriguing are efforts to reconstitute the normal fecal microbiota using stool from a healthy donor, a procedure known as fecal microbiota transplantation (FMT).[60] Although reports to date consist largely of case series, a systematic review suggests that resolution is common, occurring a 92% of cases, and adverse events are unusual.[61] One trial, which randomized 43 patients to vancomycin, vancomycin followed by bowel lavage, or a shortened (4 days) course of vancomycin followed by bowel lavage then FMT, found that 81% of patients in the FMT group had no further recurrences after transplant; of the 3 patients who failed to respond, 2 improved with a second transplant, bringing the overall response rate up to 94% 10 weeks after transplant, in comparison with a 23% to 31% response rate in the other 2 groups.[62] Two other randomized trials of FMT are in the recruitment stage at the time of writing.[63,64]

Probiotics, especially S boulardii, have also shown some potential as an adjunct to antibiotics for the treatment of recurrent CDI, although studies are small. A meta-analysis concluded that the evidence for S boulardii is favorable but weak, and additional trials are needed.[65] Fungemia from S boulardii has been reported in patients with central venous catheters, and it should be avoided in critically ill and immunocompromised patients.[66]

REFERENCES

1. Kuipers EJ, Surawicz CM. *Clostridium difficile* infection. Lancet 2008;371(9623): 1486–8.
2. Lessa FC, Gould CV, McDonald LC. Current status of *Clostridium difficile* infection epidemiology. Clin Infect Dis 2012;55(Suppl 2):S65–70.
3. Riegler M, Sedivy R, Pothoulakis C, et al. *Clostridium difficile* toxin B is more potent than toxin A in damaging human colonic epithelium in vitro. J Clin Invest 1995;95(5):2004–11.
4. McDonald LC, Killgore GE, Thompson A, et al. An epidemic, toxin gene-variant strain of *Clostridium difficile*. N Engl J Med 2005;353(23):2433–41.
5. Zilberberg MD, Shorr AF, Kollef MH. Increase in adult *Clostridium difficile*-related hospitalizations and case-fatality rate, United States, 2000-2005. Emerg Infect Dis 2008;14(6):929–31.
6. Diggs NG, Surawicz CM. *Clostridium difficile* infection: still principally a disease of the elderly. Therapy 2010;7(3):295–301.

7. Garey KW, Jiang Z-D, Yadav Y, et al. Peripartum *Clostridium difficile* infection: case series and review of the literature. Am J Obstet Gynecol 2008;199(4): 332–7.

8. Unger JA, Whimbey E, Gravett MG, et al. The emergence of *Clostridium difficile* infection among peripartum women: a case-control study of a *C. difficile* outbreak on an obstetrical service. Infect Dis Obstet Gynecol 2011;2011:267249.

9. Centers for Disease Control and Prevention CDC. Surveillance for community-associated *Clostridium difficile*—Connecticut, 2006. MMWR Morb Mortal Wkly Rep 2008;57(13):340–3.

10. Bartlett JG. Narrative review: the new epidemic of *Clostridium difficile*-associated enteric disease. Ann Intern Med 2006;145(10):758–64.

11. Owens RC, Donskey CJ, Gaynes RP, et al. Antimicrobial-associated risk factors for *Clostridium difficile* infection. Clin Infect Dis 2008;46(Suppl 1):S19–31.

12. Hensgens MP, Goorhuis A, Dekkers OM, et al. Time interval of increased risk for *Clostridium difficile* infection after exposure to antibiotics. J Antimicrob Chemother 2012;67(3):742–8.

13. Vesteinsdottir I, Gudlaugsdottir S, Einarsdottir R, et al. Risk factors for *Clostridium difficile* toxin-positive diarrhea: a population-based prospective case-control study. Eur J Clin Microbiol Infect Dis 2012;31(10):2601–10.

14. Kutty PK, Woods CW, Sena AC, et al. Risk factors for and estimated incidence of community-associated *Clostridium difficile* infection, North Carolina, USA. Emerg Infect Dis 2010;16(2):197–204.

15. Bavishi C, Dupont HL. Systematic review: the use of proton pump inhibitors and increased susceptibility to enteric infection. Aliment Pharmacol Ther 2011; 34(11–12):1269–81.

16. Howell MD, Novack V, Grgurich P, et al. Iatrogenic gastric acid suppression and the risk of nosocomial *Clostridium difficile* infection. Arch Intern Med 2010; 170(9):784–90.

17. Deshpande A, Pant C, Pasupuleti V, et al. Association between proton pump inhibitor therapy and *Clostridium difficile* infection in a meta-analysis. Clin Gastroenterol Hepatol 2012;10(3):225–33.

18. Janarthanan S, Ditah I, Adler DG, et al. *Clostridium difficile*-associated diarrhea and proton pump inhibitor therapy: a meta-analysis. Am J Gastroenterol 2012; 107(7):1001–10.

19. Kwok CS, Arthur AK, Anibueze CI, et al. Risk of *Clostridium difficile* infection with acid suppressing drugs and antibiotics: meta-analysis. Am J Gastroenterol 2012;107(7):1011–9.

20. Rodemann JF, Dubberke ER, Reske KA, et al. Incidence of *Clostridium difficile* infection in inflammatory bowel disease. Clin Gastroenterol Hepatol 2007;5(3): 339–44.

21. Issa M, Ananthakrishnan AN, Binion DG. *Clostridium difficile* and inflammatory bowel disease. Inflamm Bowel Dis 2008;14(10):1432–42.

22. Dansinger ML, Johnson S, Jansen PC, et al. Protein-losing enteropathy is associated with *Clostridium difficile* diarrhea but not with asymptomatic colonization: a prospective, case-control study. Clin Infect Dis 1996;22(6):932–7.

23. Fujitani S, George WL, Murthy AR. Comparison of clinical severity score indices for *Clostridium difficile* infection. Infect Control Hosp Epidemiol 2011;32(3):220–8.

24. Wanahita A, Goldsmith EA, Marino BJ, et al. *Clostridium difficile* infection in patients with unexplained leukocytosis. Am J Med 2003;115(7):543–6.

25. Planche T, Wilcox M. Reference assays for *Clostridium difficile* infection: one or two gold standards? J Clin Pathol 2011;64(1):1–5.

26. Planche T, Aghaizu A, Holliman R, et al. Diagnosis of *Clostridium difficile* infection by toxin detection kits: a systematic review. Lancet Infect Dis 2008;8(12): 777–84.

27. Shetty N, Wren MW, Coen PG. The role of glutamate dehydrogenase for the detection of *Clostridium difficile* in faecal samples: a meta-analysis. J Hosp Infect 2011;77(1):1–6.

28. Deshpande A, Pasupuleti V, Rolston DD, et al. Diagnostic accuracy of real-time polymerase chain reaction in detection of *Clostridium difficile* in the stool samples of patients with suspected *Clostridium difficile* infection: a meta-analysis. Clin Infect Dis 2011;53(7):e81–90.

29. Boyanton BL, Sural P, Loomis CR, et al. Loop-mediated isothermal amplification compared to real-time PCR and enzyme immunoassay for toxigenic *Clostridium difficile* detection. J Clin Microbiol 2012;50(3):640–5.

30. Cohen SH, Gerding DN, Johnson S, et al. Clinical practice guidelines for *Clostridium difficile* infection in adults: 2010 update by the Society for Healthcare Epidemiology of America (SHEA) and the Infectious Diseases Society of America (IDSA). Infect Control Hosp Epidemiol 2010;31(5):431–55.

31. Surawicz CM, McFarland LV, Greenberg RN, et al. The search for a better treatment for recurrent *Clostridium difficile* disease: use of high-dose vancomycin combined with *Saccharomyces boulardii*. Clin Infect Dis 2000;31(4):1012–7.

32. Wilcox MH, Freeman J, Fawley W, et al. Long-term surveillance of cefotaxime and piperacillin-tazobactam prescribing and incidence of *Clostridium difficile* diarrhoea. J Antimicrob Chemother 2004;54(1):168–72.

33. Climo MW, Israel DS, Wong ES, et al. Hospital-wide restriction of clindamycin: effect on the incidence of *Clostridium difficile*-associated diarrhea and cost. Ann Intern Med 1998;128(12 Pt 1):989–95.

34. Valiquette L, Cossette B, Garant M-P, et al. Impact of a reduction in the use of high-risk antibiotics on the course of an epidemic of *Clostridium difficile*-associated disease caused by the hypervirulent NAP1/027 strain. Clin Infect Dis 2007; 45(Suppl 2):S112–21.

35. Dellit TH, Owens RC, McGowan JE, et al. Infectious Diseases Society of America and the Society for Healthcare Epidemiology of America guidelines for developing an institutional program to enhance antimicrobial stewardship. Clin Infect Dis 2007;44(2):159–77.

36. Wullt M, Odenholt I, Walder M. Activity of three disinfectants and acidified nitrite against *Clostridium difficile* spores. Infect Control Hosp Epidemiol 2003;24(10): 765–8.

37. Johnson S, Gerding DN, Olson MM, et al. Prospective, controlled study of vinyl glove use to interrupt *Clostridium difficile* nosocomial transmission. Am J Med 1990;88(2):137–40.

38. Mayfield JL, Leet T, Miller J, et al. Environmental control to reduce transmission of *Clostridium difficile*. Clin Infect Dis 2000;31(4):995–1000.

39. Wilcox MH, Fawley WN, Wigglesworth N, et al. Comparison of the effect of detergent versus hypochlorite cleaning on environmental contamination and incidence of *Clostridium difficile* infection. J Hosp Infect 2003;54(2):109–14.

40. Johnston BC, Ma SS, Goldenberg JZ, et al. Probiotics for the prevention of *Clostridium difficile*-associated diarrhea: a systematic review and meta-analysis. Ann Intern Med 2012;157(12):878–88.

41. Bolton RP, Culshaw MA. Faecal metronidazole concentrations during oral and intravenous therapy for antibiotic associated colitis due to *Clostridium difficile*. Gut 1986;27(10):1169–72.

42. Kapoor K, Chandra M, Nag D, et al. Evaluation of metronidazole toxicity: a prospective study. Int J Clin Pharmacol Res 1999;19(3):83–8.

43. Nerandzic MM, Mullane K, Miller MA, et al. Reduced acquisition and overgrowth of vancomycin-resistant enterococci and Candida species in patients treated with fidaxomicin versus vancomycin for *Clostridium difficile* infection. Clin Infect Dis 2012;55(Suppl 2):S121–6.

44. Finegold SM, Molitoris D, Vaisanen ML, et al. In vitro activities of OPT-80 and comparator drugs against intestinal bacteria. Antimicrobial Agents Chemother 2004;48(12):4898–902.

45. Louie TJ, Miller MA, Mullane KM, et al. Fidaxomicin versus vancomycin for *Clostridium difficile* infection. N Engl J Med 2011;364(5):422–31.

46. Pepin J, Valiquette L, Gagnon S, et al. Outcomes of *Clostridium difficile*-associated disease treated with metronidazole or vancomycin before and after the emergence of NAP1/027. Am J Gastroenterol 2007;102(12):2781–8.

47. Zar FA, Bakkanagari SR, Moorthi KM, et al. A comparison of vancomycin and metronidazole for the treatment of *Clostridium difficile*-associated diarrhea, stratified by disease severity. Clin Infect Dis 2007;45(3):302–7.

48. Drekonja DM, Butler M, MacDonald R, et al. Comparative effectiveness of *Clostridium difficile* treatments: a systematic review. Ann Intern Med 2011;155(12): 839–47.

49. Al-Nassir WN, Sethi AK, Nerandzic MM, et al. Comparison of clinical and microbiological response to treatment of *Clostridium difficile*-associated disease with metronidazole and vancomycin. Clin Infect Dis 2008;47(1):56–62.

50. Musher DM, Aslam S, Logan N, et al. Relatively poor outcome after treatment of *Clostridium difficile* colitis with metronidazole. Clin Infect Dis 2005;40(11): 1586–90.

51. Apisarnthanarak A, Razavi B, Mundy LM. Adjunctive intracolonic vancomycin for severe *Clostridium difficile* colitis: case series and review of the literature. Clin Infect Dis 2002;35(6):690–6.

52. Markelov A, Livert D, Kohli H. Predictors of fatal outcome after colectomy for fulminant *Clostridium difficile* Colitis: a 10-year experience. Am Surg 2011; 77(8):977–80.

53. Ali SO, Welch JP, Dring RJ. Early surgical intervention for fulminant pseudomembranous colitis. Am Surg 2008;74(1):20–6.

54. Butala P, Divino CM. Surgical aspects of fulminant *Clostridium difficile* colitis. Am J Surg 2010;200(1):131–5.

55. Barbut F, Richard A, Hamadi K, et al. Epidemiology of recurrences or reinfections of *Clostridium difficile*-associated diarrhea. J Clin Microbiol 2000;38(6):2386–8.

56. Kyne L, Warny M, Qamar A, et al. Association between antibody response to toxin A and protection against recurrent *Clostridium difficile* diarrhoea. Lancet 2001;357(9251):189–93.

57. McFarland LV, Elmer GW, Surawicz CM. Breaking the cycle: treatment strategies for 163 cases of recurrent *Clostridium difficile* disease. Am J Gastroenterol 2002;97(7):1769–75.

58. Garey KW, Ghantoji SS, Shah DN, et al. A randomized, double-blind, placebo-controlled pilot study to assess the ability of rifaximin to prevent recurrent diarrhoea in patients with *Clostridium difficile* infection. J Antimicrob Chemother 2011;66(12):2850–5.

59. Curry SR, Marsh JW, Shutt KA, et al. High frequency of rifampin resistance identified in an epidemic *Clostridium difficile* clone from a large teaching hospital. Clin Infect Dis 2009;48(4):425–9.

60. Bakken JS, Borody T, Brandt LJ, et al. Treating *Clostridium difficile* infection with fecal microbiota transplantation. Clin Gastroenterol Hepatol 2011;9(12):1044–9.
61. Gough E, Shaikh H, Manges AR. Systematic review of intestinal microbiota transplantation (fecal bacteriotherapy) for recurrent *Clostridium difficile* infection. Clin Infect Dis 2011;53(10):994–1002.
62. van Nood E, Vrieze A, Nieuwdorp M, et al. Duodenal infusion of donor feces for recurrent *Clostridium difficile*. N Engl J Med 2013;368(5):407–15.
63. Oral vancomycin followed by fecal transplant versus tapering oral vancomycin. Available at: ClinicalTrials.gov. Accessed on December 15, 2012.
64. Fecal transplant for relapsing *C. difficile* infection. Available at: ClinicalTrials. gov. Accessed on December 15, 2012.
65. McFarland LV. Systematic review and meta-analysis of *Saccharomyces boulardii* in adult patients. World J Gastroenterol 2010;16(18):2202–22.
66. Enache-Angoulvant A, Hennequin C. Invasive *Saccharomyces* infection: a comprehensive review. Clin Infect Dis 2005;41(11):1559–68.

Lower Gastrointestinal Bleeding

Marcie Feinman, MD, Elliott R. Haut, MD*

KEYWORDS

- Hematochezia • Melena • Diverticulosis • Angiodysplasia

KEY POINTS

- Lower gastrointestinal bleeding is likely under-reported and remains a common causes of emergency department visits.
- Localization of bleeding is key to forming an appropriate treatment plan.
- Whether the bleeding is occult, moderate, or severe dictates the workup.
- Hemodynamically unstable patients require immediate intervention.
- Although minimally invasive techniques are often sufficient to stop the bleeding, there is still a role for surgery in certain patient populations.

INTRODUCTION

Lower gastrointestinal (GI) bleeding has an annual incidence of about 20 to 27 cases per 100,000 population in developed countries. However, it is thought that this number is falsely low because of the substantial number of patients who do not seek medical care.[1] Although lower GI bleeding is not as common as upper GI bleeding, it remains a frequent cause of hospital admissions and carries a mortality of up to 10% to 20%.

Lower GI bleeding can be classified into 3 groups based on the severity of bleeding: occult lower GI bleeding, moderate lower GI bleeding, and severe lower GI bleeding.

Patients of any age can present with occult lower GI bleeding. Because the bleed tends to be slow and chronic, patients have microcytic, hypochromic anemia. Stool guiac will be positive.

Often presenting with melena or hematochezia, moderate bleeding can occur in patients of any age. Despite the obvious bleeding, patients remain hemodynamically stable.

Patients with severe lower GI bleeding present hemodynamically unstable with heart rates greater than 100 and systolic blood pressure less than 90. They have associated low urine output and decreased hemoglobin levels. Hematochezia is

This article originally appeared in Surgical Clinics, Volume 94, Issue 1, February 2014.
Division of Acute Care Surgery, Department of Surgery, Anesthesiology/Critical Care Medicine (ACCM), Emergency Medicine, The Johns Hopkins University School of Medicine, Sheikh Zayed Tower, 1800 Orleans Street, Suite 6017, Baltimore, MD 21287, USA
* Corresponding author.
E-mail address: ehaut1@jhmi.edu

prominent. This tends to occur in elderly patients older than 65 years and has an associated mortality of 21%.[2]

BLOOD SUPPLY

Lower GI bleeding is defined as any bleed that occurs distal to the ligament of Treitz. Although the colon is the most likely source of bleeding, small bowel disease can occur. In addition, upper GI sources must always be considered in a patient who presents with bleeding per rectum.

Midgut

The midgut is defined as all structures between the foregut and the hindgut. This includes the distal duodenum, jejunum, ileum, appendix, cecum, ascending colon, hepatic flexure, and proximal transverse colon. The superior mesenteric artery (SMA) and its branches provide the blood supply to the midgut. Venous drainage is via the portal system.

Hindgut

The hindgut includes the distal one-third of the transverse colon, the splenic flexure, descending colon, sigmoid colon, and rectum. Blood supply is mainly via the inferior mesenteric artery (IMA), with rectal perfusion through the superior, middle, and inferior rectal arteries. Venous drainage is via the portal system, with the exception of the lower rectum, which drains into the systemic circulation.

The SMA and IMA are connected by the marginal artery of Drummond. This vascular arcade runs in the mesentery close to the bowel and is almost always present. As patients age, there is increased incidence of occlusion of the IMA. The left colon stays perfused, primarily because of the marginal artery (**Fig. 1**).

PATHOPHYSIOLOGY

Lower GI bleeding has multiple causes, each with its own morbidity attributed to the underlying pathophysiology. Multiple studies of the incidence and etiology of lower GI bleeding found that diverticulosis was the most common at 30%, followed by anorectal disease (14%–20%), ischemia (12%), inflammatory bowel disease (IBD) (9%), neoplasia (6%) and arteriovenous (AV) malformations (3%).[3,4]

Diverticulosis

With age, the colonic wall weakens and develops diverticula. These saclike protrusions generally occur where the penetrating vessel perforates through the circular muscle fibers, resulting in only mucosa separating the vessel from the bowel lumen. It is estimated that approximately 50% of adults over the age of 60 have radiologic evidence of diverticula, most commonly in the descending and sigmoid colon, and 20% of these patients will go on to develop bleeding. Despite the majority of diverticula being on the left side of the colon, diverticular bleeding originates from the right side of the colon in 50% to 90% of instances.[5] This bleeding stops spontaneously in the most patients; however, in about 5% of patients, the bleeding can be massive and life-threatening.

Anorectal Disease

Anorectal disease encompasses many etiologies, including hemorrhoids and anal fissures.

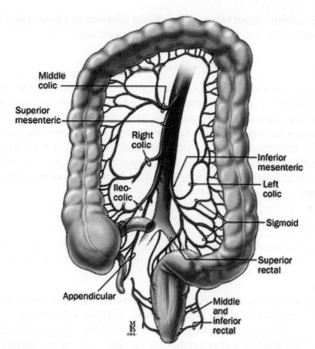

Fig. 1. Arterial blood supply of the colon and rectum. (*Courtesy of* Johns Hopkins Medicine Colorectal Center, Baltimore, MD. Available at: http://www.hopkinscoloncancercenter.org/CMS/CMS_Page.aspx?CurrentUDV=59&CMS_Page_ID=1F7C07D4-268D-4635-8975-70A594870CC8.)

Hemorrhoids

Hemorrhoids may be internal or external, although internal hemorrhoids (above the dentate line) are generally the type that cause rapid rectal bleeding. Hemorrhoids are engorged vessels in the normal anal cushions. When swollen, this tissue is very friable and susceptible to trauma, which leads to painless, bright red bleeding.

Anal fissures

Fissures begin with a tear in the anal mucosa. The tear may resolve, in which case it is an acute anal fissure, or it may persist and become a chronic anal fissure. With the passage of stool, the mucosa continues to tear and leads to bright red bleeding. Anal fissures generally occur in the midline, and any fissure off the midline should prompt a workup for an underlying etiology.

Mesenteric Ischemia

Mesenteric ischemia is caused by a mismatch in the supply and demand of oxygen at the level of the small intestine. Most commonly, this is caused by inadequate circulation to the bowel and may be embolic, thombotic, or nonocclusive (NOMI) in nature. For symptoms to occur, 2 or more vessels (celiac, SMA, or IMA) need to be affected. Cardiac disease and known atherosclerosis are big risk factors for acute mesenteric ischemia secondary to emboli or thromboses. NOMI affects critically ill patients who are vasopressor dependent. The vasoconstriction caused by these medications (especially vasopressin) results in a low-flow state to the small bowel.[6] Venous thrombosis of the visceral vessels can also precipitate an acute ischemic event.

Compromised venous return leads to interstitial swelling in the bowel wall, with subsequent impedance of arterial flow and eventual necrosis.

Ischemic Colitis

Ischemic colitis is caused by poor perfusion of the colon, which results in the inability of that area of the colon to meet its metabolic demands. It can be gangrenous or nongangrenous, acute, transient, or chronic. The left colon is predominantly affected, with the splenic flexure having increased susceptibility.[7] Intraluminal hemorrhage occurs as the mucosa becomes necrotic, sloughs, and bleeds. Damage to the tissue is caused both with the ischemic insult as well as reperfusion injury. The colon is affected from the mucosa outward, with perforation a late finding only after all layers of the colon are involved.

Inflammatory Bowel Disease

Crohn disease and ulcerative colitis are the main disease states under the heading of IBD. Both are autoimmune in nature and lead to unopposed inflammation.

Crohn disease

T cell activation stimulates interleukin (IL)-12 and tumor necrosis factor (TNF)-α, which causes chronic inflammation and tissue injury. Initially, inflammation starts focally around the crypts, followed by superficial ulceration of the mucosa. The deep mucosal layers are then invaded in a noncontinuous fashion, and noncaseating granulomas form, which can invade through the entire thickness of the bowel and into the mesentery and surrounding structures.[8] The granulomas are pathognomonic of Crohn disease; however, their absence does not exclude this diagnosis.

Ulcerative colitis

T cells cytotoxic to the colonic epithelium accumulate in the lamina propria, accompanied by B cells that secrete immunoglobulin G (IgG) and IgE. This results in inflammation of the crypts of Lieberkuhn, with abscesses and pseudopolyps.[8] Whereas Crohn disease can affect any part of the GI tract, ulcerative colitis generally begins at the rectum and is a continuous process confined exclusively to the colon.

Neoplasia

Colon carcinoma follows a distinct progression from polyp to cancer. Mutations of multiple genes are required for the formation of adenocarcinoma, including the APC gene, Kras, DCC, and p53. Certain hereditary syndromes are also classified by defects in DNA mismatch repair genes and microsatellite instability. These tumors tend to bleed slowly, and patients present with hemocult positive stools and microcytic anemia. Although cancers of the small bowel are much less common than colorectal cancers, they should be ruled out in cases of lower GI bleeding in which no other source is identified.

AV Malformation/Angiodysplasia

AV malformation

These direct connections between arteries and veins can occur in the colonic submucosa (or anywhere else in the GI tract). The lack of capillary buffers causes high pressure blood to enter directly into the venous system, making these vessels at high risk of rupture into the bowel lumen.

Angiodysplasia

Over time, previously healthy blood vessels of the cecum and ascending colon degenerate and become prone to bleeding. Although 75% of angiodysplasia cases involve the right colon, they are a significant cause of obscure bleeding and the most common cause of bleeding from the small bowel in the elderly.[9]

CLINICAL PRESENTATION

Lower GI bleeding can range from occult to massive and life threatening. The clinical findings differ based on the severity of the bleed and the underlying cause. **Table 1** consists of possible signs/symptoms/laboratory values with which patients with lower GI bleeding may present. Some things do not help figure out source—weakness, dizziness, syncope.

WORKUP AND INITIAL TREATMENT

Workup should begin with resuscitation as needed (covered more fully in the upper GI section).

Next, one should rule out an upper GI source of bleeding. Nasogastric tube (NGT) lavage should be performed in all patients with lower GI bleeding to rule out an upper GI source. In order to completely exclude an upper GI bleed, the NGT lavage must return bilious fluid without blood. Obtaining clear fluid only, while favoring a lower GI source, does not completely rule out duodenal bleeding distal to the pylorus, but proximal to the ligament of Treitz (classically a duodenal ulcer).

LOCALIZE AND STOP THE BLEEDING

Many options exist to determine where the bleeding originates from when distal to the ligament of Treitz. Which test or combination of tests to choose is determined by the patient's age, medical history, rate of bleeding, and hemodynamic stability.

Colonoscopy

Often considered the initial diagnostic modality of choice, colonoscopy can identify the origin of severe LGI bleeding in 74% to 82% of patients.[10] This invasive procedure is not without disadvantages. In order to be effective, a mechanical bowel preparation is sometimes performed, which will delay the endoscopy. A mechanical bowel preparation is not required, especially in those patients with rapid bleeding, because the blood will often act as cathartic to clean out the colon. In addition, patients require sedation, which carries its own risks. As long as patients remain stable during the bowel preparation and sedation, colonoscopy then has the advantage of not only localizing the source of bleeding, but also allowing intervention via clips, epinephrine injection, thermoregulation, or laser photocoagulation. Per the Scottish Intercollegiate Guidelines Network (SIGN) guidelines, in patients with massive lower GI bleeding, colonoscopic hemostasis is an effective means of controlling bleeding from a diverticular source when appropriately skilled providers are available.[11] Studies have looked into the timing of colonoscopy to attempt to ascertain if early endoscopy has any benefit. A randomized, controlled trial found that urgent colonoscopy (defined as within 8 hours of presentation) had improved diagnosis but not improved outcomes as compared to standard colonoscopy (within 48 hours of presentation).[12]

Table 1
Clinical presentation of lower GI bleeding

	History	Physical Examination	Laboratory Findings
Diverticulosis	Can have bloating or cramping, afebrile, often symptomatic	Hematochezia (brisk bleed/left colon) or melena (slow bleed/right colon), no abdominal tenderness	Decreased hemoglobin, possible microcytic hypochromic anemia (chronic occult bleed)
Crohn disease	Crampy abdominal pain, diarrhea, steatorrhea, fatigue, weight loss, arthritis, eye complaints, skin disorders, renal stones	Stool guaiac positive, abdominal tenderness, possible right lower quadrant mass, possible enterocutaneous fistula, possible anal fissure/fistula	Microcytic hypochromic anemia, B12 deficiency, elevated C-reactive protein (CRP)/erythrocyte sedimentation rate (ESR), increased white blood cells (WBCs)
Ulcerative colitis	Colicky abdominal pain, urgency, tenesmus, incontinence, diarrhea or constipation (if distal disease)	Gross blood on rectal examination, abdominal tenderness, peripheral edema, muscle wasting	Anemia, elevated ESR, low albumin, elevated fecal lactoferrin, possible elevated alkaline phosphatase
Mesenteric ischemia	Pain out of proportion to examination (periumbilical), nausea/vomiting, bloody diarrhea, weight loss, food avoidance	Minimal findings, no peritonitis, stool guaiac positive	Increased WBCs, increased lactate, metabolic acidosis, possible elevated amylase
Ischemic colitis	Mild-to-moderate abdominal pain (lateral), bloody diarrhea	Abdominal tenderness (left greater than right), gross blood on rectal examination	Increased WBCs, elevated lactate, amylase, creatine phosphokinase (CPK) and lactate dehydrogenase (LDH), metabolic acidosis, anemia
Hemorrhoids	Painless bleeding, itching, mild incontinence, history of cirrhosis	Prolapsed hemorrhoids, gross blood on rectal examination, stigmata of liver disease	Iron deficiency anemia (if chronic), possible elevated liver function tests/coagulopathy
Anal fissure	Tearing pain with bowel movements, perianal pruritis	Severe pain on rectal examination, bright red blood	Often normal
Neoplasia	Abdominal pain, distention, decreased caliber of stool, tenesmus, rectal pain, weight loss	Palpable mass, abdominal tenderness, guiac-positive stool, rectal mass on direct rectal examination (DRE), pallor	Microcytic hypochromic anemia, possible elevated carcinoembryonic antigen
AV malformation/angiodysplasia	Painless rectal bleeding	Asymptomatic, hematochezia, or melena	Anemia

Nuclear Scintigraphy

This diagnostic modality can detect bleeding rates between 0.1 and 0.5 cc/min. Considered 10 times more sensitive than mesenteric angiography for detecting bleeding, nuclear scintigraphy is a sensitive diagnostic tool (86% sensitivity). However, the specificity is only 50%. One study by Ng and colleagues[13] determined that time to positivity of a nuclear medicine scan helped guide further treatment. If a blush was seen within 2 minutes of starting the scan, there was a positive predictive value of 75% on angiography. Conversely, if the blush occurred beyond 2 minutes, this was associated with a negative predictive value of 93% for angiography. In addition to low specificity, nuclear scintigraphy has several other disadvantages. These include the lack of ability to intervene during the study, as well as the fact that patients need to be actively bleeding at the time of the test to have a positive result. Because of this, many authors advocate using nuclear scintigraphy as a screening modality only to determine which patients would benefit from mesenteric angiography. While not a strong recommendation, the SIGN guidelines suggest considering nuclear scintigraphy to assist in localizing lower GI bleeding in patients with recent hemorrhage.[11]

Angiography

Angiography can be used when colonoscopy fails to localize a bleeding source, or when bleeding is so brisk as to preclude colonoscopy as a useful diagnostic modality. Requiring a minimum bleed of 0.5 cc/min, angiography has the benefit of being both diagnostic and potentially therapeutic in brisk bleeds. Interventions include selective vasopressin infusions and superselective angioembolization. Generally, the SMA is investigated first, because much lower GI bleeding arises from the right colon. This is followed by the IMA next and the celiac trunk last, if necessary. The disadvantages of angiography include a low sensitivity (only about 30%–47%) and the requirement of a substantial amount of active bleeding at the time of the study in order to be positive. However, if the patient does have brisk active bleeding, emergency angiography and vasopressin infusion have been shown to improve operative morbidity, mortality, and outcome.[14] In patients with massive lower GI bleeding, if colonoscopy fails to identify and control the site of hemorrhage, transarterial embolization is recommended.[11]

Surgical Intervention

Emergency surgery may be needed to control bleeding in about 10% to 25% of patients in whom nonoperative management is unsuccessful or unavailable.[15] Indications for emergent surgery include hemodynamic instability with active bleeding, persistent recurrent bleeding, or transfusion requirement of greater than 6 units of packed red blood cells (PRBCs) in 24 hours with active bleeding.[10] Patients requiring ten or more units of PRBCs in 24 hours have a significantly greater mortality than patients who receive less than 10 units of blood (45% vs 7%).[16] Therefore, the commonly accepted transfusion trigger to perform surgery for a lower GI bleed is 6 units of PRBCs to avoid the mortality associated with giving more blood and delaying definitive management. If emergency surgery is required, definitive localization of the bleeding site is ideal, because segmental colonic resection is preferred. However, segmental resection should be avoided unless the source is definitely identified, because this operation is associated with high rebleeding, morbidity, and mortality rates. If the bleed cannot be localized, a subtotal colectomy is the recommended procedure. Bleeding caused by tumors should be resected with the appropriate oncologic procedure to ensure adequate margins and lymph nodes in the specimen.

OBSCURE BLEEDING

Although the colon is by far the most likely source of lower GI bleeding, the small bowel can also be affected. This part of the GI tract has traditionally been difficult to evaluate; however, many new modalities are available for visualization. Wireless capsule endoscopy is the most widely used for diagnosis of small bowel bleeding. Although it does not have therapeutic capabilities, capsule endoscopy is noninvasive and allows visualization of the complete small bowel, leading to improved diagnosis over alternative modalities.[17] Other options for diagnosis of a small bowel source of bleeding are push enteroscopy or double balloon enteroscopy. Despite the potential therapeutic advantage of enteroscopy, the invasive nature of the procedure and the ability to only evaluate the most proximal 60 cm of jejunum make these options less attractive than capsule endoscopy. Surgical management of massive occult lower GI bleeding may include the use of intraoperative enteroscopy. Intraoperative Enteroscopy (IOE) remains indicated when: (1) small bowel lesions have been identified by a preoperative work-up; (2) lesions cannot be managed by angio-embolization and/or endoscopic methods, or when surgery is required for complete treatment (ie, small bowel tumors), and (3) bleeding cannot be localized during surgical explorations. The ability of IOE to identify bleeding lesions is good and has been shown to be equal to the video capsule endoscopy diagnostic yield, with a higher sensitivity than push–pull enteroscopy.[18] However, this invasive procedure carries a 16.8% morbidity and should only be used if all other methods fail.[19]

SUMMARY

Although not as common as upper GI bleeding, bleeding that originates distal to the ligament of Treitz remains a frequent cause of hospital admissions, with a significant associated morbidity and mortality. Workup should focus on stabilization of the patient primarily, followed by localization and cessation of the bleed. Various modalities exist for these purposes and should be chosen based on patient presentation and severity of the bleeding. Although incredible advances have been made in minimally invasive options for treatment of lower GI bleeds, surgery remains a viable option for patients who remain unstable despite adequate resuscitation and for those who fail more conservative treatments.

REFERENCES

1. Talley NJ, Jones M. Self-reported rectal bleeding in a United States community: prevalence, risk factors, and health care seeking. Am J Gastroenterol 1998; 93(11):2179–83.
2. Longstreth GF. Epidemiology and outcome of patients hospitalized with acute lower gastrointestinal hemorrhage: a population-based study. Am J Gastroenterol 1997;92(3):419–24.
3. Ghassemi KA, Jensen DM. Lower GI bleeding: epidemiology and management. Curr Gastroenterol Rep 2013;15:333.
4. Gayer C, Chino A, Lucas C, et al. Acute lower gastrointestinal bleeding in 1,112 patients admitted to an urban emergency medical center. Surgery 2009;146(4): 600–6 [discussion: 606–7].
5. Meyers MA, Alonso DR, Gray GF, et al. Pathogenesis of bleeding colonic diverticulosis. Gastroenterology 1976;71(4):577–83.
6. Chang RW, Chang JB, Longo W. Update in management of mesenteric ischemia. World J Gastroenterol 2006;12(20):3243–7.

7. Theodoropoulou A, Koutroubakis IE. Ischemic colitis: clinical practice in diagnosis and treatment. World J Gastroenterol 2008;14(48):7302-8.
8. Thoreson R, Cullen JJ. Pathophysiology of inflammatory bowel disease: an overview. Surg Clin North Am 2007;87(3):575-85.
9. Regula J, Wronska E, Pachlewski J. Vascular lesions of the gastrointestinal tract. Best Pract Res Clin Gastroenterol 2008;22(2):313-28.
10. Vernava AM III, Moore BA, Longo WE, et al. Lower gastrointestinal bleeding. Dis Colon Rectum 1997;40(7):846-58.
11. Scottish Intercollegiate Guidelines Network (SIGN). Management of acute upper and lower gastrointestinal bleeding. A national clinical guideline. SIGN Publication; no. 105. Edinburgh (Scotland): Scottish Intercollegiate Guidelines Network (SIGN); 2008.
12. Green BT, Rockey DC, Portwood G, et al. Urgent colonoscopy for evaluation and management of acute lower gastrointestinal hemorrhage: a randomized controlled trial. Am J Gastroenterol 2005;100(11):2395-402.
13. Ng DA, Opelka FG, Beck DE, et al. Predictive value of technetium Tc 99m-labeled red blood cell scintigraphy for positive angiogram in massive lower gastrointestinal hemorrhage. Dis Colon Rectum 1997;40(4):471-7.
14. Browder W, Cerise EJ, Litwin MS. Impact of emergency angiography in massive lower gastrointestinal bleeding. Ann Surg 1986;204(5):530-6.
15. Chalasani N, Wilcox CM. Etiology and outcome of lower gastrointestinal bleeding in patients with AIDS. Am J Gastroenterol 1998;93(2):175-8.
16. Bender JS, Wiencek RG, Bouwman DL. Morbidity and mortality following total abdominal colectomy for massive lower gastrointestinal bleeding. Am Surg 1991;57:536-41.
17. Ell C, Remke S, May A, et al. The first prospective controlled trial comparing wireless capsule endoscopy with push enteroscopy in chronic gastrointestinal bleeding. Endoscopy 2002;34(9):685-9.
18. Hartmann D, Schmidt H, Bolz G, et al. A prospective two-center study comparing wireless capsule endoscopy with intraoperative enteroscopy in patients with obscure GI bleeding. Gastrointest Endosc 2005;61:826-32.
19. Bonnet S, Douard R, Malamut G, et al. Intraoperative enteroscopy in the management of obscure gastrointestinal bleeding. Dig Liver Dis 2013;45(4):277-84.

Modern Management of Hemorrhoidal Disease

Jason F. Hall, MD, MPH[a,b],*

KEYWORDS

- Hemorrhoids • Nonoperative management • Hemorrhoidectomy
- Internal hemorrhoids • External hemorrhoids • Prolapsing hemorrhoids
- Thrombosed hemorrhoids

KEY POINTS

- Most hemorrhoidal complaints can be managed nonoperatively.
- Symptomatic internal hemorrhoids typically cause rectal bleeding.
- Symptomatic external hemorrhoids typically cause thrombosis and pain.
- Providers should be familiar with several different techniques to address hemorrhoidal complaints.
- Rubber band ligation is generally helpful in addressing hemorrhoidal bleeding that has not improved with nonoperative treatment.
- Excisional hemorrhoidectomy is effective in managing prolapsing or recurrent hemorrhoidal disease.

INTRODUCTION

Complaints secondary to hemorrhoidal disease have been treated by health care providers for at least 4000 years (**Table 1**).[1] John of Ardene (1307–1390), a surgeon in the English Middle Ages, reportedly stated: "The common people call them piles, the aristocracy call them hemorrhoids, the French call them figs—what does it matter so long as you can cure them?"[2] Most hemorrhoidal presentations can be managed nonoperatively. When hemorrhoidal symptoms do not respond to medical therapy, procedural intervention is recommended. A firm grasp of anorectal anatomy is essential for choosing the appropriate method of treatment. This article reviews the anatomy and pathophysiology of hemorrhoidal disease and the most commonly used techniques for the nonoperative and operative palliation of hemorrhoidal complaints.

This article originally appeared in Gastroenterology Clinics, Volume 42, Issue 4, December 2013.

Disclosures: The author has no relevant disclosures.

[a] Department of Colon and Rectal Surgery, Lahey Clinic, 41 Mall Road, Burlington, MA 01805, USA; [b] Department of Surgery, Tufts University School of Medicine, 145 Harrison Avenue, Boston, MA 02111, USA

* Department of Colon and Rectal Surgery, Lahey Clinic, 41 Mall Road, Burlington, MA 01805.

E-mail address: jason.f.hall@lahey.org

Clinics Collections 7 (2015) 603–616

http://dx.doi.org/10.1016/j.ccol.2015.06.040

Table 1
Clinical classification of hemorrhoidal pathology

	Location/Size	Symptoms
First degree	Bulge into anal canal	Painless bleeding
Second degree	Exit the anal canal with defecation Reduce spontaneously	Painless bleeding Pruritus
Third degree	Prolapse from anal canal with defecation Require manual reduction	Painless bleeding Pruritus Mucous/fecal leakage
Fourth degree	Permanent prolapse from anal canal Not reducible	Pain Bleeding Mucous/fecal leakage

ANATOMY AND PATHOPHYSIOLOGY

Hemorrhoids are specialized, vascular cushions located in the anal canal. Hemorrhoids are typically clustered into three anatomically distinct cushions located in the left lateral, right anterolateral, and right posterolateral anal canal (**Fig. 1**). They are found in the submucosal layer and are considered sinusoids because they do not typically have a muscular wall.[3] Hemorrhoids are held in the anal canal by Treitz muscle, a submucosal extension of the conjoined longitudinal ligament. The fibers seem to act as a support lattice not only for hemorrhoids but for other important structures in the anal canal. Some authors have reported a loss of these support structures with aging, perhaps explaining the increased incidence of hemorrhoidal complaints with age.[4]

Hemorrhoidal structures are typically described as internal hemorrhoids or external hemorrhoids. Internal hemorrhoids are proximal to the dentate line and have visceral innervation. For this reason, internal hemorrhoids generally do not present with pain as

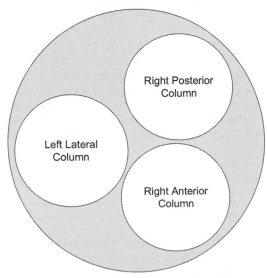

Fig. 1. Classic anatomic relationship of hemorrhoidal columns with patient in prone position.

an initial complaint. More often, patients with internal hemorrhoids complain of painless bleeding. Internal hemorrhoids generally are spanned by the anal transitional zone, and therefore can be covered by columnar, squamous, or basaloid cells. External hemorrhoids are located below the dentate line in the distal third of the anal canal. External hemorrhoids are covered by anoderm (squamous epithelium). Because of their somatic innervation, external hemorrhoids are more likely to present with pain.

Hemorrhoids are thought to enhance anal continence and may contribute 15% to 20% of resting anal canal pressure.[5] They also complete closure of the anus and may enhance control of defecation. Because hemorrhoids have sensory innervation, they also relay important data regarding the quality and composition (gas, liquid, stool) of intrarectal contents.

Because hemorrhoids represent collections of sinusoids, intra-abdominal pressure phenomena are easily manifested. Development of hemorrhoidal disease is likely associated with activities that increase in intra-abdominal pressure. This increase may be secondary to straining, excessive time spent on the toilet, or constipation. Other etiologic factors that can cause hemorrhoidal irritation include diarrhea and dehydration. Women in the third trimester of pregnancy commonly report hemorrhoidal swelling caused by increased intravascular volume and the estrogen sensitivity of hemorrhoidal tissues.

PHYSICAL EXAMINATION

Patients with anorectal complaints should be examined in a comprehensive and systematic fashion. The examination begins with inspection of the perianal skin. Often this is the only examination necessary because the pathology may be evident on the perianal skin. Often thrombosed external hemorrhoids are evident externally and can be identified because they are covered with anoderm. They commonly have a hint of visible clot underneath the surface of the anoderm (**Fig. 2**). These can be differentiated from prolapsed internal hemorrhoids, which are not covered with squamous epithelium, but rather columnar mucosa (**Fig. 3**).

Digital rectal examination can exclude the presence of palpable masses within the anal canal. Valuable information about the tone, contractile strength, and bulk of the anal sphincter mechanism can also be gained through digital examination.

Anoscopy is usually performed to inspect the anal canal mucosa and can often identify thrombosed internal hemorrhoids, fissures, condyloma, and the internal openings of fistula tracts, among other anorectal pathology. Rigid or flexible proctoscopy can evaluate the rectum for more proximal causes of bleeding, such as proctitis or rectal neoplasms.

HEMORRHOIDAL CLASSIFICATION

Hemorrhoids are normal structures and therefore they are only treated if they become symptomatic. They are commonly classified as first-, second-, third-, or fourth-degree hemorrhoids. First degree hemorrhoids simply represent hemorrhoids bulging into the anal canal but not out of the anal canal. Patients with this level of hemorrhoidal disease typically present with painless bleeding. Often this can be recurrent and ephemeral, occurring on a few selected days over the course of months.

Second-degree hemorrhoids are hemorrhoids that prolapse out of the anal canal with defecation but spontaneously reduce. Patients with second-degree hemorrhoids often complain of painless bleeding and perianal itching caused by chronic moisture secreted by the anal canal mucosa.

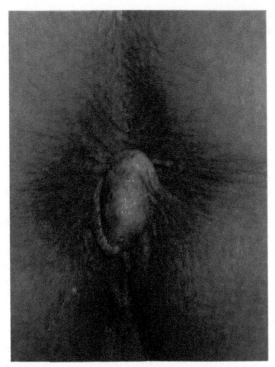

Fig. 2. Classic appearance of a thrombosed external hemorrhoid.

Third-degree hemorrhoids represent hemorrhoids that have prolapsed out of the anal canal and that require manual reduction. Often patients need to reduce the hemorrhoids several times per day or after every bowel movement. Patients with third degree hemorrhoids may report a history of bleeding with defecation; pain (likely caused by local ischemia); and mucus drainage.

Fourth-degree hemorrhoids are commonly referred to as incarcerated hemorrhoids **(Fig. 4**A). In this situation, hemorrhoids are permanently prolapsed outside of the anal canal and cannot be reduced manually. These patients typically present with bleeding

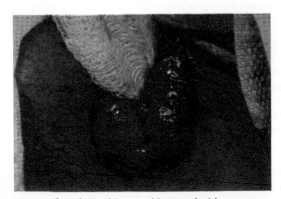

Fig. 3. Classic appearance of prolapsed internal hemorrhoids.

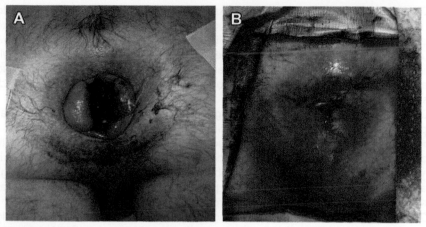

Fig. 4. (A) Grade 4 hemorrhoids. (B) Appearance of the anus after excisional hemorrhoidectomy.

and severe pain or discomfort. Many patients in this category require urgent surgical intervention (**Fig. 4**B).

NONOPERATIVE TREATMENT
Diet and Lifestyle Modifications

First- and second-degree hemorrhoidal disease can generally be treated with nonoperative measures. The primary goal of nonoperative treatment is to reverse the pathophysiologic trigger of hemorrhoidal disease and to reduce symptoms. In most patients, this therapy involves reduction of the intra-abdominal pressure transmitted to the hemorrhoidal vessels during bowel movements. Some patients require adjuncts to investigate unexplained constipation or diarrhea, which may have stimulated hemorrhoidal disease.

The mainstay of nonoperative hemorrhoidal treatment is to increase fiber and water consumption. Several studies document that fiber supplementation can reduce symptoms and bleeding, although this effect may take several weeks to manifest.[6,7] Patients should also be counseled on other lifestyle modifications, including the avoidance of prolonged sitting or straining on the toilet, perianal hygiene, and avoiding triggers of constipation or diarrhea.

Topical and Oral Agents

There are several over-the-counter medications that purport to reduce hemorrhoidal symptoms. Most of these treatment are aimed at providing symptomatic relief rather than truly altering the underlying pathophysiology of the disease. The various preparations include several medications including local anesthetics, vasoactive agents, corticosteroids, antibiotics, and lubricants. Although these treatments are plentiful, data regarding their efficacy are sparse.

Vasoconstrictive medications can be applied to the anal canal to alter the vascular channels supplying the hemorrhoidal tissues. Vasocontriction would theoretically reduce the size and perhaps secretions from hemorrhoidal tissues. One widely available commercial example is Preparation-H (Pfizer). This medication consists of petroleum, mineral oil, and 0.25% phenylephrine.[8]

Other authors have described effective use of nitrates for patients with hemorrhoids and elevated anal canal pressures. Although effective, treatment with topical nitrates was associated with a high incidence of nitrate-associated headaches.[9] Patients with acutely thrombosed internal or external hemorrhoids can sometimes be treated with topical calcium channel blockers, such as nifedipine.[10] These agents likely reduce spasm in the internal sphincter leading to manual or autoreduction of hemorrhoidal tissues.

Calcium dobesilate is a vaosactive drug used in the management of diabetic retinopathy and venous insufficiency. Calcium dobesilate's mechanism of action is thought to be related to decreasing tissue edema by altering vascular permeability and platelet aggregation. Menteş and colleagues[11] randomized 29 patients with symptomatic hemorrhoids to calcium dobesilate and a high-fiber diet or to a high-fiber diet alone. Eighty-six percent of patients treated with calcium dobesilate described cessation of bleeding and improvement in perianal irritation.

Oral flavinoids are also used in the management of hemorrhoidal disease. Flavinoids are a class of venotonic agents that also can alter vascular permeability and reduce tissue edema. Their mechanism of action is unclear but they are used in Europe and Asia for the treatment of hemorrhoidal disease.[11] A recent Cochrane review examined the use of oral phlebotonics including flavinoids and calcium dobesilate in the management of hemorrhoidal disease. Phelobotonics exhibited a remarkable treatment effect in favor of their use when the outcomes of pruritus, bleeding, discharge or leakage, and overall symptom improvement were compared with a control group.[12] These compounds have not gained wide acceptance in the United States.

Office Procedures

Several office procedures are available for the management of symptomatic hemorrhoids. These include infrared coagulation, sclerotherapy, cryotherapy, and rubber band ligation. All of the available techniques rely on tissue destruction and resultant tissue fixation caused by fibrosis.

Rubber band ligation

Rubber band ligation is most often used to treat first- and second-degree hemorrhoids. Certain third-degree hemorrhoids also can be treated with rubber band ligation. A rubber band is placed around the hemorrhoid above the dentate line (**Fig. 5**), causing localized ischemia in the intervening tissue. A portion of the hemorrhoid and the rubber band are passed in several days during defecation. The resultant fibrosis causes fixation of the remaining hemorrhoidal tissues. This prevents further prolapse and bleeding.

Several instruments are commercially available for application of the rubber bands. Suction ligators allow the surgeon to draw in the hemorrhoidal tissue using wall suction. The rubber band is applied with the same device; this approach is advantageous because it allows the surgeon to position an anoscope with the nondominant hand and apply the rubber band with the other hand. Other devices require the operator to grasp the hemorrhoidal pile with forceps and apply the rubber band with the other hand (**Fig. 6**). These types of devices require an assistant to hold the anoscope while the surgeon is applying the rubber band. This technical disadvantage is balanced by the fact that one can usually band more tissue with the latter device.

Hemorrhoidal banding is effective in controlling bleeding in greater than 90% of cases.[13] There are several rare complications of banding. These complications include bleeding, vasovagal response, pain, urinary retention, and rarely pelvic sepsis.

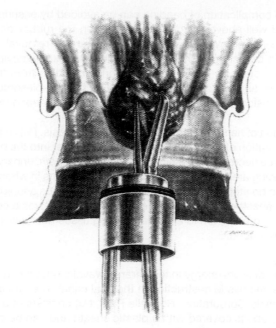

Fig. 5. The internal hemorrhoid is grasped above the dentate line in preparation for place-ment of a rubber band at that level. (*From* Corman M, Nicholls RJ, Fazio VW, et al. Corman's colon and rectal surgery. 5th edition. Philadelphia: Lippincott Williams & Wilkins; 2004; with permission.)

Rubber bands are commonly placed for intermittent bleeding. Increased bleeding after placement of a rubber band ligature is a frequent complaint and usually self-limited. A few patients may experience delayed bleeding after the rubber band cuts through the hemorrhoidal tissue (7–10 days). This is usually a one-time event; how-ever, rarely the bleeding can be massive and require examination under anesthesia and ligation of the offending hemorrhoidal pile.

A   **B**

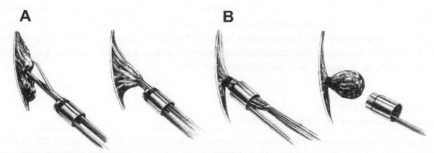

Fig. 6. (*A*) Care must be taken to elevate the hemorrhoidal tissues off of the underlying in-ternal sphincter. (*B*) The rubber band is placed at the base of the hemorrhoidal tissues using the applicator. This ultimately results in ischemic necrosis of the hemorrhoid. Ultimately, this process leads to scarring and fixation of the remaining hemorrhoidal tissues. (*From* Corman M, Nicholls RJ, Fazio VW, et al. Corman's colon and rectal surgery. 5th edition. Philadelphia: Lippincott Williams & Wilkins; 2004; with permission.)

Severe pain as a complication of banding can be avoided by ensuring that the rubber band is placed well above the dentate line. When the rubber band is correctly placed, need for early removal because of pain is rare. If removal of the band is necessary, this can be accomplished with a knife or hook. Removing the band in an office setting can often be accompanied by brisk bleeding from the traumatized hemorrhoidal tissues, and one should be prepared for this troublesome complication. Having a good bedside assistant, suction, and dilute epinephrine available are essential.

A rare complication of hemorrhoidal banding is pelvic sepsis. Pelvic sepsis typically results from incorporation of the underlying internal sphincter into the band, leading to more extensive tissue necrosis and infection. Symptoms of pain, urinary retention, and fever following banding are hallmarks of pelvic sepsis. Patients in whom the diagnosis is suspected should be started on broad-spectrum intravenous antibiotics and urgent examination under anesthesia should be performed. This involves a complete examination of the anus and perineum to exclude evolving tissue necrosis, and all necrotic tissues should be debrided.

Infrared coagulation

Infrared coagulation delivers energy in the infrared wavelength spectrum. This energy causes thrombosis and tissue destruction in the anal canal. The energy delivery system (IRC2100; Redfield Corporation, Rochelle Park, NJ) consists of a light generator and a probe. The probe is covered with a plastic sheath and can be applied through an anoscope. A 1- to 1.5-second pulse delivers the appropriate amount of energy.[14] The operator aims to apply the infrared energy above the dentate line because this area is insensate. When patients are randomized to infrared coagulation versus rubber band ligation, several studies suggest that rubber band ligation is associated with more postprocedural pain.[15,16]

Cryotherapy

Cyrotherapy involves treating the offending hemorrhoidal tissues with a liquid nitrogen probe. This procedure leads to swelling and subsequent necrosis of the surrounding tissues. This technique is time consuming and requires special equipment, and has therefore not gained wide acceptance.[2]

Sclerotherapy

Sclerotherapy typically involves injecting a sclerosing agent into the submucosa. This then causes fibrosis of the surrounding tissues. This technique was first described in the nineteenth century,[17] although now it is typically performed with a phenol-based solution. Sclerotherapy can be effective in the short term, although its effects do not tend to be long lasting.[14] Complications of sclerotherapy include bacteremia, pelvic sepsis, prostatic abscess, and necrotizing fasciitis.[18,19]

OPERATIVE THERAPY
Operative Management of Hemorrhoids

Surgical hemorrhoidectomy is typically offered to patients who have failed office procedures, who have large external hemorrhoids, or who have combined internal/external hemorrhoids that are symptomatic (grades III–IV).[20] Coagulopathic patients requiring definitive control of bleeding are also candidates for operative therapy.[21] Operative approaches to hemorrhoids generally can be grouped into three categories: (1) excisional hemorrhoidectomy, (2) stapled hemorrhoidopexy, and (3) Doppler-guided transanal devascularization.

Preparation for Surgery

We generally use a similar preoperative approach for all of anorectal surgery. Patients self-administer an enema on the morning of surgery. Mechanical bowel preparation is seldom necessary unless we are planning concomitant colonoscopy.

Although there are several anesthetic options including general and spinal anesthesia, we generally use local anesthesia or sedation. Patients are usually sedated with propofol and/or midazolam. We find this approach facilitates faster recovery and discharge.[22]

Proper positioning of the patient is essential in anorectal surgery. We most commonly use the prone-jackknife position. The buttocks are retracted laterally with tape for better exposure. The lithotomy or lateral decubitus positions are also viable options based on surgeon experience and comfort level.

Excisional Hemorrhoidectomy

Excisional hemorrhoidectomy can be broadly classified into closed (or Ferguson) type, open (or Milligan-Morgan) type, circumferential, or Whitehead type. The Ferguson and Milligan-Morgan techniques of hemorrhoidectomy are essentially the same and only differ on whether the anal mucosa and anoderm are reapproximated after ligation of the hemorrhoidal pedicle.

Division of tissues during excisional hemorrhoidectomy can be accomplished by a variety of means, including a scalpel, scissors, monopolar cauterization, bipolar energy, and ultrasonic devices.[23–25] The available literature does not bear out any advantage of any particular approach.[26,27] Surgeons should be familiar with several different techniques and approaches.

Ferguson

Ferguson or closed hemorrhoidectomy is the most common form of hemorrhoidectomy performed in the United States.[20,28] This type of hemorrhoidectomy is performed by using a hemostat or Kelly clamp to tent up the external hemorrhoid at the anal verge (**Fig. 7**A). A curvilinear incision is made from the distal end (close to the anoderm) to the proximal portion of the hemorrhoid. It is important to have a long smooth incision for proper closure and to avoid "dog ears." The hemorrhoidal tissue is then dissected free from the underlying sphincter muscles (see **Fig. 7**B). During this portion of the case it is essential to stay in the submucosal plane. Dissecting outside of this plane either leads to excessive bleeding if one is too close to the hemorrhoidal column, or injury to

A   **B**

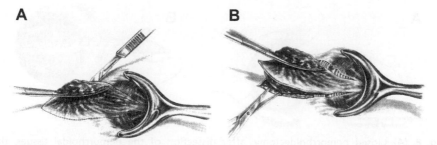

Fig. 7. (A) Closed hemorrhoidectomy: a hemostat or Kelly clamp to tent up the external hemorrhoid at the anal verge. (B) Closed hemorrhoidectomy: the hemorrhoidal tissue is then dissected free from the underlying sphincter muscles. (*From* Corman M, Nicholls RJ, Fazio VW, et al. Corman's colon and rectal surgery. 5th edition. Philadelphia: Lippincott Williams & Wilkins; 2004; with permission.)

internal sphincter if one is too close to the internal sphincter. Generally, if the dissection is performed correctly a healthy sphincter muscle can be identified at the base of the dissection (**Fig. 8**A). After the base of the hemorrhoid is reached, the pedicle of the hemorrhoid is ligated and the hemorrhoidal tissue is amputated. One of the stitches used to ligate the pedicle should be left long because this suture can be used to close the wound in a running fashion (see **Fig. 8**B). As the stitch is run toward the anoderm small bites of the underlying muscle are taken to obliterate the dead space. This stitch is also locked to ensure hemostasis. Once the anoderm is reached, a simple running stitch is used.

Milligan-Morgan or open hemorrhoidectomy
This technique was described by Milligan and Morgan, and is more commonly performed in the United Kingdom.[20,29] The steps are essentially the same as a Ferguson hemorrhoidectomy with the exception that the hemorhhoidectomy wound is not closed. Several studies have examined the outcomes of open and closed approaches to hemorrhoidectomy in patients with grade 3 and 4 disease. A closed technique was associated with less pain and better wound healing.[30,31]

Whitehead procedure
The general concept behind a Whitehead hemorrhoidectomy is the circumferential excision of hemorrhoidal tissues followed by advancement of the anal canal mucosa to close the defect. Rectangular or trapezoidal flaps are developed in the distal anal canal. A similar flap is developed more cephalad that contains the hemorrhoidal tissue. The hemorrhoidal tissue is excised, and more distal flap is advanced up into the anal canal. This flap is often pexied to the internal sphincter for added security. Finally, the flap is anastomosed to the mucosa above.[32] The procedure is not commonly performed because of its relative complexity compared with excisional hemorrhoidectomy, but also because of the potential long-term complications, especially anal ectropion. There have been several modifications of the procedure to improve operative results.[33–35]

Outcomes of excisional hemorrhoidectomy
A recent meta-analysis found that the long-term outcomes of excisional hemorrhoidectomy were superior to those of office procedures. Other authors have demonstrated that when compared with rubber band ligation excisional hemorrhoidectomy is more effective at achieving complete remission of hemorrhoidal symptoms.[36]

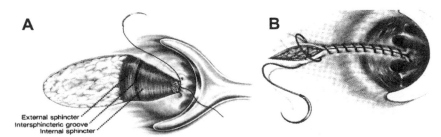

Fig. 8. (*A*) Closed hemorrhoidectomy: after dissection of the hemorrhoidal tissues, the sphincter muscles can be visualized. In the open or Milligan-Morgan technique the incision is left open to granulate through secondary intention. (*B*) Closed hemorrhoidectomy: the wound is closed in a running fashion. (*From* Corman M, Nicholls RJ, Fazio VW, et al. Corman's colon and rectal surgery. 5th edition. Philadelphia: Lippincott Williams & Wilkins; 2004; with permission.)

Patients undergoing excisional hemorrhoidectomy are less likely to require multiple treatments. Excisional hemorrhoidectomy had higher associations with certain complications, such as anal stenosis and postoperative hemorrhage. Excisional hemorrhoidectomy was also associated with an increased incidence of incontinence to flatus, although this result did not reach statistical significance.[36]

Stapled Hemorrhoidopexy

Stapled hemorrhoidopexy was first described as a treatment of mucosal prolapse. Subsequently its use was expanded to the treatment of hemorrhoids.[37,38] The procedure is most useful for the treatment of bleeding and/or prolapsing internal hemorrhoids in patients with relatively confluent/circumferential disease. It has no effect on external hemorrhoids and therefore its use is somewhat limited.

A circular anal dilator is sutured to the perianal skin to secure it in place. During this process the internal hemorrhoidal component is maximally reduced. A purse-string suture is placed 2 to 4 cm above the dentate line, at the base of the hemorrhoidal columns. Correct placement of this suture is critical to prevent placement of the staple line too close to the dentate line, which can result in chronic pain (**Fig. 9**). It is also essential that the purse-string be placed in the submucosal layer. If stitches are placed too deep, one can cause injury to the internal sphincter resulting in increased rates of fecal incontinence.[39,40]

The stapler head is inserted through the purse-string and secured. The stapler is closed while maintaining moderate tension on the purse-string. The stapler is then fired and opened revealing a staple line above the hemorrhoidal tissue. Although some hemorrhoid tissue may be included in the segment of mucosa that is excised, stapled hemorrhoidectomy functions to prevent prolapse of the hemorrhoids by pexying them in the anal canal.

Outcomes of stapled hemorrhoidopexy

Two recent meta-analyses demonstrated no significant differences between stapled hemorrhoidopexy and conventional hemorrhoidectomy when the outcomes of

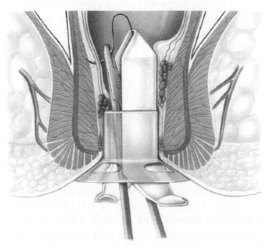

Fig. 9. Stapled hemorrhoidopexy: a pursestring is placed 2 to 4 cm above the dentate line. A specialized stapler is used to then remove redundant hemorrhoidal tissues and pexy the remaining hemorrhoids. (*From* Sardinha TC, Corman ML. Hemorrhoids. Surg Clin North Am 2002;82(6):1153–67; with permission.)

urgency, pruritus, and pain were examined. The stapled technique was also associated with a higher chance of long-term recurrence.[41,42] Although stapled hemorrhoidopexy is associated with several unique complications (ie, rectovaginal fistula, staple line bleeding, chronic pain), overall complication rates are similar to those of excisional hemorrhoidectomy. A meta-analysis of almost 2000 patients found the complication rates to be 20.2% for stapled hemorrhoidopexy versus 25.2% for conventional hemorrhoidectomy ($P = .06$).[42]

Doppler-Guided Transanal Hemorrhoid Devascularization

This technique involves suture ligation of each hemorrhoidal column without resection. The feeding vessels of each hemorrhoidal column are identified using a Doppler probe. This technique has been marketed as a less painful alternative to excisional hemorrhoidectomy.

The transanal hemorrhoid devascularization kit includes a patented anoscope. The anoscope is assembled and inserted into the anal canal. The anoscope is used to identify the signal of artery supplying each hemorrhoidal column, usually at the top of the hemorrhoidal column. Once the artery is identified, it is then ligated using a 0 Vicryl suture. The anoscope and Doppler are then used to confirm the disappearance of the arterial signal. The same stitch is then used to oversew the hemorrhoidal column.[43]

Outcomes of Doppler-guided transanal hemorrhoid devascularization

Doppler-guided or -assisted hemorrhoidal ligation has been reported to be effective in 90% of patients, with recurrence rates ranging from 10% to 15%.[44–46] Other authors found that recurrences are more common when this technique is applied to grade IV hemorrhoids.[47]

SUMMARY

Symptomatic hemorrhoids are a commonly occurring problem. There are a variety of surgical and nonoperative options for management of hemorrhoidal disease. Grade 1 and 2 hemorrhoids can generally be managed with nonoperative measures. Grade 3 and 4 hemorrhoids are generally managed with procedure interventions. The experienced anorectal surgeon should have a variety of techniques at her or his disposal.

REFERENCES

1. Parks AG. De haemorrhois. A study in surgical history. Guys Hosp Rep 1955;104: 135–56.
2. Hulme-Moir M, Bartolo DC. Disorders of the anorectum. Gastroenterol Clin North Am 2001;30:183–97.
3. Thomson WH. The nature of haemorrhoids. Br J Surg 1975;62:542–52.
4. Haas PA, Fox TA Jr. Age-related changes and scar formations of perianal connective tissue. Dis Colon Rectum 1980;23:160–9.
5. Lestar B, Pennickx F, Kerremans R. The composition of anal basal pressure. An in vivo and in vitro study in man. Int J Colorectal Dis 1989;4:118–22.
6. Alonso-Coello P, Mills E, Heels-Ansdell D, et al. Fiber for the treatment of hemorrhoids complications: a systematic review and metaanalysis. Am J Gastroenterol 2006;101:181–8.
7. Moesgaard F, Nielsen ML, Hansen JB, et al. High fiber diet reduces bleeding and pain in patients with hemorrhoids: a double-blind trial of Vi-Siblin. Dis Colon Rectum 1982;25:454–6.

8. Lohsiriwat V. Hemorrhoids: from basic pathophysiology to clinical management. World J Gastroenterol 2012;18(17):2009–17.
9. Tjandra JJ, Tan JJ, Lim JF, et al. Rectogesic (glyceryl trinitrate 0.2%) ointment relieves symptoms of haemorrhoids associated with high resting anal canal pressures. Colorectal Dis 2007;9:457–63.
10. Perrotti P, Antropoli C, Molino D, et al. Conservative treatment of acute thrombosed external hemorrhoids with topical nifedipine. Dis Colon Rectum 2001;44: 405–9.
11. Menteş BB, Görgül A, Tatlicioğlu E, et al. Efficacy of calcium dobesilate in treating acute attacks of hemorrhoidal disease. Dis Colon Rectum 2001;44:1489–95.
12. Perera N, Liolitsa D, Iype S, et al. Phlebotonics for haemorrhoids. Cochrane Database Syst Rev 2012;(8):CD004322.
13. Su MY, Chiu CT, Wu CS, et al. Endoscopic hemorrhoidal ligation of symptomatic internal hemorrhoids. Gastrointest Endosc 2003;58:871–4.
14. Halverson A. Hemorrhoids. Clin Colon Rectal Surg 2007;20(2):77–85.
15. Poen AC, Felt-Bersma RJ, Cuesta MA, et al. A randomized controlled trial of rubber band ligation versus infra-red coagulation in the treatment of internal haemorrhoids. Eur J Gastroenterol Hepatol 2000;12(5):535–9.
16. Marques CF, Nahas SC, Nahas CS, et al. Early results of the treatment of internal hemorrhoid disease by infrared coagulation and elastic banding: a prospective randomized cross-over trial. Tech Coloproctol 2006;10(4):312–7.
17. Goligher JC. Surgery of the anus, rectum and colon. 4th edition. London: Bailliere Tindall; 1980. p. 93–135.
18. Guy RJ, Seow-Choen F. Septic complications after treatment of haemorrhoids. Br J Surg 2003;90:147–56.
19. Adami B, Eckardt VF, Suermann RB, et al. Bacteremia after proctoscopy and hemorrhoidal injection sclerotherapy. Dis Colon Rectum 1981;24:373–4.
20. Rivadeneira DE, Steele SR, Ternent C, et al, on behalf of the Standards Practice Task Force of The American Society of Colon and Rectal Surgeons. Practice parameters for the management of hemorrhoids (revised 2010). Dis Colon Rectum 2011;54(9):1059–64.
21. Singer M. Hemorrhoids. In: Beck DE, Roberts PL, Saclarides TJ, et al, editors. The ASCRS textbook of colon and rectal surgery. 2nd edition. New York: Springer; 2011. p. 175–202.
22. Read TE, Henry SE, Hovis RM, et al. Prospective evaluation of anesthetic technique for anorectal surgery. Dis Colon rectum 2002;45(11):1553–8.
23. Gencosmanoglu R, Sad O, Koc D, et al. Hemorrhoidectomy: open or closed technique? A prospective, randomized clinical trial. Dis Colon Rectum 2002;45:70–5.
24. Arbman G, Krook H, Haapaniemi S. Closed vs. open hemorrhoidectomy—is there any difference? Dis Colon Rectum 2000;43:31–4.
25. Abo-hashem AA, Sarhan A, Aly AM. Harmonic scalpel compared with bipolar electro-cautery hemorrhoidectomy: a randomized controlled trial. Int J Surg 2010;8:243–7.
26. Chung CC, Ha JP, Tai YP, et al. Double-blind, randomized trial comparing Harmonic scalpel hemorrhoidectomy, bipolar scissors hemorrhoidectomy, and scissors excision: ligation technique. Dis Colon Rectum 2002;45:789–94.
27. Nienhuijs S, de Hingh I. Conventional versus LigaSure hemorrhoidectomy for patients with symptomatic hemorrhoids. Cochrane Database Syst Rev 2009;(1):CD006761.
28. Ferguson JA, Mazier WP, Ganchrow MI, et al. The closed technique of hemorrhoidecomy. Surgery 1971;70(3):480–4.

29. Milligan ET, Morgan CN, Jones LE. Surgical anatomy of the anal canal and the operative treatment of hemorrhoids. Lancet 1937;2:119–24.
30. You SY, Kim SH, Chung CS, et al. Open vs. closed hemorrhoidectomy. Dis Colon Rectum 2005;48(1):108–13.
31. Sanchez C, Chinn BT. Hemorrhoids. Clin Colon Rectal Surg 2011;24(1):5–13, 23.
32. Whitehead W. The surgical treatment of haemorrhoids. Br Med J 1882;1(1101): 148–50.
33. Burchell MC, Thow GB, Manson RR. A "modified Whitehead" hemorrhoidectomy. Dis Colon Rectum 1976;19:225–32.
34. Barrios G, Khubchandani M. Whitehead operation revisited. Dis Colon Rectum 1979;22:330–2.
35. Khubchandani M. Results of Whitehead operation. Dis Colon Rectum 1984;27: 730–2.
36. Shanmugam V, Thaha MA, Rabindranath KS, et al. Systematic review of randomized trials comparing rubber band ligation with excisional haemorrhoidectomy. Br J Surg 2005;92(12):1481–7.
37. Pescatori M, Favetta U, Dedola S, et al. Transanal stapled excision for rectal mucosal prolapse. Tech coloproctol 1997;1:96–8.
38. Longo A. Treatment of hemorrhoid disease by reduction of mucosa and hemorrhoid prolapse with a circular-suturing device: a new procedure. In: Proceedings of the 6th World Congress of Endoscopic Surgery. Rome (Italy): 1998. p. 777–84.
39. Ng KH, Chew MH, Eu WK. Modified stapled haemorrhoidectomy: a suggested improved technique. ANZ J Surg 2008;78:394–7.
40. Pigot F, Dao-Quang M, Castinel A, et al. Low haemorrhoidopexy staple line does not improve results and increases risk for incontinence. Tech Coloproctol 2006; 10:329–33.
41. Nisar PJ, Acheson AG, Neal KR, et al. Stapled hemorrhoidopexy compared with conventional hemorrhoidectomy: systematic review of randomized controlled trials. Dis Colon Rectum 2004;47:1837–45.
42. Tjandra JJ, Chan MK. Systematic review on the procedure for prolapse and hemorrhoids (stapled hemorrhoidopexy). Dis Colon Rectum 2007;50:878–92.
43. Morinaga K, Hasuda K, Ikeda T. Novel therapy for internal hemorrhoids: ligation of the hemorrhoidal artery with a newly devised instrument (Moricorn) in conjunction with a Doppler Flowmeter. Am J Gastroenterol 1995;90(4):610–3.
44. Ratto C, Donisi L, Parello A, et al. Evaluation of transanal hemorrhoidal dearterialization as a minimally invasive therapeutic approach to hemorrhoids. Dis Colon Rectum 2010;53:803–11.
45. Felice C, Privitera A, Ellul E, et al. Doppler-guided hemorrhoidal artery ligation: an alternative to hemorrhoidectomy. Dis Colon Rectum 2005;48:2090–3.
46. Faucheron JL, Gangner Y. Doppler-guided hemorrhoidal artery ligation for the treatment of symptomatic hemorrhoids: early and three-year follow-up results in 100 consecutive patients. Dis Colon Rectum 2008;51:945–9.
47. Giordano P, Overton J, Madeddu F, et al. Transanal hemorrhoidal dearterialization: a systematic review. Dis Colon Rectum 2009;52:1665–71.

Printed and bound by CPI Group (UK) Ltd, Croydon, CR0 4YY

03/10/2024

01040399-0010